Operative Techniques in
Breast Surgery, Trunk, Reconstruction and Body Contouring

Operative Techniques in Breast Surgery, Trunk, Reconstruction and Body Contouring

Joseph J. Disa, MD, FACS

EDITOR

Vice Chair of Clinical Activities
Department of Surgery
Attending Surgeon
Memorial Sloan Kettering Cancer Center
Professor of Surgery
Weill Medical College of Cornell University
New York, New York

Kevin C. Chung, MD, MS

EDITOR-IN-CHIEF

Chief of Hand Surgery, Michigan Medicine
Director
University of Michigan Comprehensive Hand Center
Charles B. G. de Nancrede Professor of Surgery
Professor of Plastic Surgery and Orthopaedic Surgery
Assistant Dean for Faculty Affairs
Associate Director of Global REACH
University of Michigan Medical School
Ann Arbor, Michigan

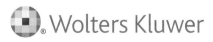

Philadelphia • Baltimore • New York • London
Buenos Aires • Hong Kong • Sydney • Tokyo

Executive Editor: Brian Brown
Development Editor: Ashley Fischer
Editorial Coordinator: John Larkin
Marketing Manager: Julie Sikora
Senior Production Project Manager: Alicia Jackson
Senior Designer: Joan Wendt
Artist/Illustrator: Body Scientific International
Senior Manufacturing Coordinator: Beth Welsh
Prepress Vendor: SPi Global

Printed in China

Cataloging-in-Publication Data available on request from the Publisher.
ISBN 978-1-4963-4809-8

shop.lww.com

Contributors

Jeffrey A. Ascherman, MD
Thomas S. Zimmer Professor of
  Reconstructive Surgery at CUMC
Site Chief, Division of Plastic Surgery
Columbia University Medical
New York, New York

Fadi Bakal, MD
Plastic Surgery Department
Brussels University Hospital
Vrije Universiteit Brussel
Brussels, Belgium

Devra B. Becker, MD, FACS
Associate Professor
Department of Plastic Surgery
Chief of Plastic Surgery, UPMC
  Passavant
Director of Wound Healing Services,
  UPMC Passavant
Department of Plastic Surgery
University of Pittsburgh Medical Center
Pittsburgh, Pennsylvania

Maureen Beederman, MD
Resident
Section of Plastic and Reconstructive
  Surgery
Department of Surgery
The University of Chicago Medicine
Chicago, Illinois

Charles E. Butler, MD, FACS
Professor and Chairman
Department of Plastic Surgery
The University of Texas MD Anderson
  Cancer Center
Houston, Texas

Bradley Calobrace, MD
CaloAesthetics Plastic Surgery Center
CaloSpa
Louisville, Kentucky

Chris A. Campbell, MD, FACS
Associate Professor
Department of Plastic Surgery
University of Virginia
Charlottesville, Virginia

Jennifer Capla, MD
Plastic Surgeon
Private Practice
Department of Plastic Surgery
Northwell–Lenox Hill Hospital
New York, New York

Bernard W. Chang, MD
Chief of Plastic Surgery
Mercy Medical Center
Baltimore, Maryland

Ming-Huei Cheng, MD, MBA, FACS
Professor
Division of Plastic Reconstructive
  Microsurgery
Department of Plastic & Reconstructive
  Surgery
Chang Gung Memorial Hospital
Taoyuan City, Taiwan

Pierre M. Chevray, MD, PhD
Houston Methodist
Institute for Reconstructive Surgery
Associate Professor
Weill Cornell Medical College
Adjunct Associate Professor
Baylor College of Medicine
Program Director
Houston Methodist Plastic Surgery
  Residency
Houston, Texas

Carrie K. Chu, MD, MS
Assistant Professor
Department of Plastic Surgery
The University of Texas MD
  Anderson
Cancer Center
Houston, Texas

Mark W. Clemens, MD, FACS
Associate Professor
Department of Plastic Surgery
MD Anderson Cancer Center
University of Texas
Houston, Texas

Zachary J. Collier, MD
Division of Plastic & Reconstructive
  Surgery
Department of Surgery
USC Keck School of Medicine
Los Angeles, California

Brendan Collins, MD
Attending Physician and Microsurgical
  Fellowship Director
Mercy Medical Center
Baltimore, Maryland

Amy S. Colwell, MD, FACS
Associate Professor, Harvard Medical
  School
Division of Plastic Surgery
Massachusetts General Hospital
Boston, Massachusetts

Kasandra Dassoulas, MD
Richmond Aesthetic Surgery
Midlothian, Virginia

Joseph J. Disa, MD, FACS
Vice Chair of Clinical Activities
Department of Surgery
Attending Surgeon
Memorial Sloan Kettering Cancer
  Center
Professor of Surgery
Weill Medical College of Cornell
  University
New York, New York

Gregory A. Dumanian, MD
Lucille and Orion Stuteville Professor
  of Surgery
Chief of Plastic Surgery
Feinberg School of Medicine
Northwestern University
Chicago, Illinois

Sean M. Fisher, MD
Plastic and Reconstructive Surgery
  Resident
University of Washington
Seattle, Washington

Jordan D. Frey, MD
Resident
Hansjörg Wyss Department of Plastic
  Surgery
NYU Langone Health
New York, New York

Katherine M. Gast, MD, MS
Assistant Professor of Surgery
Plastic and Reconstructive Surgery
Medical Director, Comprehensive
  Gender Services Program
University of Wisconsin
Madison, Wisconsin

David Gerth, MD
Plastic Surgery
MOSA Surgery
Miami Beach, Florida

Paul A. Ghareeb, MD
Fellow
Division of Plastic and Reconstructive
Surgery
Emory University School of
Medicine
Atlanta, Georgia

Nicholas Haddock, MD
Associate Professor
Department of Plastic Surgery
University of Texas Southwestern
Dallas, Texas

Eric G. Halvorson, MD
Halvorson Plastic Surgery
Asheville, North Carolina

Moustapha Hamdi, MD, PhD
Professor and Chairman of Plastic
Surgery Department
Brussels University Hospital–Vrije
Universiteit Brussel
Brussels, Belgium

Alexes Hazen, MD, FACS
Associate Professor
NYU Langone Health
New York, New York

Peter Henderson, MD, MBA
Assistant Professor of Surgery
Division of Plastic and Reconstructive
Surgery
Icahn School of Medicine at
Mount Sinai
New York, New York

Jung-Ju Huang, MD
Associate Professor
Plastic and Reconstructive Surgery
Chang Gung Memorial Hospital
Chang Gung University
Linkou, Taiwan

John Hulsen, MD
Clinical Fellow, Aesthetic and
Reconstructive Breast Surgery
Division of Plastic and Reconstructive
Surgery
Massachusetts General Hospital/
Harvard Medical School
Boston, Massachusetts

Dennis J. Hurwitz, BS, MD
Clinical Professor of Plastic Surgery
Plastic Surgery
University of Pittsburgh Medical
Center
Attending Plastic Surgeon UPMC
Magee-Womens Hospital Surgery
University of Pittsburgh Medical
Center
Pittsburgh, Pennsylvania

Amir Inbal, MD
Section of Plastic and Reconstructive
Surgery
Department of Surgery
University of Chicago Medical
Center
Chicago, Illinois

Jeffrey E. Janis, MD, FACS
Professor of Plastic Surgery,
Neurosurgery, Neurology, and
Surgery
Chief of Plastic Surgery
University Hospitals
Ohio State University Wexner Medical
Center
Columbus, Ohio

Sahil K. Kapur, MD
Assistant Professor
Department of Plastic Surgery
The University of Texas MD Anderson
Cancer Center
Houston, Texas

Nolan Karp, MD
Professor of Plastic Surgery
New York University School of
Medicine
New York, New York

Ibrahim Khansa, MD
Division of Plastic and Maxillofacial
Surgery
Children's Hospital Los
Angeles
Los Angeles, California

**Hana Farhang Khoee, MD, MSc,
FRCSC**
Adjunct Professor
Department of Surgery
Schulich School of Medicine &
Dentistry
Western University
London, Ontario, Canada
Plastic, Reconstructive, and Aesthetic
Surgeon
Department of Surgery
Windsor Regional Hospital
Windsor, Ontario, Canada

Jeff J. Kim, MD
Resident Physician, PGY6
Section of Plastic and Reconstructive
Surgery
Department of Surgery
The University of Chicago Medical
Center
Chicago, Illinois

Gabriel M. Kind, MD
Attending Staff
Division of Microsurgery
Department of Plastic Surgery
California Pacific Medical Center
San Francisco, California
Associate Clinical Professor
Division of Plastic and Reconstructive
Surgery
Department of Surgery
University of California–San Francisco
San Francisco, California
Clinical Instructor
Department of Surgery (Plastic &
Reconstructive Surgery)
Stanford School of Medicine
Stanford University Medical Center
Palo Alto, California

Jennifer A. Klok, MD, MSc
Associate Staff
Division of Plastic Surgery
Department of Surgery
Peterborough Regional Health Centre
Peterborough, Ontario, Canada

Bill Kortesis, MD, FACS
Co-owner and Partner
Hunstad/Kortesis/Bharti Cosmetic
Surgery
Huntersville, North Carolina

Jeffrey H. Kozlow, MD, MS
Associate Professor (Clinical Track)
Section of Plastic Surgery
University of Michigan
Ann Arbor, Michigan

Theodore A. Kung, MD
Assistant Professor of Surgery
Section of Plastic and Reconstructive
Surgery
University of Michigan
Michigan Medicine
Ann Arbor, Michigan

William M. Kuzon, Jr, MD, PhD
Reed O. Dingman Collegiate Professor
of Plastic Surgery
Section of Plastic Surgery
University of Michigan
Chief of Surgery
VA Ann Arbor Healthcare
Ann Arbor, Michigan

David L. Larson, MD
Professor Emeritus
Department of Plastic Surgery
Medical College of Wisconsin
Milwaukee, Wisconsin
Accreditation Field Representative
Accreditation Council for Graduate
Medical Education
Chicago, Illinois

Albert Losken, MD, FACS
William G. Hamm Professor of Plastic
Surgery, Program Director
Emory Division of Plastic and
Reconstructive Surgery
Atlanta, Georgia

Ryan P. Ter Louw, MD
Plastic Surgeon
Muskegon Surgical Associates
Muskegon, Michigan

Alan Matarasso, MD, FACS
Clinical Professor of Surgery
Hofstra University/Northwell School of
Medicine
President-Elect
American Society of Plastic Surgeons,
Executive Committee & Board of
Directors
Past President, the Rhinoplasty Society
& Chair Board of Trustees, & 2016-
2017 Traveling Professor
Past President, New York Regional
Society of Plastic Surgeons & Chair
Board of Trustees

Chet Mays, MD
Private Practice
CaloAesthetics Plastic Surgery
Center
Louisville, Kentucky

Alexander F. Mericli, MD
Assistant Professor
Department of Plastic Surgery
MD Anderson Cancer Center
University of Texas
Houston, Texas

Joseph Michaels, MD
Private Practice
North Bethesda, Maryland
Assistant Professor of Plastic Surgery
Department of Plastic Surgery
John Hopkins Medicine
Baltimore, Maryland

Lauren M. Mioton, MD
Resident Physician
Division of Plastic and Reconstructive
Surgery
Northwestern University
Chicago, Illinois

Arash Momeni, MD
Assistant Professor of Surgery
Director, Clinical Outcomes
Research
Ryan-Upson Scholar in Plastic and
Reconstructive Surgery
Division of Plastic & Reconstructive
Surgery
Stanford University Medical Center
Palo Alto, California

Adeyiza O. Momoh, MD
Associate Professor of Plastic Surgery
Program Director, Integrated Plastic
Surgery Residency
University of Michigan
Ann Arbor, Michigan

**Peter Neligan, MB, FRCS(I), FRCSC,
FACS**
Professor of Surgery
Director, Center for Reconstructive
Surgery
University of Washington Medical
Center
Seattle, Washington

Ajani G. Nugent, MD
Assistant Professor
Division of Plastic and Reconstructive
Surgery
Department of Surgery
Miller School of Medicine
University of Miami
Miami, Florida

**Adrian S. H. Ooi, MBBS, MMed
(Surgery), MRCS, FAMS (Plastic
Surgery)**
Consultant Plastic Surgeon
Department of Plastic, Reconstructive
and Aesthetic Surgery
Singapore General Hospital
SingHealth Head & Neck Disease
Center
SingHealth
Singapore, Singapore

Julie E. Park, MD
Assistant Professor
Section of Plastic & Reconstructive
Surgery
University of Chicago Medical Centre
Department of Surgery
The University of Chicago Medicine &
Biological Sciences
Chicago, Illinois

Chad A. Purnell, MD
Resident Physician
Division of Plastic Surgery
Feinberg School of Medicine
Northwestern University
Chicago, Illinois

**Charalambos "Babis"
Rammos, MD, FACS**
Assistant Professor of Surgery
Division of Plastic Surgery
Department of Surgery
Vice Chairman of Research
Department of Surgery
College of Medicine
University of Illinois
Peoria, Illinois

Edward C. Ray, MD, FACS
Assistant Professor of Surgery
Chair, Microsurgery Advisory
Committee
Division of Plastic & Reconstructive
Surgery
Cedars-Sinai Medical Center
Los Angeles, California

David J. Rowe, MD, FACS
Assistant Professor, Plastic Surgery
MetroHealth Medical Center
Cleveland, Ohio

J. Peter Rubin, MD
Endowed Professor and Chair
Department of Plastic Surgery
University of Pittsburgh
Pittsburgh, Pennsylvania

Christopher J. Salgado, MD
Professor and Interim Chief of Plastic
Surgery
Division of Plastic Surgery
Medical Director of the LGBTQ Center
for Wellness
Gender and Sexual Health
Department of Surgery
University of Miami Miller School of
Medicine/Jackson Memorial Hospital
System
Miami, Florida

Ann R. Schwentker, MD
Associate Professor of Pediatric Plastic
and Craniofacial Surgery
Cincinnati Children's Hospital Medical
Center
Program Director, Plastic Surgery
University of Cincinnati
Cincinnati, Ohio

Deana Shenaq, MD
Resident
Section of Plastic & Reconstructive
Surgery
Department of Surgery
University of Chicago Medical
Centre
Section of Plastic and Reconstructive
Surgery
The University of Chicago Medicine &
Biological Sciences
Chicago, Illinois

Michele A. Shermak, MD, FACS
Associate Professor of Plastic
Surgery
Johns Hopkins Department of Plastic
Surgery
Baltimore, Maryland
Private Practice Plastic Surgery
Lutherville, Maryland

Wesley N. Sivak, MD, PhD
Fellow
Department of Plastic Surgery
University of Pittsburgh
Pittsburgh, Pennsylvania

Darren M. Smith, MD
Plastic Surgeon, Aesthetic
    Surgeon
New York, New York

David H. Song, MD, MBA, FACS
Physician Executive Director
MedStar Health
Plastic & Reconstructive Surgery
Professor and Chairman
Department of Plastic Surgery
Georgetown University
Washington, District of Columbia

Scott Spear, MD†
Founding Chair
Department of Plastic Surgery
Georgetown University Hospital
Washington, District of Columbia

Dhivya R. Srinivasa, MD
Resident
Plastic and Reconstructive Surgery
University of Michigan
Ann Arbor, Michigan

John T. Stranix, MD
Chief Resident
Hansjörg Wyss Department of Plastic
    Surgery
NYU Langone Health
New York, New York

Louis L. Strock, MD
Assistant Clinical Professor
Department of Plastic Surgery
University of Texas Southwestern
    Medical Center
Dallas, Texas
Private Practice
Fort Worth, Texas

Sergey Y. Turin, MD
Resident Physician
Division of Plastic and Reconstructive
    Surgery
Feinberg School of Medicine
Northwestern University
Chicago, Illinois

Katie E. Weichman, MD
Assistant Professor of Surgery
Department of Surgery
Albert Einstein School of Medicine/
    Montefiore Medical Center
Bronx, New York

Eric J. Wright, MD
Reconstructive and Aesthetic Breast
    Fellow
Division of Plastic Surgery
Harvard Medical School
Massachusetts General Hospital
Boston, Massachusetts

Liza C. Wu, MD, FACS
Chief of Microsurgery
PENN Plastic Surgery
Professor of Surgery
University of Pennsylvania
Philadelphia, Pennsylvania

Essie Kueberuwa Yates, MD
Plastic & Reconstructive Surgeon
Yates Institute of Plastic Surgery
Lauderdale, Florida

Toni Zhong, MD, MHS, FRCS(C)
Associate Professor
Departments of Surgery and Surgical
    Oncology
University of Toronto
Fellowship Director
Division of Plastic and Reconstructive
    Surgery
University of Toronto
Plastic Surgeon–Scientist
Belinda Stronach Chair of UHN
    Breast
Cancer Reconstructive Surgery
Director of the UHN Breast
    Reconstruction Program
University Health Network
Mount Sinai Hospital
Toronto, Ontario, Canada

Yasmina Zoghbi, MD
Resident
Division of Plastic Surgery
Department of Surgery
Icahn School of Medicine at Mount
    Sinai
New York, New York

Terri A. Zomerlei, MD
Clinical Instructor House Staff
                Columbus, Ohio

Preface

Reconstruction of trunk defects illustrates the application of innovative reconstructive principles. Breast reconstruction for conditions, such as cancer treatment, augmentation, and reduction, is essential to women's health. Other trunk problems such as hernias, body contouring procedures after weight loss, or buttock deformities tax the creativity of the surgeon to design an operation for the problem and to fit the patient.

The authors were selected based on their expertise in diagnosing the anatomic concerns and to articulate surgical treatments of each body region of the trunk by referring to principles in an illustrative approach. Each operation is described in a step-by-step fashion with professional sketches to highlight essential components of the operation so that the procedure can be conducted safely to yield predictable outcomes.

I am grateful for the interest in our textbooks. I have worked with Dr. Disa the editor of this volume and all the outstanding experts in this field to create an encyclopedic offering that will enhance your practices in an efficient learning module. I hope you enjoy reading this textbook from cover to cover. Thank you for your interest and support.

Kevin C. Chung, MD, MS
Chief of Hand Surgery, Michigan Medicine
Director, University of Michigan Comprehensive Hand Center
Charles B. G. de Nancrede Professor of Surgery
Professor of Plastic Surgery and Orthopaedic Surgery
Assistant Dean for Faculty Affairs
Associate Director of Global REACH
University of Michigan Medical School
Ann Arbor, Michigan

Contents

[†] Deceased

Video Clips

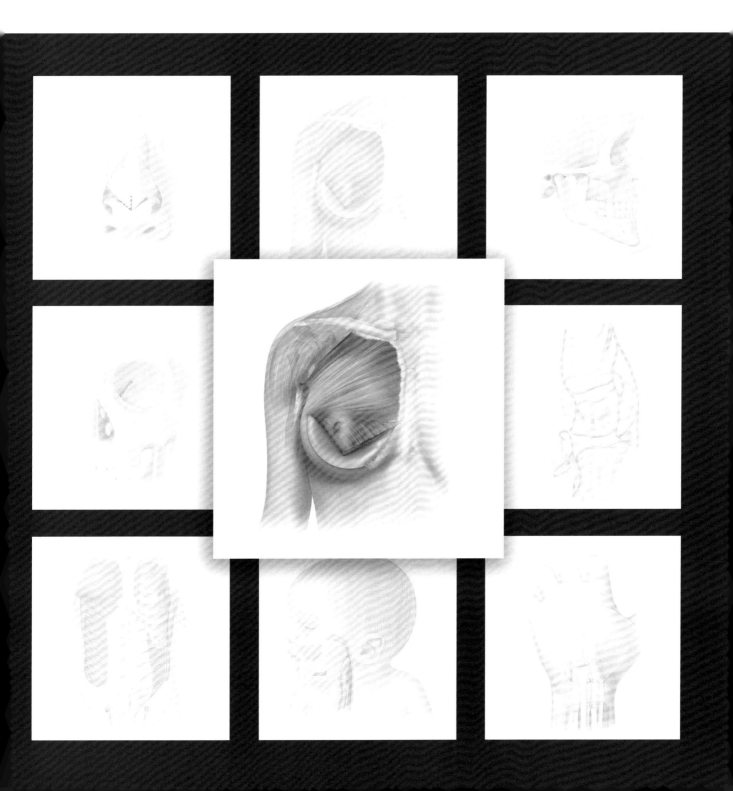

PART **1**
Plastic Surgery of the Breast

Section I: Augmentation Mammoplasty

Transaxillary Breast Augmentation

Louis L. Strock

DEFINITION

- Hypomastia. This patient requested that she have a procedure to enlarge her breasts in a conservative way. She also stated that she preferred to have her breast implants placed in a way that would allow her to avoid incisions on her breasts (**FIG 1A,B**).

ANATOMY

- To manage the request of this patient, the level and shape of the inframammary fold (IMF) will be lowered with the aid of endoscopic assistance. The pectoralis major muscle and overlying fascia will be divided according to external markings and correlated with internal muscle anatomy.

PATIENT HISTORY AND PHYSICAL FINDINGS

- This patient is a 34-year-old woman who presented for breast augmentation after having had three children. She requested that her breasts be enlarged to a small C cup, with as soft a feel as possible. Her examination was remarkable for mild asymmetry, thin tissue, and large nipple size. Her breast base width measurement was 11 cm, and pinch thickness measurements were 1.5 cm laterally, superiorly, and medially. She was also noted to have extremely large nipples that she requested to have reduced at the time her breast implants were placed (**FIG 2**).

SURGICAL MANAGEMENT

Preoperative Planning

- Preoperative planning centered on the choice of breast implant type in the context of her aesthetic goals and tissue type. She preferred the feel and intermediate projection of a Mentor MemoryGel smooth wall, round,

moderate plus profile silicone gel device. Other options considered included the same device type in moderate and high profile versions, and a moderate height, moderate projection shaped highly cohesive gel device. She stated preference of a partial subpectoral plane of placement over a subfascial approach. Incision choices offered to this patient included inframammary and transaxillary, with the latter preferred by the patient to attempt to avoid incisions visible on her breasts. Nipple reduction was requested by the patient, to be performed following completion of the breast augmentation procedure and access incision closure.

Equipment

- A standard HD endoscopic tower and camera are used in this procedure. This equipment is identical to that used for any subspecialty that utilizes an endoscopic tower and camera. The endoscope that is preferred is a 10-mm 30-degree angled scope, that is intended to fit correctly into the Emory Endoscopic retractor (**FIG 3**). A cautery handle with a suction end is used, and holds a cautery tube with a spatulated end. This is the basis for the dissection at the heart of this procedure. Additionally, 4-prong Freeman skin hooks, 2 mirror image Agris-Dingman dissectors, a 1-in fiberoptic retractor with suction port, facelift scissors, and two 1-in short Deaver retractors make up the instrument set for the procedure.[1]

Positioning

- The patient is positioned with the arms out ninety degrees and straightened on armboards. All equipment, cords, and tubing are directed toward the feet of the patient in the midline. This allows for ease of transition during the procedure for device placement on either side. There is adequate

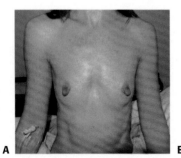
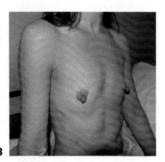

FIG 1 • A,B. Preoperative photos showing thin tissue patient. She has minimal breast volume, poor inframammary fold definition, and distinctly large nipples.

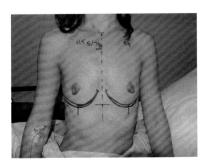

FIG 2 • Frontal markings show plan to lower the inframammary fold to accommodate dimensions of device to be used.

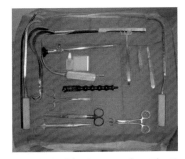

FIG 3 • Instrument tray used for the procedure. The Emory Endoscopic retractor is with paired 10-mm 30-degree-angled endoscope. The cautery handle has a suction port in back, and a hub for hollow cautery rods with spatulated ends. The author prefers mirror image J-shaped rods, but other variants are available. Four-prong skin hooks, two mirror image Agris-Dingman dissectors, two 1-in. Deaver retractors, facelift scissors, and Adson-Brown forceps complete the set.

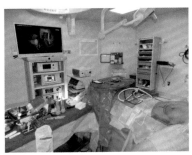

FIG 4 • All equipment is positioned at the foot of the bed, including the endoscopic tower. All cords are kept in a central position to prevent having to move them during the procedure, regardless of which side is being augmented. The patient is positioned with the arms out at 90 degrees. The endoscopic portion of the procedure is performed with the surgeon above the shoulder.

separation of the anesthesia equipment from the head and shoulders of the patient to allow the surgeon to stand above the shoulder on each side during the endoscopic tissue release portion of the procedure on each side (**FIG 4**).

Approach

- The procedure can be performed adequately in this patient with use of inframammary or transaxillary approaches for incision access. The periareolar approach is more difficult given the relatively small size of the areola in this patient. Her thin tissue makes a partial subpectoral, or dual plane, approach preferred to maximize soft tissue cover over the implants.

◼ Incision and Initial Dissection

- An S-shaped incision was planned, centered in the axillary apex (**TECH FIG 1**). This incision pattern was selected because it allows for a long functional length in a patient with a narrow area of hair-bearing skin in the axilla. The long portion of the incision was marked within the longest existing skin crease. The anterior extension is placed to stay behind the posterior aspect of the pectoralis major muscle. This is critical to keep the incision hidden during recovery. A cross-hatch is made centrally to facilitate skin closure. The incision is made through the hair-bearing skin to the subcutaneous tissue. The anterior skin flap is raised in an anterior direction toward the lateral edge of the pectoralis major muscle. The skin flap is kept thin to avoid entry into the axillary contents. This helps to avoid damage to the intercostobrachial nerve. Once the lateral border of the pectoralis major muscle is identified, its fascia is incised, and the subpectoral space is entered under direct vision. A finger sweep technique is used to further develop the separation between the pectoralis major and pectoralis minor muscles.

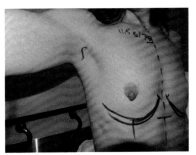

TECH FIG 1 • In this patient, an S-shaped incision was planned. This incision design was used due to the narrow width of the segment of hair-bearing skin. This design permits a longer functional length to attempt to minimize potential damage to the device during placement, and minimize ultimate incision visibility during recovery.

TECHNIQUES

T E C H N I Q U E S

■ Optical Cavity

- Once the entry between the incision and the space between the pectoralis major and minor muscles has been defined, the endoscopic retractor is introduced. Once correctly positioned, the 10-mm 30-degree-angled endoscope is brought into the operative field and placed into the retractor sheath. The camera head on the endoscope is checked for proper orientation, a critical step to ensure safety with the technique. The suction cautery is then used to create an optical cavity from the undersurface of the pectoralis major muscle (**TECH FIG 2A**). Staying on the undersurface of the muscle allows for variations in rib cage anatomy

to not be a problem. This is performed in a uniform fashion to create optimal visualization of the pectoralis major muscle in preparation for the muscle release. The author feels that using the cautery to create the optical cavity is critical to avoid significant blood staining of tissues that can otherwise make endoscopic tissue dissection difficult. *The key to this procedure is to avoid bleeding in the tissue pocket!* (**TECH FIG 2B–D**). Though the initial descriptions of this procedure advocated use of the Agris-Dingman dissectors, the author has found that the occasional bloody outcome from that approach can be avoided with use of the cautery to create the optical cavity.[2]

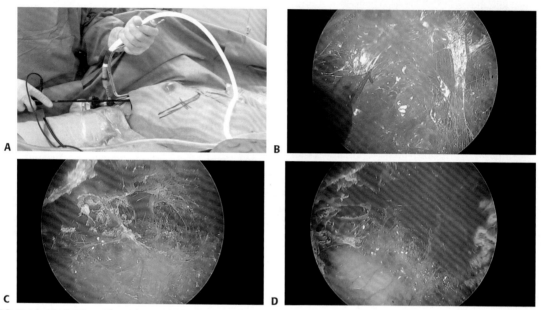

TECH FIG 2 • A. The endoscopic equipment is used in a way that ensures proper orientation of the endoscopic tower. The camera head is checked to confirm correct alignment and orientation for the endoscopic dissection. The suction cautery allows for successful smoke evacuation, vital to correct endoscopic visualization. **B–D.** Endoscopic view of the entry into the subpectoral space. Note areolar plane and lack of anatomic markings. Orientation on this right sided dissection is as follows: left is medial, right is lateral, the rib cage is inferior, and the pectoralis major muscle is superior. The optical cavity is created using the cautery off the undersurface of the pectoralis major muscle. The entire base of the pectoralis major muscle is dissected to complete creation of the optical cavity.

■ Pectoralis Major Muscle Release

- Successful creation of an optical cavity facilitates release of the pectoralis major muscle. The first step to release of the pectoral muscle is to correlate internal anatomy with external landmarks. This is the key step to the technical control needed to control the level and shape of the IMF (**TECH FIG 3A–D**). An advantage of the axillary approach is that, when performed as described, the surgeon has a direct and clear view of the pectoralis major muscle and fascial layers that cannot be matched with an inframammary approach. Additionally, the incision itself has no bearing on the IMF or the level it is placed.
- In the patient shown, the plan was to lower the IMF. The initial muscle release is performed to divide the muscle at a level several millimeters above the existing IMF, medial to lateral, again carefully correlating external landmarks to internal anatomy. Transillumination can be very helpful in confirming that the muscle has been divided at the desired level. Once this has been confirmed, the cautery is used

to dissect in a very controlled and limited fashion in a plane superficial to the lower muscle cuff. Because of the magnification of the endoscope, limited tissue cuts make powerful and significant changes in the area of the IMF. Transillumination can again be used to confirm that the release is to the desired level of the new IMF. The muscle edges of the upper and lower cuffs are inspected and contacted with the cautery if any bleeding points are noted. *It is of critical importance that overdissection be avoided!* (**TECH FIG 3E–G**) Additionally, it is critical to understand that when planning to lower the IMF, the actual *release of the pectoralis major muscle should never be below the existing IMF*, as such a release will consistently result in a double bubble deformity. If the goal is to maintain the IMF at the same level without change, then the pectoralis major should be divided at a level 1.5 to 2 cm above the existing IMF. When properly performed, visual clarity afforded by the endoscope allows for the prepectoral fascia to be divided or maintained as needed.

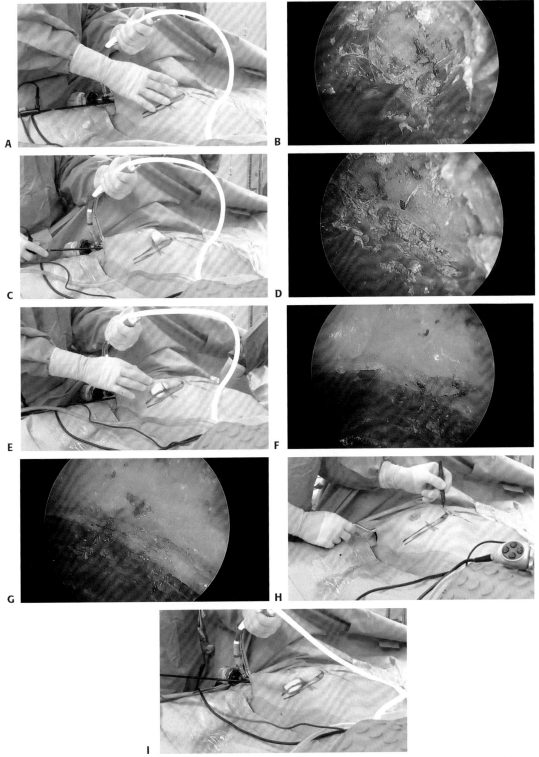

TECH FIG 3 • A. The start of the release of the pectoralis major muscle is based on correlating external markings with internal anatomy. **B,C.** The release level is just above the existing level of the IMF. The correct level can also confirmed by transillumination, as shown. **D.** The completion of the initial release is shown. **E.** Transillumination confirms the IMF level from the initial dissection, and then after the fold is lowered in a precise manner. The lateral portion of the tissue pocket is underdissected intentionally at this stage. **F,G.** The IMF is lowered by dissection just superficial to the prepectoral fascia of the lower muscle cuff. This is shown before **(F)** and after **(G)** the controlled release, performed to match external markings. Note that small cuts performed in this way are needed to lower the IMF, and that any overrelease is difficult to correct with this approach and should be aggressively avoided! **(H).** The adequacy of the periphery of the dissection is checked with the aid of Agris-Dingmandissectors, placed in a way to avoid excessive contact with the underlying ribs. **I.** The endoscopic equipment is used to make any final refinements and to check hemostasis prior to device placement. The device selection is made at this time so that the dimensions of the pocket are refined to match the dimensions of the device to be placed.

- The Agris-Dingman dissectors are then used to confirm the adequacy of the peripheral extent of the dissection (**TECH FIG 3H**). They are used in a way to minimize contact with rib periosteum. They are not used to manipulate the muscle at this point in the procedure.

- The endoscopic retractor and endoscope are reintroduced to recheck for optimal hemostasis and complete any refinements of the soft tissue release in preparation for device placement (**TECH FIG 3I**). On completion of this, the endoscope is removed and retractor is used as a conduit for placement of preferred irrigation solutions.

■ Device Placement

- Selection of the specific device to be used can now proceed according to surgeon preference. It is the author's preference to make this decision at the time of pocket refinement so that the dimensions of the tissue pocket can fit the width of the device as closely as possible. It is also the author's preference that once the device is selected, the packaging is opened on the back table and handled by the surgeon only with new gloves. Antibiotic solution is placed into the implant container, after which the device is placed into an insertion sleeve (**TECH FIG 4A**). Although the procedure can be performed without this, it seems appropriate that this simple measure can help decrease contact between the device and the skin and subcutaneous tissues, including hair-bearing skin, to attempt to lessen exposure of the device to bacteria during placement.

- After placement, the correct position of the device vertically in the tissue pocket is confirmed with the patient placed in a sitting position. Additionally, the fit of the implant to the width of the pocket is checked, so that the posterior aspect of the device lies flat against the rib cage and the anterior surface is flat against the muscle and breast tissue in the dual plane. Any adjustments are made as needed (**TECH FIG 4B–F**). If a shaped implant has been used, the vertical position must be confirmed carefully, because these devices are not able to be manipulated postoperatively in the same way that smooth devices can be. Additionally, correct orientation of the device must be checked by inspection of the upper device landmarks available, which varies between manufacturers. A fiberoptic retractor is used for this purpose.[3,4]

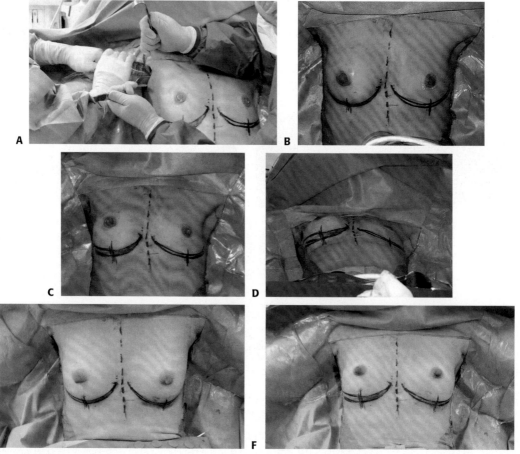

TECH FIG 4 • A. In preparation for device placement, two 1-in. Deaver retractors are used to open access to the tissue tunnel. One is placed parallel to the clavicle and one parallel to the lateral rib cage to maximize the opening. An insertion sleeve is used to assist in placement and to minimize device contact with skin and subcutaneous tissues. **B–D.** Photos are shown following placement of the first device in the three positions used to confirm that the device is placed to the level of the modified IMF and to confirm the overall adequacy of appearance. Note that the pocket fits the implant precisely. **E,F.** Following placement of the second device, the appearance of the second side is confirmed and overall symmetry is checked.

TECHNIQUES

■ Closure and Dressings

- After completion of the second side, a fiberoptic retractor is used for inspection of the upper tissue pocket. After meticulous hemostasis has been obtained, the upper pocket is irrigate with saline solution. The deep dermis is closed using 3-0 PDS, followed by 5-0 plain gut (**TECH FIG 5A**). The axillary skin closure must be secure given its exposure to repetitive movement and perspiration.

- One inch Microfoam (3M Corporation) tape is used to reinforce the level and shape of the IMF. This tape reinforcement also pushes tissue swelling away from the IMF area.
- Gauze is placed over the incision followed by 4-inch Microfoam tape. This is important to generate pressure over the axilla to discourage fluid collections and keep the devices as low as placed in the operating room (**TECH FIG 5B**).

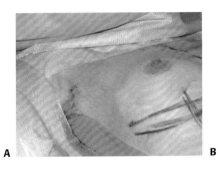 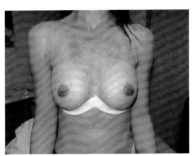

TECH FIG 5 • **A.** Incision is closed in a multilayer fashion. **B.** Initial postoperative visit 1 day following procedure. Tape along the IMF, placed at the conclusion of the procedure is in place to help stabilize the shape and level of the IMF.

A   **B**

PEARLS AND PITFALLS

Incision design	■ Anterior extension of incision must be planned to *not extend beyond the posterior border of the pectoralis major muscle.*
Incision to pectoralis major muscle	■ A thin skin flap is raised anteriorly from the incision until the lateral border of the pectoralis major muscle is identified.
Entry into the subpectoral space	■ The lateral pectoralis major muscle fascia is incised allowing entry into the space deep to the pectoralis major and above the pectoralis minor muscle. A finger sweep is used to aid in identifying the space clearly.
Optical cavity creation	■ Cautery dissection is used to create a uniform space, or optical cavity, first developing the areolar plane *just deep to the pectoralis major.* This is continued until the entire undersurface of the pectoralis major can be clearly delineated, in preparation for the muscle release.
Pectoralis major muscle release	■ The initial cut into the pectoralis major muscle is made just above the existing IMF, confirmed and controlled by *correlating external landmarks to internal anatomy.* ■ This correlation must be rechecked repeatedly. ■ The IMF is then lowered by dissection just superficial to the prepectoral fascia of the lower muscle cuff.
Postoperative dressing	■ Pressure is placed to address the soft tissue tunnel used for device placement, to prevent the device from moving upward in the early postop period.

POSTOPERATIVE CARE

- Postoperative pressure dressing is removed 1 to 3 days after the procedure. The tape reinforcement of the IMF is kept in place for 1 week (**FIG 5**).
- Patients are encouraged to begin controlled arm movement the day after the procedure.
- Patients are free to begin nonimpact aerobic exercise after 1 week. That includes unlimited cycling. All aerobic exercise can resume after 2 weeks.

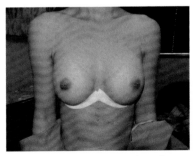

FIG 5 • Second postoperative visit at 1 week confirms excellent shape. The tape along the IMF is removed but additional support from a tight underwire bra is used to help stabilize the IMF.

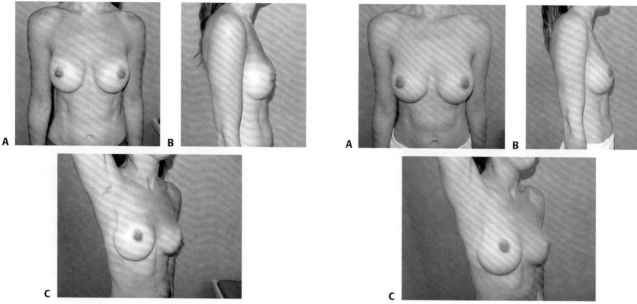

FIG 6 • A–C. Postoperative photos at 6 months.

FIG 7 • A–C. Postoperative photos at 18 months.

OUTCOMES

- Postoperative photos are shown on postoperative intervals. Photos are shown of frontal, oblique, lateral, and axillary incision at 6 months (**FIG 6**) and 18 months (**FIG 7**).[5]

COMPLICATIONS

- Complications associated with the procedure are those of breast augmentation.
- Unique to this version of breast augmentation is the potential for the device to shift back up into the soft tissue tunnel used for placement. Only after this aspect of care has been mastered, in addition to technique for creation of the tissue pocket, can shaped devices be used with this approach. If textured/shaped implants shift upward during the recovery period, it is not likely that they can be returned to the correct position.

REFERENCES

1. Price CI, Eaves FF, Nahai F, Jones G, Bostwick J. Endoscopic transaxillary subpectoral breast augmentation. *Plast Reconstr Surg.* 1994;94(5):612-619.
2. Strock LL. Transaxillary endoscopic silicone gel breast augmentation. *Aesthetic Surg J.* 2010;30(5):745-755.
3. Huang GJ, Wichmann, JL, Mills DC. Transaxillary subpectoral augmentation mammoplasty: a single surgeon's 20-year experience. *Aesthetic Surg J.* 2011;31(7):781-801.
4. Gryskiewicz J, LeDuc R. Transaxillary nonendoscopic subpectoral augmentation mammoplasty: a 10-year experience with gel vs. saline in 2000 patients- with ling-term patient satisfaction measured by the Breast-Q. *Aesthetic Surg J.* 2014;34(5):696-713.
5. Strock LL. Commentary on: "Transaxillary endoscopic breast augmentation using shaped gel implants". *Aesthet Surg J.* 2015;35(8): 962-964.

Breast Augmentation: Subglandular, Subfascial, and Submuscular Implant Placement

CHAPTER 2

Chet Mays and Bradley Calobrace

DEFINITION

- A critical choice in breast augmentation is where to place the implant pocket.
  - Subglandular
  - Subfascial
  - Submuscular (for purposes of this paper, submuscular refers to below the pectoralis major)
- Implant choice, size, and location are based on a variety of patient qualities.
- A biodimensional analysis is essential in determining the optimal implant type, size, and pocket location. There are many methods of evaluation. The High Five system described by Tebbetts is a systematic approach that illustrates the most important aspects of evaluation, including the following:[24]
  - Base width of breast
  - Base width of implant
  - Nipple to fold distance
  - Estimate of final implant volume
  - Pocket determination based on skin pinch thickness

Subglandular Implant

- The subglandular implant is deep to the breast tissue and superficial fascia, but superficial to the deep pectoralis fascia, coming to rest on the inframammary fold (**FIG 1**).
- The subglandular pocket has long been regarded as the most natural pocket.[2]
- The advantages of subglandular implant placement include the following:
  - It avoids implant deformation or distortion that can be seen in the subpectoral position
  - Enhances the improvement in the constricted or ptotic breast
  - Allows an easier dissection plane
  - Decreased postoperative discomfort
  - Allows access to the inframammary fold (IMF) as the superficial and deep fascial components merge
- There are some disadvantages of the subglandular pocket, which include the following:
  - Pocket with the least soft tissue coverage to disguise the implant
  - Increased visibility or palpability of implant with wrinkling or rippling
  - Higher capsular contracture rate
  - Less support and stabilization of the implants, especially shaped devices, compared to subfascial or submuscular pockets

Subfascial Implant

- Advantages to placing the implant in a subfascial pocket (**FIG 2**) include the following:[1,3;23]
  - It avoids implant deformation or distortion (animation deformity) that can be seen in the subpectoral position.
  - This position provides additional soft tissue coverage between the implant and the skin as compared to the subglandular pocket.
  - Fascia provides additional support to minimize implant edge visibility and palpability seen most commonly with subglandular placement.
  - Fascia provides support of implant especially in the upper pole minimizing excess implant movement and potential rotation with shaped implants.
  - Less postoperative pain as compared to submuscular placement
  - Fascia provides a distinct layer separating the implant from the overlying breast parenchyma.
- The disadvantages of a subfascial pocket include the following:
  - Less soft tissue coverage compared to submuscular coverage

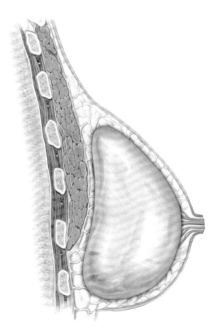

FIG 1 • Subglandular implant placement is deep to the breast tissue but superficial to the pectoralis fascia.

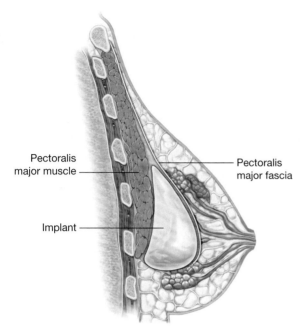

FIG 2 • Subfascial implant placement is deep to the breast tissue and the pectoralis major fascia but superficial to the muscle.

- More challenging dissection to separate deep pectoral fascia from underlying muscle while keeping fascia intact.
- Higher rate of capsular contracture compared to submuscular

Submuscular Implant

- Advantages to placing the implant in a submuscular pocket (**FIG 3**) as compared to placement in the subglandular or subfascial pocket include the following:
  - Lower capsular contracture rates[1,4]

- Enhanced coverage of the implant
- Reduced issues with wrinkling
- Sloping natural upper pole
- Enhanced support for the breast implant
- Enhanced radiographic imaging with mammogram[5,22]
- The disadvantages of a submuscular pocket include the following:
  - Animation deformity
  - Increased risk of implant superior malposition with waterfall deformity
  - Increased postoperative pain
  - Limited expansion of the lower pole of breast (required to expand constricted and ptotic breasts)
- The most significant attribute of the submuscular pocket is in providing maximum soft tissue coverage for the implant. The widespread use of saline implants and wrinkling issues led to surgeons looking for improved implant coverage. After the moratorium on silicone was lifted, surgeons in the United States continued to use the submuscular pocket with mostly smooth and to a limited extent textured silicone implants.[6]

ANATOMY

- An understanding of the breast blood and nerve supply is critical when performing breast surgery (**FIG 4AB**).
- Muscular attachments are shown in **FIG 4C**.
- The breast is a skin appendage contained within layers of the superficial fascia.
  - The superficial layer of this fascia is near the dermis and is not distinct from it.
  - The deep layer of the superficial fascia is more distinct and is identifiable on the deep surface of the breast when the breast is elevated in a subglandular augmentation mammoplasty.

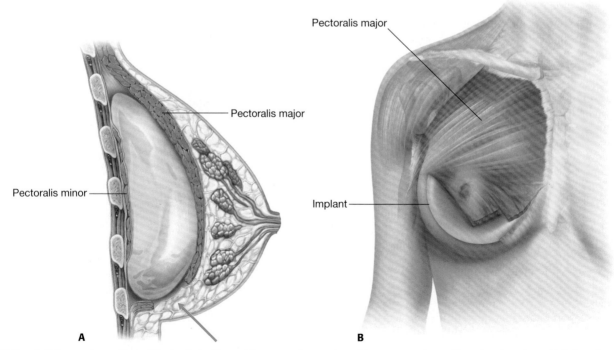

FIG 3 • **A.** Submuscular position of the implant with overlying pectoralis muscle and breast parenchyma. Note that the released inferior edge of the pectoralis major allows lower pole expansion (*arrow*). **B.** Anterior view of the implant placement below the pectoralis major.

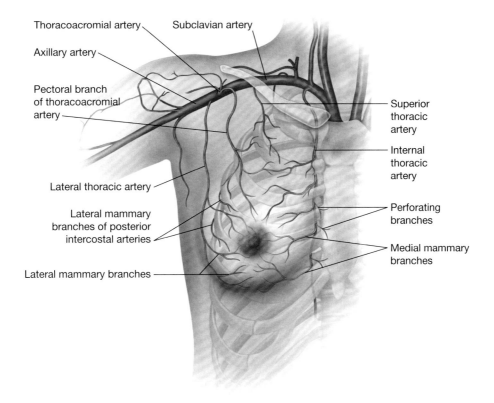

A

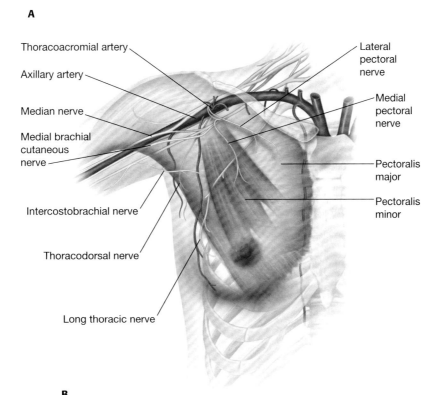

B

FIG 4 • **A.** Arterial blood supply of the breast. **B.** Nerve branches supplying the breast.

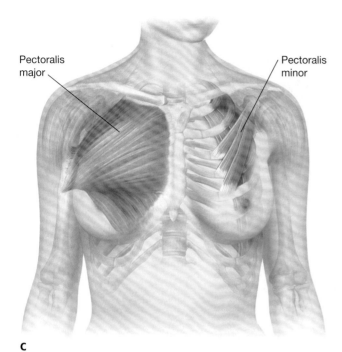

Pectoralis major

Pectoralis minor

C

FIG 4 (Continued) • **C.** Muscular attachments to the chest. The pectoralis major is removed on the right side of the picture revealing the underlying pectoralis minor.

- There is loose areolar tissue between the deep layer of the superficial fascia and the fascia to cover the pectoralis major that and to cover the adjacent rectus abdominis, serratus anterior, and external oblique muscles.
- The deep pectoralis fascia has its origin on the clavicle and sternum, extending toward the lateral border of the muscle to form the axillary fascia (**FIG 5**).
  - It continues down to cover the latissimus dorsi muscle, rectus abdominis, serratus anterior, and external oblique.

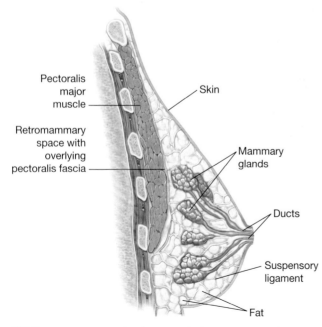

Pectoralis major muscle

Skin

Retromammary space with overlying pectoralis fascia

Mammary glands

Ducts

Suspensory ligament

Fat

FIG 5 • Breast anatomy showing pectoralis fascia posterior to the breast tissue.

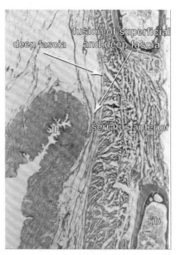

FIG 6 • Histologic slide of the inframammary fold (IMF) showing the superficial and deep fascia fusing together.[7]

- The subfascial pocket is deep to this deep pectoral fascia but superficial to the underlying muscle.
  - This fascia is thin and more fragile in the lower two-thirds of the pectoralis muscle and becomes denser and substantial in the upper third of the muscle.
- The thin fascia in the lower aspects of the breast can make the initial subfascial dissection more challenging, which becomes easier as the dissection proceeds toward the upper pectoralis muscle.
- The deep fascia overlying the pectoralis and the deep layer of the superficial fascia underlying the breast unite with the dermis to form the IMF (**FIG 6**).[7]

PATIENT HISTORY AND PHYSICAL FINDINGS

- Initial consultation should evaluate the patient's goals and anticipated results with the breast augmentation.
- A thorough history and physical should be done to identify any risk factors for the procedure, including bleeding or clotting disorders.
- Any history of breast lumps, masses, or breast disease should be elicited.
- A family history is required.
- In planning for optimal implant pocket selection, it is important to determine the desired appearance or "look" the patient is seeking.
  - The submuscular pocket is more likely to create a smooth, sloping upper pole with minimal roundedness in the upper pole.
  - A patient desiring a more rounded upper pole with a more obvious "implant appearance" with implant shape visibility may prefer a subglandular implant, provided there is adequate soft tissue coverage.
  - The subfascial approach can provide a compromise between the two; the implant will be in a plane similar to the subglandular, but the additional fascia layer will minimize implant edge visibility and palpability that can be seen with the subglandular pocket.
- The preoperative exam of the breast augmentation patient will guide the surgeon's implant selection and pocket placement. The physical exam measurements should include the following (**FIG 7**):

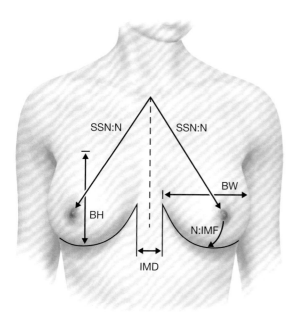

FIG 7 • Necessary physical exam breast measurements.

- Breast width (BW)
- Sternal notch to nipple (SSN:N)
- Breast height (BH)
- Nipple to IMF (N:IMF) at rest and under maximal stretch.
- Upper pole pinch (UPP), medial pinch (MP), and lateral pinch (LP)
- Intermammary distance (IMD)

Pinch Test

- A key point of the exam is the upper pole pinch test.
  - A pinch test of less than 2 cm indicates the need for a submuscular placement of the implant to avoid noticeable rippling (**FIG 8A**).
  - If the pinch test is more than 2 cm (1 cm of soft tissue thickness), the patient is a candidate for a subglandular or subfascial pocket (**FIG 8B**). (The deep fascial layer will provide additional coverage over the implant to allow for subfascial placement.)
- Implant selection impacts adequacy of soft tissue coverage. Keep in mind the thinner the soft tissue, the greater the risk of implant palpation and rippling.
  - Some implants are prone to more wrinkling, including underfilled saline implants and textured devices.
  - We require a pinch test of more than 2 cm if placing the implant subfascially or subglandularly, where the soft tissue coverage is firm and good quality.

- If the soft tissue coverage is lax and poor quality or if the implant selected is deemed at risk for wrinkling, a pinch test greater than 3 cm is more reliable in providing adequate coverage and minimizing the risk of rippling.
- Adequate soft tissue coverage in the upper pole in a subglandular augmentation will camouflage the transition between the breast and implant, aiding to a smooth natural upper pole.
- The deep fascia overlying the implant in the subfascial pocket will provide additional support and coverage in the upper pole and minimize the implant edge visibility, which can be seen if implants are placed in the subglandular pocket with limited upper pole coverage.
- If the patient prefers a full, rounded upper pole with an obvious transition between her implant and soft tissue, a subglandular implant would be preferred even if the pinch test is less than 2 cm.
  - One must have a discussion regarding visible and palpable rippling of the implant if placing the implant subglandular and the pinch test is less than 2 cm.
- Capsular contracture can be reduced by using a textured implant in the subglandular position, but one must consider the risks of rippling with textured implant in a patient with inadequate upper pole coverage with a pinch test of less than 2 cm.[1]

Physical Assessment

- Assess for all asymmetries, including breast volume, IMF, nipple-areolar complex (NAC), and chest wall.
- Chest wall (skeletal and muscle) abnormalities or asymmetries are often underappreciated and can significantly alter the final result (**FIG 9**).[8]
  - Pectus excavatum occurs occasionally, whereas pectus carinatum and Poland syndrome are rare.[9]
  - Central deformities are typically ameliorated sufficiently by breast augmentation alone.
  - Deep pectus excavatum deformities can be treated simultaneously with a custom solid silicone implant made from a plaster mold, although most patients decline this option.
  - Poland syndrome (absence of sternal head of pectoralis muscle) is best addressed with subglandular augmentation as the sternal head of the pectoralis major muscle is absent. When more severe, more extensive adjunctive procedures, such as tissue expansion, fat grafting, and latissimus muscle transfer, may be required.[10]
  - Hemithorax asymmetry due to differences in shape, protrusion, or regression can create an uneven breast foundation, suggesting different size implants despite equivalent breast volumes.

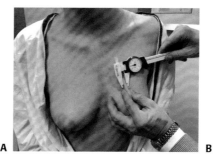 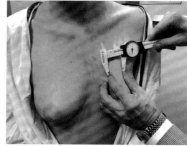

FIG 8 • **A.** Upper pole pinch test less than 2 cm and **(B)** more than 2 cm.

A   B

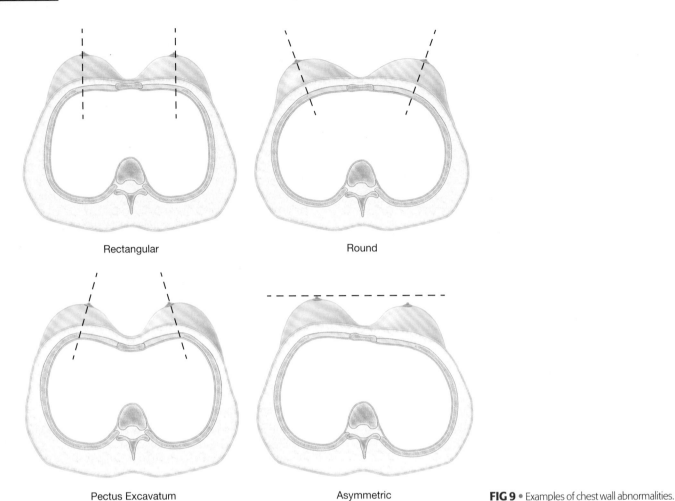

Rectangular   Round

Pectus Excavatum   Asymmetric

FIG 9 • Examples of chest wall abnormalities.

- Unilateral prominence of the chest wall is often associated with scoliosis (**FIG 10**).
- Subtle unilateral pectoralis hypertrophy should not affect subglandular or subfascial implant placement, but it could affect subpectoral placement and overall implant projection.

IMAGING

- Screening mammography per the American College of Surgeons is recommended for patients over 40 years of age.
- Many plastic surgeons recommend a baseline mammogram at 35 or older prior to a breast augmentation, especially if a family history is present.
- Any additional diagnostic studies are guided by the preoperative exam.

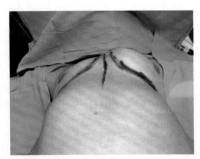

FIG 10 • Left chest wall prominence compared to the right chest wall.

- Any palpable mass requires evaluation, usually with a diagnostic ultrasound and/or mammogram.

SURGICAL MANAGEMENT

- The preoperative evaluation and decision-making are a critical step in achieving optimal outcomes in breast augmentation.
- Capsular contracture is the leading indication for revision breast surgery after a breast augmentation and every effort should be made during planning and execution to minimize the risk of capsular contracture postoperatively. Placement of breast implants in the submuscular pocket has consistently demonstrated reduction in capsular contracture rates compared with the other pocket choices.[1,4]
- Validated steps to reduce this risk include the following:
    - Nipple shields[11]
    - No-touch technique[12]
    - Use of an insertion sleeve[13]
    - Pocket irrigation with triple antibiotics[14]
    - Inframammary incisions[4]
    - Use of textured implants[1,4]

Preoperative Planning

Incision

- The decision on incision placement is based on a variety of variables:
    - Patient and surgeon preferences
    - Anatomic considerations

- Implant type and size
- Issues of capsular contracture, breast-feeding, and NAC sensation
- There are many potential advantages of the inframammary approach, including the following:
  - Well-hidden scar in the fold of the breast
  - Incisional length is unlimited, thus can accommodate any and all implant choices
  - Excellent visualization for dissection of the implant pocket
  - The ability to control the IMF position during incision closure
  - Can be used for any complication revision
  - Lower capsular contracture
  - Minimal issue of a scar contracture creating deformity
  - Potentially less nipple sensation changes
- Potential disadvantages of the inframammary incision include the following:
  - The scar is located on the breast
  - Scar may be more visible if breast fold is absent or if the scar becomes pigmented
  - Must determine final IMF position preaugmentation and place scar precisely in planned new fold.
  - Scar position more vulnerable to irritation from the bra
- There are many potential advantages of the periareolar approach, including the following:
  - Scar can be camouflaged in the areolar border
  - Direct visualization and access into the breast pocket
  - Can lower the IMF to any location without predetermining location
  - Central access allows use in most revision cases with optimal visualization and access to the upper pole of the breast
  - Access for parenchymal breast scoring in constricted breast deformities
- Potential disadvantages of the periareolar incision include the following:
  - The scar is located on the breast
  - Access is through a tunnel and may limit visualization in dense, heavy breasts
  - Cannot use if areolae are too small
  - Poor scarring possible and can create significant deformities
  - IMF control sutures not possible when IMF is lowered
  - Transection of breast ducts may increase bacterial contamination
  - Potentially higher capsular contracture rates[15]
- Good candidates for the inframammary approach may include the following:
  - Small areola
  - When controlling IMF is desired
  - Indistinct areolar border
  - Desire for no scar on the breast
  - Potentially when placing larger implants
  - Desire future breast feeding as interference with lactation has been implicated with periareolar incision.[5]
  - Concerns with nipple sensation, although no strong data to support this concern.[3,16]
- Good candidates for the periareolar approach may include the following:
  - Very distinct areolar borders present

- When areola large enough to accommodate implant and avoid implant trauma
- When performing a concurrent mastopexy
- Indistinct or absence of IMF to hide scar
- When lowering IMF (IMF position does not need to be predetermined)
- Treatment of tuberous breasts (parenchymal scoring, IMF lowering)
- The incision should be as small as possible but large enough to dissect the pocket and place the implant without distorting or injuring the device.
  - Incision length ranges include 3 to 4.5 cm for saline implants, 4 to 6 cm for silicone round implants, and 4.5 to 7 cm for shaped cohesive silicone implants.[17]
  - The length of the incision would be smaller with saline than with silicone implants. Factors requiring increased incision length include the following:
    - Implant volume
    - Implant texture
    - Silicone compared to saline
    - Increased gel cohesiveness (silicone gel firmness)
    - Increase implant projection
    - Shaped implants (cohesiveness and gel distribution)
- When using the periareolar approach, the incision is made around the areola and the dissection is carried inferiorly the appropriate distance to accommodate the selected breast implant.
  - However, when the approach is through an IMF incision, the final position of the fold postaugmentation must be predetermined so the incision can be placed accurately in that location.
  - Before surgery, the IMF is identified and marked in the sitting position (**FIG 11A**). To determine the true IMF position, the breast is autorotated inferiorly to identify the inferior extent of the attachments of the IMF (**FIG 11B**).
- The distance measured from the nipple to the true fold under maximal stretch assesses the amount of lower pole skin available to accommodate the selected implant.
- The amount of lower pole skin required and the ultimate position of the fold is a function of many factors, including the type of implant (saline vs silicone, round vs shaped), size of implant, pocket location, and the strength and stability of the soft tissue of the lower pole.
- An acceptable standard that can be used is to follow the guidelines that an implant with a base diameter of 11 cm requires 7 cm, a base diameter of 12 cm requires 8 cm, and a base diameter of 13 cm requires 9 cm from nipple to fold.[18]
- Another useful method of estimating fold position is based on implant height and projection and can be used for round or shaped implants[17]:
  - Optimal nipple to IMF distance = (1/2 implant projection) + (1/2 implant height)
  - IMF lowering = (optimal nipple to IMF distance) – (measured nipple to IMF distance)
- If the measured nipple to fold distance is less than the desired or optimal distance, the fold will need to be lowered.
- Keep in mind that textured and smooth implants have different effect on the lower pole skin and fold over time. A larger smooth implant will lead to more stretch on the lower pole compared to a smaller or textured implant.

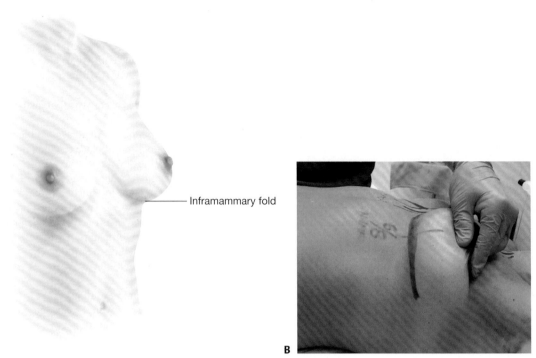

A   **B**

FIG 11 • A. The inframammary fold is a natural boundary where the chest and the breast meet. **B.** Autorotation of the breast. N:IMF is 6 cm at rest. N:IMF is 8 cm on stretch/autorotation.

Pocket Control

- Pocket control is key and begins during preoperative markings to design the pocket size necessary to accommodate the selected implant.
- Controlling the pocket involves placement of the IMF, defining the medial and lateral pocket margins.
  - This creates the desired cleavage and prevents lateral migration or malposition of the implant.
- Whereas smooth implants often are designed with a larger pocket to allow for implant mobility and perceived softness, pocket design should be more limited when using a textured implant.
  - Excess movement can lead to irritation and seroma formation.
- When using a shaped textured implant, a controlled pocket is even more essential to minimize the risk of implant rotation postoperatively.
  - This requires defining the lateral, medial, and inferior as well as the superior border and limiting the pocket to only what is required to accommodate the shaped device.
  - The implant and pocket should ultimately have a "hand-in-glove" fit.[19]

Positioning

- Patients are placed on the operating room table in the supine position.
- The arms are secured to the arm board at approximately 45 degrees to stabilize the patient in the upright position. Actual arm placement is between 45 and 60 degrees (**FIG 12**).
- Some surgeons place the arms directly by the patient's side.
- Having the arms abducted to 90 degrees should be avoided because this does not allow the breasts to be in a relaxed position when sitting the patient up to check adequacy of implant placement and soft tissue redraping.

Approach

- Before surgical preparation, 50 mL of a local field block of 1/4% lidocaine, 1/8% bupivacaine, and 1:400 000 epinephrine is injected into breast (Table 1).
- A 20-mL syringe with a 22-gauge spinal needle is used to inject the anesthetic into the dermis along the planned incision line, deep to the dermis along the IMF, the medial pectoral border, the anterior axillary line, and deep to the breast parenchyma, in a fanning fashion throughout the area of planned pocket creation (**FIG 13**).
  - These injections provide assistance not only in operative hemostasis but also in the management of postoperative pain.
  - This is less important in the subglandular augmentation as postoperative pain is significantly less than with a submuscular augmentation.

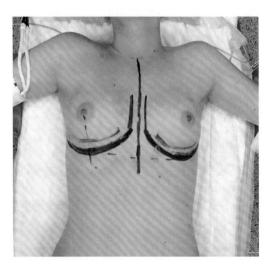

FIG 12 • Arms abducted at approximately 45 to 60 degrees in supine position.

Table 1 Breast Local Anesthetic Formula

Drug	Amount
½% lidocaine plain	25 mL
½% lidocaine/1:200 000 epinephrine	25 mL
½% bupivacaine/1:200 000 epinephrine	25 mL
Injectable saline	25 mL
Total concentration: ¼% lidocaine, 1/8% bupivacaine, 1:400 000 epinephrine	100 mL

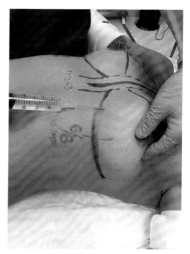

FIG 13 • Breast infusion with 20-cc syringe and a 22-gauge spinal needle.

■ Subglandular and Subfascial Placement

- The distinction between the subglandular and the subfascial plane is subtle and opinions differ on whether it is of clinical importance.
- The common aspect is both involve dissection superficial to the muscle and avoid both, the animation deformity associated with the muscle and the limitation the muscle plays on the ability of the implant to expand the breast envelope.

Inframammary Fold Incision

- A variety of incisional approaches to the subglandular, subfascial, or submuscular pocket are possible, the inframammary fold (IMF) being the most common.
  - This incision is performed the same for both subglandular or subfascial pockets.
- After determining the IMF position (either the native true fold position or the planned lowered position), a paramedian line is drawn through the center of the breast and bisects the newly drawn IMF.
- The incision's medial extent begins 1 cm medial to the paramedian line and extends laterally for the appropriate distance, as previously described based on the implant type (**TECH FIG 1A**).
  - The incision is made with a no. 15 blade through the skin to the mid-dermis (**TECH FIG 1B**).

- Dissection is then carried out with electrocautery through the skin and subcutaneous tissue, beveling superiorly while rotating the breast off of the chest wall.
- Once dissection has been carried superiorly for 1 cm, the dissection is carried through the superficial fascia and toward the chest wall.
- The beveling preserves a small cuff of superficial fascia at the incision, which ensures the fold is not inadvertently lowered and also provides a cuff of Scarpa fascia that will prove useful during closure (**TECH FIG 1C**).
- As dissection proceeds toward the chest wall, a constant upward retraction of the breast tissue is maintained, exposing the pectoralis major with its overlying fascia (**TECH FIG 1D**).
  - The upward retraction of the breast tissue is key, as the suspensory ligaments of the breast concomitantly elevate the muscle to expose the muscle edge.
  - The only distinguishing characteristic is at the level of the IMF incision, dissection begins over the pectoralis fascia for the subglandular pocket or deep to the fascia for a subfascial pocket.
  - The elevation of the subglandular pocket is superficial to the pectoralis fascia, and the elevation of the subfascial is deep to the breast and fascia, but superficial to the muscle.

TECHNIQUES

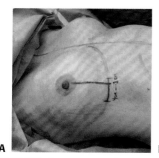
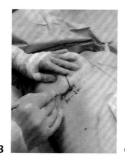
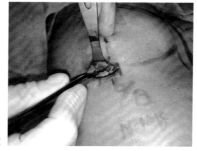
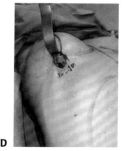

A **B** **C** **D**

TECH FIG 1 • **A.** Paramedian line drawn from the nipple to the IMF. Note the 5 cm incision length. **B.** 5-cm inframammary incision. **C.** Cuff of Scarpa fascia. **D.** Upward rotation of the breast with retractor exposes the underlying pectoralis muscle.

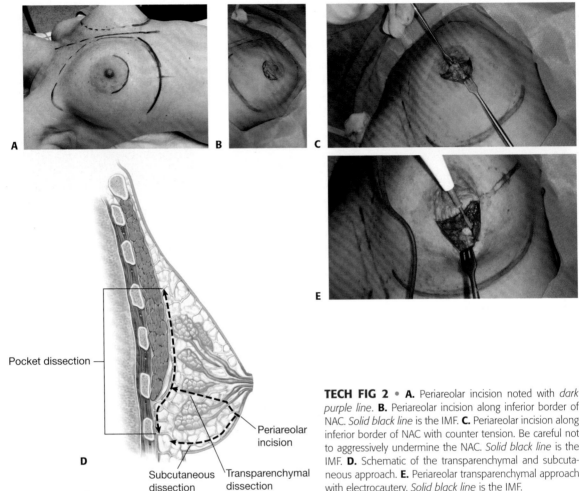

TECH FIG 2 • A. Periareolar incision noted with *dark purple line*. **B.** Periareolar incision along inferior border of NAC. *Solid black line* is the IMF. **C.** Periareolar incision along inferior border of NAC with counter tension. Be careful not to aggressively undermine the NAC. *Solid black line* is the IMF. **D.** Schematic of the transparenchymal and subcutaneous approach. **E.** Periareolar transparenchymal approach with electrocautery. *Solid black line* is the IMF.

Periareolar Incision

- Development of the periareolar incision differs slightly based on either subglandular or subfascial implant placement is intended. The differences are distinguished below.
- The planned incision location is marked directly on the border of the inferior areolar and breast skin with a series of dots.
- The dots are used instead of a line for more accurate visualization of the exact areolar border.
- It is most important to follow the exact outline of the areolar border even if irregular because any deviation off the border to smooth the incision outline leads to a more visible scar (**TECH FIG 2A**).
- The planned incision should extend equidistance medial and lateral from the midline but not to exceed half of the circumference of the areola.
- With the skin placed under tension by the assistant, the incision is made precisely on the areolar border with a no. 15 blade through the skin to the mid-dermis (**TECH FIG 2B**).
- Dissection then proceeds through the deep dermis and breast parenchyma with electrocautery.
- The skin edges are retracted inferiorly and superiorly, and dissection is carried down through the parenchyma toward the pectoralis fascia (**TECH FIG 2C**).

- The dissection should be directed in an inferior direction to ensure that the nipple-areolar complex (NAC) is not inadvertently undermined during dissection and the blood supply compromised.
- Dissection proceeds either directly through the breast tissue (transparenchymal) to the pectoralis fascia or inferiorly under the skin (subcutaneous) until the fascia is reached at the fold. The authors prefer the transparenchymal approach (**TECH FIG 2D,E**).

Subglandular Pocket

- With the subcutaneous periareolar approach (like the IMF approach), the breast elevation and pocket creation begins at the fold and proceeds superiorly in the subglandular plane.
- The IMF is a fusion of the deep fascia attached to the pectoralis and the superficial fascia of the breast.
  - Care is taken to prevent disruption of the IMF as the breast is elevated off the pectoralis fascia.
- If the transparenchymal periareolar approach is used, the dissection is directed through the breast down to the pectoralis fascia.
  - The subglandular pocket is then developed as an inferior flap and superior flap with its overlying breast tissue, creating a continuous pocket superficial to the pectoralis muscle fascia.

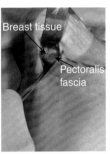
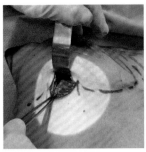

TECH FIG 3 • A. Elevation of the overlying breast tissue with underlying pectoralis muscle and fascia. **B.** Subglandular pocket with pectoralis muscle/fascia visible posterior to the pocket.

- If the fold is inadvertently disrupted and the IMF lowering is not planned, the fold must be controlled with deep fascial sutures at the time of incision closure.
- Continued upward retraction of the breast will elevate the breast and its underlying superficial fascia as a single unit, leaving the deep pectoralis fascia attached to the muscle.
- The dissection is carried superiorly, medial and lateral to create the desired pocket (**TECH FIG 3**).

Subfascial Pocket

- With the subcutaneous periareolar approach (like the IMF approach), the breast elevation and pocket creation begins at the fold and proceeds superiorly in the subfascial plane.
- The IMF is a fusion of the deep fascia attached to the pectoralis and the superficial fascia of the breast.
  - Care is taken to prevent disruption of the IMF as the breast and underlying pectoralis fascia are elevated off the underlying pectoralis muscle.
- If the transparenchymal periareolar approach is used, then dissection is directed through the breast down to the pectoralis fascia.
  - The subfascial pocket is then developed as an inferior flap and superior flap of fascia with its overlying breast tissue, creating a continuous pocket superficial to the pectoralis muscle but beneath the fascia.
- If the fold is inadvertently disrupted and the IMF lowering is not planned, the fold must be controlled with deep fascial sutures at the time of incision closure.
- The inferior extent of the pectoralis fascia is thin and elevation is best carried out with the cut current of the electrocautery. The superior fascia is thicker and more developed providing more easily dissected plane.
- Continued upward retraction of the breast will elevate the fascial plane.
- The fascia is left attached to the overlying breast tissue and elevated as a single unit.
- The dissection is carried superiorly, medial and lateral to create the desired pocket (**TECH FIG 4**).

Pocket Control

- As with any breast augmentation, pocket control is key.
- Avoid overdissection of the pocket laterally to optimize medial projection of the implant and minimize lateralization of the implant.
  - Subglandular implants have less lateral drift compared with submuscular implants because they lack

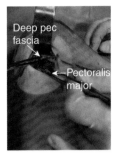

TECH FIG 4 • Creation of the subfascial plane. The deep pectoralis fascia is elevated with the breast tissue exposing the underlying pectoralis major muscle.

the lateral action of the forceful pectoralis muscle contraction.
  - As one carries the subglandular dissection medially, the midline can quickly be violated due to the lack of sternal muscle attachments that usually limit the dissection in the submuscular plane.
  - The fascia is adherent to the underlying pectoralis muscle as the sternum is approached in the subfascial dissection and will provide some limitation to medial overdissection compared to the subglandular pocket.
  - Overdissection can lead to implant medialization and the potential for postoperative symmastia. This is especially true when the chest wall is concave or slanting medially. Special caution with limited medial dissection is warranted in these cases.
- Remember if IMF lowering is needed, the dissection is in the subglandular pocket, as the attachments creating the fold are superficial to the deep pectoral fascia.[20]

Implant Placement

- Once dissection is complete, the pocket is irrigated with triple antibiotic solution (1 g cefazolin sodium, 80 mg gentamicin, 50 000 units bacitracin mixed in 500 mL of normal saline) and hemostasis is assessed (**TECH FIG 5A**).
  - The authors as a personal preference generally remove bacitracin and add betadine solution (50 cc) to the irrigation mixture if no allergy exists.[14]
- The implants are soaked in the irrigation solution before insertion. Gloves are changed and rinsed with the irrigation solution to remove any residue.
- In the authors' practice, the implant is placed into the pocket with the assistance of an insertion sleeve such as the Keller funnel (**TECH FIG 5B**).
  - The opening of the funnel should be cut large enough to allow easy egress of the implant through the funnel. This is confirmed by passing the implant with irrigation solution through the funnel before insertion.
  - The implant orientation is confirmed in the funnel, and a maneuver of squeezing the implant through the funnel with pressure exerted on the back of the funnel slips the implant into the breast pocket.
  - These maneuvers provide a "no-touch" technique, which has been associated with lower capsular contracture rates.[13]

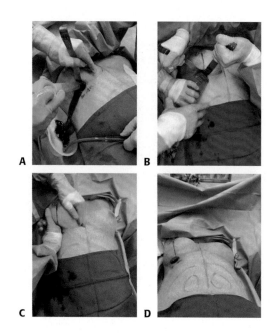

TECH FIG 5 • A. Irrigation of breast pocket prior to implant placement. **B.** Insertion of breast implant into subglandular pocket with Keller funnel. **C.** Hand-assisted implant pocket assessment and breast tissue redraping. **D.** Note the pocket control and the medial projection of the implant in the supine position.

- Once the implant is in the pocket, a finger-assisted assessment and manipulation of the implant within the pocket is necessary to confirm its proper placement and assure appropriate redraping of the breast parenchyma over the implant (**TECH FIG 5C**).
  - This maneuver is especially important with textured devices, as these implants are less mobile and less likely to stretch the pocket and, thus, a distortion or wrinkling of the implant in a tight pocket may be permanent if not resolved before closure.
  - Repeated removal and insertions of the implant should be avoided to minimize implant or incision damage, potential contamination, and pocket over-dissection. This is especially important with shaped implants, as a stretched pocket from over manipulation could lead to implant rotation postoperatively (**TECH FIG 5D**).

Pocket Closure

- Before incision closure, the patient should be placed in the upright position to assess implant position, fold position, and symmetry (**TECH FIG 6A**).
- The inframammary approach is useful to control the fold position during the final closure.

- The cuff of superficial Scarpa fascia that was preserved during the initial incision is used to secure the fold during closure.
- If the IMF structure is stable, and was not violated or lowered during the pocket formation, reapproximation of the superficial fascia during closure is usually adequate.
- If the fold is mobile from inherent weakness or was disrupted with fold lowering, the pocket closure should include stabilization of the fold.
  - Fold stabilization is accomplished by incorporating the deep fascia in the closure.
  - The Scarpa fascia cuff is sutured to the deep fascia in the lower incisional edge during the closure of the IMF (**TECH FIG 6B**).
  - Both the periareolar and inframammary incision are closed in three layers: deep fascia/parenchyma (2-0 Vicryl running), deep dermis (4-0 PDS interrupted), and subcuticular (4-0 PDS running) (**TECH FIG 6C**).
  - Periareolar incisional closures do not stabilize the fold structure as it does with an IMF incision closure.
  - If using a textured device, the implant must be seated at the desired position at the base of the breast pocket because it is less likely to settle in the pocket postoperatively as can be seen with smooth breast implants (**TECH FIG 6D**).

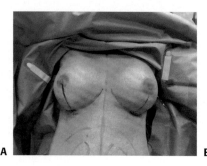
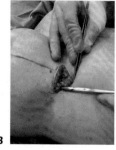

TECH FIG 6 • A. Patient sitting upright prior to final closure to assess for symmetry and final aesthetic result. **B.** Fold stabilization with a 2-0 Vicryl incorporating the deep fascia in the Scarpa fascial closure.

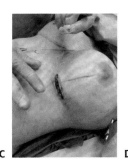
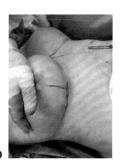

TECH FIG 6 (Continued) • **C.** Image of the final closure incorporating superficial Scarpa fascia and deep fascia as one consistent layer without the presence of an incisional step off. **D.** Downward pressure on the implant/breast demonstrates a locked and stable IMF.

◼ Submuscular (Subpectoral) Implants

Inframammary Fold Incision

- Although the submuscular pocket can be accessed by any incision (periareolar, inframammary, transaxillary, transumbilical), the most common approach is through the inframammary incision.
- After determining the IMF position (either the native true fold position or the planned lowered position), a paramedian line is drawn through the center of the breast and bisects the newly drawn IMF.
- The incision's medial extent begins 1 cm medial to the paramedian line and extends laterally for the appropriate distance, as previously described based on the implant type (see **TECH FIG 1A**).
  - The incision is made with a no. 15 blade through the skin to the mid-dermis (see **TECH FIG 1B**).
- Dissection is then carried out with electrocautery through the skin and subcutaneous tissue, beveling superiorly while rotating the breast off of the chest wall.
- Once dissection has been carried superiorly for 1 cm, the dissection is carried through the superficial fascia and toward the lateral pectoral border deep on the chest wall.
- The beveling preserves a small cuff of superficial fascia at the incision, which ensures that the fold is not inadvertently lowered and also provides a cuff of fascia that will prove useful during closure (see **TECH FIG 1C**).
- Dissection is carried down toward the chest wall while maintaining a constant upward retraction of the breast tissue, ultimately exposing the lateral edge of the pectoralis muscle.
  - The upward retraction of the breast tissue is key as the suspensory ligaments of the breast will concomitantly elevate the muscle (see **TECH FIG 1D**).
- It is imperative to not cut the muscle unless you can elevate the muscle off the chest wall.
  - Inability to elevate the muscle most likely indicates that the identified muscle is actually not the pectoralis, but rather the serratus, rectus, or an intercostal muscle.
  - Dissection through an intercostal could lead to penetration of the pleural space and pneumothorax.
- Once the lateral border of the pectoralis is identified, the fascia is incised to expose the underlying muscle. Continued upward retraction of the breast will elevate the lateral border, allowing further dissection and placement of the retractor beneath the overlying pectoralis muscle.

Periareolar Incision

- The planned incision location is marked directly on the border of the inferior areolar and breast skin with a series of dots. The dots are used instead of a line to allow more accurate visualization of the exact areolar border.
- It is most important to follow the exact outline of the areolar border even if irregular as any deviation off the border in order to smooth the incision outline leads to a more visible scar.
- The planned incision should extend equidistance medial and lateral from the midline but not to exceed half of the circumference of the areola (see **TECH FIG 2A**).
- With the skin placed under tension by the assistant, the incision is made precisely on the areolar border with a 15 blade through the skin to the mid-dermis.
  - Dissection then proceeds through the deep dermis and breast parenchyma with electrocautery (see **TECH FIG 2B,C**).
- The skin edges are retracted inferiorly and superiorly, and dissection is carried down through the parenchyma toward the pectoralis fascia.
- The dissection should be directed in an inferior direction to insure that the NAC is not inadvertently undermined during dissection and blood supply compromised.
- Dissection proceeds either directly through the breast tissue (transparenchymal) to the pectoralis fascia or inferiorly under the skin (subcutaneous) until the fascia is reached at the fold. The authors prefer the transparenchymal approach (see **TECH FIG 2D**).
- With the subcutaneous periareolar approach (like the IMF approach), the breast elevation and pocket creation begins at the fold and proceeds superiorly in the subpectoral pocket.
- The IMF is a fusion of the deep fascia attached to the pectoralis and the superficial fascia of the breast (see **FIG 6**). Take care to prevent disruption of the IMF as the breast and pectoral fascia are elevated.
- If creating a subpectoral dual plane pocket, dissection proceeds subcutaneously or transparenchymal down to the lateral border of the pectoralis muscle.
- If accessing the submuscular pocket, the lateral border of the pectoralis is identified and the fascia is incised to expose the underlying muscle. Continued upward retraction of the breast will elevate the lateral border, allowing further dissection and placement of the retractor beneath the overlying pectoralis muscle

TECHNIQUES

- When creating the submuscular pocket, it is imperative to not cut the muscle unless it can be elevated off the chest wall.
- Inability to elevate the muscle most likely indicates that the identified muscle is actually not the pectoralis, but rather the serratus, rectus, or an intercostal muscle.
  - Dissection through an intercostal could lead to penetration of the pleural space and pneumothorax.

Pocket Dissection

- After the subpectoral space is entered, dissection is carried upward centrally to the superior extent of the pocket.
- Dissection is then carried laterally just superficial to the pectoralis minor until the lateral border of the pocket is reached.
  - Keep lateral dissection of the pocket to a minimum with the cautery because the breast/nipple neural supply from the lateral cutaneous nerves can be inadvertently cut.
  - Blunt dissection of the lateral edge of the pocket decreases the chance of nerve transection.
- Carry the dissection inferiorly along the lateral border of the pocket, identifying and staying superficial to the serratus muscle until the inferior extent of the pocket at the IMF is reached.

- Avoid overdissection of your pocket laterally to facilitate optimal medial projection of the implant.
- The pectoralis is then released along the planned IMF, staying 1 cm superior to the fold to account for caudal muscle descent.
- Dissection directly at the fold will often lead to a fold that is lower than planned as the muscle retracts inferiorly (**TECH FIG 7A**).
- As the dissection is carried medially along the IMF, it is critically important to stop it at the most medial extent along the sternum (**TECH FIG 7B**).
  - Preservation of the most caudal attachment of the pectoralis muscle at the *transition point* (TP) along the sternum is critical to minimize the chance of window shading of the pectoralis with subsequent medial implant exposure and animation deformities (**TECH FIG 7C,D**).
  - A *transition zone* (TZ) of tapered muscle release connects the transition point to the main body of medial pectoral muscle along the sternum.
- The extent of the pocket is completed by defining the medial pectoral border and dividing all of the accessory slips of pectoralis muscle that insert along the ribs, preserving only the main body of the muscle as it inserts along the sternum.

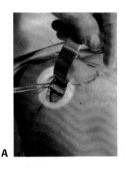 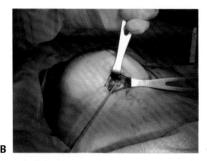 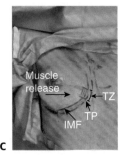

A   B   C

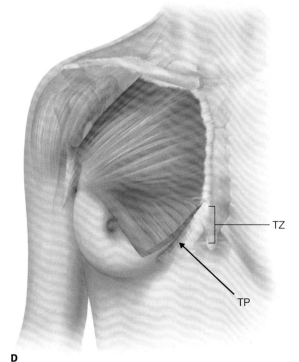

D

TECH FIG 7 • A. Inferior/lateral border of the pectoralis major after it was released along the IMF. **B.** Inferior release of the pectoralis major heading medially toward the sternum. **C.** Transition zone (*TZ*) and transition point (*TP*). Dashed line reveals pectoralis muscle release medially up to the TP. Solid line represents the inframammary fold (*IMF*). **D.** Schematic demonstrating the release of the pectoralis off of the chest wall to the transition point (*TP*). Notice the transition zone (*TZ*) which is a zone of thinning of the muscle at the caudal end of the sternum just medial to the TP.

- Dividing these muscle slips with electrocautery instead of blunt dissection improves postoperative cleavage and maintains hemostasis. Although completely dividing all accessory slips is required to achieve maximal cleavage, division of the main body of medial pectoralis muscle should be preserved, other than conservative thinning at the transition zone, to minimize the risk of postoperative wrinkling or implant show.
- This division of the inferior pectoralis muscle just above the IMF during initial pocket dissection creates a level 1 dual plane. Thus, all subpectoral pockets where the muscle is released inferiorly are actually dual-plane pockets, as the segment between the caudal edge of the divided muscle and the IMF is subglandular.[21]
  - The level of dual plane required varies, and each surgery can be tailored to provide the optimal level based on soft tissue requirements and implant selection.
  - The greater the amount of breast parenchyma or breast laxity, the greater the level of dual plane.
  - It is this creation of a lower pole subglandular pocket that allows for an optimal breast-implant interface and soft tissue redraping.
  - Failure to optimize the breast-implant interface can lead to a waterfall deformity, with the breast sliding off of the implant.
- When submuscular, IMF lowering can be more challenging as it is tempting to carry the dissection under the muscle inferiorly to lower the fold.
- The dissection along the chest wall at the level of the fold is deep to the suspensory ligament structures that create the IMF.
- IMF lowering in the subpectoral pocket requires transitioning into a more superficial plane above the pectoralis fascia to lower the IMF.[20]
- Dissection deep to the pectoral fascia will likely result in a lowered fold with persistence of the fold structure, resulting in a double-bubble deformity.
  - This is more likely when dissection begins from above, such as a periareolar or transaxillary approach.
- When using an IMF incision, the dissection below the native fold begins in the subcutaneous plane until the pectoralis muscle is reached, resulting in appropriate obliteration of the native fold at the correct level.

Implant Placement

- The implants are bathed in the irrigation solution before insertion. Gloves are changed and rinsed with the irrigation solution to remove any residue (see **TECH FIG 5A**).
- In the authors' practice, the implant is placed into the pocket with the assistance of an insertion sleeve such as the Keller funnel (see **TECH FIG 5B**).
  - The opening of the funnel should be cut large enough to allow easy egress of the implant through the funnel. This is easily confirmed by passing the implant with irrigation solution through the funnel prior to pocket insertion.

- The implant orientation is then confirmed in the funnel, and a maneuver of squeezing the implant through the funnel with gentle pressure exerted on the back of the funnel allows the implant to slip effortlessly into the breast pocket.
- These maneuvers provide a "no-touch" technique, which has been associated with lower capsular contracture rates.[12,13]
- Once the implant is in the pocket (see **FIG 3A**), a finger-assisted assessment and manipulation of the implant within the pocket is necessary to confirm its proper placement and ensure appropriate redraping of the breast parenchyma over the implant (see **TECH FIG 5C**).
  - This maneuver is especially important with textured devices, as these implants are less mobile and less likely to stretch the pocket and, thus, a distortion or wrinkling of the implant in a tight pocket may be permanent if not resolved before closure.
- Repeated removal and insertions of the implant should be avoided to minimize implant or incision damage, potential contamination, and pocket overdissection.
  - This approach is especially important with shaped implants, as a stretched pocket from overmanipulation could lead to implant rotation postoperatively.

Pocket Closure

- Before incision closure, the patient should be placed in the upright position to assess implant position, fold position, and symmetry, and the adequacy of the dual plane (see **TECH FIG 6A**).
- The IMF approach for submuscular implant placement is useful to control the fold position during the final closure. The cuff of superficial Scarpa fascia that was preserved during the initial incision is used to secure the fold during closure.
  - If the IMF structure is stable and has not been violated or lowered during the procedure, reapproximation of the superficial fascia during closure is usually adequate.
  - If the fold is mobile and unstable from either inherent weakness or from disruption during fold lowering, the pocket closure should include stabilization of the fold.
    - Fold stabilization is accomplished by incorporating the deep fascia in the closure.
    - The Scarpa fascia cuff is sutured to the deep fascia in the lower incisional edge during the closure of the IMF (see **TECH FIG 6B,C**).
- Both the periareolar and inframammary incision are closed in three layers: deep fascia/parenchyma (2-0 Vicryl running), deep dermis (4-0 PDS interrupted), and subcuticular (4-0 PDS running).
- If using a textured device, the implant must be seated at the desired position at the base of the breast pocket because it is less likely to settle in the pocket postoperatively as can be seen with smooth breast implants (see **TECH FIG 6D**).

PEARLS AND PITFALLS

Live by the pinch	■ A pinch test of less than 2 cm should guide the surgeon away from subglandular and subfascial pocket creation. ■ Implants that are more prone to rippling (eg, textured implants, saline implants) or poor quality soft tissue might require an even thicker soft tissue coverage and a pinch test of more than 3 cm may be warranted.
Avoid midline overdissection	■ No muscle sternal attachments encountered in subglandular or subfascial plane. Symmastia prevention is important.
Control the fold	■ If IMF is mobile, disrupted or lowered, the closure must incorporate the deep fascia to secure the fold.
Reduce capsular contracture risk	■ Textured implants in the subglandular/subfascial pocket, no-touch technique, nipple shields, pocket irrigation with triple antibiotics, insertion sleeve, submuscular implant pocket, inframammary incision, and cohesive-shaped implants.
Pocket control	■ Precise pocket dissection to minimize malposition, rotation, lateral drift.
Periareolar incision	■ Avoid undermining the NAC to minimize disruption of the blood supply to the nipple.
Subfascial pocket entry	■ Use the cut current to facilitate elevation of the thin fascia. Fascia thickens as you move superiorly.
Submuscular pocket entry	■ If you cannot lift the muscle (pectoralis major) off the chest wall, *do not* cut it.
Respect the transition point and zone	■ Divide pectoralis muscle 1 cm above the fold to the transition point, thin along the transition zone, and release only accessory muscle slips along sternum to prevent wrinkling and window shading of muscle.
Optimize submuscular dual plane	■ Place implants submuscular and create a subglandular pocket in the lower pole with a dual plane to optimize breast tissue-implant relationship.

POSTOPERATIVE CARE

■ Incisions are covered with Steri-strips.
■ Contour tape is placed along the fold and lateral breast.
■ Breasts are wrapped with a Kerlix and Ace wrap for 24 hours.
■ For textured implants, a breast band is worn for 1 week.
■ Early range of motion, beginning in the recovery room, is initiated for all patients, which includes shoulder rolls in both directions in addition to elevation of the arms outward to the sides and over the head.
■ With smooth devices, implant massage begins postoperatively on day 4 and includes displacing the implant upward and downward in the pocket, crossing the arms and pulling the implants inward to create cleavage, and downward pressure on the implants to stretch the lower pole.
■ With textured implants, both round and shaped, limited arm movement other than range of motion is recommended for the first week.
■ Implant massage with textured implants is contraindicated, because the textured surface can irritate the pocket and potentially create serous fluid around the implant. Likewise, the implants are placed in a controlled pocket with the implant positioned appropriately at the base of the pocket; displacement could lead to implant malposition or, in the case of shaped devices, rotation of the implant.
■ Patients are allowed to resume wearing regular bras after 4 weeks but should continue with sports bras during bedtime for an additional 2 to 4 weeks to limit lateral implant movement during pocket formation.
■ Normal activity resumes within a few days after surgery, but exercise and high-impact activity should be delayed for 3 to 4 weeks for subfascial and subglandular implants and 4 to 6 weeks for submuscular implants.
■ If a variety of smooth and textured (round or shaped) breast implants are being used within a practice, it is extremely important to communicate to ancillary staff the type of device placed with each patient to initiate the appropriate postoperative protocol, as inappropriate instructions can lead to postoperative problems such as seromas, malposition, and rotational deformities.

■ Whereas smooth implants often seem high initially and often require downward massage and the use of breast bands or bandeaus, textured devices that are appropriately seated in the base of the breast pocket should only occasionally require such maneuvers.
■ Whereas smooth implants will seem more mobile and softer in the first few weeks after surgery in comparison with textured devices, the textured implants will soften with modest movement often present after 4 to 6 weeks.

OUTCOMES

■ Preoperative and postoperative photos of bilateral subglandular breast augmentation are shown in **FIG 14**.

COMPLICATIONS

■ Capsular contracture
■ Infection
■ Malposition (symmastia, double-bubble, lateral drift, superior malposition with waterfall) (**FIG 15**)

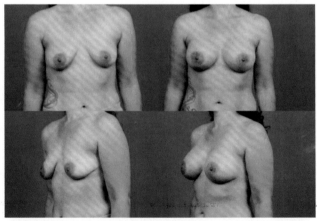

FIG 14 • Preoperative and postoperative photos of a 31-year-old woman who underwent bilateral subglandular breast augmentation through an IMF incision, with 355 cc moderate profile textured implants.

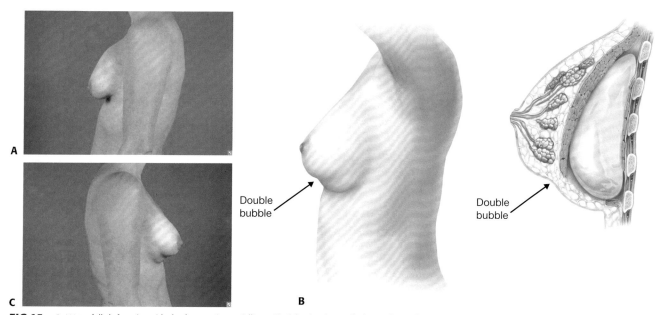

FIG 15 • A. Waterfall deformity with the breast tissue falling off of the implant. Black curvilinear line represents the breast-implant interface. **B, C.** Double-bubble deformity resulting from overdissection deep to the pectoralis major muscle attachments on the chest.

- Double capsule/seroma
- Nipple and breast sensation changes
- Implant failure (leak rupture, fracture)
- Implant extrusion
- Neuropraxia
- Poor scarring

REFERENCES

1. Stevens WG, Nahabedian MY, Calobrace MB, et al. Risk factor analysis for capsular contracture: a 5-year Sientra study analysis using round, smooth and textured implants for breast augmentation. *Plast Reconstr Surg.* 2013;132(5):1115-1123.
2. Strasser EJ. Results of subglandular versus subpectoral augmentation over time: one surgeon's observations. *Aesthet Surg J.* 2006;26:45-50.
3. Okwueze MI, Spear ME, Zwyghuizen AM, et al. Effect of augmentation mammoplasty on breast sensation. *Plast Reconstr Surg.* 2006;117(1):73-83.
4. Namnoum JD, Largent J, Kaplan HM, et al. Primary breast augmentation clinical trial outcomes stratified by surgical incision, anatomical placement and implant device type. *J Plast Reconstr Aesthet Surg.* 2013;66(9):1165-1172.
5. Michalopoulos K. The effects of breast augmentation surgery on future ability to lactate. *Breast J.* 2007;13(1):62-67.
6. Calobrace MB, Kaufman DL, Gordon AE, et al. Evolving practices in augmentation operative techniques with Sientra HSC round implants. *Plast Reconstr Surg.* 2014;134(suppl 1):57S-67S.
7. Muntan CD, Sundine MJ, Rink RD, et al. Inframammary fold: a histological reappraisal. *Plast Reconstr Surg.* 2000;105:549-556.
8. Gabriel A, Fritzsche S, Creasman C, et al. Incidence of breast and chest wall asymmetries: 4D photography. *Aesthet Surg J.* 2011;31:506-510.
9. Rohrich RJ, Hartley W, Brown S. Incidence of breast and chest wall asymmetry in breast augmentation: a retrospective analysis of 100 patients. *Plast Reconstr Surg.* 2006;118(7 suppl):7S-13S.
10. Hodgkinson DJ. The management of anterior chest wall deformity in patients presenting for breast augmentation. *Plast Reconstr Surg.* 2002;109:1714-1723.
11. Wixtrom RN, Stutman RL, Burke RM, et al. Risk of breast implant bacterial contamination from endogenous breast flora, prevention with nipple shields, and implications for biofilm formation. *Aesthet Surg J.* 2012;32:956-963.
12. Mladick RA. "No-touch" submuscular saline breast augmentation technique. *Aesthetic Plast Surg.* 1993;17:183-192.
13. Flugstad NA et al. Does implant insertion with a funnel decrease capsular contracture? A preliminary report. *Aesthet Surg J.* 2016;36(5):550-556.
14. Adams WP, Rios JL, Smith S. Enhancing patient outcomes in aesthetic and reconstructive breast surgery using triple antibiotic breast irrigation: six-year prospective clinical study. *Plast Reconstr Surg.* 2006;118(suppl 7):46S-52S.
15. Wiener TC. Relationship of incision choice to capsular contracture. *Aesthetic Plast Surg.* 2008;32(2):303-306.
16. Mofid MM, Klatsky SA, Singh NK, Nahabedian MY. Nipple-areola complex sensitivity after primary breast augmentation: a comparison of periareolar and inframammary incision approaches. *Plast Reconstr Surg.* 2006;117(6):1694.
17. Calobrace MB. Teaching breast augmentation. *Clin Plast Surg.* 2015;42:493-504.
18. Teitelbaum S. The inframammary approach to breast augmentation. *Clin Plast Surg.* 2009;36:33-43.
19. Hammond DC. Technique and results using Memory-Shape implants in aesthetic and reconstructive) breast surgery. *Plast Reconstr Surg.* 2014;134(suppl 3):16S-26S.
20. Schusterman MA. Lowering the inframammary fold. *Aesthet Surg J.* 2004;24:482-485.
21. Tebbetts JB. Dual plane breast augmentation: optimizing implant-soft-tissue relationships in a wide range of breast types. *Plast Reconstr Surg.* 2001;107:1255-1272.
22. Handel N. The effects of silicone implants on the diagnosis, prognosis, and treatment of breast cancer. *Plast Reconstr Surg.* 2007;120(7):81S-93S.
23. Munhos AM, Gemperli R, Goes JCS. Transaxillary subfascial augmentation mammoplasty with anatomic form-stable silicone implants. *Clin Plast Surg.* 2015;42:565-585.
24. Tebbetts JB, Adams WP. Five critical decisions in breast augmentation using five measurements in 5 minutes: the high five decision support process. *Plast Reconstr Surg.* 2005;116:2005-2016.

Breast Augmentation Plane: Dual Plane

CHAPTER 3

Bill Kortesis and Charalambos "Babis" Rammos

DEFINITION

- According to the American Society for Aesthetic Plastic Surgery (ASAPS) 2016 statistics, breast augmentation was the second most common aesthetic surgical procedure performed in the USA, with approximately 311 000 procedures performed.[1]
- A thorough physical examination of the prospective breast augmentation candidate is imperative.
- Any asymmetry of breast size, nipple position, and inframammary fold is documented.
- The most commonly used implant locations are partial subpectoral and subfascial.
- A combination of two pocket locations in the same breast (dual plane) can address the implant-soft tissue dynamics that may occur.

ANATOMY

- In dual plane augmentation, the implant lies partially behind the pectoralis major muscle, and partially behind the breast parenchyma (in dual planes simultaneously).[2]
- The parenchyma-muscle interface is specifically altered, and a specific group of pectoralis major muscle origins are totally divided.
  - The inferior origins of the muscle are only divided without any division of the sternal attachments.
  - A plane between the parenchyma and the anterior surface of the muscle is formed to a varying degree, resulting in three different types of dual plane: type I, type II, and type III.

PATHOGENESIS

- Micromastia occurs as a developmental phenomenon either as primary mammary hypoplasia or due to chest wall pathology such as Poland syndrome.
- It may also present as an involutional process, due to weight loss or after pregnancy and lactation.
- Micromastia may lead to a negative body image and have a negative effect on quality of life.

PATIENT HISTORY AND PHYSICAL FINDINGS

- Goals and expectations of the patient are discussed in detail during consultation.
- A thorough personal and family history is performed focusing on:
  - History of any breast disease and breast cancer
  - History of pregnancy
  - Desire for future pregnancy
  - Mammogram: Screening mammogram is obtained for any patient over 35 years old.

- Physical examination focuses on:
  - Current height and weight
  - Current breast size and desired breast size
  - Palpation for any breast masses, lymph nodes, or nipple discharge
  - Observation of breast ptosis and degree of ptosis, and the need for synchronous mastopexy
  - Observation of chest wall and breast asymmetries, such as differences in inframammary fold height, nipple-areola complex (NAC) height, breast volume, and breast shape

IMAGING

- The authors use the VECTRA 3D imaging and simulation system for all patients interested in breast augmentation. The device takes a three-dimensional photograph that can then be visualized in the monitor, with the addition of breast measurements.
  - Differences between the two breasts, such as breast volume and sternal notch to nipple distance, can be depicted (**FIG 1**).

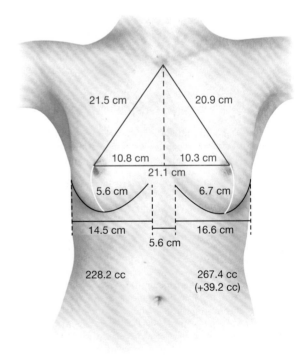

FIG 1 • Three-dimensional photograph of a 27-year-old female using the VECTRA 3D imaging device. Breast measurements are shown. Differences between right and left breast in terms of volume and sternal notch to nipple distance are recorded.

- Using different implant shapes and sizes, the surgeon produced a simulated postsurgical result, allowing the patients to have a visual image of the outcome. It has been shown that the use of the VECTRA 3D imaging system may provide a high degree of accuracy for breast volume (90%) and contour (98.4%).[3]

SURGICAL MANAGEMENT

- The main objectives of breast augmentation are as follows:
  - Enhancement of breast shape and volume
  - Improving self-esteem and quality of life.[4] A prospective analysis using the BREAST-Q showed that breast augmentation is associated with high patient satisfaction and significant improvements in quality of life.[5]

Preoperative Planning

- Breast measurements
  - Breast width at its widest point
  - Nipple to inframammary fold (N-IMF) distance
  - Sternal notch to nipple distance
  - Breast height
- Assessment of breast parenchyma and skin
  - Elasticity: This is performed with deflection of the skin, and observation for resistance.
  - Pinch test: This is performed at the superior and medial portion of the breast, between the examiner's thumb and index finger. A result of less than 2 cm is most of the times an indication for placement of the implant in the subpectoral plane.
- Choice of implant volume. Sizers are placed in a bra and compared to the images obtained by the three-dimensional imaging.
- The patient is marked preoperatively in the upright standing position (**FIG 2**).
  - Midline, from sternal notch to xiphoid
  - Inframammary fold
  - Superior, medial, and lateral borders of the breast. The medial borders are marked 1.5 cm lateral to the midline, so as to prevent synmastia.
  - Breast meridian
  - Incision. For an inframammary approach, the marking is placed below the inframammary fold, centered at the breast meridian, most often 4 cm in length, 2 cm medial and 2 cm lateral to the meridian.

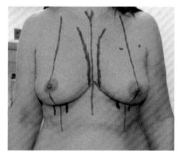

FIG 2 • The markings are made in the preoperative area and reviewed with the patient.

Positioning

- The patient is brought to the operating room and placed in the supine position on the operating table with the arms extended up to 90 degrees and well secured to the arm boards. Both shoulders should be at the same height.

Approach

- Inframammary incision placement
  - Wide exposure, better visualization
  - Easier manipulation of the inframammary fold position
  - Easier placement of the implant
- Submuscular pocket and retromammary plane creation
- Dual plane augmentation[6] (**FIG 3**).
  - Type I dual plane: Complete division of pectoralis major muscle origin across the inframammary fold, stopping at the medial aspect, with no separation of the parenchyma-muscle interface
    - Most routine breasts
    - All of the parenchyma should be above the inframammary fold
    - Minimally stretched lower pole envelope. Areola to inframammary fold distance under stretch between 4 and 6 cm
    - Maximal muscle cover over the implant, compared to all types

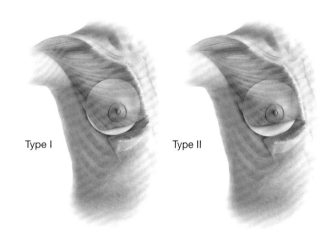

Type I   Type II

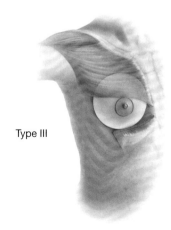

Type III

FIG 3 • Dual-plane augmentation techniques. The inferior origins of the pectoralis major muscle are disinserted, with preservation of the sternal origins. The more cephalad the dissection between the muscle and the parenchyma, the more cephalad the retraction of the pectoralis muscle.

- Type II dual plane: Complete division of pectoralis major muscle origin across the inframammary fold, stopping at the medial aspect, with synchronous retromammary pocket plane formation to the level of the inferior border of the areola
  - Lower pole envelope more stretched, areola to inframammary fold distance under stretch between 5.5 and 6.5 cm
  - Most of the parenchyma should be above the inframammary fold.
  - Mobile breast tissue over the pectoralis muscles
- Type III dual plane: Complete division of pectoralis major muscle origin across the inframammary fold, stopping at the medial aspect, with synchronous retromammary pocket plane formation to the level of the superior border of the areola
  - Markedly stretched lower pole envelope, areola to inframammary fold distance under stretch between 7 and 8 cm
  - Most of the parenchyma lies below the inframammary fold.

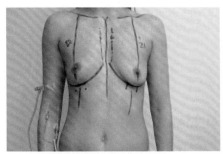

FIG 4 • Preoperative markings of a 25-year-old female undergoing breast augmentation. Dual plane technique type I was used on the right breast, and dual plane technique type II on the left. The lower pole envelope of the right breast is minimally stretched, compared to the more stretched lower envelope on the left breast.

  - Breast parenchyma slides off the surface of the pectoralis.
  - Constricted lower poles
- The same patient may benefit from different types of dual plane augmentation on the two breasts (**FIG 4**).

■ Inframammary Approach With a Smooth Round Silicone Implant, Partial Subpectoral Placement, and Dual Plane Type II Placement

Incision and Dissection

- Tegaderm is placed on top of the nipple-areola complex (NAC).
- Local anesthesia containing a mix of lidocaine and Marcaine with epinephrine is injected into the marked incision and as a breast block.
- The inframammary incision is made sharply through the dermis and the superficial layer of the fat until the Scarpa fascia is encountered.
- A double skin hook is placed followed by an Army-Navy retractor and dissection is continued with Bovie electrocautery cephalad with care not to violate the Scarpa fascia.
- The breast tissue is divided, and the pectoralis muscle fascia is identified.
- Suprafascial dissection is carried accordingly to create a type II dual plane dissection.
- After dual plane dissection, the pectoralis muscle is grasped and divided till the areolar space under the muscle is identified.
  - A lighted retractor is then placed below the pectoralis major muscle and strong upward traction is placed so as to separate the pectoralis major from the pectoralis minor muscle (**TECH FIG 1**).
  - The initial fiber incision is made medially, where pectoralis major is absent.
- Pocket dissection is performed with the monopolar electrocautery and there is no use of blunt dissection.
- Submuscular dissection proceeds from medial to lateral in a clockwise fashion for the left breast and in

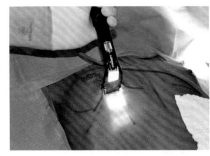

TECH FIG 1 • Dual plane dissection type II is performed before proceeding with pocket creation. Use of a lighted retractor to separate the pectoralis major from the pectoralis minor muscle.

an anticlockwise fashion for the right breast, until the pocket is of appropriate size.
  - Care is taken to avoid any contact with the ribs so as to decrease postoperative pain.
- Care is taken to disinsert the medial origin of the pectoralis major muscle so as to achieve adequate expansion of the lower pole.
  - Care is taken to not disinsert the sternal fibers of the muscle.
- Meticulous hemostasis is achieved.

Implant Insertion and Closure

- Tester gel implants are inserted, and the patient is placed in the upright seated position. If there are areas for additional dissection, these are marked.
- The pockets are irrigated with triple antibiotic solution.
- The formal implants are then placed in a sterile manner using the no-touch technique.
  - The implant is transferred to the Keller funnel avoiding any contact with the operating table or the surgeon's gloves (**TECH FIG 2A**).

- A Deaver retractor is used by the assistant to facilitate placement of the implant (**TECH FIG 2B**).
- Closure is performed in three layers:
  - 2-0 Vicryl is used for the breast parenchyma (**TECH FIG 2C,D**).
- 4-0 Monocryl is used for interrupted deep dermal sutures, followed by a running subcuticular 4-0 Monocryl suture.
- The patient is placed again in an upright seated position for final assessment (**TECH FIG 2E**).

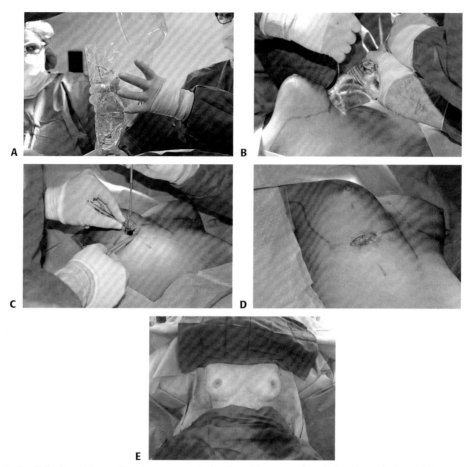

TECH FIG 2 • **A,B.** The Keller funnel is used for placement of the implants. The no-touch technique is used. There is direct transfer of the implant to the funnel without touching the implant. **C.** Deeper layer that will be closed is grasped with forceps. **D.** Closure of the deeper breast tissue is performed before skin closure. **E.** Patient at the seated upright position with the implants in place.

PEARLS AND PITFALLS

Hemostasis	■ Meticulous hemostasis should be achieved to avoid postoperative hematoma and an inflammatory response that may lead to capsular contracture.
Pectoralis muscle	■ The most medial fibers of the pectoralis major muscle should be released to avoid a constricted lower pole. Carefully not to disinsert the sternal fibers as that can lead to window-shading and decreased implant coverage.
Dual plane	■ Advantage of increasing implant and breast parenchyma interface, expanding the lower pole, and allowing for changes of the nipple-areolar complex.
Implant placement	■ The no-touch technique is used at all times, to avoid implant contamination.
Dissection	■ Dissection should be accurate to accommodate the implant and overdissection should be avoided at all times.
Ribs	■ Contact with the ribs should be avoided, so as to decrease postoperative pain.

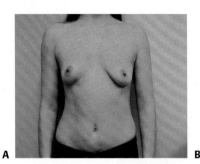 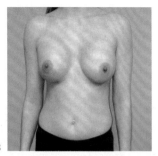

FIG 5 • A. Preoperative frontal view of a 25-year-old woman with micromastia. **B.** Patient 1 month after submuscular breast augmentation with a 345-mL smooth round implant with moderate projection. Dual plane augmentation type I was performed on the right, and dual plane augmentation type II was performed on the left.

POSTOPERATIVE CARE

- Patients are discharged at the same day of surgery after they recover in the postoperative anesthesia care unit.
- Postoperative medications
  - Oral analgesics
  - Seven-day course of oral antibiotics
- Paper tape is used to cover the incisions.
- A soft bra is used.
- Activity
  - Patients are instructed to avoid heavy lifting, no more than 10 lb, for 10 days.
  - Light exercise is permitted starting postoperative day 1. Additional exercises such as arm abduction and arm elevation are encouraged, to achieve stretching of the pectoralis major muscle and accelerate recovery by decreasing pain.
- Patients may shower on postoperative day 1.
- Manual massage for round implant starts as soon as tolerated by the patient with the aim to prevent capsular contracture.
- Follow-up appointments are scheduled for day 1, 1 week, 3 weeks, 3 months, 6 months, and 1 year.

OUTCOMES

- A clinical example of a patient with inframammary breast augmentation with smooth round silicone implants and dual plane augmentation is shown in **FIG 5**.

COMPLICATIONS

- Hematoma formation is rare and ranges from 0.5% to 1%.
- Infection is rare and occurs in less than 1% of the patients.

- Double-bubble deformity may occur due to violation of Scarpa fascia at the level of the inframammary fold, with subsequent caudal migration of the implant in relationship to the breast mound.
- The cause of capsular contracture is inflammation, which in turn may be due to tissue trauma, bacteria, and blood.
  - The use of the Keller funnel has been shown to lead to a statistically significant reduction in the incidence of reoperations performed due to capsular contracture within 12 months of primary breast augmentation.[7]

REFERENCES

1. American Society for Aesthetic Plastic Surgery. Cosmetic Surgery National Data Bank Statistics. *Aesthet Surg J.* 2017;37(suppl 2):1-29.
2. Adams WP Jr, Mallucci P. Breast augmentation. *Plast Reconstr Surg.* 2012;130(4):597-611.
3. Roostaeian A, Adams WP Jr. Three-dimensional imaging for breast augmentation: is this technology providing accurate simulations? *Aesthet Surg J.* 2014;34:857-875.
4. Swanson E. Prospective outcome study of 225 cases of breast augmentation. *Plast Reconstr Surg.* 2013;131:1158-1166.
5. Alderman AK, Bauer J, Fardo D, Abrahamse P, Pusic A. Understanding the effect of breast augmentation on quality of life: prospective analysis using the BREAST-Q. *Plast Reconstr Surg.* 2014;133:787-795.
6. Tebbetts JB. Dual plane breast augmentation: optimizing implant-soft tissue relationships in a wide range of breast types. *Plast Reconstr Surg.* 2001;107:1255-1272.
7. Flugstad NA, Pozner JN, Baxter RA, et al. Does implant insertion with a funnel decrease capsular contracture? A preliminary report. *Aesthet Surg J.* 2016;36(5):550-556.

Breast Augmentation With Round and Anatomic Implants

Bill Kortesis and Charalambos "Babis" Rammos

CHAPTER 4

DEFINITION

- Round implants are most commonly used in the United States.
  - They are symmetrical in height and width and have varying projections for a given volume, typically designated as low, moderate, high profile, and extra high.
    - The more the projection increases for a fixed volume, the more the width of the device decreases (**FIG 1A**).
  - Round implants may be smooth or textured and may be filled with either saline or silicone gel.
    - Fourth and fifth generation round silicone devices, currently used in the market, are designed with thinner shells and a more cohesive gel.
- Anatomic (shaped) implants have become an important alternative for breast augmentation.
  - Shaped implants are textured to reduce movement and can have differences in height, projection, and width.
    - They have greater projection in the caudal portion and less projection in the cephalic portion (**FIG 1B**), mimicking the natural shape of the breast.
  - The more cohesive and dense silicone gel (fifth generation) allows the implant to maintain its shape, and resist the natural forces exerted by the soft tissue envelope.
  - Orientation markings on the device position it properly in the breast pocket.

ANATOMY

- The breast extends from the 2nd or 3rd rib down to the 6th or 7th rib (cephalad to caudad) and from the lateral sternum to the anterior axillary line (medial to lateral).
- The major blood supply to the breast is from the internal mammary artery.
- Lateral and anterior branches of the second through sixth intercostal nerves provide innervation to the skin overlying the breast.

PATHOGENESIS

- Micromastia occurs as a developmental phenomenon either as primary mammary hypoplasia or due to chest wall pathology such as Poland syndrome.
- It may also present as an involutional process, due to weight loss or after pregnancy and lactation.
- Micromastia may lead to a negative body image and have a deleterious effect on quality of life.
- According to the American Society for Aesthetic Plastic Surgery (ASAPS) 2015 statistics, breast augmentation was the second most common aesthetic surgical procedure performed, with approximately 306 000 cases.[1]

PATIENT HISTORY AND PHYSICAL FINDINGS

- Goals and expectations of the patient are discussed in detail during consultation.
- A thorough personal and family history is performed.
  - History of any breast disease and breast cancer
  - History of pregnancy
  - Desire for future pregnancy
  - Mammogram: Screening mammogram is obtained for any patient over 35 years of age.
- Physical examination
  - Current height and weight
  - Current breast size and desired breast size
  - Palpation for any breast masses, lymph nodes, or nipple discharge
  - Observation of breast ptosis and degree of ptosis, and the need for synchronous mastopexy

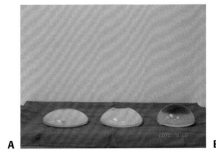
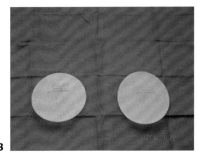

FIG 1 • A. Lateral view of a moderate projection (*left*), full projection (*center*), and extra full projection (*right*) 400 mL smooth round silicone gel implant. As the projection increases, the height and the width of the device decrease. **B.** Moderate height, full projection (*left*) and full height, full projection (*right*) anatomic 420-mL gel implants as seen from above.

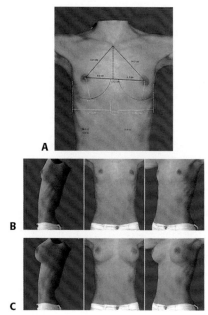

FIG 2 • Three-dimensional photograph of a 24-year-old female using the VECTRA 3D imaging device. **A.** Breast measurements. **B.** Preoperative frontal, lateral, and oblique views. **C.** Simulated images obtained using a 320-mL shaped implant.

- Observation of chest wall and breast asymmetries, such as differences in inframammary fold height, nipple-areolar complex height, breast volume, and breast shape

IMAGING

- The authors use the VECTRA 3D imaging and simulation system for all patients interested in breast augmentation. The device takes a 3D photograph that can then be visualized in the monitor, with the addition of breast measurements (**FIG 2A,B**).
- Using different implant shapes and sizes, a simulated postsurgical result is produced, allowing the patients to have a visual image of the outcome (**FIG 2C**).
- The use of the VECTRA 3D imaging system provides a high degree of accuracy for breast volume (90%) and contour (98.4%).[2]

SURGICAL MANAGEMENT

- Main objectives of breast augmentation:
  - Enhancement of breast shape and volume
  - Improve self-esteem and quality of life.[3] A prospective analysis using the BREAST-Q showed that breast augmentation is associated with high patient satisfaction and significant improvements in quality of life.[4]
- Main indications for use of a round implant:
  - Desire for a fuller look
  - Good skin quality and overall breast anatomy
  - Concerns about device rotation
- Main indications for use of an anatomic implant:
  - Thin patients with little breast volume. In this patient population, the final shape of the breast will be determined by the device itself.
  - Patients with deficiency at the inferior pole
  - Patients with chest height-width disproportions, such as patients who have a very long, but not very wide chest, or have a very wide, but not very long chest.

- Patients with breast asymmetries. By using a variety of heights, widths, and projections, these asymmetries may be overcome.
- Patients who do not want a full round upper pole appearance.
- Main factors to consider when using shaped implants rather than round implants:
  - Incision length needs to be slightly longer because of the filling material traits.
  - Orientation: Precise placement of the implant is critical as disorientation will lead to distortion of the breast shape.
  - Implant height needs to be chosen wisely to avoid overfilling or underfilling of the upper pole of the breast.
  - Lowering the inframammary fold is important.
    - Different methods have been described for the projected postoperative inframammary fold, including those by Caplin.[5]
      - The authors prefer to use the nipple to inframammary fold at stretch and the implant width (Table 1).
- For either type of implant, the main steps of the procedure are the same:
  - Make the incision and aim cephalad with attention not to violate Scarpa fascia.
  - Create a dual plane.
  - Identify the pectoralis major muscle edge and incise.
  - Create a subpectoral pocket with care not to elevate the pectoralis minor muscle.
  - Place tester implants (sizers).
  - Exchange tester implants for the formal implants.
  - Close the wound in layers.

Preoperative Planning

- At the time of consultation
  - Breast measurements
    - Breast width at its widest point.
    - Nipple to inframammary fold (N-IMF) distance.
    - Sternal notch to nipple distance.
    - Breast height.
  - Assessment of breast parenchyma and skin
    - Elasticity: This is performed with deflection of the skin, and observation for resistance.
    - Pinch test: This is performed at the superior and medial portion of the breast, between the examiner's thumb and index finger. A result of less than 2 cm is usually an indication for placement of the implant in the subpectoral plane.
  - Choice of implant volume. Sizers are placed in a bra and compared to the images obtained by the 3D imaging.

Table 1 Calculations for Lowering the Inframammary Fold for Anatomic Implants

Breast Implant Width	Nipple to Fold Distance[a]
11.0 cm	7.0 ± 0.5 cm
11.5 cm	7.5 ± 0.5 cm
12.0 cm	8.0 ± 0.5 cm
12.5 cm	8.5 ± 0.5 cm
10.0 cm	9.0 ± 0.5 cm
13.5 cm	9.5 ± 0.5 cm
14.0 cm	10.0 cm[b]

[a]Under maximal stretch.
[b]No more than 10 cm.

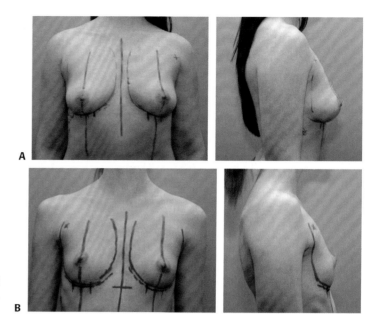

FIG 3 • The markings are made in the preoperative area and reviewed with the patient. **A.** Markings for round implants. **B.** Markings for shaped implants.

- Preoperatively, the following markings are made with the patient in the upright standing position (**FIG 3**):
  - Midline, from sternal notch to xiphoid
  - Inframammary fold
    - For anatomic implants, the projected postoperative fold position is based on the aforementioned measurements.
  - Superior, medial, and lateral borders of the breast. The medial borders are marked 1.5 cm lateral to the midline, so as to prevent synmastia
  - Breast meridian
  - Marking of the incision
    - For round implants using an inframammary approach, the marking is placed below the inframammary fold, centered at the breast meridian, most often 4 cm in length, 2 cm medial, and 2 cm lateral to the meridian.
    - For shaped implants using an inframammary approach, the marking is placed at the expected postoperative inframammary fold, centered at the breast meridian, most often 5 cm in length, 2.5 cm medial, and 2.5 cm lateral to the meridian.

Positioning

- The patient is brought to the operating room and placed in the supine position on the operating table with the arms extended up to 90 degrees and well secured to the arm boards.
- The shoulders should be at the same height.

Approach

- Incision placement
  - Inframammary
    - Placement of the incision at the inframammary fold for round implants and at the expected postoperative inframammary fold for anatomic implants.
    - Wide exposure, better visualization
    - Easier manipulation of the inframammary fold position
    - Easier placement of the implant
  - Periareolar
    - Incision is made at the inferior border of the areola
    - Scar generally heals well
    - Wide exposure
    - Approach involves either dissecting straight down through the breast or creating a lower breast flap to the level of the inframammary fold.
  - Transaxillary
    - Incision is placed at the axilla, lateral to the edge of the pectoralis major muscle
    - Hidden scar, not close to the breast
    - More challenging pocket dissection
    - Natural-appearing results have been reported with this approach and the use of shaped implants.[6]
- Pocket
  - Partial subpectoral
    - Submuscular pocket is created with release of the lateral border of the pectoralis major attachments and its inferomedial attachments.
    - Lower part of the implant is covered by the underside of the breast, and superior part of the implant is covered by the pectoralis major muscle.
  - Subglandular
    - Pocket is created between the underside of the breast and the anterior fascia of the pectoralis muscle.
    - Less technically challenging
  - Subfascial
    - Pocket is created between the anterior fascia of the pectoralis major muscle and the muscle itself.
    - Additional coverage of the implant provided by the fascial layer.
- With either type of implant, the authors most often use the inframammary approach, with placement of the implant in a partial subpectoral plane, and creation of a dual plane.
  - Alternatively, implants can be placed in the subfascial plane.

TECHNIQUES

■ Inframammary Approach With Partial Subpectoral Placement and Dual Plane Creation

Incision and Dissection

- Tegaderm is placed on top of the nipple-areolar complex (**TECH FIG 1A**).
- Local anesthesia containing a mix of lidocaine and Marcaine with epinephrine is injected into the marked incision and as a breast block.
- The inframammary incision is made sharply through the dermis and the superficial layer of the fat until Scarpa fascia is encountered (**TECH FIG 1B**).
- A double skin hook is placed followed by an Army Navy retractor, and dissection is continued with bovie electrocautery cephalad with care taken not to violate Scarpa fascia (**TECH FIG 1C**).
- The breast tissue is divided, and the pectoralis muscle fascia is identified (**TECH FIG 1D,E**).

- Suprafascial dissection is carried accordingly to create a dual plane dissection (**TECH FIG 1F**).
- After dual plane dissection, the pectoralis muscle is grasped and divided till the areolar space under the muscle is identified.
  - A lighted retractor is then placed below the pectoralis major muscle, and strong upward traction is placed so as to separate the pectoralis major from the pectoralis minor muscle.

Pocket Creation

- Pocket dissection is performed with the monopolar electrocautery and without use of blunt dissection.
- Submuscular dissection proceeds from medial to lateral in a clockwise fashion for the left breast and in an anticlockwise fashion for the right breast, until the pocket is of appropriate size.
  - Care is taken to avoid any contact with the ribs so as to minimize postoperative pain.

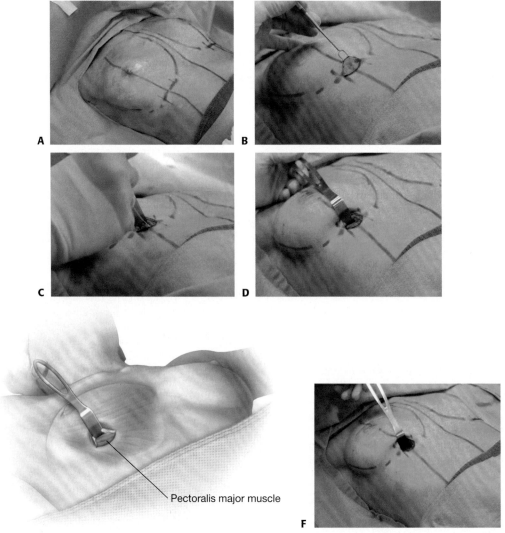

Pectoralis major muscle

TECH FIG 1 • A. Tegaderm is applied over the nipple-areolar complex. **B.** Inframammary incision made to the level of Scarpa fascia. **C.** Dissection continues in a cephalad direction. **D,E.** After breast tissue division, the pectoralis major muscle is encountered. **F.** Dual plane dissection is performed before proceeding with pocket creation.

TECHNIQUES

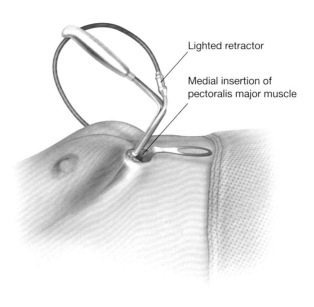

Lighted retractor

Medial insertion of
pectoralis major muscle

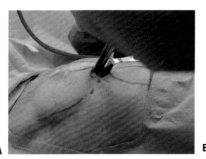

A   **B**

TECH FIG 2 • A,B. The medial origin of the pectoralis major muscle is identified and will be incised to achieve lower pole expansion.

- The medial origin of the pectoralis major muscle is disinserted so as to achieve adequate expansion of the lower pole (**TECH FIG 2**).
- Meticulous hemostasis is achieved.

Implant Placement

- Tester implants are placed and the patient is placed in the upright seated position (**TECH FIG 3A**).
  - If there are areas for additional dissection, these are marked.
- The pockets are irrigated with triple antibiotic solution.
- The formal implants are then placed in a sterile manner using the no-touch technique.
  - The packaging is opened, and the implant is transferred to the Keller funnel, avoiding any contact with

the operating table or the surgeon's gloves (**TECH FIG 3B–D**).
- A Deaver retractor is used by the assistant to facilitate placement of the implant (**TECH FIG 3E**).

Completion

- Closure is performed in three layers:
  - 2-0 Vicryl is used for the breast parenchyma (**TECH FIG 4A,B**)
  - 4-0 Monocryl for interrupted deep dermal sutures, followed by a running subcuticular 4-0 Monocryl suture (**TECH FIG 4C**)
- The patient is placed again in an upright seated position for final assessment (**TECH FIG 4D**).
- Paper tape is placed over the incisions (**TECH FIG 4E**).

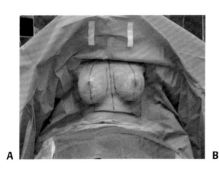

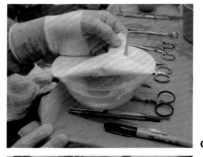

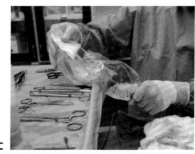

A   **B**   **C**

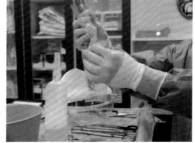

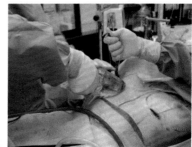

TECH FIG 3 • A. Patient in the upright seated position with tester gel implants placed. **B–E.** The no-touch technique incorporating the Keller funnel is used for placement of the implants.

D   **E**

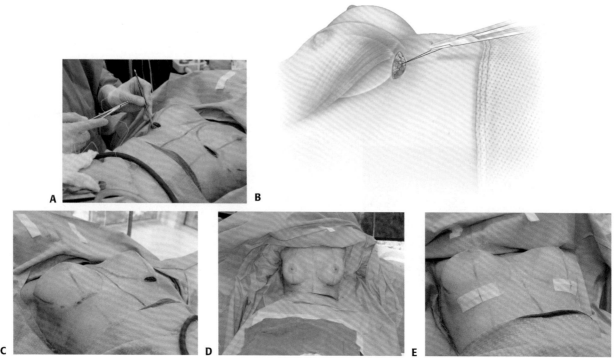

TECH FIG 4 • A. Deeper layer that will be closed is grasped with forceps. **B.** Closure of the deeper breast tissue is performed before skin closure. **C.** Skin closure is performed. **D.** Patient at the seated upright position with the formal implants in place. **E.** Paper tape placed over the incisions.

▪ Inframammary Approach with Subfascial Placement

- The technique is similar to the partial subpectoral technique in terms of marking, incision placement, implant insertion, and closure.

- The difference pertains to the pocket dissection.
  - The pocket is created between the anterior fascia of the pectoralis major muscle and the muscle itself, providing an additional layer of coverage for the implant.
  - The pocket is dissected laterally to the lateral edge of the pectoralis major muscle.

PEARLS AND PITFALLS

Hemostasis	▪ Meticulous hemostasis should be achieved to avoid postoperative hematoma and an inflammatory response that may lead to capsular contracture.
Pectoralis muscle	▪ The most inferior medial fibers of the pectoralis major muscle should be released to avoid a constricted lower pole.
Dual plane	▪ Advantage of increasing implant and breast parenchyma interface, expanding the lower pole, and allowing for changes of the nipple-areolar complex.
Implant orientation	▪ Proper orientation of shaped implants is verified to avoid distortion of the shape of the breast.
Implant placement	▪ The no-touch technique is used at all times, to avoid implant contamination, and excessive force is avoided to prevent damage of the device.
Incision placement	▪ For round implants, the inframammary incision should be placed slightly lower in regard to the inframammary fold, to avoid a high rising scar onto the breast.
Projected inframammary fold	▪ Lowering of the inframammary fold for anatomic-shaped implants is performed as needed based on preoperative measurements.
Dissection	▪ Dissection should be accurate to accommodate the implant, and overdissection should be avoided at all times.
Ribs	▪ Contact with the ribs should be avoided, so as to decrease postoperative pain.

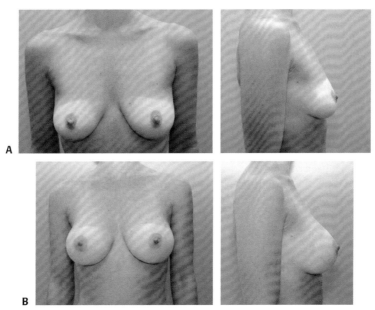

FIG 4 • A. Preoperative frontal and lateral views of a 38-year-old woman with micromastia (above). **B.** Images obtained at 3-month follow-up after subfascial breast augmentation with a 300-mL smooth round implant with moderate projection.

POSTOPERATIVE CARE

- Patients are discharged at the same day of surgery after they recover in the postoperative anesthesia care unit.
- Postoperative medications include oral analgesics and a 7-day course of oral antibiotics.
- A soft bra is used.
- Patients are instructed to avoid heavy lifting, no more than 10 lb, for 10 days.
  - Light exercise is permitted starting postoperative day 1. Additional exercises, such as arm abduction and arm elevation, are encouraged to achieve stretching of the pectoralis major muscle and to accelerate recovery by decreasing pain.

- Patients may shower in postoperative day 1.
- Manual massage
  - For round implants, manual massage of the implant starts as soon as tolerated by the patient with the aim to prevent capsular contracture.
  - For anatomic implants, no manual massage is performed.
- Follow-up appointment is scheduled for day 1, 1 week, 3 weeks, 3 months, 6 months, and 1 year.

OUTCOMES

- Clinical examples of patients with breast augmentation with round and anatomic implants are shown in **FIGS 4** and **5**, respectively.

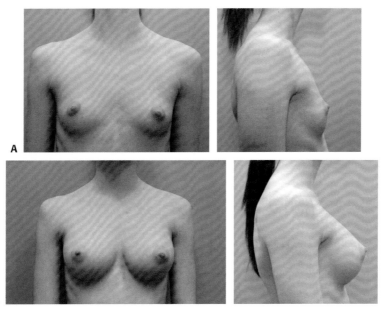

FIG 5 • A. Preoperative frontal and lateral views of a 24-year-old woman with micromastia. **B.** Images obtained at 3-month follow-up after submuscular breast augmentation with a 255-mL moderate height, full projection–shaped implant.

COMPLICATIONS

- Hematoma formation is rare and ranges from 0.5% to 1%.
- Infection is rare and occurs in less than 1% of the patients.
- Double-bubble deformity may occur due to violation of Scarpa fascia at the level of the inframammary fold, with subsequent caudal migration of the implant in relationship to the breast mound.
  - Rotation rate with the use of anatomic implants has been reported to be less than 2.5% at 6 years.[7]
- The cause of capsular contracture is inflammation, which in turn may be due to tissue trauma, bacteria, and blood.
  - The use of the Keller funnel has been shown to lead to a statistically significant reduction in the incidence of reoperations performed due to capsular contracture within 12 months of primary breast augmentation.[8]
  - Shaped, highly cohesive implants have lower rates of capsular contracture.[9]
- Anatomic implants have low rates of rupture.[10]

REFERENCES

1. American Society for Aesthetic Plastic Surgery. 2015 Cosmetic Surgery National Data Bank Statistics. ASAPS http://www. surgery.org/sites/default/files/Stats2015.pdf
2. Roostaeian A, Adams WP Jr. Three-dimensional imaging for breast augmentation: is this technology providing accurate simulations? *Aesthet Surg J.* 2014;34:857-875.
3. Swanson E. Prospective outcome study of 225 cases of breast augmentation. *Plast Reconstr Surg.* 2013;131:1158-1166.
4. Alderman AK, Bauer J, Fardo D, et al. Understanding the effect of breast augmentation on quality of life: prospective analysis using the BREAST-Q. *Plast Reconstr Surg.* 2014;133:787-795.
5. Caplin DA. Indications for the use of MemoryShape breast implants in aesthetic and reconstructive breast surgery: long-term clinical outcomes of shaped versus round silicone breast implants. *Plast Reconstr Surg.* 2014;134(3 suppl):27S-37S.
6. Sim HB, Sun SH. Transaxillary endoscopic breast augmentation with shaped gel implants. *Aesthet Surg J.* 2015;35:952-961.
7. Hammond DC, Migliori MM, Caplin DA, et al. Mentor contour profile gel implants: clinical outcomes at 6 years. *Plast Reconstr Surg.* 2012;129:1381-1391.
8. Flugstad NA, Pozner JN, Baxter RA, et al. Does implant insertion with a funnel decrease capsular contracture? A preliminary report. *Aesthet Surg J.* 2016;36:550-556.
9. Maxwell GP, Van Natta BW, Murphy DK, et al. Natrelle style 410 form-stable silicone breast implants: core study results at 6 years. *Aesthet Surg J.* 2012;32:709-717.
10. Heden P, Bronz G, Elberg JJ, et al. Long-term safety and effectiveness of style 410 highly cohesive silicone breast implants. *Aesthetic Plast Surg.* 2009;33:430-436.

Female to Male Transgender Breast Surgery

Ann R. Schwentker

CHAPTER 5

DEFINITION

- Transgender person: individuals who identify with a gender that is distinct from their assigned sex at birth.
- Gender dysphoria: emotional stress caused by differences between a person's assigned sex and his/her gender identity.
- Transition: a period of formal transformation of one's gender identity that may include changing name, clothing, preferred pronouns, gender-affirming hormones, and/or surgery.
- Female to male, trans man: a person assigned female gender at birth who identifies as male.
- Male to female, trans woman: a person assigned male gender at birth who identifies as female.

ANATOMY

- The anatomy may vary widely, depending on the patient's body habitus.
- All patients have excess glandular breast tissue. Other factors that influence surgical planning include the following:
  - Whether or not there is areolar enlargement
  - Nipple position
  - The amount of skin excess

PATIENT HISTORY AND PHYSICAL FINDINGS

- The World Professional Association for Transgender Health (www.wpath.org) has published a Standards of Care manual that should be consulted in determining an individual's suitability for surgery. In particular, it is desirable that patients be supported by a mental health professional to manage their dysphoria.
- Thorough breast exam including any masses, asymmetry, nipple/areolar size and position, ptosis, and skin excess.
- The importance of nipple sensation to the patient should be assessed. All available techniques may reduce or eliminate nipple sensation and erectile function[1] and make breast-feeding impossible, which may dissuade some patients.

IMAGING

- Any masses should be imaged and worked up as for a female with a breast mass.
- Patients who above age 45 should have a preoperative mammogram. It is not possible to remove 100% of breast tissue with this procedure, and patients should discuss with their medical doctors whether postoperative mammograms are necessary.

NONOPERATIVE MANAGEMENT

- Many patients begin transitioning by wearing binders. These can cause chafing and intertrigo, which should be treated prior to surgery.
- Patients may experience significant breast gland involution after starting testosterone therapy. Although this is not sufficient to avoid surgery, it may alter the surgical plan in small-breasted patients.

SURGICAL MANAGEMENT

- Insurance coverage for transgender surgery is variable. Comorbidities that may increase the chance of insurance coverage for surgery include the following:
  - Breast cancer, breast mass, or BRCA positivity
  - Fibrocystic disease with documented intractable pain
  - Intertrigo
  - Symptoms of macromastia

Preoperative Planning

- Patients with small areolae and very small (A cup) breasts may be candidates for periareolar mastectomy.
- If there is significant skin excess, a breast amputation will almost always be preferable.

Positioning

- The patient is positioned supine with the arms at 90 degrees and securely wrapped to arm boards (**FIG 1**). The table is placed so that the patient can be moved to a seated position during surgery.

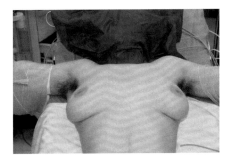

FIG 1 • Intraoperative positioning.

TECHNIQUES

■ Periareolar Mastectomy

- This results in fewer scars but makes it more difficult to control nipple size and position.
- If the areola is small, a semicircular infra-areolar incision is made. This may also be made within the areola to further camouflage the scar.[2]
- If the areola is enlarged or there is slight skin excess, a periareolar donut is designed and de-epithelialized, with a full-thickness semicircular incision inferiorly.
- 3 to 4 mm of breast tissue is preserved on the deep surface of the areola for blood supply. This dissection is performed sharply.

- The remainder of the breast gland is separated from the subcutaneous tissue using primarily blunt dissection at the level of the breast capsule. The gland may also be detached from the pectoralis fascia on its deep surface using blunt dissection.
- Hemostasis is obtained, and a closed suction drain is placed.
- The incision is closed by gathering the skin around the areola to position the nipple inferiorly and laterally, using absorbable sutures.

■ Breast Amputation With Free Nipple Grafts

- The large inframammary scar may be positioned at the inferior border of the pectoralis, and the free nipple grafts allow control of nipple size and position.
- The nipple is removed as a 28 × 22 mm (or desired shape/size) oval full-thickness skin graft, thinned, and placed on moist gauze.
- The inferior incision is marked just below the inframammary fold to be sure that the retaining ligaments are removed because the fold is a distinctly female structure. It is horizontal medially and can curve superiorly in its lateral portion to follow the curve of the pectoralis major muscle.
- The superior incision is marked by pulling the breast down over the inframammary fold and transposing the fold anteriorly, taking care to remove all areolar tissue.
- The incision should not be extended too far medially or laterally, as extra dog ears can be addressed with

tailoring or an in-office local procedure at a later date. Ideally, the incision is the width of the pectoralis muscle.
- The breast gland is removed as in a mastectomy, dissecting at the level of the breast capsule, preserving all subcutaneous fat and the pectoralis fascia. Dissection proceeds up to the clavicle.
- The inferior skin flap is undermined if necessary and advanced to align with the inferior border of the pectoralis major muscle. This both hides the scar and decreases tension on the final closure.
- The incisions are closed over drains, advancing the dog ears toward the middle of the breasts to shorten the scars.
- The nipple position is marked using paper patterns with the patient in the seated position.
- The nipple location is de-epithelialized, and the nipples sutured into position with long Vicryl sutures and fast-absorbing gut.
- The nipples are dressed with tie-over xeroform bolsters.

PEARLS AND PITFALLS

Nipple position	▪ Male nipples vary widely in size and position but are typically oval (wider transversely), lower, and more lateral than female.[3] ▪ It can be helpful to have patients bring a photo of their ideal nipple size/shape/position for planning purposes.
Hematoma/seroma	▪ Closed suction drains are used until drainage decreases. ▪ Compression (ACE or binder) is used for 6 weeks. ▪ Lifting is limited for 6 weeks.
IMF incision placement	▪ It is critical to remove the skin and ligaments of the IMF to avoid the depression that will result if this is simply released from the fascia and advanced. ▪ The inferior incision can then be advanced as in a reverse abdominoplasty to allow the incision to align precisely with the inferior border of the pectoralis muscle, which camouflages the scar.
Biopsy	▪ The removed tissue is biologically female breast tissue and as such should always be sent for pathologic examination.

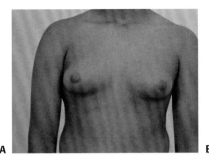 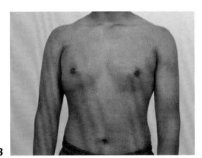

FIG 2 • **A.** Preoperative photograph. Note small areolae and breasts with limited skin excess. **B.** Postoperative photograph of same patient 1 year after periareolar mastectomy. No areolar reduction was performed. Note the mild hypertrophic scar on the right, which later underwent revision.

POSTOPERATIVE CARE

- Drains remain until drainage decreases below 30 cc in two consecutive 24-hour periods.
- Nipple bolsters are left for 10 to 14 days. The nipples are then treated with Bacitracin and large Band-Aids for another week or until scabbing resolves. Scar massage begins at 4 weeks.
- A circumferential ACE bandage is used for 1 week, and then, patients may transition to binder or spandex undershirt.
- Lifting and upper body exercise are strictly limited for the first 6 weeks. Thereafter, bulking up the pectoralis muscles is strongly encouraged, as it assists with camouflaging the scars.

OUTCOMES

- Satisfaction in this patient population is generally high[1,4] (**FIGS 2** to **4**).

- Minor revisions (scar revision, nipple revision, dog ears) are commonly required.[3,4]

COMPLICATIONS

- Hematoma requires urgent return to the operating room and evacuation.[3]
- Seroma may often be treated with aspiration and compression. The skin flaps are anesthetic for several weeks, and this is well tolerated.
- Nipple loss is extremely rare and generally results from premature loss of bolsters. Either tattooing or nipple reconstruction may be performed.
- Hypertrophic scarring is managed with scar massage, Kenalog injection, and/or revision as indicated.

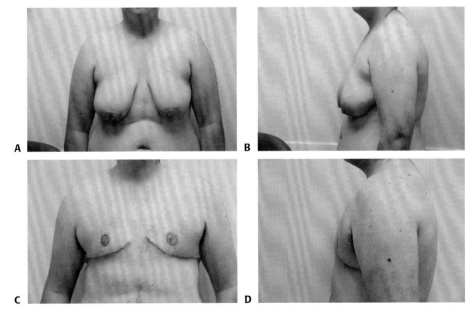

FIG 3 • **A,B.** Preoperative photograph. Note large, heavy, pendulous breasts with enlarged areolae. **C,D.** Postoperative photograph of same patient 4 months after breast amputation with free nipple grafts.

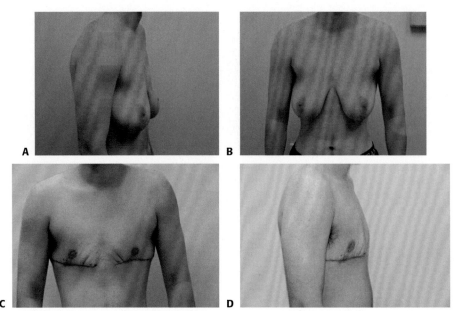

FIG 4 • A,B. Preoperative photograph. Note pendulous breasts with significant skin excess. **C,D.** Postoperative photograph of same patient 1 month after breast amputation with free nipple grafts. Note that wrinkling of the medial dog ears has not yet resolved in this early photograph.

REFERENCES

1. Nelson L, Whallett EJ, McGregor JC. Transgender patient satisfaction following reduction mammaplasty. *J Plast Reconstr Aesthet Surg.* 2009;62(3):331-334.
2. Atiyeh BS, Chahine F, El-Khatib A, et al. Gynecomastia: simultaneous subcutaneous mastectomy and areolar reduction with minimal inconspicuous scarring. *Aesthetic Plast Surg.* 2015;39(6):916-921.
3. Beer GM, Budi S, Seifert B, et al. Configuration and localization of the nipple-areola complex in man. *Plast Reconstr Surg.* 2001;108(7):1947-1952.
4. Berry MG, Curtis R, Davies D. Female-to-make transgender chest reconstruction: a large consecutive, single-surgeon experience. *J Plast Reconstr Aesthet Surg.* 2012;65(6):711-719.

Section II: Mastopexy

Mastopexy: Periareolar, Vertical, and Wise Pattern

Ryan P. Ter Louw and Scott Spear[†]

DEFINITIONS

- Ptosis of the breast is described by the Regnault classification (**FIG 1**).
  - Grade 1: minor ptosis; the nipple is at the level of the inframammary fold, above the lower contour of the gland.
  - Grade 2: moderate ptosis; the nipple is below the level of the inframammary fold, above the lower contour of the gland.
  - Grade 3: major ptosis; the nipple is below the level of the inframammary fold, at the lower contour of the gland.
- Mastopexy—*masto* meaning breast, *pexy* meaning to lift or fixate.
- Periareolar mastopexy results in a scar camouflaged in the junction of the pigmented areolar and unpigmented breast skin.
  - Concentric mastopexy, eccentric, "donut" mastopexy
- Vertical or circumvertical mastopexy results in a scar camouflaged in the junction of the pigmented areolar and unpigmented breast skin with a vertical extension along the breast meridian down toward the inframammary fold.
  - There may be a transverse scar as well if there is too much skin to be tailored in the circumareolar and vertical components.
- Wise pattern mastopexy is planned from the outset to result in a scar around the areola, a vertical extension along the breast meridian down to the inframammary fold, with a horizontal scar hidden in the inframammary fold.

ANATOMY

- The arterial supply of the breast is predominantly based off internal mammary perforators and the lateral thoracic artery.
- Sensation to the nipple is derived from the 4th posterior intercostal nerve.
- Cooper ligaments suspend the breast, originating on the pectoralis fascia and inserting into the dermis of the breast.
- The borders of the breast:
  - Superior—clavicle
  - Inferior—inframammary fold
  - Lateral—latissimus muscle
  - Medial—sternum

PATHOGENESIS

- Decreased elasticity of breast tissue with aging
- Hormone-induced inflation and deflation of breast tissue
- Stretch of Cooper ligaments
- Deflation of breast envelope following breast feeding

PATIENT HISTORY AND PHYSICAL FINDINGS

- History
  - Current cup size, height, and weight
  - Childbearing, breast-feeding, and future family planning
  - Personal and familial cancer history
  - Prior breast surgery, biopsies, radiation
  - Date of last mammogram
- Examination[1]
  - Regnault classification of ptosis
  - Soft tissue evaluation: skin laxity, density of glandular tissue
  - Soft tissue masses, axillary lymphadenopathy, nipple discharge
  - Critical measurements
    - Nipple to sternal notch
    - Nipple to inframammary fold
    - Breast width
    - Nipple to midline
    - Areolar diameter
    - Patient weight, height, and bra size
  - Symmetry of nipple position and breast size should be noted and mentioned to the patient in the initial consultation. If present before surgery, asymmetry will persist postoperatively to some degree.
  - Chest wall deformities as well as the presence or absence of pectoralis major and latissimus muscles should be noted.

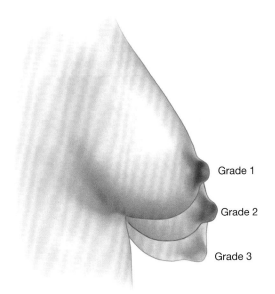

Grade 1

Grade 2

Grade 3

FIG 1 • Regnault classification of breast ptosis. Grade 1: nipple-areolar complex at the level of the inframammary fold. Grade 2: nipple-areolar complex below the level of the inframammary fold. Grade 3: nipple-areolar complex at the lowest portion of the breast.

[†]Deceased

IMAGING

- A yearly screening mammogram is recommended beginning at age 40, or 10 years earlier than a primary relative's diagnosis of breast cancer.

DIFFERENTIAL DIAGNOSIS

- Tuberous breast deformity
- Pseudoptosis

SURGICAL MANAGEMENT

Preoperative Planning[2-4]

- Preoperative planning in the mastopexy patient is critical for obtaining an aesthetic result.

- Mastopexies have been the source of a disproportionate amount of litigation, so the surgeon should not take these operations lightly. Understanding the indications and limitations for each type of mastopexy will aid in avoiding trouble.
- Periareolar mastopexy is most useful in patients who need limited movement of the nipple-areolar complex.
  - It allows for movement of the nipple-areola complex approximately 2 cm. Attempting to move the nipple more than 2 cm will result in flattening of the breast mound.
  - Periareolar mastopexy is ideal for grade 0 or 1 ptosis, glandular ptosis, or in the setting of combined augmentation mastopexy (**FIG 2A,B**).
- Vertical mastopexy is a versatile operation that allows the surgeon to resite the nipple, regardless of the degree of ptosis, while reshaping the breast mound and tailoring the skin envelope (**FIG 2C–F**).

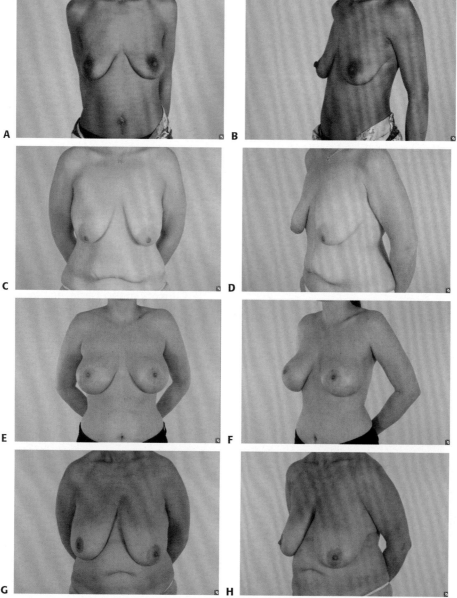

FIG 2 • A,B. Preoperative photographs of an ideal patient for periareolar mastopexy with grade 1 ptosis and deflated breast parenchyma. **C,D.** Preoperative photographs of a patient with grade 2 breast ptosis with planned vertical mastopexy and augmentation mammaplasty. **E,F.** Preoperative photos of a patient before undergoing revision mastopexy for treatment of pseudoptosis. **G,H.** Preoperative photos of patient with grade 2 ptosis and asymmetry after mild weight loss. She requested mastopexy while maintaining breast volume.

- Wise pattern mastopexy is typically reserved for patients with significant skin redundancy that do not want a decrease in breast volume (**FIG 2G,H**).
  - Patients with nipple to inframammary fold distance of 12 cm or greater may be good candidates for this procedure, with the trade-off of an additional horizontal scar under the breast.
  - In vertical mastopexies, the decision to incorporate a horizontal incision is a function of removing dog ears at the IMF. The true Wise pattern mastopexy requires marking and committing to the surgical incisions with the patient in the standing position.
  - The entire Wise pattern incision pattern can be de-epithelialized to maintain breast volume.

Positioning

- The patient should be positioned supine on the operating room table with the hips at the flexion point of the bed to facilitate the sitting position intraoperatively.
- The arms may be tucked at the patient's side or out on arm boards but should be secured and padded adequately.

Periareolar Mastopexy

Planning and Markings

- The concentric or donut mastopexy is indicated for patients with minimal or grade 1 breast ptosis.
- The surgeon should not attempt to achieve an aggressive movement of the nipple-areolar complex with this technique as it may excessively flatten the contour of the breast, produce a dilated widened areola, or result in poor circumareolar scarring.
  - The concentric mastopexy should be applied only to patients with reasonably aesthetic nipple position within the minimally ptotic breast.
  - If the nipple is not within the breast meridian, eccentric or crescentic mastopexy should be considered.
- The patient is marked in the anatomic standing position, with arms at the sides.
- The midline, inframammary fold, and breast meridian are marked.
- The overall breast symmetry and NAC are assessed.
- The proposed nipple position is transposed from the IMF to the anterior breast skin.
- The outer mastopexy circumference is typically marked freehand (**TECH FIG 1A**).
  - The outer markings skirt the edges of the areola medially and laterally.
  - The critical upper and lower limits of the typically oval outer periareolar pattern are determined superiorly by the desired new upper border location for the superior edge of the areola and inferiorly by the length of skin

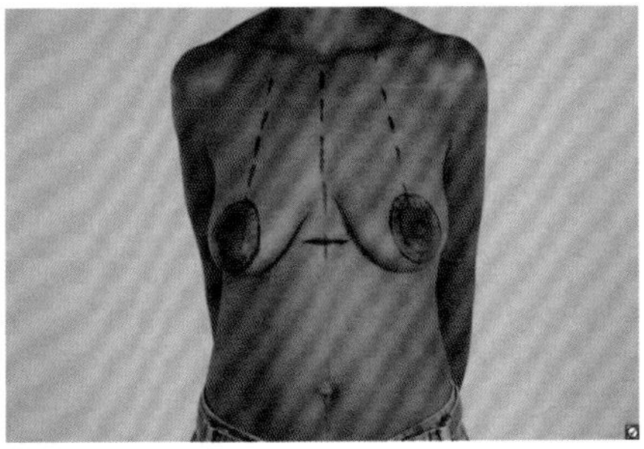

A

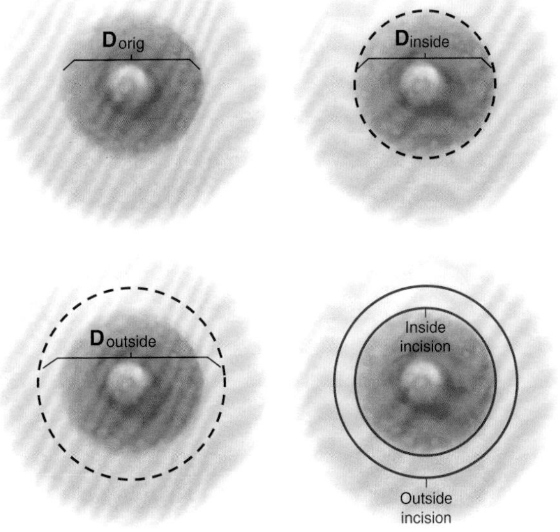

B

RULE 1: $D_{outside} \leq D_{orig} + (D_{orig} - D_{inside})$

RULE 2: $D_{outside} \leq 2 \times D_{inside}$

RULE 3: $D_{final} = 1/2\,(D_{outside} + D_{inside})$

TECH FIG 1 • A. Markings begin by identifying the midline, inframammary fold, and breast meridian for each breast. The estimated degree of nipple elevation is marked at the 12 o'clock position, addressing any asymmetry in nipple height that may be present. Finally, the outer diameter of the new nipple areolar border is drawn, with the skin to be de-epithelialized shaded in *red*. **B.** Three rules to aid preoperative planning of periareolar mastopexies. (Adapted from Spear SL, Kassan M, Little JW. Guidelines in concentric mastopexy. *Plast Reconstr Surg.* 1990;85(6):961–966.)

desirable to leave between the lower edge of the areola and the IMF (typically 5–8 cm depending on the size of the breast)

- The inner pattern is usually drawn as a round circle using a "cookie cutter" pattern of 38 to 42 mm.
- Basic guidelines for concentric mastopexy described by Spear et al.[5] provide guidelines for nipple-areolar marking (**TECH FIG 1B**).
  - First and most importantly: Diameter outside – diameter original should be equal to or less than (diameter original – diameter inner), meaning it is preferable to remove more pigmented skin than unpigmented skin.
  - Second: Diameter outside should ideally be no more than two times the diameter inside.
  - Third: Diameter final = ½ (diameter outside + diameter inside).

Incisions and Closure

- A 38- or 42-mm cookie cutter is used to mark the proposed nipple-areola diameter with the assistant applying mild tension.

- The inner circle is incised first, followed by the outer circle for efficiency in using the applied counter-tension.
- The remaining donut (often eccentric) is de-epithelialized with a no. 10 or 15 blade. The nipple blood supply is adequate from underlying parenchymal perforators in the native breast unless there is an implant behind the breast. Thus, a full-thickness skin incision may be made circumferentially.
  - Limited superficial circumferential subcutaneous undermining with electrocautery can be performed to decrease tension with closure.
- Closure needs to be carefully done and meticulous and is performed with each suture bite directly opposite to the previous other side to equally distribute areolar tissue along the larger outer diameter.
- If areolar widening is a concern, a carefully placed permanent purse string or wagon wheel (eg, Gore-Tex) suture may be used.
- Mild periareolar wrinkling is common in the immediate postoperative period, but routinely settles in 1 to 2 months.
  - Severe wrinkling or puckering implies poor closure technique or overly aggressive skin excision.

■ Vertical Mastopexy

Planning and Markings[6,7]

- The addition of a vertical incision to the mastopexy significantly increases its utility.
  - Vertical mastopexy can adequately correct all grades of ptosis.

- The patient should be marked in the standing position and should begin with midline, IMF, and breast meridian (**TECH FIG 2A,C,F**).
- The breast meridian marking should be carried inferiorly onto the patient's abdomen, as it will aid in placement of the vertical mastopexy markings (**TECH FIG 2B**).

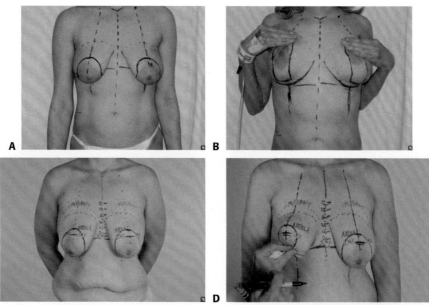

TECH FIG 2 • Preoperative marking photographs of a vertical mastopexy in a patient with grade 2 ptosis. **A.** The markings begin with midline, breast meridian, and inframammary folds. Next, the vertical mastopexy incision is marked by placing the superior most part of the keyhole incision approximately 2 cm above proposed nipple position or the IMF. **B.** The inferior part of the vertical incision stops 2 cm above the IMF. **C–E.** Preoperative markings for a third patient, who was undergoing vertical mastopexy with augmentation. **C.** Preoperative markings begin with marking the midline, breast meridian, the inframammary fold, and the proposed nipple position. The upper border of the breast tissue marked with the *dotted black line*. The proposed location of the upper border of the implant is estimated 8 to 10 cm below the clavicle. **D.** Moderate tension is placed on the breast skin to cone the breast and estimate the width of skin to be excised from the vertical extent of the vertical mastopexy.

TECHNIQUES

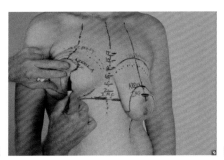
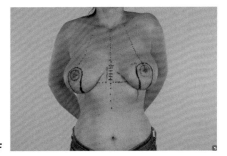

TECH FIG 2 (Continued) • **E.** After the pinch test, the vertical incision is then drawn and stops 2 cm above the inframammary fold. **F.** Preoperative markings for in a different patient undergoing vertical revision mastopexy for treatment of pseudoptosis begin with midline, breast meridian, and inframammary folds in *black marker*. Midline 1-cm increments are marked from IMF in the superior direction to aid with improving symmetry of nipple position. Finally, the vertical mastopexy is incision marked with the inferior most point stopping 2 cm above the IMF.

- The proposed nipple position is transposed from the IMF to a comparable point on the front of the breast bilaterally.
  - The new nipple position should then be measured for symmetry.
  - Periareolar markings can be drawn with the aid of a keyhole or freehand.
  - The vertical component is marked by medial and lateral displacement of the breast (**TECH FIG 2D,E**). By gently displacing the breast laterally, the medial vertical incision can be marked at the breast meridian. Likewise, the breast is displaced medially, and the lateral vertical incision can be marked at the breast meridian.
- If the patient is also undergoing augmentation, the proposed upper border of the implant is marked as well, as shown in **TECH FIG 2C–E**.

Incisions and Closure

- A vertical mastopexy incision popularized by Lejour is described here.[3,8]
- First, a 38- or 42-mm cookie cutter is used to mark the nipple.

- It is incised with a no. 10 or 15 blade followed by incision of the outer periareolar marking (**TECH FIG 3A**).
- The incision is carried to the level of the dermis.
- The intervening skin segment is de-epithelialized with preservation of the subdermal plexus (**TECH FIG 3B**).
- The vertical incisions can then be carried out through the dermis.
  - When glandular rearrangement is planned, electrocautery is used to vertically incise the glandular tissue to the level of the chest wall.
  - The gland is then elevated off of the chest wall from medial to lateral.
- Attention is then paid to creating skin flaps in the plane between breast parenchyma and subcutaneous fat along the vertical mastopexy incision.
- Medial and lateral glandular pillars have been created and may be used for autoaugmentation of the breast (**TECH FIG 3C**).
  - Rotation of the medial or lateral glandular pillar in the subglandular plane moves the ptotic breast tissue to a more aesthetically pleasing position.

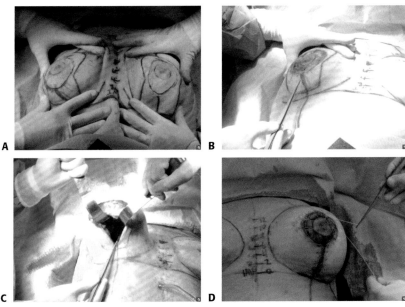

TECH FIG 3 • **A.** Intraoperative photograph following nipple incision guided by 42-mm cookie cutter. Incision around nipple with 42-mm cookie cutter and incision around the planned periareolar de-epitelized portion. **B.** Intraoperative photograph after de-epithelialization. The remainder of the skin within vertical mastopexy incision may be excised just below level of the dermis. **C.** Medial and lateral parenchymal pillars are created to allow for autoaugmentation of the breast. **D.** Demonstration of a periareolar wagon wheel Gore-Tex suture technique to prevent widening of the nipple-areolar complex.

- The pillars are then approximated with 2-0 PDS to shape the breast mound. The skin is approximated with staples, and the patient is brought to sitting position on the operating room table for visual inspection.
- The periareolar incision may be closed with a regular or interlocking pursestring Gore-Tex suture if areolar widening is a concern (**TECH FIG 3D**).

Other Techniques

- The standard vertical mastopexy relies upon glandular pillars and skin for support. The Graf technique uses a chest wall–based, inferior glandular flap to augment the upper pole.

- The glandular flap is passed through a sling of superficial two-thirds of pectoralis muscle to provide further support.
- Its utility and longevity are well described by Graf et al.[9]
- Acellular dermal matrix (ADM) is well established in the setting of breast reconstruction. ADM is yet another option for providing support to the glandular pillars, or it can be used in lieu of the pectoralis loop for support in the Graf procedure.
  - The parenchymal pillars are sewn together with absorbable suture.
  - Then ADM is fashioned to the lower pole under mild tension to help support the breast mound (**TECH FIG 4**).

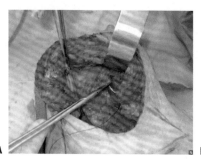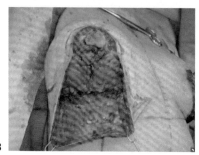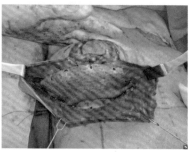

TECH FIG 4 • A. Intraoperative view of medial and lateral pillars being sutured together with absorbable monofilament suture. **B.** Intraoperative view demonstrating medial and lateral pillars sutured together. **C.** The pillars are supported with an inferior sling of acellular dermal matrix to prevent the recurrence of pseudoptosis or "bottoming out."

■ Wise Pattern Mastopexy

Planning and Markings

- The planned inverted T incision pattern allows for resection of redundant skin and glandular tissue in patients with more significant ptosis.
  - This technique is similar to the Wise pattern used in reduction mammaplasty, with the goal to primarily reshape the breast mound, rather than reducing the volume.
- The patient is marked in the anatomic standing position, with arms at the sides (**TECH FIG 5**).

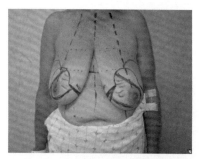

TECH FIG 5 • Preoperative markings for Wise pattern mastopexy begin by marking the midline, breast meridian, upper border of the breast, and inframammary folds in *black marker*. The inframammary fold is then transposed anteriorly onto the breast skin to estimate nipple placement. This is represented by the *lower horizontal dotted black line*. The keyhole breast template is used to mark new nipple diameter and vertical incision, also in *black marker*. The *red marker* represents the dermoglandular pedicle, which will be de-epithelialized to maintain nipple blood supply.

- The midline, inframammary fold, and breast meridian are marked, and overall breast symmetry and NAC is assessed.
- The proposed nipple position is transposed from the IMF bilaterally. The top of the proposed areola is marked 2 cm above the new nipple position. The keyhole marker is used to trace the periareolar incision.
- The breast is displaced medially and laterally to help determine the width of the inverted T incision.
- The choice of glandular pedicle supporting the NAC varies by the size and shape of each breast.
  - The senior author prefers a broad superior dermoglandular or superomedial dermoglandular pedicle supported by the internal mammary artery perforators.
- The vertical incision length, planned areola-to-fold distance, varies with breast size.
  - Areola-to-fold distances typically range from 6 to 9 cm in length.
  - The wider the breast, the longer the vertical component must be to create adequate lower pole breast volume.
  - Making the areola-to-fold distance too small tethers the lower portion of the breast, creating a wide and boxy contour.
- The nipple is generally marked with a 42-mm cookie cutter.
- With the assistant placing the breast on tension, the nipple incision is made with a no. 15 blade.
- The remainder of the breast incisions are made.
- When planning a Wise pattern mastopexy, the horizontal excisions are marked in the standard reduction mammaplasty fashion.

Incisions and Closure

- If committed to a Wise pattern mastopexy, all incisions may be carried out with a scalpel.
- To preserve breast volume, the entire Wise pattern incision can be de-epithelialized (**TECH FIG 6A,B**).
- In similar fashion, medial and lateral pillars are created with electrocautery (**TECH FIG 6C,D**).
  - Once the pillars are created, they are used to autoaugment the breast in a retroglandular plane (**TECH FIG 6E**).
  - The excess central inferior wedge of tissue may be mobilized and transposed superiorly based upon a medial, lateral, or inferior pedicle if volume autoaugmentation is desired.
    - The two medial and lateral pillars are stabilized with internal absorbable sutures.
- The skin is tailored closed with a skin stapler to assess symmetry, and the patient is moved to the sitting position on the operating room table for final assessment and adjustments.
- Incision closure is performed in the standard fashion with buried monofilament absorbable sutures.
- A closed suction drain may be left in place and removed at or after the first postoperative visit.

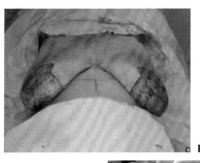
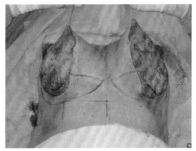
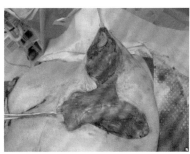
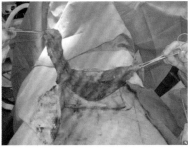
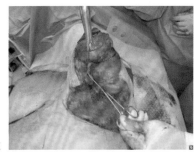

TECH FIG 6 • A. The nipple incision is carried out after measurement with a 38- to 45-mm cookie cutter. In contrast to a breast reduction, all the skin within the Wise pattern is de-epithelialized. **B.** The breast are retracted superiorly with skin hooks to allow de-epithelialization of the inferior Wise pattern skin. **C.** After the lower pole skin has been removed, incisions are carried through the breast tissue to chest wall. This develops lateral and medial pillars. (The later pillar is shown here in the retractor.) **D.** The medial and lateral pillars are displayed here. **E.** The medial and lateral pillars are tucked under the dermoglandular pedicle supporting the nipple to provide autoaugmentation.

PEARLS AND PITFALLS

Periareolar mastopexy[10]	■ Do not attempt to move the nipple-areolar complex more than 2 cm as it will flatten the breast. ■ Use the three concentric mastopexy rules described by Spear et al. to avoid complications. ■ Superficially undermine surrounding breast skin flaps for tension-free closure. ■ Mastopexy should be performed after augmentation in a combined procedure, as augmentation will decrease the amount of skin resection necessary.
Vertical mastopexy[8,11,12]	■ This technique may be combined with augmentation. If augmentation mastopexy is planned, augmentation should be performed first. The subpectoral or subglandular plane may be initially accessed through the vertical incision or the inframammary incision. ■ The vertical incision should stop 2 cm above the IMF to avoid disrupting the fold. The excess gathered skin will settle in 2–3 months or the excess can be trimmed with a dog ear correction in the IMF. ■ Tailor tacking the vertical incision closed and sitting the patient supine are useful in assessing the initial result and symmetry. ■ If the outer marked areolar diameter is significantly larger than the inner areolar diameter, a blocking suture is useful to prevent areolar enlargement or scar widening. ■ More aggressive mastopexy with a planned excision in the fold can be performed in patients with excessive skin laxity or cases without simultaneous augmentation.
Wise pattern mastopexy	■ Reserved for grade 3 ptosis or breast requiring significant skin redundancy. ■ Medial and lateral de-epithelialized skin flaps may be used to provide upper pole autoaugmentation. ■ Use the inframammary fold or most projected point of the breast for ideal nipple placement to avoid malposition, particularly a high-riding nipple. ■ Maintain an adequate dermoglandular pedicle in high-grade ptosis to prevent nipple-areolar necrosis.

POSTOPERATIVE CARE

- Compressive surgical bra
- No strenuous upper body exercise activity for 4 to 6 weeks
- Surgical drains typically not needed
- 24 hours or less of perioperative antibiotics
- Occlusive dressing for 48 hours

OUTCOMES

- Mastopexy is an operation with a steep learning curve, and special attention should be paid to preoperative planning and patient selection (**FIG 3**).
- Patient and surgeon expectations should be discussed to ensure agreement on a realistic result.

- When properly planned and executed, mastopexy has high satisfaction rates.
  - However, patients with significant ptosis, diabetes, obesity, tobacco use, or prior radiation should be approached with caution.

COMPLICATIONS

- Bleeding, infection, dehiscence, delayed wound healing
- Nipple-areolar necrosis in the previously irradiated or augmented breast
- Areolar widening, hypertrophic or widened scar
- Asymmetry
- Nipple malposition

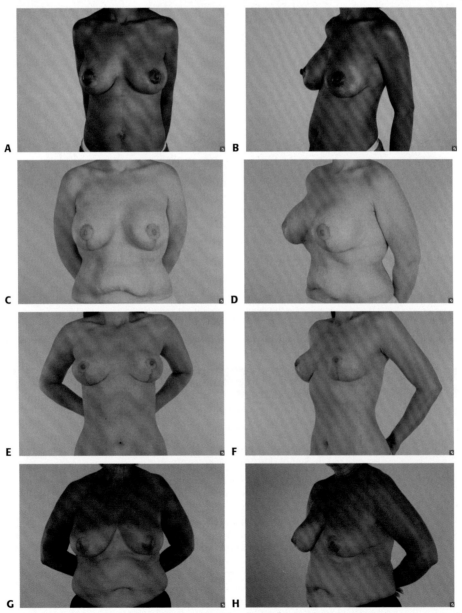

FIG 3 • A,B. Postoperative photos of the patient in **FIG 2A,B** after periareolar mastopexy show an improved upper pole breast slope and skin envelope with resolution of ptosis. **C,D.** Postoperative photos of the patient in **FIG 2C,D** after vertical mastopexy and augmentation. **E,F.** Postoperative photos of the patient in **FIG 2E,F** after revision vertical mastopexy using acellular dermal matrix for treatment of pseudoptosis. **G,H.** Postoperative photos of the patient in **FIG 2G,H** about 6 months after Wise pattern mastopexy.

ACKNOWLEDGMENT

Dr Ter Louw dedicates this chapter to the memory of Scott L. Spear, MD, FACS, who passed away during its preparation. Founding Chair of the Georgetown University Hospital Department of Plastic Surgery, Washington, DC, Dr Spear was an innovator, a skilled and thoughtful surgeon, a mentor to many, and a dedicated husband, father, and friend.

REFERENCES

1. De Mey A, Greuse M, Azzam C. The evolution of mammaplasty. *Eur J Plast Surg.* 2005;28:213-217.
2. Lassus C. New refinements in vertical mammaplasty. *Chir Plast.* 1981;6:81-86.
3. Lejour M. Vertical mammaplasty: update and appraisal of late results. *Plast Reconstr Surg.* 1999;104:771.
4. Benelli L. A new periareolar mammaplasty: the "round block" technique. *Aesthetic Plast Surg* 1990;14:93-100.
5. Spear SL, Kassan M, Little JW. Guidelines in concentric mastopexy. *Plast Reconstr Surg.* 1990;85(6):961-966.
6. Rohrich RJ, Thornton JF, Jakubietz RG, et al. The limited scar mastopexy: current concepts and approaches to correct breast ptosis. *PlastReconstr Surg.* 2004;114(6):1622-1630.
7. Lai HMJ, Lam T. A mathematical design in creating the new nipple-areolar complex in vertical mammaplasty. *Plast Reconstr Surg Glob Open.* 2014;2:e177.
8. Lejour M. Vertical mammaplasty early complications after 250 personal consecutive cases. *Plast Reconstr Surg.* 1999;104:764.
9. Graf R, Ricardo Dall Oglio Tolazzi A, Balbinot P, et al. Influence of the pectoralis major muscle sling in chest wall-based flap suspension after vertical mammaplasty: ten-year follow-up. *Aesthet Surg J.* 2016;36(10):1113-1121.
10. Gruber RP, Jones HW Jr. The "donut" mastopexy: indications and complications. *Plast Reconstr Surg.* 1980;65(1):34-38.
11. Berthe JV, Massaut J, Greuse M, et al. The vertical mammaplasty: a reappraisal of the technique and its complications. *Plast Reconstr Surg.* 2003;111:2192.
12. Beer GM, Spicher I, Cierpka KA, et al. Benefits and pitfalls of vertical breast reduction. *Br J Plast Surg.* 2004;57:12.

7

CHAPTER

Section III: Reduction Mammaplasty

Reduction Mammaplasty

Peter Henderson and Joseph J. Disa

DEFINITION

- Breast hypertrophy can be a physically and socially debilitating condition that frequently leads women to seek surgical intervention. Macromastia is defined as symptomatic breast tissue less than 1500 g, and gigantomastia is defined as symptomatic breast tissue greater than 1500 g.
- Reduction mammoplasty has two elements: skin excision pattern and parenchymal excision/pedicle design. With few exceptions, these two elements are independent variables that can be combined in any manner. The vertical-only skin excision pattern and the superomedial pedicle design are increasingly commonly used, and are often combined, especially in patients in whom the maintenance of upper pole projection is important, and the degree of ptosis/excess skin is not excessive.

ANATOMY

- The boundaries of the breast are commonly considered to be the clavicle cranially, the inframammary fold caudally, the sternum medially, and the lateral/anterior aspect of the latissimus muscle laterally. The tail of Spence extends from the upper outer quadrant into the axilla (**FIG 1**).
- The blood supply to the breast is from perforators from the internal mammary (thoracic) artery and vein, as well as the thoracoacromial and lateral thoracic vessels.
- The breast is innervated by the 4th through 6th intercostal nerves.
- In females, the areola is usually round and 38 to 40 mm.
- Breast ptosis is most commonly graded on the Regnault scale (**FIG 2**). Grade 0 (no ptosis) indicates that the nipple sits cranially to the IMF. Grade 1 indicates that the nipple sits at the level of the IMF. Grade 2 indicates that the nipple sits caudal to the IMF but not at the caudal-most point of the breast. Grade 3 indicates that the nipple sits at the caudal-most point of the breast. Pseudoptosis is when the nipple sits at or above the IMF, but there is excessive breast tissue below the IMF (this has a characteristic "bottomed out" appearance).
- Common, clinically relevant breast measurements include nipple-sternal notch and nipple-IMF distances.
- Bra sizes are an imperfect way to gauge breast size (not in the least because most women do not wear the correct size bra). The convention is that the "number" in the breast size is the circumference of the chest wall (measured just caudal to the breast). The "cup" size is indicated by a letter, with each letter's position in the alphabet indicating the increased number of inches that are measured when the circumference

around the breasts is measured (eg, "32B" means that the chest wall circumference is 32 in., and the circumference around the breasts is 34 in.).

PATHOGENESIS

- Breast hypertrophy is a congenital disorder that frequently is exacerbated by weight gain. Especially in young patients, it can be due to increased end-organ responsiveness to estrogen.

NATURAL HISTORY

- In addition to being socially debilitating in young patients, breast hypertrophy can progress to physical ailments, including "notching" of the shoulders due to the bra straps, neck and upper back pain, and intertriginous infections.

PATIENT HISTORY AND PHYSICAL FINDINGS

- Detailed patient and family history of breast disease is crucial (including benign tumors, malignancy, screening, etc.), and information regarding any prior radiation treatment and the operative reports from any prior breast procedures (most notably partial mastectomy/"lumpectomy" or prior breast reduction) should be obtained.

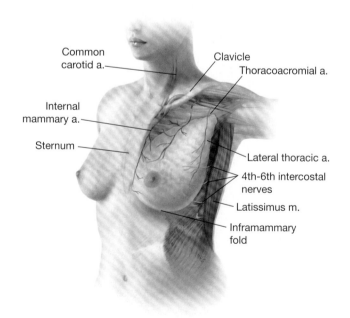

Common carotid a.
Clavicle
Thoracoacromial a.
Internal mammary a.
Sternum
Lateral thoracic a.
4th-6th intercostal nerves
Latissimus m.
Inframammary fold

FIG 1 • Breast anatomy.

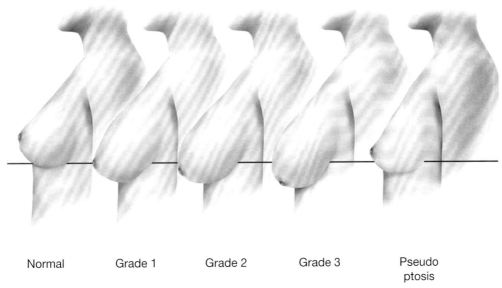

FIG 2 • Regnault scale for breast ptosis.

| Normal | Grade 1 | Grade 2 | Grade 3 | Pseudo ptosis |

- Factors relevant to lifetime estrogen exposure, such as age at menarche, menopause (if applicable), number of pregnancies, and use of birth control medications, are also important.
- Breast-feeding history (including plans for future childrearing) is mandatory.
- Nicotine use should be carefully investigated; most surgeons will not perform this elective procedure on anyone who has smoked in the past 2 to 4 weeks.
- Personal importance of erogenous breast sensitivity should be discussed, as decreased or complete absence of nipple sensation is a possible consequence.
- Symptoms related to breast hypertrophy (should notching, back pain, intertriginous infections, and difficulties with personal hygiene) should be noted.
- Physical exam should note any asymmetry between breasts, complete bimanual examination for masses in both breasts and bilateral axillae, and appropriate breast measurements (nipple-sternal notch, nipple-IMF).

IMAGING

- In patients who are of an age when standard, surveillance breast imaging is recommended (40–50 years, depending on the recommending agency), and mammography should always be performed prior to any breast reduction procedure. Many surgeons will obtain surveillance imaging prior to reduction regardless of age, though this practice is not formally endorsed.

DIFFERENTIAL DIAGNOSIS

- Though unlikely, the possibility of a large breast mass must be considered when a patient is evaluated for presumed breast hypertrophy.

NONOPERATIVE MANAGEMENT

- Weight loss may lead to a small incremental improvement in symptoms but rarely is significant enough to sufficiently alleviate symptoms.
- Liposuction is a reasonable approach in a very small subset of patients (namely those with excessive breast volume without ptosis).

SURGICAL MANAGEMENT

Preoperative Planning

- It is important that a frank discussion occur between surgeon and patient regarding each patient's wishes for postoperative breast size. This will rarely have a significant impact on the type of procedure performed but will impact the amount of breast tissue excised.

Positioning

- Patient should be positioned supine on the operating room table.
- Because the patient will be flexed at the waist in order to "sit upright" during the procedure, secure the arms (usually out, on arm boards) and head, and ensure that the patient's waist is appropriately positioned relative to the break in the table.

Approach

- Options for skin excision patterns include the "Wise pattern" ("anchor" or "inverted T") and vertical-only ("mosque"). Options for parenchymal excision/pedicle design include superior, superomedial, medial, inferior, central mound, lateral, and bipedicle (among others).[1]

■ Vertical, Superomedial Pedicle Reduction Mammaplasty

- Inject wetting solution into the inferomedial and infero-lateral portions of the resection specimen (what would be the medial and lateral parts of the "anchor" in the traditional Wise pattern excision).
- Mark the neo-areola with a nipple sizer ("cookie cutter"); most surgeons use 42 mm.
- Incise partial-thickness dermis of the pedicle and the circumareolar incision.
- Place the breast tourniquet.
- De-epithelialize the pedicle (taking care not to inadvertently undermine the nipple-areola complex).
- Incise full-thickness dermis around the pedicle.
- Remove the breast tourniquet.
- Incise the breast parenchyma straight down to the chest wall, taking care not to undermine the pedicle.
- Incise full-thickness dermis to the rest of the skin incisions.

- Undermine the inferomedial and inferolateral corners just below the dermis (many surgeons will use curved Mayo scissors, especially if wetting solution has been injected).
- Remove the skin/fat/breast parenchyma specimen as one single piece.
- Irrigate and ensure hemostasis.
- Weigh specimens.
- Rotate the pedicles (clockwise on the right breast and counterclockwise on the left breast) to ensure that they rest comfortably in a tension-free manner.
- Place "pillar stitches" between the resulting medial and lateral pillars through the breast parenchyma (with or without the overlying dermis).
- Assess for symmetry, with potential interventions for insufficient symmetry being the excision of additional tissue and altering the pillar stitches.
- Use of closed-suction drains is typically unnecessary.
- Close the skin in the deep dermal and subcuticular positions.[2–4]

■ Central Mound Reduction Mammaplasty

Markings

- Preoperative markings should be done in the upright or sitting position (**TECH FIG 1A-C**).
  - The most reliable location for the nipple-areola complex is with the superior border at the level of the inframammary fold (this provides better results than a predetermined nipple-sternal notch distance, or the midhumeral point).
- It is advisable to initially mark a vertical-only skin excision pattern (later a horizontal component can be excised if needed).

- Nipple sizers (usually 42 mm) are used to define the new borders of the areola (if at all possible, remove all additional areolar tissue to prevent unsightly pigmented skin at closure lines).

Excision of Parenchyma

- Incise the circumareolar and vertical-only skin excision markings, and de-epithelialize all tissue besides the newly defined nipple-areola complex.
- Excise as much breast parenchyma inferior to the nipple-areola complex as necessary in order to achieve the desired breast size (**TECH FIG 2A-C**).
  - The central tenet of the central mound technique is to maintain a pedicle directly from the nipple-areola complex to the underlying pectoralis major muscle;

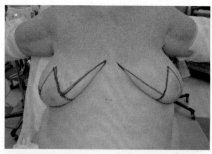
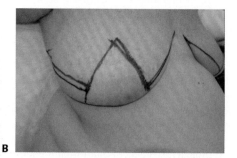
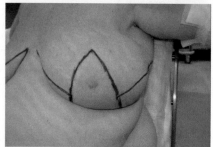

TECH FIG 1 • Markings for central mound breast reduction using the Wise pattern.

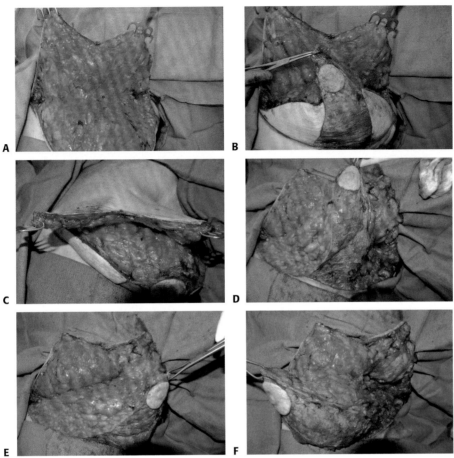

TECH FIG 2 • A–C. Skin flaps of appropriate thickness to maintain adequate vascularity are elevated off the gland laterally, medially, and superiorly. **D–F.** The footprint of the breast is left attached to the muscle and is not undermined.

therefore, do not undermine the nipple-areola complex in the course of removing excess breast parenchyma (**TECH FIG 2D-F**).

■ If necessary, skin flaps medial, superior, and lateral to the nipple-areola complex can be created in order to allow for the necessary mobility to transpose the nipple-areola complex into its final position near the level of the inframammary fold. This is done in a manner angling away from the nipple-areola complex (thereby creating a "cone" with the nipple-areola complex at the apex). The parenchyma of the skin flaps should be at least 2 cm thick to maximize vascularity.

■ Excision of the breast parenchyma leads to the creation of medial and lateral "pillars," which are sutured together with deeply placed, heavy, slowly absorbable sutures.

Completion

■ The patient is flexed at the waist to "sit up."

■ At this point, the breast is examined to determine whether there is sufficient excess skin and/or breast parenchyma to warrant the excision of a horizontal wedge of tissue. If so, the markings should be made such that the closure will fall at the level of the inframammary fold. If

no further breast parenchymal excision is warranted, the skin can be removed by de-epithelialization alone. If the patient would benefit from the excision of additional breast parenchyma, then the horizontal wedge can be taken as a full-thickness segment.

■ The tissue is irrigated and hemostasis is ensured.

■ Closed-suction drains can be placed, depending on surgeon preference.

■ The areola is inset to its new location, and the skin is closed (**TECH FIG 3**).

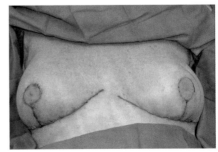

TECH FIG 3 • Intraoperative appearance after gland and nipple-areola repositioning.

PEARLS AND PITFALLS

Skin excision pattern	▪ When the vertical-only skin excision pattern is attempted, the amount of excess skin at the inferior portion of the vertical wound should be examined. A mild amount of "bunching" can be tolerated, as it usually "settles out" over the first 6 months. A moderate or significant amount of excess skin should be excised in a transverse direction, essentially converting the "vertical-only" skin excision pattern into a Wise pattern.
Nicotine use	▪ Nicotine use (either in cigarettes or in nicotine patches) significantly increases the risk of NAC ischemia, fat necrosis, and other wound healing complications. The nicotine metabolite cotinine can be detected in the urine, and a point-of-care test can be performed in the preoperative area immediately prior to the scheduled operation if concern exists.
Parenchymal excision	▪ Efforts should be made to minimize the amount of parenchymal tissue removed underlying the final location of the NAC (superior and lateral to the pedicle); overresection can lead to poor NAC projection.

POSTOPERATIVE CARE

▪ Bras that provide maximal support (and do not contain any rigid components like underwire) should be worn for the first 2 to 4 weeks.

▪ If closed-suction drains were used, they will likely be able to be removed in 1 to 7 days.

▪ Nipple-areola complex ischemia/necrosis is a rare but dreaded complication that should be checked for regularly in the immediate to early postoperative period (creation of a pedicle that is sufficiently wide and thick can significantly reduce the risk of this happening). If NAC ischemia is thought to present in the early postoperative period, periareolar sutures can be removed, undoing the inset and potentially releasing any ischemia-inducing configuration.

OUTCOMES

▪ Most patients are satisfied following breast reduction procedures (**FIG 3**).

▪ Use of superomedial pedicle is thought to maximize upper pole fullness and reduce the likelihood of pseudoptosis ("bottoming out") that is thought to occur more frequently with an inferior pedicle design.

▪ Nipple sensation is rarely absent, but usually decreased relative to the preoperative baseline. Occasionally, nipple sensation is increased postoperatively due to decrease stretch/tension once the excess weight/volume has been removed.

▪ Ability to breast-feed is impaired in approximately 40% of patients.

COMPLICATIONS

▪ Hematoma can occur, but risk can be minimized if hemostasis is diligently attempted.

▪ Seroma can occur and can usually be addressed with percutaneous drainage.

▪ Fat necrosis can be a consequence of parenchymal ischemia. It usually softens (if not completely resolves) in a matter of months, but sometimes requires surgical excision.

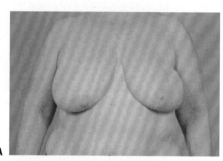

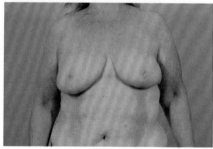

FIG 3 • **A.** Patient preoperatively. **B.** Three years after breast reduction.

▪ NAC ischemia is rare but can potentially lead to necrosis and complete loss of the NAC.

▪ Alterations in nipple sensation or breast-feeding ability are not uncommon, and the patient should be counseled in the preoperative period as to the possibility of this occurring.

REFERENCES

1. Antony AK, Yegiyants SS, Danielson KK, et al. A matched cohort study of superomedial pedicle vertical scar breast reduction (100 breasts) and traditional inferior pedicle Wise-pattern reduction (100 breasts): an outcomes study over 3 years. *Plast Reconstr Surg* 2013;132:1068-1076.
2. Hall-Findlay EJ. Pedicles in vertical breast reduction and mastopexy. *Clin Plast Surg.* 2002;29(3):379-391.
3. Spear SL, Davison SP, Ducic I. Superomedial pedicle reduction with short scar. *Semin Plast Surg.* 2004;18(3):203-210.
4. Van Deventer PV, Graewe FR. The blood supply of the breast revisited. *Plast Reconstr Surg.* 2016;137(5):1388-1397.

Inferior Pedicle

Paul A. Ghareeb and Albert Losken

DEFINITION

- Reduction mammaplasty remains one of the most commonly performed operations by plastic surgeons.
- Inferior pedicle reduction mammaplasty is one of the most widely used reduction techniques because it is easy to learn, is safe, and has reproducible outcomes.[1]
- This technique was described and refined in the 1970s by Ribiero, Robbins, Georgiade, and Courtiss and Goldwyn.[2,3]
- Is most commonly utilized with a Wise pattern (inverted T) skin excision.
- The inferior pedicle reduction technique is extremely versatile and can be used in almost any reduction procedure. We have found it to be useful in patients with long nipple to notch distances and those with large anticipated reduction specimens.
- The complication rates for inferior pedicle reductions have been shown to be equivalent for small and large (greater than 1000 g) reductions, making this technique particularly useful when treating gigantomastia.[4]

ANATOMY

- Borders of the breast
  - Superiorly: clavicle
  - Medially: sternum
  - Inferiorly: superior border of rectus fascia
  - Laterally: anterior border of latissimus
- Blood supply
  - Intercostal perforators
    - Primary blood supply to the inferior pedicle
  - Internal mammary perforators
  - Lateral thoracic artery
  - Thoracoacromial artery
- Innervation
  - Intercostal sensory branches
    - The fourth intercostal sensory nerve provides the majority of sensation to the nipple-areolar complex (NAC).
    - The sensory branches course just above pectoralis fascia before piercing the breast parenchyma to supply the overlying skin and nipple. It is important to maintain a layer of breast tissue over the pectoralis when performing reduction mammaplasty to prevent damage to these nerves.

PATIENT HISTORY AND PHYSICAL FINDINGS

- Focused history
  - Current brassiere size and desired size after mammaplasty is important to determine with the patient preoperatively in order to guide goals and expectations.
  - Symptoms of macromastia and any interventions attempted must be elucidated and recorded preoperatively.
  - History of childbirth, breast-feeding, and desire to have further children are important to discuss. With the inferior pedicle technique, most women maintain the ability to breast-feed postoperatively but should be counseled on this during the consultation.
  - Mammographic history if applicable, as well as family history of breast disease or cancer.
  - A history of smoking should be discussed prior to any reduction, and patients should be counseled to stop smoking at least 1 month prior to reduction mammaplasty due to the significantly increased risk of wound healing complications.
- Physical exam
  - Examine the overall breast shape, asymmetries, previous scars, and estimate breast size in grams. Always examine for breast masses and nipple sensation. Record breast measurements including sternal-notch-to-nipple and nipple-to-inframammary fold distances.
    - Patients considered to be good candidates for an inferior pedicle reduction often times have long nipple to notch and nipple to IMF distances, which can both be easily addressed with this technique. Furthermore, patients with boxy-appearing breasts can be shaped effectively with the skin excision.
  - Evaluate existing ptosis utilizing the Regnault classification.
  - Note any additional axillary tissue laterally that would not be resected with standard reduction mammaplasty. This is often an area that the patient assumes will be treated with standard reduction procedures but must be counseled that this is an additional area that must be treated.

IMAGING

- Mammography is recommended for women who meet screening criteria.
- No other routine imaging is required preoperatively.

SURGICAL MANAGEMENT

Preoperative Planning

- Preoperative markings are critical to the success of any breast reduction.
- The patient is examined in the standing position, with her arms resting to either side.
- The midline is marked first from sternal notch to the umbilicus.

- The true breast meridian is then marked on each side from the midclavicular line down onto the abdominal wall. Note that this may not always align with the position of the NAC.
- Pitanguy point is then identified and marked by placing one's fingers underneath the breast at the inframammary fold and curling them forward to be palpated by the opposite hand. This allows the surgeon to determine the final resting position of the NAC. This is approximately 21 cm from the sternal notch but can vary depending on the body and breast shape.
  - It is important to mark this point correctly at the IMF. By marking too high, one may produce a "sunny side up" nipple, which points upward, or a "snoopy deformity" by placing the nipple too far inferiorly.
- The vertical limbs of the Wise pattern are then created approximately 7 cm in length on each side, starting at Pitanguy point and coursing inferiorly. A McKissock keyhole tool may be used for the purpose of creating the vertical limbs, but we prefer to use the medial and lateral distraction technique. In this fashion, the breast is distracted medially and laterally, and the vertical limb is drawn in continuity with the superior and inferior breast meridian markings.
  - The distance between the base of the vertical limbs correlates with the final change in breast base diameter.
- The horizontal markings are then drawn to connect the vertical limbs to the inframammary fold marking at the medial and lateral most aspects of the breast.
  - The horizontal takeout can be tailored as short or long as necessary to achieve the desired outcome. The markings are typically carried out further for larger resections or boxy-appearing breasts, whereas in smaller reductions, can be achieved with a shorter horizontal scar.
  - The IMF marking is made just above the level of the existing IMF. It can be preserved at the inverted T–junction if viability of the upper flaps is a concern.
- After the markings have been completed, they should be compared to the contralateral side to ensure symmetry. In asymmetric reductions, this may be difficult to assess.
- **FIG 1** demonstrates the standard preoperative markings for an inferior pedicle reduction.

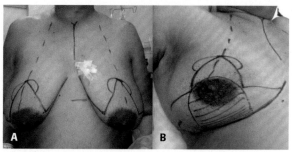

FIG 1 • **A,B.** Preoperative markings for the inferior pedicle Wise pattern reduction in a patient undergoing bilateral oncoplastic reduction for a left breast cancer.

Positioning

- The patient is placed supine on the operating room table and is positioned to be able to sit up if necessary.
- The arms are extended on arm boards, taking care not to over extend and distort the breast. They are secured with standard straps and soft padded wraps to facilitate placing the patient in the upright position.
- The breasts are prepped and draped to include the sternal notch, clavicles, and lateral most aspects of the breast and axilla. For unilateral procedures, the contralateral breast is exposed to be examined during the procedure.

Approach

- At the start of the procedure, the planned inferior pedicle is designed from the inframammary fold incision along the breast meridian to include a 1-cm cuff of tissue surrounding the NAC. The base of the pedicle should be 8 to 10 cm in width to ensure proper vascularity of the NAC. This is kept wider in bigger reductions with longer pedicles.
- The NAC is then marked by sight or with a cookie cutter at 40 to 44 mm, and the final nipple position is planned and marked at the apex of the vertical limbs. No tension is applied to the NAC while marking to reduce the likelihood of creating an unnatural final appearance.
- A line approximately 1 cm above the inframammary fold is marked for the inferior aspect of the Wise pattern. This is performed to avoid disrupting the dense attachments of the fold.

■ Incision

- The nipple is incised sharply with a knife through the epidermis only.
- The remainder of the Wise pattern markings and the planned inferior pedicle are then incised sharply, and the pedicle is de-epithelialized with a large curved Mayo scissors or a no. 10 blade (**TECH FIG 1**).
  - It is helpful to place a towel around the base of the breast and secure tightly with a clamp to maintain appropriate tension for de-epithelialization.
  - Linear partial-thickness incisions through the epidermis with a scalpel can further assist with de-epithelialization with scissors.

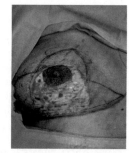

TECH FIG 1 • The Wise pattern has been incised and the inferior pedicle de-epithelialized.

Dissection

- The superior flaps are then developed up toward the breast base. The extent of dissection depends on the size of the breasts and the pedicle and is limited if possible. These are generally created approximately 1 in. thick to maintain upper pole fullness and to ensure vascularity to the overlying skin (**TECH FIG 2B**).
  - The nondominant hand is typically placed under the breast, and the parenchyma is grasped and rolled inferiorly over the hand to provide tension for dissection when an assistant is unavailable to retract.
- Once the superior flaps have been created, the dermoglandular pedicle is developed straight down to the chest wall. The pedicle should not be undermined in order to prevent nipple necrosis.
  - The "two finger" dissection technique is useful when developing the pedicle to provide tension. The nondominant index and long fingers are used to spread the parenchyma, and the tissue is divided with cautery.

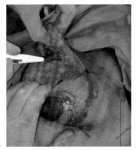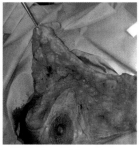

TECH FIG 2 • A,B. The superior flaps are elevated first. These are kept relatively thick to ensure enough superior pole fullness and to help prevent bottoming-out.

This allows the surgeon to retract for him or herself, which is the best way to ensure that the pedicle is not being undermined.
  - The pedicle is kept wider at the base to ensure optimal vascularity.

Resection

- The medial resection is then carried out. Care is taken initially to leave some breast tissue at the medial aspect of the excision to maintain medial fullness. This is examined after tailor tacking, and further resection can be carried out if required.
- The superior and lateral areas are then resected, and the entire specimen is handed off en bloc to be weighed (**TECH FIG 3**). The breast parenchyma is kept superiorly if possible to maintain upper pole fullness. However, we will typically over-resect the lateral aspect of the reduction due to the common presence of additional axillary tissue. This can be further treated with liposuction if necessary.
- The inferior corners of the vertical limbs are then brought down and secured at the breast meridian marking to form the inverted T, and the rest of the breast is tailor-tacked with staples to evaluate shape and symmetry. Additional resection can be performed at this time to achieve a satisfactory result.

- Often times, there remains excess skin that can be removed. This is often found at the vertical component but can also occur at the medial or lateral horizontal incision. Appropriate tailor tacking at this point in the procedure is important to identify these areas for further resection.

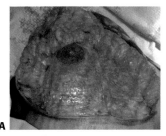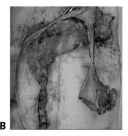

TECH FIG 3 • A. The inferior pedicle is demonstrated after medial and lateral resection has been carried out. **B.** The resected specimen is demonstrated. Note that the majority of resected tissue is from the lateral aspect of the breast.

Suturing

- Internal shaping sutures are not generally used in our practice but can be considered based upon surgeon preference.
- If the final NAC position was not previously marked and incised, this may now be done so. It is often helpful to sit the patient up to ensure that the NAC is symmetrically placed at the point of maximal projection on

the breast mound. This is often measured at 4 to 5 cm from the inframammary fold to the inferior aspect of the NAC.
  - A suture can be used in a pendulum fashion to ensure symmetric positioning of the nipple.
- Drains are not typically used in our reduction procedures but may be considered based on surgeon preference.

TECHNIQUES

- The inverted T junction is closed first with an external 3-0 monofilament suture in half-buried horizontal mattress fashion. The T junction at the NAC base is next closed in similar fashion, followed by the rest of the incisions. The incisions are closed with 3-0 monofilament suture in interrupted deep dermal fashion, followed by a running subcuticular stitch with 3-0 or 4-0 monofilament suture (**TECH FIG 4**). Mastisol and Steri-Strips are then placed over the incisions, and padding is placed over the breasts. A supportive surgical brassiere is placed in the operating room at the completion of the case.

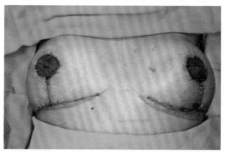

TECH FIG 4 • The final on-table result after closure and inset of the NAC. The inferior T junction is closed with an external half-buried horizontal mattress suture. In this case, the left side (oncologic side) was kept bigger in anticipation for radiation therapy.

PEARLS AND PITFALLS

Markings and incision	■ The preoperative markings are key to achieving a successful outcome in reduction mammaplasty. ■ Mark and incise the inframammary fold incision approximately 1 cm above the true IMF to avoid disrupting the fold. ■ The horizontal incision can be made as long or short as necessary to properly shape the breast.
Flaps and pedicle	■ One can choose whether to develop the superior flaps or pedicle first, but in our experience, it is easier to develop the flaps first and then to use the "two finger" technique to develop the pedicle. This technique for pedicle development can be utilized for other pedicle types as well. ■ The surgeon must be aware of the pedicle at all times when performing the resection. Avoiding undermining of the pedicle is critical to a safe procedure. ■ Developing thicker superior flaps will prevent flattening of the upper pole and further protect against bottoming out.
NAC	■ Leave a layer of breast parenchyma over the pectoralis fascia to avoid damaging the sensory nerves to the nipple. ■ The NAC should never be placed too high or too medial, because this creates an unnatural look and may be difficult to conceal in a bathing suit or brassiere. ■ The NAC should be observed for signs of ischemia or congestion prior to completion of the procedure. In rare circumstances, conversion to a free nipple graft can be performed for salvage if the NAC is felt to be nonviable.

POSTOPERATIVE CARE

- The vast majority of reduction mammoplasties in our practice are performed on an outpatient basis and are seen back in the office within 2 weeks for a routine postoperative appointment.
- The patient is kept in a supportive surgical bra or wireless sports bra at all times except when showering for the first 4 to 6 weeks. Once all of their incisions have healed, they are cleared to begin wearing a bra with underwiring.

OUTCOMES

- Satisfaction rates with reduction mammaplasty are among the highest in any area of plastic surgery, with approximately 95% of patients stating they would do it again if given the choice.[5,6] Several reports using validated questionnaires have determined reproducible improvement in both

physical and psychosocial symptoms postoperatively.[5,7] Furthermore, reduction surgery has been found to be a stimulus for further weight loss and blood glucose control in motivated patients.[8]

- The reoperation rates for reduction mammaplasty are approximately 8% to 9%.[9] Most of these cases are for scar revision, although some patients require revision for fat necrosis or other causes.
- Postoperative results are demonstrated in **FIGS 2** and **3**.

COMPLICATIONS

- The overall complication rate for reduction mammaplasty ranges widely from 5.1% to 45% in the literature.[6,9–11] Most complications are mild in nature and can be treated conservatively.
- Wound healing problems are the most common complication of Wise pattern reduction mammaplasty. This most

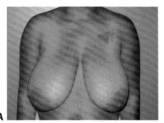 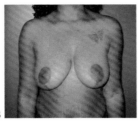

FIG 2 • **(A)** Preoperative and **(B)** postoperative result of a 27-year-old female who underwent inferior pedicle reduction mammaplasty. An inferior pedicle was chosen for easier inset. A superior or superomedial pedicle would have been fairly long and harder to appropriately reduce. Her nipple to notch measurements were 34.5 cm on the right and 34 cm on the left, while her nipple to IMF measurements were 16 on the right and 17 on the left. Final resection volumes were 1088 g on the right and 959 g on the left.

commonly occurs at the inferior T junction, and in almost all cases may be treated conservatively with Silvadene or moist wet to dry dressings with resolution.

- To avoid necrosis at the T junction, one must take care to avoid shearing the skin edges from the underlying breast tissue and excessive tension on the closure at this area.
- Bottoming out, which refers to the development of excess lower pole tissue and stretching over time, is a phenomena that can occur with inferior pedicle reductions. There have been several techniques presented to prevent this, but at the current time, we do not routinely perform any additional maneuvers to avoid this.
- Hematomas, fat necrosis, and infectious complications are relatively common following reduction mammaplasty. Most can be treated conservatively, but some patients will require surgical intervention.

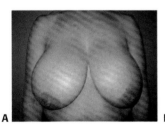 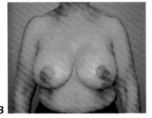

FIG 3 • **(A)** Preoperative and **(B)** postoperative result of a 54-year-old female who underwent inferior pedicle reduction mammaplasty. In this case, most of the breast volume was carried superiorly, and therefore, an inferior pedicle was chosen. Her nipple-to-notch measurements were 33 cm on the right and 32 cm on the left, while her nipple-to-IMF measurements were 16 cm bilaterally. Her final resection volumes were 801 g on the right and 706 g on the left.

- Nipple-areola complex sensation is often affected following reduction mammaplasty. The greatest degree of sensitivity change persists in the early preoperative period, but most patient have improved or normal sensation at 6 months postoperatively.[12] Theoretically, the inferior pedicle technique leaves more branches of the fourth intercostal nerve to the NAC intact, possibly providing some benefit when compared to other pedicle types.
- Nipple ischemia and necrosis is a rare but unfortunate complication of any reduction mammaplasty procedure. The overall risk of either partial or full necrosis is approximately 3.6%.[11] Partial-thickness loss can be treated conservatively with Silvadene and dressing changes, whereas full-thickness defects must often be debrided and primarily closed for optimal results. Depigmentation can occur after partial-thickness loss, especially in darker colored areolas.

REFERENCES

1. Rohrich RJ, Gosman AA, Brown SA, et al. Current preferences for breast reduction techniques: a survey of board-certified plastic surgeons 2002. *Plast Reconstr Surg.* 2004;114:1724-1733.
2. Courtiss EH, Goldwyn RM. Reduction mammaplasty by the inferior pedicle technique. An alternative to free nipple and areola grafting for severe macromastia or extreme ptosis. *Plast Reconstr Surg.* 1977;59:500-507.
3. Georgiade NG, Serafin D, Morris R, et al. Reduction mammaplasty utilizing an inferior pedicle nipple areolar flap. *Ann Plast Surg.* 1979;3:211-218.
4. Hunter J, Ceydeli A. Correlation between complication rate and tissue resection volume in inferior pedicle reduction mammaplasty: a retrospective study. *Aesthetic Surg J.* 2006;26:153-156.
5. Gonzalez M, Glickman L, Aladegbami B, Simpson R. Quality of life after breast reduction surgery: a 10-year retrospective analysis using the Breast Q Questionnaire: does breast size matter? *Ann Plast Surg.* 2012;69:361.
6. Dabbah A, Lehman JA, Parker MG, et al. Reduction mammaplasty: an outcome analysis. *Ann Plast Surg.* 1995;35:337-341.
7. Coriddi M, Nadeau M, Taghizadeh M, Taylor A. Analysis of satisfaction and well-being following breast reduction using a validated survey instrument: the BREAST-Q. *Plast Reconstr Surg.* 2013;132:285.
8. Singh K, Pinell X, Losken A. Is reduction mammaplasty a stimulus for weight loss and improved quality of life? *Ann Plast Surg.* 2010;64(5):585-587.
9. Manahan M, et al. An outcomes analysis of 2142 breast reduction procedures. *Ann Plast Surg.* 2015;74:289.
10. Fischer J, Cleveland E, Shang E, et al. Complications following reduction mammaplasty. *Aesthet Surg J.* 2014;34:66-73.
11. Cunningham B, Gear A, Kerrigan C, Collins E. Analysis of breast reduction complications derived from the BRAVO study. *Plast Reconstr Surg.* 2005;115:1597.
12. Hamdi M, Greuse M, Mey A, Webster M. A prospective quantitative comparison of breast sensation after superior and inferior pedicle mammaplasty. *Br J Plast Surg.* 2001;54:39-42.

9

CHAPTER

Breast Reduction With Free Nipple Graft

Paul A. Ghareeb and Albert Losken

DEFINITION

- Reduction mammaplasty is one of the most commonly performed operations in plastic surgery.
- Free nipple graft reduction was first reported by Thorek in 1922.[1]
- This technique is typically reserved for patients at high risk for nipple loss, in patients who wish to be smaller than what can be achieved by preserving the nipple on a pedicle, and in those who are at increased anesthetic risk.
- The nipple may be preserved with the areola as a composite graft or may be harvested by itself with subsequent tattooing of the areola.

ANATOMY

- Borders of the breast:
  - Superiorly: Clavicle
  - Medially: Sternum
  - Inferiorly: Superior border of rectus fascia
  - Laterally: Anterior border of latissimus
- Blood supply:
  - Intercostal perforators
  - Internal mammary perforators
  - Lateral thoracic artery
  - Thoracoacromial artery

PATIENT HISTORY AND PHYSICAL FINDINGS

- Focused history:
  - Current brassiere size and desired size after mammaplasty is important to determine with the patient preoperatively.
    - Free nipple graft reduction is a good option in patients who wish to be smaller than what can be achieved with a pedicled reduction.
  - Symptoms of macromastia and any interventions should be documented.
  - History of breast-feeding and the desire to have further children are important to discuss.
    - Patients undergoing free nipple graft reduction should be counseled about the inability to breast-feed postoperatively, as this may affect their decision to undergo this procedure until childbearing is complete.
  - Mammographic history if applicable, as well as family history of breast disease or cancer.
  - A history of smoking should be discussed prior to any reduction, and patients should be counseled to stop smoking at least 1 month prior to reduction mammaplasty due to the significantly increased risk of wound healing complications.

- Physical exam:
  - Examine the overall breast shape, asymmetries, previous scars, and estimate breast size in grams. Examine for breast masses and nipple sensation. Record breast measurements including sternal notch to nipple and nipple to inframammary fold distances.
  - Evaluate existing ptosis utilizing the Regnault classification.
  - Note any additional axillary tissue laterally that would not be resected with standard reduction mammaplasty. This area must be pointed out preoperatively so that patients understand where the limit of resection will be.

IMAGING

- Mammography is recommended for women who meet screening criteria.

SURGICAL MANAGEMENT

Preoperative Planning

- Patients who are good candidates for free nipple graft reduction include the following:
  - Patients who are at increased risk for nipple necrosis, including patients with gigantomastia (where greater than 2000 g of tissue per breast is expected to be resected)
  - Patients who would like to be smaller than what a pedicled reduction can provide
  - Patients with medical comorbidities who would not tolerate a longer operation, as the free graft technique is significantly shorter
  - Patients who are smokers or who have other comorbidities whereby breast amputation is safer than having undermined Wise pattern flaps
- Furthermore, any breast reduction where the NAC is felt to be nonviable may be converted to a free nipple graft.
- The surgical markings are performed in the preoperative holding area, with the patient standing and arms resting on each side.
- We typically utilize a Wise pattern skin excision pattern when performing a free nipple graft procedure for optimal shaping of the skin envelope (**FIG 1**). Our technique for marking is described in detail in the Inferior Pedicle chapter.

Positioning

- The patient is placed supine on the operating room table, with arms extended on arm boards and secured with soft roll. It is important not to extend the arms too far, as this may distort the breast shape.
- The patient is positioned at the break of the bed, so that she may be placed in the upright position if necessary.

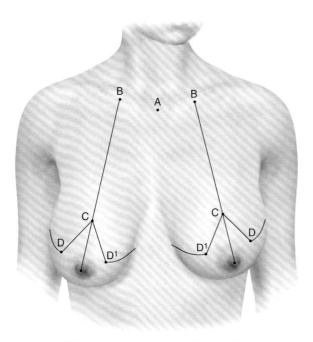

FIG 1 • Wise pattern skin excision markings.

Approach

- The method of nipple graft to be performed is determined by the patient's skin color and quality, scarring, and desires.
  - We feel that tattooing of the areola oftentimes produces superior results as compared with the free nipple-areolar graft, especially in patients with darker skin who are at risk for depigmentation. However, in patients who do not wish to undergo future tattooing, the areola should be grafted.
- If the entire nipple-areolar complex is to be grafted, the nipple is marked with a cookie cutter at approximately 40 to 44 mm.
- If the nipple is to be harvested with subsequent tattooing of the areola, then the nipple base is marked.
- The standard Wise pattern markings are re-marked, with the inframammary fold incision marked at 1 cm above the actual fold. This is to preserve the dense attachments present in this area.
- The resection pattern is based on breast amputation techniques, with the majority of the reduction specimen taken out as a wedge at the inferior pole of the breast.
  - Many other techniques have been described for resection of breast tissue, including the creation of dermoglandular flaps to provide improved projection. However, we feel that with a conservative resection and preservation of superior and central breast tissue with minimal undermining, adequate shape can be created.

- If the initial surgical plan is to perform a free nipple graft, then the nipple is harvested first (**TECH FIG 1A**).
- After the nipple is harvested, the inferior breast tissue is resected in a wedge-shaped pattern, making sure to preserve enough tissue superiorly to maintain adequate breast projection.
  - The Wise pattern markings are incised sharply.
  - The resection is typically started at the superior aspect of the breast.
  - At first, minimal tissue is resected from the vertical component of the Wise pattern. This is maintained to ensure adequate projection and can always be resected later if necessary.
  - Once the horizontal component of the Wise pattern is reached, the dissection is aimed inferiorly toward the fold and carried down to the chest wall (**TECH FIG 1B**).
    - It is easy to over-resect with this technique. It is important to aim caudally when performing the initial resection and not to undermine the superior breast flaps. More tissue can always be resected if necessary after the initial specimen is removed.
- After the resection has been carried out, the remaining inferior breast tissue is tucked superiorly and the breast is tailor-tacked and examined for shape and symmetry.
- If required, additional tissue may be resected prior to closure. Oftentimes, excess fullness remains laterally and should be excised.
- If the skin envelope is felt to be too loose, additional skin can be resected from the vertical components. By excising more lateral vertical skin, the lateral aspect of the breast can be advanced medially to provide a more defined lateral breast border.
  - Once adequate shape has been obtained, the incisions are closed with a 3-0 monofilament absorbable suture in deep dermal fashion, followed by a running subcuticular stitch.

- Drains are not typically used in our practice.
- Another option is to attempt an inferior or central mound and if it seems as though the pedicle is too long or the nipple appears congested or poorly perfused, it can be converted to a shorter glandular mound and free nipple or nipple areolar graft.
  - It is important not to commit to a keyhole reduction pattern if a graft is anticipated.
- Free nipple and areolar grafting
  - The NAC is incised sharply with a knife and harvested as a full-thickness graft.
  - Once the breast has been reduced and all incisions have been closed, the point of maximal projection is marked with the cookie cutter at 40 to 44 mm. This area is then de-epithelialized.
  - After adequate thinning with a scissor on the back table, the graft is then secured to the recipient bed with a 4-0 or 5-0 absorbable suture (**TECH FIG 1C**).
  - A xeroform and cotton-ball tie-over bolster is then used to secure the graft.
- Free nipple grafting
  - The nipple is transected at the base sharply with a knife.
  - After the reduction is complete, the point of maximal projection is marked.
  - Two small rectangular flaps are lifted in a horizontal fashion to provide for increased contact between the nipple and recipient bed (**TECH FIG D–F**).
  - The nipple graft is then placed between the flaps and is secured at the base.
  - The edges of the nipple are trimmed, and the flaps are sutured to the nipple edges with a 5-0 absorbable suture to allow for maximal graft survival.
  - A Telfa nonstick dressing is applied to the nipple and secured with Steri-Strips to act as a bolster.

TECHNIQUES

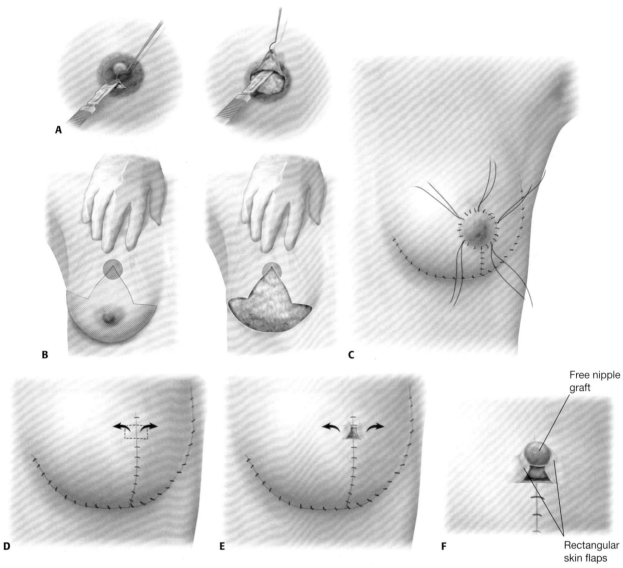

TECH FIG 1 • **A.** The nipple-areola complex is sharply removed with a no. 10 blade. It is then thinned on the back table to an appropriate depth for grafting. **B.** (*Left*) The proposed area of breast tissue to be excised is marked. (*Right*) The tissue is removed, making sure to leave enough tissue superiorly and centrally with minimal undermining. **C.** The nipple is inset with a 5-0 absorbable suture after final closure is achieved. A Xeroform tie-over bolster is utilized to maintain graft position for 1 to 2 weeks. **D.** After closure of the reduction incisions, two small rectangular flaps are designed to allow placement of the nipple graft. **E.** Elevation of the rectangular flaps. **F.** Insetting of the nipple graft within the rectangular flaps to allow for maximal nipple graft revascularization and take.

PEARLS AND PITFALLS

Skin excision	▪ Wise pattern skin excision pattern is well suited for free nipple graft reduction.
Nipple graft technique	▪ The nipple can be grafted alone, or the nipple-areolar complex can be grafted as a unit. ▪ Often grafting the nipple alone with subsequent tattooing is optimal but involves an additional step and cost.
Do not over-resect	▪ It is easy to over-resect tissue. Be sure to leave enough tissue behind to adequately shape the breast.
Bolstering	▪ The bolster should be left in place for 1 to 2 weeks to maximize graft take.
Improving projection	▪ An inferior dermoglandular flap can be created if needed to augment projection.

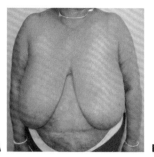 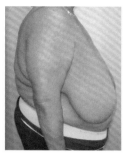 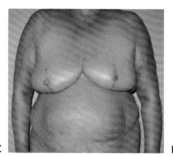 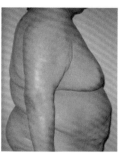

FIG 2 • **A,B.** Preoperative photos of a 54-year-old female presenting with gigantomastia. Her nipple-to-notch measurements were 51 cm on the right and 50 cm on the left. Her nipple-to-fold measurement was 20 cm bilaterally. **C,D.** Postoperative results after free nipple-only reduction with a Wise pattern skin excision, before ultimate tattooing of the areola. The resection specimens weighed 2102 g on the left and 2126 g on the right.

POSTOPERATIVE CARE

- The vast majority of reduction mammoplasties in our practice are performed on an outpatient basis. Patients undergoing free nipple graft reduction are instructed to maintain the bolster dressing until their follow-up appointment. This is removed in the office approximately 10 to 14 days postoperatively, and the graft is assessed. A protective dressing is then kept on for an additional 2 weeks.
- The patient is kept in a supportive surgical brassiere or wireless sports brassiere at all times except when showering for the first 4 to 6 weeks. Once the incisions have healed, she is cleared to begin wearing a brassiere with underwiring.

OUTCOMES

- Pre- and postoperative photos of free nipple graft reductions are shown in **FIGS 2** and **3**.
- Reduction mammaplasty is one of the most satisfying procedures performed by plastic surgeons, with approximately 95% of patients willing to undergo the procedure again when surveyed.[2,3]
- Reoperation rates for reduction mammaplasty are around 8% to 9%. Most of these are for scar revisions, although rarely they may include other causes.[4]
- Nipple sensitivity and erectile function may be preserved to some degree, but in certain situations may be lost completely.[5]

- With the free nipple graft technique, the ability to breast-feed is lost. Patients must be counseled on this prior to the operation.

COMPLICATIONS

- Overall complication rates following breast reduction vary widely in the literature, from 5.1% to 45%.[6-8] Most of these complications are minor and may be treated conservatively.
- Complications following free nipple breast reduction are likely less common than other techniques, because the length of the procedure is often shorter and there is minimal undermining and repositioning of breast tissue.
- Wound healing complications are often lower in free nipple reductions, owing to decreased undermining.[9] This is most often treated with local wound care, but in some cases debridement and closure or skin grafting may be necessary.
- Partial or full graft loss is extremely uncommon in our practice but can occur. Severe cases may be treated with debridement and delayed nipple reconstruction.
- Hypopigmentation may occur and is more troublesome in patients with darker skin (**FIG 4**). Patients should be counseled on this prior to surgery, and free nipple-only grafts with subsequent tattooing should be considered in these patients.
- When free nipple-areolar grafts undergo hypopigmentation, it is difficult to correct this with tattooing.

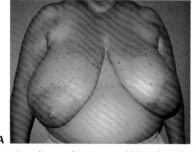 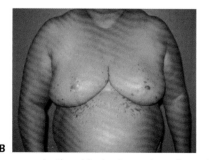

FIG 3 • **A,B.** Pre- and postoperative photos of a 61-year-old female with gigantomastia. She wished to be much smaller and did not have a preference for nipple sensibility or function. Her nipple-to-notch measurements were 42 cm on the right and 41 cm on the left. Her nipple-to-fold measurements were 23 cm on the right and 20 cm on the left. She underwent a free nipple-only reduction with a Wise pattern skin excision. The total amount of tissue excised was 2300 g on the right and 1900 g on the left.

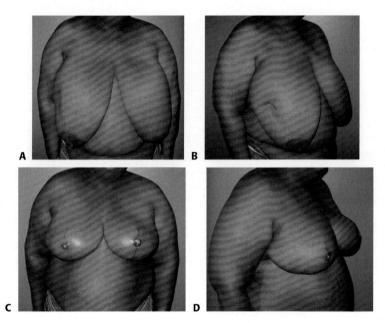

FIG 4 • A,B. Preoperative photos of a 29-year-old female with a right breast scar. Her nipple-to-notch measurements were 47 cm on the right and 50 cm on the right. Her nipple-to-IMF distances were 26 cm on the right and 20 cm on the left. **C,D.** Postoperative photos after bilateral free nipple reduction using a Wise pattern skin excision, before areolar tattooing. The amount of tissue resected was 2350 g on the right and 2250 g on the left. She developed some hypopigmentation of the grafts bilaterally.

REFERENCES

1. Thorek M. Possibilities in the reconstruction of the human. *NY Med J.* 1922;116:572-575.
2. Gonzalez M, Glickman L, Aladegbami B, Simpson R. Quality of life after breast reduction surgery: a 10-year retrospective analysis using the breast Q questionnaire: does breast size matter? *Ann Plast Surg.* 2012;69:361.
3. Dabbah A, Lehman JA, Parker MG, et al. Reduction mammaplasty: an outcome analysis. *Ann Plast Surg.* 1995;35:337-341
4. Manahan M, et al. An outcomes analysis of 2142 breast reduction procedures. *Ann Plast Surg.* 2015;74:289.
5. Ahmed O, Kolhe P. Comparison of nipple and areolar sensation after breast reduction by free nipple graft and inferior pedicle techniques. *Br J Plast Surg.* 2000;53:126-129.
6. Fischer J, Cleveland E, Shang E, et al. Complications following reduction mammaplasty. *Aesthet Surg J.* 2014;34:66-73.
7. Manahan M. et al. An outcomes analysis of 2142 breast reduction procedures. *Ann Plast Surg.* 2015;74:289.
8. Cunningham B, Gear A, Kerrigan C, Collins E. Analysis of breast reduction complications derived from the BRAVO study. *Plast Reconstr Surg.* 2005;115:1597.
9. Hawtof DB, Levine M, Kapetansky DI, Peiper D. Complications of reduction mammaplasty: comparison of nipple-areolar graft and pedicle. *Ann Plast Surg.* 1989;23:3-10.

Gynecomastia

10

John T. Stranix and Alexes Hazen

DEFINITION

- Gynecomastia refers to benign, excessive enlargement of parenchymal tissue in the male breast. The etiology of gynecomastia is multifactorial, often idiopathic, and affects up to 40% to 50% of men.[1]

ANATOMY

- In gynecomastia, the excess glandular tissue is typically centered under the nipple-areola complex (NAC), with a predominantly fibrous component (**FIG 1**).
  - Pseudogynecomastia refers to diffuse fatty enlargement of the male breast related to obesity and demonstrates a predominance of adipose vs fibrous tissue.
- Normal male breasts are flat in appearance with mild fullness around the NAC.
- The male NAC diameter is normally 2 to 4 cm (mean 2.8 cm) and centered on the midclavicular line over the fourth intercostal space. Mean sternal notch to nipple distance is 20 cm.
- The pectoralis muscle provides superior fullness to the anterior male chest that transitions inferiorly to flat tissue over the lower chest at the level of the inframammary fold (IMF).
  - A well-defined IMF results in a more feminine breast appearance.

PATHOGENESIS

- Benign proliferation of male breast parenchyma occurs due to a relative increase in the ratio of free estrogen to androgen locally in the breast.[2]
- Physiologic gynecomastia occurs in newborns (circulating maternal estrogens), adolescents (excess plasma estradiol during early stages of puberty), and men after age 65 (decreased testosterone production).
  - Neonatal and pubertal gynecomastia are typically self-limiting and usually resolve over several months to years.
- Pathologic gynecomastia can result from various metabolic (cirrhosis, renal failure), endocrine (hypogonadal state, hyperthyroidism), oncologic (adrenal or testicular tumors), or congenital (Klinefelter syndrome) disorders.
- Pharmacologic gynecomastia has been linked to a number of medications and occurs by several known mechanisms; however, direct mechanisms have not been identified for all associated medications.[3]
- Gynecomastia does not increase the risk of male breast cancer development compared to the normal male population.
  - Patients with Klinefelter syndrome, however, have up to a 50 times increased risk of developing breast cancer.[4] Due to the elevated oncologic risk in this population, an excisional technique should be used to provide a specimen for pathology analysis.

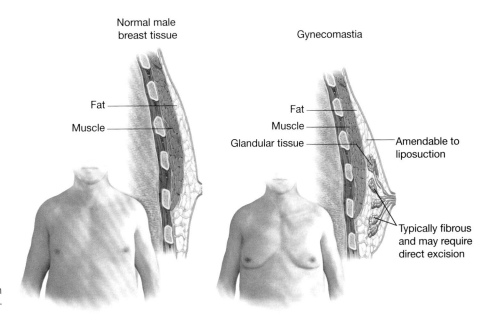

Normal male breast tissue

Gynecomastia

Fat
Muscle

Fat
Muscle
Glandular tissue

Amendable to liposuction

Typically fibrous and may require direct excision

FIG 1 • Cross-sectional depiction of normal male chest anatomy compared to gynecomastia.

PATIENT HISTORY AND PHYSICAL FINDINGS

- Clinical evaluation of enlarged male breasts begins with a detailed history and review of symptoms, focusing on elucidating known causes of gynecomastia and differentiation from pseudogynecomastia and tumor.
  - History should include age, onset and duration of enlargement, breast symptoms (pain, tenderness, discharge), medications, alcohol or recreational drug use, and social/psychological effects of breast enlargement. Past medical, surgical, family, and reproductive history should also be obtained.
  - Signs/symptoms of liver disease, malnutrition, kidney failure, hyper- or hypothyroidism, weight changes, adrenal disease, and malignancy.
- Physical examination
  - Breasts should be assessed for symmetry, nipple abnormalities, glandular or fat predominance, skin excess, degree of ptosis, and nodules or masses. Approximately 50% of gynecomastia is bilateral.[1] Axillary and supraclavicular lymph node basins should be examined in the setting of a suspicious mass.
  - Glandular tissue in gynecomastia is characterized by mobile, rubbery subareolar breast tissue.
  - Masses or nodules with abnormal firmness, overlying skin changes, eccentric location, or associated nipple discharge should raise concern for breast carcinoma.
  - Secondary sexual characteristics should be examined: body hair distribution, muscle mass, penile development, and testicular size, consistency, and symmetry.
  - Signs of systemic disease should also be evaluated: thyromegaly, exophthalmos, hepato- or splenomegaly, abdominal masses, ascites or cirrhotic stigmata, visual fields, cranial nerves, and fundoscopy.

IMAGING AND OTHER DIAGNOSTIC STUDIES

- Laboratory or radiographic studies are not necessary in most cases of gynecomastia.
- Mammography, and possibly biopsy, is indicated if findings on physical examination are consistent with a breast neoplasm.
- Testicular ultrasound should be obtained in the setting of prepubertal bilateral gynecomastia, evidence of under-virilization, and/or a testicular mass.[5] Endocrine labs are also appropriate in this situation; consider karyotype if Klinefelter syndrome is possible.
- Laboratory testing should be directed by abnormalities identified on history and physical exam.

DIFFERENTIAL DIAGNOSIS

- Physiologic
- Drug-induced
- Hypogonadism
- Tumors
- Systemic
- Congenital
- Familial
- Miscellaneous
- Idiopathic

NONOPERATIVE MANAGEMENT

- The majority of patients with new-onset gynecomastia are best managed with reassurance and observation for 12 to 18 months.[1,6]

- No detectable abnormality is found in up to 60% of patients on initial evaluation.[5]
- Correction of underlying causes should be performed: discontinue offending medications, correct hormonal imbalances, address metabolic or endocrine disorders.
- Medical therapy with testosterone and aromatase inhibitors has had limited success. Treatment with tamoxifen, however, has been shown to result in gynecomastia regression in recent randomized trials.[1]

SURGICAL MANAGEMENT

- Surgical intervention should be considered for patients with a diagnosis of symptomatic gynecomastia of duration greater than 12 months.
  - Due to irreversible fibrosis of hypertrophic breast tissue that develops 6 to 12 months after the onset of gynecomastia, medical treatments beyond that stage are unlikely to result in significant regression.[1,7]
- Surgical treatment of gynecomastia has evolved to become increasingly less invasive through the use of liposuction and endoscopy; however, more severe cases often require open techniques with a higher scar burden.
- Multiple classification systems have been developed to guide surgical management. The system devised by Rohrich et al.[7] classified gynecomastia based on breast size and degree of ptosis.

Preoperative Planning

- In addition to standard components of informed consent, the preoperative consultation must include a discussion of scar burden/location, possible need for direct excision of residual subareolar fibrous tissue, as well as the potential for undercorrection requiring a second-stage procedure.
  - Even patients with only mild gynecomastia may have a residual fibrous component that is not amenable to liposuction and requires excision.
- Preoperative markings are performed with the patients in the upright sitting or standing position.
- Prophylactic antibiotics covering skin flora are administered prior to skin incision.

Positioning

- Surgery is performed under general anesthesia as an outpatient procedure.
- Patients are positioned supine with arms abducted and secured to padded, adjustable arm boards. The hips are centered over the bed break, and the patient is secured with a safety strap.
  - Intraoperative assessment of adequate/symmetric resection requires sitting the patients fully upright in the operating room and they should be secured in a manner that enables this to be safely accomplished.
- Sequential compression devices are applied to the lower extremities.
- The entire anterior chest is prepped into the field to allow intraoperative symmetry assessment. Chest hair is removed with electric clippers as needed.

Approach

- Patients with mild to moderate glandular hypertrophy (grades I and II) rarely have significant skin excess. Definitive treatment with suction-assisted lipectomy, power-assisted liposuction (PAL), and/or ultrasound-assisted liposuction (UAL) is frequently possible; direct excision of residual subareolar fibrous tissue may be required.[7,8]

- UAL is often associated with improved skin retraction, making it a more effective treatment modality for gynecomastia than conventional liposuction alone.[9]
- PAL has been shown to reduce operative fatigue and improve control in chest wall contouring.[10]

- Patients with more severe gynecomastia and/or ptosis (grades III and IV) typically require resection of excess skin and possibly NAC repositioning.
  - Our preference is to perform redundant skin excision along the IMF.
  - In extreme cases, breast amputation with free nipple grafting may be necessary.

■ Ultrasound-Assisted Liposuction

Markings

- With the patient standing, the IMF, breast boundaries, and planned incision sites along the lateral IMF are marked.
- Concentric topographic marks centered over the most prominent area of the breast may also be drawn to assist with liposuction.
- An inferior semicircular periareolar incision may be included if direct excision is anticipated.

Liposuction

- Use a no. 11 blade to make bilateral breast stab incisions along the lateral IMF.
  - Additional stab incisions (periareolar, upper anterior axilla) may improve cross-hatching and undermining/disruption of the IMF.
- Systematically infiltrate all treatment areas in multiple layers with wetting solution using a 3.0-mm cannula with a 1:1 ratio of infiltrate to estimated aspirate (superwet technique).
  - Wetting solution consists of 1 L of lactated Ringer solution containing 1 cc of 1:1000 epinephrine and 30 cc of 1% lidocaine.
- Perform UAL on a high energy level using a 3.0- to 5.0-mm cannula connected to a standard surgical aspirator. Unlike traditional liposuction, the intermediate and immediate subdermal adipose layers are targeted to achieve maximal skin retraction using a careful bimanual technique with constant and deliberate passes in a radial fashion (**TECH FIG 1**). Routine skin protection measures should be used to prevent thermal injury.
  - Concentrate additional passes through the dense fibrous tissue in the subareolar region; consider increasing the energy level if needed for greater effect in this area.
  - Completely undermine and disrupt the IMF to achieve a smooth transition from the breast to the upper abdomen.
  - Use extreme caution when suctioning the adherent zone over the superolateral pectoralis muscle (only minimally for contouring if necessary).
  - Primary treatment end points are loss of tissue resistance or blood in the aspirate.
- Convert to standard liposuction or PAL using a 3.0- to 5.0-mm cannula to evacuate residual emulsified fat in the deep and intermediate layers in performing final contouring.

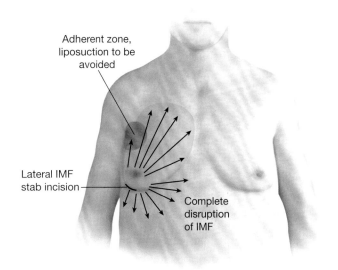

TECH FIG 1 • Depiction of liposuction technique. Lateral IMF access incision and *black arrows* depict passes of the cannula. The area to be liposuctioned is shown in *blue*. The superolateral adherent zone over the pectoralis major is shown as a *red circle* that should be avoided by the cannula. Inferiorly, the cannula is used to disrupt the IMF and allow for a smooth contour onto the upper abdomen.

Removal of Persistent Tissue

- Often dense subareolar tissue persists despite target liposuction (not uncommon even in mild gynecomastia), requiring morcellation or direct excision.
- Arthroscopic shaver morcellation, using a standard orthopedic arthroscopic system connected to an endoscopic shaver cannula with a rotating dentated cutting tip.[11]
  - The arthroscopic shaver cannula is inserted through the lateral IMF stab incision with the dentated opening on the tip directed away from the skin.
  - With the cannula oscillation speed set between 4000 and 6000 rpm, the shaver is repeatedly passed through the residual subareolar fibrous tissue until the desired result is achieved.
- Direct excision through an inferior semicircular periareolar incision (**TECH FIG 2**).
  - An inferior periareolar incision is made with a no. 15 blade that can be extended to encompass the entire inferior half of the areola if necessary.
  - Cautery is used to circumferentially dissect out the readily palpable firm glandular tissue. Roughly 1 cm of immediately subareolar glandular tissue should be left to avoid a depression or saucer deformity.

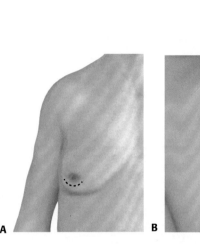
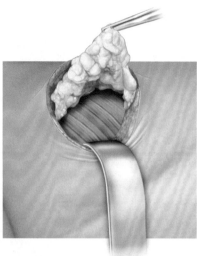

TECH FIG 2 • A. Location of periareolar incision for direct excision of glandular tissue. **B.** Dense fibrous tissue not amenable to liposuction is excised directly.

■ Redundant Skin Excision

Markings

- With the patient standing, the IMF, midclavicular line, and breast boundaries are marked.
- A horizontal ellipse is drawn with its inferior aspect, following the IMF.
- The superior line of the ellipse is drawn to mark the area of planned skin excision based on the amount of skin laxity.
- Following completion of parenchymal liposuction, the patient should be positioned sitting upright on the operating table to assess the breast skin envelope and degree of excess/ptosis.
- Mark the IMFs bilaterally again. This will serve as the inferior border of the ellipse for skin excision.

- Along the length of the IMF, use the pinch test to determine the width of the ellipse needed to remove the excess skin and close under minimal tension. Mark the superior border of the ellipse to be excised accordingly.

Excision and Completion

- Incise the marked ellipse through the dermis and remove the excess skin using cautery in a subcutaneous plane.
  - This exposure provides an excellent opportunity to confirm complete disruption of the IMF as well. Any residual bands or attachments should be divided with cautery.
- After hemostasis is obtained, place a closed suction drain with a remote egress laterally.
- Reapproximate skin with resorbable buried deep dermal sutures and a running subcuticular stitch.

■ Breast Amputation With Free Nipple Grafting

Markings

- With the patient standing, the IMF, midclavicular line, and sternal notch are marked.
- Similar to the excess skin excision pattern described, a horizontal ellipse is drawn with its inferior aspect following the length of the IMF.
- Because of the severe ptosis requiring mastectomy, the superior line of the ellipse is drawn to mark the area of planned skin excision based on the amount of skin laxity and includes the NAC (**TECH FIG 3**).

Tissue Excision

- Infiltrate the breast parenchyma and planned incisions (**TECH FIG 4A**) with a dilute solution of 0.5% lidocaine with 1:200 000 epinephrine.
- Outline the NAC and excise it as a full-thickness graft. Debride any fat from the underside of the graft and store it in saline-soaked gauze.

- Incise the superior aspect of the ellipse through dermis using a no. 15 blade.
- Elevate the superior breast skin and subcutaneous tissue in the superficial fascial plane similar to a mastectomy flap, using cautery, knife, or scissors as preferred (**TECH FIG 4B**).

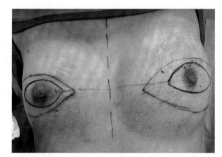

TECH FIG 3 • Grade III gynecomastia with preoperative markings for mastectomy with free nipple grafting. Inner ellipse excised to make defatting the free nipple graft easier, and the planned skin excision (*outer ellipses*) is resected parallel to IMF and estimated by pinch test.

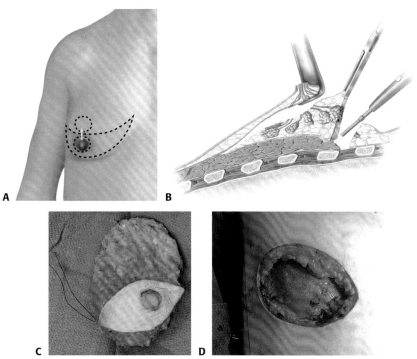

TECH FIG 4 • **A.** Planned incisions for subcutaneous mastectomy with free nipple grafting. The subcutaneous tissue shown in *green* is excised. The scar is placed along the level of the IMF. **B.** The breast tissue is elevated off the pectoralis fascia. **C.** Mastectomy specimen with short stitch marking superior and long stitch lateral. Notice how far superiorly the glandular resection extends. **D.** Resulting defect after mastectomy, which is closed in layers.

- Once the superior aspect of the breast tissue is reached, it is elevated off the pectoralis fascia from superior to inferior until reaching the level of the IMF and the inferior aspect of the ellipse.
- Ensure that the superior and inferior skin flaps of the ellipse will close without tension, and then incise the inferior aspect of the ellipse and remove the breast tissue (**TECH FIG 4C,D**).
- Confirm hemostasis and close the new IMF incision primarily in layers.
- Repeat the same procedure on the contralateral side.

Nipple Grafting

- Draw the new NAC position as a 3-cm-wide oval centered in the midclavicular line over the fourth intercostal space.

- Once satisfied with nipple position and symmetry, de-epithelialize the 3-cm ovals.
- Trim the free nipple grafts to fit with the nipples centered on the oval and secure using 4-0 chromic suture on a taper needle (**TECH FIG 5A**).
- Apply bolster dressings of cotton soaked with mineral oil and wrapped in Xeroform gauze. Secure these with silk sutures over bilateral NACs (**TECH FIG 5B**).
  - These bolsters remain in place for 5 to 7 days postoperatively.

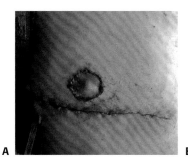
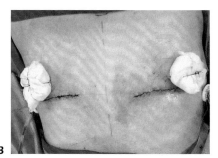

TECH FIG 5 • **A.** Free nipple grafts are inset over de-epithelialized area above the IMF incision. **B.** Bolsters applied to free nipple grafts for 5 to 7 days.

PEARLS AND PITFALLS

Subglandular excision	■ Consider excising residual subareolar fibrous tissue at the time of UAL using either the arthroscopic shaver or direct excision technique. ■ Maintain 1 cm of subcutaneous tissue under NAC to avoid a saucer deformity.
Liposuction technique	■ Focus UAL on the subdermal adipose tissue to achieve maximal skin retraction. ■ Avoid suctioning the adherent area over the superolateral pectoralis muscle. ■ Completely undermine/disrupt the IMF to create a smooth inferior chest transition.
Intraoperative assessment	■ In order to adequately evaluate the surgical result, sit the patient upright on the operating table following resection to ensure satisfactory contour and symmetry.
Revisions	■ Wait more than 6 months for maximal skin retraction prior to performing resection of residual excess skin/tissue.
Duration of gynecomastia	■ Gynecomastia present for more than 12 months is unlikely to resolve spontaneously due to parenchymal fibrosis and typically requires surgical intervention.
Postoperative care	■ Chest compression dressings should be worn continuously for 2 weeks postoperatively.

POSTOPERATIVE CARE

■ Except in rare instances of extremely large resections, these cases are performed as ambulatory procedures with patients going home the same day.

■ Patients are instructed to wear a chest compression garment or Ace wrap for 2 weeks postoperatively. This maintains pressure on the chest to minimize hematoma and seroma formation.

■ Closed suction drains are placed only for procedures that include more than liposuction. These are typically removed at the first postoperative visit.

■ Postoperative follow-up visits are scheduled at 1 week, 4 weeks, and 4 to 6 months.

■ Patients who underwent UAL-only resection should be re-evaluated around 6 months to allow time for skin retraction before determining the need for revision with excision of excess skin and residual parenchymal tissue.[7,8]

OUTCOMES

■ Gynecomastia reduction surgery outcomes show high overall patient satisfaction rates. Overall complication rates range from 14.5% to 53% with hematoma being the most common.[12–14] Hematoma rates appear higher in open subcutaneous mastectomies (11%–16%), compared to cases treated with liposuction alone (1%).[9,12–14] Inadequate resection with the need for revision is the most common long-term complication.[7,8]

COMPLICATIONS

■ Hematoma
■ Seroma
■ Infection
■ Inadequate resection
■ Poor scarring
■ Contour deformity/asymmetry
■ Sensory changes

ACKNOWLEDGMENT

The authors thank our research coordinator, Grace Poudrier, for her significant contribution to this chapter. We sincerely appreciate her hard work and dedication.

REFERENCES

1. Braunstein GD. Clinical practice. Gynecomastia. *N Engl J Med.* 2007;357:1229-1237.
2. Mathur R, Braunstein GD. Gynecomastia: pathomechanisms and treatment strategies. *Horm Res.* 1997;48:95-102.
3. Deepinder F, Braunstein GD. Drug-induced gynecomastia: an evidence-based review. *Expert Opin Drug Saf.* 2012;11:779-795.
4. Hultborn R, Hanson C, Kopf I, et al. Prevalence of Klinefelter's syndrome in male breast cancer patients. *Anticancer Res.* 1997;17:4293-4297.
5. Bowers SP, Pearlman NW, McIntyre RC Jr, et al. Cost-effective management of gynecomastia. *Am J Surg.* 1998;176:638-641.
6. Johnson RE, Murad MH. Gynecomastia: pathophysiology, evaluation, and management. *Mayo Clin Proc.* 2009;84:1010-1015.
7. Rohrich RJ, Ha RY, Kenkel JM, Adams WP Jr. Classification and management of gynecomastia: defining the role of ultrasound-assisted liposuction. *Plast Reconstr Surg.* 2003;111:909-923.
8. Brown RH, Chang DK, Siy R, Friedman J. Trends in the surgical correction of gynecomastia. *Semin Plast Surg.* 2015;29:122-130.
9. Wong KY, Malata CM. Conventional versus ultrasound-assisted liposuction in gynaecomastia surgery: a 13-year review. *J Plast Reconstr Aesthet Surg.* 2014;67:921-926.
10. Lista F, Ahmad J. Power-assisted liposuction and the pull-through technique for the treatment of gynecomastia. *Plast Reconstr Surg.* 2008;121:740-747.
11. Prado AC, Castillo PF. Minimal surgical access to treat gynecomastia with the use of a power-assisted arthroscopic-endoscopic cartilage shaver. *Plast Reconstr Surg.* 2005;115:939-942.
12. Colombo-Benkmann M, Buse B, Stern J, Herfarth C. Indications for and results of surgical therapy for male gynecomastia. *Am J Surg.* 1999;178:60-63.
13. Li CC, Fu JP, Chang SC, et al. Surgical treatment of gynecomastia: complications and outcomes. *Ann Plast Surg.* 2012;69:510-515.
14. Petty PM, Solomon M, Buchel EW, Tran NV. Gynecomastia: evolving paradigm of management and comparison of techniques. *Plast Reconstr Surg.* 2010;125:1301-1308.

Section IV: Breast Reconstruction for Partial Mastectomy Defects
Partial Breast Reconstruction With Local Tissue Rearrangement

Moustapha Hamdi

DEFINITION

- The treatment of breast cancer is an evolving field. Different modalities are continuously being developed to maximize patient survival while minimizing the treatment's morbidity.[1-5]
- Currently, the two main options for the management of primary breast cancer are total mastectomy and lumpectomy/quadrantectomy with radiation.[1-5]
- Studies have shown that women diagnosed at early stages of invasive breast cancer have equivalent outcomes when they are treated with lumpectomy and radiation therapy or modified radical mastectomy.[2-5]
- Oncoplastic surgery is a combination of breast conservative surgery and an immediate partial breast reconstruction.[6]
- This chapter reviews partial breast reconstruction after partial mastectomy.

ANATOMY[7]

The Blood Supply

- The blood supply of the breast is a rich anastomotic network derived from the axillary, internal thoracic (internal mammary), and two intercostal arteries.
- Multiple factors can influence how robust each of these sources of inflow may be (age, endocrine activity, overall health, systemic diseases, eg, diabetes/atherosclerosis, smoking, radiotherapy).
- The major inflow sources, from medial to lateral, are the internal mammary segmental perforators, the intercostal perforators, the thoracoacromial perforators, and the external mammary artery.
- The anteromedial and anterolateral intercostal perforators are major contributors to the vascularization of the nipple-areola complex (NAC).
- The venous drainage is a dual system: a superficial subdermal plexus, which eventually meets up in the deep system, and a deep system, which accompanies the mentioned arterial system.

The Nerve Supply

- The medial and central breast sensations come from the second through the sixth anteromedial intercostal nerves.
- The nipple-areola sensation is contributed by the third, fourth, and fifth anteromedial and anterolateral intercostal nerves.
- Careful consideration of the nerve supply helps to maximize nipple sensation. When pedicled flaps (see Chapter 22) are passed into partial mastectomy defects, the tunnel should be created high enough to avoid lateral denervation to the breast.

PATIENT HISTORY AND PHYSICAL FINDINGS

- Breast and plastic surgeons must have a thorough understanding of breast anatomy, physiology, and the qualities of an aesthetically pleasing breast shape.
- Surgeons performing the oncoplastic approach should consider the aesthetic subunits when planning cosmetic quadrectomies, resections, and reconstructions.
- Also, knowledge of the anatomical landmarks, breast proportions, and shape is essential to achieve a pleasing outcome.
- Preoperative evaluation of the patient and her breasts must be standard and detailed.
- The examination must include the following:
  - Evaluation of breast skin, elasticity, thickness, scars, and any defining marks such as tattoos, stretch marks, contour irregularities, and previous breast surgery should be taken into account when planning breast-conserving therapy (BCT).
  - Palpation for masses or abnormalities in the breast parenchyma, nipple inspection, and detailed documentation of breast sensation are integral.
  - Breast shape, grade of ptosis, and size are determinants of success in surgical treatment.
- The base and width of the breast, the width of the NAC, the height of the nipple, and the distance from the sternal notch, midline and inframammary crease, must be recorded in detail.
- Any natural breast asymmetry should be pointed out to the patient before surgery.
- Different body types, skin laxity, and fat distribution are important factors in the decision-making process.

SURGICAL MANAGEMENT

Oncological Approach

- Indications: Most early-stage cancers (T1 and T2 cancers with or without nodal involvement) are indicated for BCT.[6,8]
- Contraindications: Patients with a high probability for recurrence, especially those with multicentric disease, those who are pregnant or have collagen vascular disease, or those who have a history of prior radiation therapy.[6,8]

- Relative contraindications include the following:
  - Patients with a high probability of subsequent cancers (BRCA mutations)
  - Patients who are likely to have a poor cosmetic result, which includes patients with a high tumor/breast ratio
  - Medially and inferiorly based tumors
  - Tumors that require removal of the NAC

Clinical Approach

- The success of this procedure depends on the size of the cancer, the anatomical position, and the volume of resection needed to achieve clear margins in relation to the volume of the breast.
- The choice of the technique used depends on many factors, including the extent of resection, the time of surgery, the breast size and tumor location, and patient preferences.
- Preoperatively, incision lines and preservation of the NAC should be discussed with the oncologic surgeon and patient.
- The estimation of the defect size after tumor resection and breast size/tumor ratio is a guideline to the choice of the reconstructive method (**FIG 1**).
- Immediate correction of asymmetry by a contralateral mastopexy or reduction should also be discussed (Table 1).
- There are two basic types of surgery techniques in partial breast reconstruction: volume displacement and volume replacement.
  - Volume displacement techniques refer to advancement, rotation, or transposition of large local breast flaps into the smaller created defect, redistributing the volume loss. The dissection involves the advancement of a full-thickness segment of breast fibroglandular tissue to fill the dead space. Volume displacement procedures and surgical scars are optimal when combined with mastopexy-reduction techniques. The tumor is excised within the planned markings of the reduction specimen in medium, large, or ptotic breasts, and the remaining parenchyma is sufficient enough to reshape the breast mound.
  - Volume replacement techniques are technically more difficult and are used in small to moderate-size breasts or when the tumor/breast ratio is large and the remaining breast tissue is insufficient for the rearrangement and the replacement of the defect. Volume replacement with the use of nonbreast local or distant flaps provides both tissue for the filling of the glandular defect and the skin deficiency of the reconstructed breast (see Chapter 22).

Table 1 Important Considerations in Partial Breast Reconstruction

1.	Incision lines
2.	Nipple-areola preservation
3.	Estimation of defect size after tumor resection
4.	Reconstructive method depending on breast size/tumor size ratio
5.	Consider delayed immediate reconstruction if doubt about margins
6.	Status of contralateral breast: no surgery vs mastopexy/reduction or prophylactic mastectomy

Preoperative Planning

- The patient is preferably marked before surgery. The breast size, tumor size, and location as well as the final defect size are estimated.
- Good communication between teams, oncological and reconstructive, if this is being performed by a two-team approach
- It is important to understand the importance of blood supply to the nipple, placement of skin incisions, and have an understanding of breast aesthetics.
- It is equally important that the reconstructive surgeon realize the size and location of the tumor, importance of margin status, and locoregional control.
- Both surgeons should review the radiographic imaging and discuss the anticipated defect location and defect size, as well as whether or not the resection would include skin.
- This will assist with determination of the most appropriate glandular pedicle required to maintain nipple viability and reshape the mound.
- Anticipate a backup plan, as occasionally the defect is different to that anticipated, and an alternative approach is required. The incisions for the tumor resection are chosen from an oncological aspect but in the most aesthetically pleasing fashion.
- Planning of skin incisions and parenchymal excisions follow templates using reduction mammaplasty and mastopexy techniques.
- The pattern can be rotated laterally or medially to fit the location of the tumor. The choice of the pedicle is related to the tumor location (Table 2).
- Tumors involving the lower pole are the most easily treated because this region is removed during most reduction techniques.

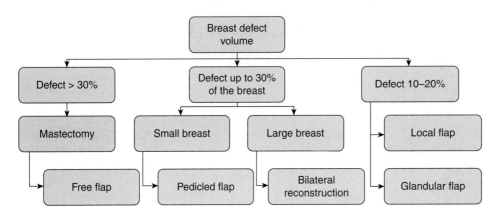

FIG 1 • An algorithm to partial breast reconstruction.

Table 2 Choice of Pedicle Based upon Location of the Defect

Location of the Defect	Choice of Pedicle
Inferior, inferomedial, or inferolateral	Superior, superomedial or superolateral pedicle
Superior	Inferior or centroinferior pedicle
Superomedial	Superolateral pedicle with an inferocentral component to fill the defect
Superolateral	Superomedial pedicle with an inferocentral component to fill the defect
Central	Inferior pedicle

- A similar mammoplasty technique is performed on the contralateral breast to match the size and shape of the tumor-affected breast.
- If radiation is planned, consider keeping the tumor-affected breast about 10% larger in size compared to the contralateral remodeled breast because some shrinking and volume changes of the radiated breast are likely to occur.
- However, immediate partial reconstruction should be delayed if the surgeon is uncertain about the margins or tumor extension (eg, tumors with large in situ component) despite the preoperative radiological assessment. A *delayed immediate reconstruction* can still be performed within a few days after the definitive margins become known.

■ Tumor Resection

- Tumor removal is performed in the usual fashion using safe and effective oncological principles.[9,10]
- Intraoperative margin assessment could include radiographical imaging, macroscopic assessment, frozen section, or touch cytology.

- We have found that patient selection, cavity sampling, and generous resection further reduce the incidence of positive margins.
- The cavity is then clipped for postoperative surveillance and guidance for radiation boosts to the tumor bed if required.

■ Principles of Rearrangement Techniques[6]

- For nipple pedicle choice, the shortest pedicle will maximize nipple viability and allow additional glandular manipulation without worrying about nipple compromise.
- As a general rule, if the pedicle points to or can be rotated into the defect, it can be used (Table 2).

- When it is not possible to preserve the nipple, either because of the size of the breasts or because of the location of the tumor, options include amputation and free nipple graft, or nipple reconstruction at a later date.
- The pedicle is de-epithelialized and dissected enough to allow rotation into the proposed nipple position (**TECH FIG 1**).

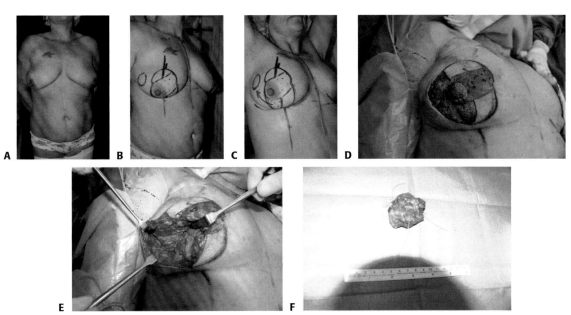

TECH FIG 1 • A 48-year-old patient who was a candidate for BCT for a T2 tumor over the superolateral quadrant. **A.** Preoperative view shows ptotic breasts. **B.** The surgical plan consisted of a vertical scar mammaplasty with a superomedial pedicle technique. **C.** A glandular flap extension was planned to fill the defect in the lateral quadrant after tumor removal. **D.** The pedicle was deepithilized. **E.** The lumpectomy was done through the lateral mammoplasty incision. **F.** The tumor was oriented and sent to the pathology analysis.

TECHNIQUES

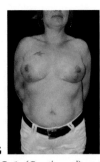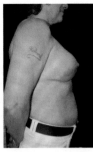

TECH FIG 1 (Continued) • **G.** The result: front view showed a good breast symmetry. **H.** The result: a lateral view showed a good breast contour without any deformity.

- If the defect is removed within the reduction specimen, it is then adequately filled through glandular displacement with the pedicle or remaining glandular tissue (**TECH FIG 2**).

- If it is thought that additional glandular flaps are required to fill the dead space, a decision is made based on what tissue is available:
  - *Single pedicle technique:* If the defect can be filled by rotating an extended portion of the original nipple pedicle, this is often the technique of choice. This works well for smaller defects in women with smaller or moderate-sized breasts, or when tissue can be taken with the pedicle from a less cosmetically sensitive area and rotated to fill a defect.
  - *Secondary pedicle technique:* This is used in larger defects with large breasts if the primary pedicle or residual parenchyma is not sufficient. A second pedicle is designed to fill the dead space separate from the nipple pedicle.
- Glandular shaping is performed using absorbable sutures where necessary, and the skin is then redraped over the mound.
- Drains are used if the defect is in communication with the axillary dissection.

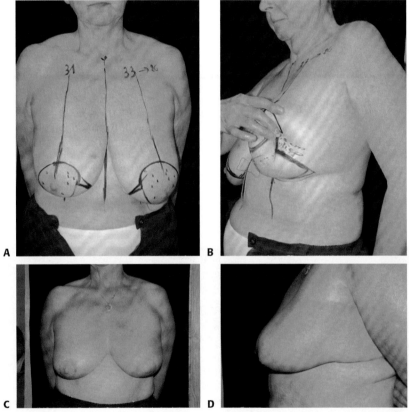

TECH FIG 2 • A 64-year-old patient who was diagnosed with T2 ductal carcinoma of the left breast. A 3-cm tumor was located in the infero-lateral quadrant. An inverted-T mammaplasty with superior pedicle was planned in order to perform a quadrantectomy with immediate partial reconstruction and contralateral remodeling for symmetrization. **A.** Preoperative view shows the mammaplasty markings. **B.** The quadrantectomy was planned within the inverted-T mammaplasty pattern. **C,D.** The result after radiotherapy at 1 year postoperatively.

PEARLS AND PITFALLS

Timing	▪ Delayed partial breast reconstruction should be considered in every situation where tumor margins could not be adequately determined preoperatively.
Marking	▪ The contralateral nondiseased side should be designed to be a bit higher to anticipate the long-term breast sagging. ▪ The affected breast (cancer side should be marked to end up with larger volume comparing to the contralateral breast to anticipate postoperative irradiation effect).
Tumorectomy	▪ Tumor specimen should be clearly oriented for pathology. ▪ Posttumorectomy defect should be marked by surgical clips.
Pedicles	▪ Avoid large tissue detachment in high-risk patients. ▪ Avoid dead space, especially in the lower breast.
Follow-up	▪ Close collaboration and communication between plastic surgery, radiologist, and oncologist is mandatory to discuss breast changes after breast rearrangement surgery.

POSTOPERATIVE CARE

- Patients receive VTE prophylaxis during the time of relative immobilization.
- Patients leave the hospital when the drains are removed, which is in average 1 to 2 days.
- A sports bra is applied for 4 weeks postoperatively.
- Adjuvant irradiation of the breast, if indicated, can be started at 6 weeks postreconstruction. Adjuvant chemotherapy can start 3 weeks postoperatively.

OUTCOMES AND COMPLICATIONS

- The 5-year survival of partial mastectomy with radiation is not statistically different when compared to mastectomy alone in patients with stage I or II breast cancer.[2–5]
- The 5-year incidence of in-breast tumor recurrence was higher in the lumpectomy and radiation patients compared to the quadrantectomy and radiation patients (8.1% vs 3.1%).[2,3]
  - In lumpectomy, the goal is tumor excision with clear surgical margins.
  - In quadrantectomy, a wide excision is performed with an additional 1 to 2 cm or even more of healthy parenchyma around the tumor, including skin and underlying muscle fascia.
- The majority of local recurrences occur at the site of initial tumor excision (57% to 88%) or in the same breast quadrant (22% to 28%).[11]
- The presence of DCIS at the surgical margin is associated with the identification of residual DSIC in 40% to 82% of re-excised specimens and is correlated with margin widths of 41% at 1 mm, 31% at 1 to 2 mm, and 0% with 2 mm of clearance.[3]
- A recent meta-analysis showed lower positive margins after oncoplastic surgery (12%) compared to breast conservative surgery without oncoplastic reconstruction (21%).[12]
- Local recurrences were also lower after oncoplastic surgery (4.2% compared to 7% with BCT alone).[12–14]
- Approximately 10% to 30% of patients are dissatisfied with the aesthetic result after partial mastectomy with radiation.[15,16]
- Oncoplastic surgery or partial breast reconstruction allows for wider tumor resection with aesthetic favorable outcomes and lower positive margins.[15–21]
- Incorporating a reduction mammoplasty with partial mastectomy can potentially be a complex procedure.[22,23]

- The aesthetic outcome was considered good or very good in 81% of patients.[12,18–21]
- Recent literature, however, suggests that early complications are similar to mere reduction mammoplasty. In a review by Spear et al., none of the complications significantly interfered with healing, radiation, chemotherapy, or the quality of the result.[22,23]

REFERENCES

1. Winchester DP, Cox JD. Standards for diagnosis and management of invasive breast carcinoma. *CA Cancer J Clin*. 1998;48:83-107.
2. Veronesi U, Cascinelli N, Mariani L, et al. Twenty-year follow-up of a randomized study comparing breast-conserving surgery with radical mastectomy for early breast cancer. *N Engl J Med*. 2002;347: 1227-1232.
3. Patani N, Khaled Y, Al Reefy MK. Ductal carcinoma in-situ: an update for clinical practice. *Surg Oncol*. 2011;20:e23-e31.
4. Fisher B, Anderson S, Bryant J, et al. Twenty-year follow-up of a randomized trial comparing total mastectomy, lumpectomy, and lumpectomy plus irradiation for the treatment of invasive breast cancer. *N Engl J Med*. 2002;347:1233-1241.
5. Huston TL, Simmons RM. Locally recurrent breast cancer after conservative therapy. *Am J Surg*. 2005;189:229-235.
6. Losken A, Hamdi M. Partial breast reconstruction: current perspectives. *Plast Reconstr Surg*. 2009;124(3):722-736.
7. van Deventer PV, Graewe FR. The blood supply of the breast revisited. *Plast Reconstr Surg*. 2016;137(5):1388-1397.
8. Hamdi M, Wolfli J, Van Landuyt K. Partial mastectomy reconstruction. *Clin Plast Surg*. 2007;34(1):51-62.
9. Vicini FA, Recht A. Age at diagnosis and outcome for women with ductal carcinoma-in-situ of the breast: a critical review of the literature. *J Clin Oncol*. 2002;20(11):2736-2744.
10. Dillon MF, Hill AD, Quinn CM, et al. A pathologic assessment of adequate margin status in breast-conserving therapy. *Ann Surg Oncol*. 2006;13(3):333-339.
11. Osborne MP, Borgen PI, et al. Salvage mastectomy for local and regional recurrence after breast conserving operation and radiation therapy. *Surg Gynecol Obstet*. 1992;174:189-194.
12. Losken A, Dugal C, Styblo T, Carlson G. A meta-analysis comparing breast conservation therapy alone to the oncoplastic technique. *Ann Plast Surg*. 2014;72(2):145-149.
13. Fehlauer F, Tribius S, et al. Long-term radiation sequelae after breast-conserving therapy in women with early-stage breast cancer: an observational study using the LENT-SOMA scoring system. *Int J Radiat Oncol Biol Phys*. 2003;55(3):651-658.
14. Eaton B, Losken A, Okwan-Duodu D, et al. Local recurrence patterns in breast cancer patients treated with oncoplastic reduction mammoplasty and radiotherapy. *Ann Surg Oncol*. 2014;21:93-99.

15. Berrino P, Campora E, Santi P. Postquadrantectomy breast deformities; classification and techniques of surgical correction. *Plast Reconstr Surg.* 1987;79(4):567-572.

16. Clough K, Kroll S, Audretsch W. An approach to the repair of partial mastectomy defects. *Plast Reconstr Surg.* 1999;104(2):409-420.

17. Mcculley SJ, Macmillan RD. Therapeutic mammaplasty—analysis of 50 consecutive cases. *Br J Plast Surg.* 2005;58(7):902-907.

18. Munhoz A, Montang E, et al. Critical analysis of reduction mammaplasty techniques in combination with conservation breast surgery for early breast cancer treatment. *Plast Reconstr Surg.* 2006;117(4): 1091-1103.

19. Fitoussi AD, Berry MG, Fama F, et al. Oncoplastic breast surgery for cancer: analysis of 540 consecutive cases (outcomes article). *Plast Reconstr Surg.* 2010;125:454-462.

20. Song HM, Styblo TM, Carlson GW, Losken A, The use of oncoplastic reduction techniques to reconstruct partial mastectomy defects in women with ductal carcinoma in situ. *Breast J.* 2010;16(2): 141-146.

21. Kronowitz SJ, Kuerer HM, Buchholz TA, et al. A management algorithm and practical oncoplastic surgical techniques for repairing partial mastectomy defects. *Plast Reconstr Surg.* 2008;122(6): 1631-1647.

22. Spear LS, Pelletiere CV, et al. Experience with reduction mammaplasty combined with breast conservation therapy in the treatment of breast cancer. *Plast Reconstr Surg.* 2003;111(3):1102-1109.

23. Losken A, Schaefer TG, Newell M, Styblo TM, The impact of partial breast reconstruction using reduction techniques on postoperative cancer surveillance. *Plast Reconstr Surg.* 2009;124(1):9-17.

Local Flaps in Partial Breast Reconstruction

Moustapha Hamdi and Fadi Bakal

DEFINITION

- Partial breast reconstruction is an area of evolving interest with improving surgical techniques; it is indicated in breast conservation therapy (BCT), which is on its own a popular treatment option for women with breast cancer.[1,2] The rate of its use has increased from 40% in 1991 to 60% in 2002 when compared with mastectomy, and that trend continues to rise.[1]
- Oncoplastic surgery within multidisciplinary approach is standard in BCT.
- The oncoplastic surgical approach allowed surgeons to tailor the techniques to prevent deformities, minimize involved margins, and reduce the potential for local recurrence.
- Partial breast reconstruction with pedicled flap is alternative to mastectomy in selected patients as such in patients with a high tumor/breast size ratio.
- Every case requiring partial breast reconstruction should be addressed within a multidisciplinary approach.
- Pedicled perforator flaps provide adequate partial breast reconstruction with minimal donor-site morbidity.

ANATOMY

- The latissimus dorsi (LD) flap has a constant anatomy.[3–5] The blood supply of the latissimus dorsi comes from a terminal branch of the subscapular artery. The subscapular artery runs about 5 cm before dividing into the scapular circumflex and thoracodorsal arteries.
- The thoracodorsal artery gives off one or two branches to the serratus anterior muscle and one branch to the skin (**FIG 1**).
- Perforating vessels from the intercostal and lumbar arteries supply the muscle and overlying skin.[11,12]

PATIENT HISTORY AND PHYSICAL FINDINGS

- Breast and plastic surgeons must have a thorough understanding of breast anatomy and physiology and the qualities of an aesthetically pleasing breast shape.
- Surgeons performing the oncoplastic approach should consider the aesthetic subunits when planning cosmetic quadrantectomies, resections, and reconstructions.[3]
- Also, knowledge of the anatomical landmarks, breast proportions, and shape is essential to achieve a pleasing outcome.
- Preoperative evaluation of the patient and her breasts must be standardized and detailed.

- The examination must include the following:
  - Evaluation of breast skin, elasticity, thickness, scars, and any defining marks such as tattoos, stretch marks, contour irregularities, and previous breast surgery should be taken into account when planning BCT.

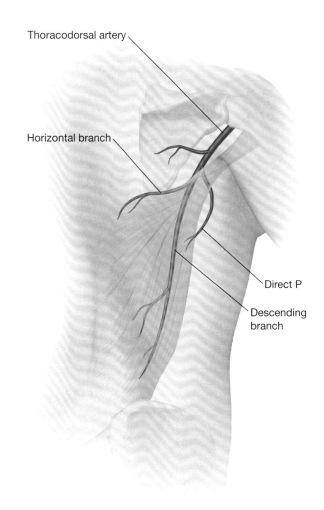

FIG 1 • The TD vessels most commonly divide into five branches, but two are dominant muscular branches: the transverse branch, and the lateral or vertical branch. Both branches give musculocutaneous perforator to the skin. A direct branch can also be found, which courses anteriorly around the LD muscle toward the skin.

- Palpation for masses or abnormalities in the breast parenchyma, nipple inspection, and detailed documentation of breast sensation are integral.
  - Breast shape, grade of ptosis, and size are determinants of success in surgical treatment.
- The base and width of the breast, the width of the NAC, the height of the nipple, and the distance from the sternal notch, midline, and inframammary crease must be recorded in detail.[4]
- Any natural breast asymmetry should be pointed out to the patient before surgery.
- Different body types, skin laxity, and fat distribution are important factors in the decision-making process.

SURGICAL MANAGEMENT

- Depending on the location and the size of the breast defect, different flaps can be used for partial mastectomy reconstruction based on the thoracodorsal-serratus, intercostal, or superior epigastic vessels.[2–18]
- A small lateral defect can easily be closed with a skin rotation flap or lateral thoracic axial skin flap. However, most of these flaps become unavailable when axillary lymph node dissection is performed.
- Lateral breast defects are usually reconstructed using a flap based on the thoracodorsal system. The LD musculocutaneous flap is the most commonly used.
- Currently, perforator flaps are more often used to spare muscle function.
  - The pedicled perforator flaps mostly used by us for partial breast reconstruction, classified according to the basic nutrient arteries and recommended by the "Gent" Consensus update in 2002,[6] are
    - Thoracodorsal artery perforator (TDAP) flap
    - Serratus anterior artery perforator (SAAP) flap
    - Intercostal artery perforator (ICAP) flap
    - Superior epigastric artery perforator (SEAP)
- A similar skin paddle to the classical LD musculocutaneous flap can be raised on perforators either from the thoracodorsal or intercostal vessels.

Types of Flaps

TDAP Flap

- The TDAP flap is based on perforators originating from the descending (vertical) or horizontal branches of the thoracodorsal vessels (see **FIG 1**; **FIG 2**). Anatomic studies on cadavers have reported the presence of 2 to 3 musculocutaneous perforators from the vertical branch.[7–9]
- The proximal perforator enters the subcutaneous plane obliquely 8 to 10 cm distal to the posterior axillary fold and 2 to 3 cm posterior to the anterior border of the muscle. The second perforator is found 2 to 4 cm distally to the first one.
- Occasionally, a direct cutaneous perforator arising from the thoracodorsal vessel passes around the anterior border of the muscle, making flap harvesting easier (see **FIG 1**).
- There may not be always a single reliable perforator for the TDAP flap, due to anatomical variations. In this case, the surgeon must be aware and prepared to modify the flap dissection intraoperatively, as a muscle-sparing TDAP flap.

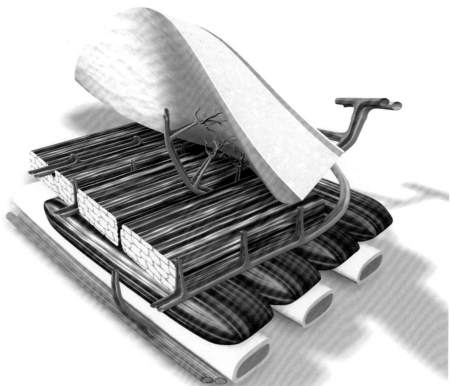

A

FIG 2 • Illustrations show: TDAP flap with musculocutaneous perforators **(A)**.

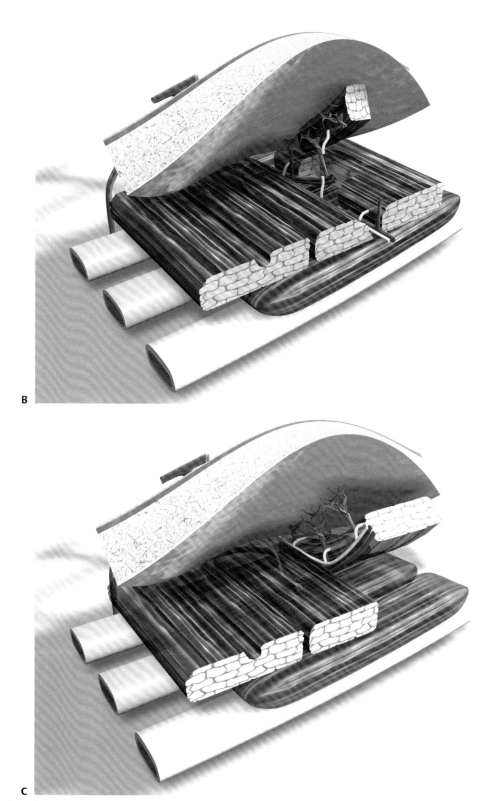

B

C

FIG 2 (Continued) • **B.** TDAP flap with perforator still attached to 4 × 2 cm muscle segment (muscle-sparing TDAP type I). **C.** TDAP flap raised on the descending branches and its perforators (muscle-sparing TDAP flap type II). Reprinted from Hamdi H, et. al. Pedicled perforator flaps in breast reconstruction: a new concept. *Br J Plast Surg*. 2004;57(6):531-539, with permission from Elsevier.

- The TDAP flaps are classified as follows[9]:
  - TDAP flap, when no muscle component is included in the flap.
  - TDAP-MS-I, where a small segment of muscle (4 × 2 cm) is kept attached to the back of the perforator vessels. The muscle segment protects the perforator from excessive tension and provides more freedom in flap positioning (**FIG 2B**).
  - TDAP-MS-II is indicated when multiple but small perforators are encountered. A larger segment, up to 5 cm wide along the anterior border of the LD muscle together with the descending branch of the thoracodorsal vessels, is then included within the flap in order to ensure maximal blood supply to the skin paddle (**FIG 2C**).

ICAP Flap

- The ICAP flap is based on perforators, arising from the intercostal vessels.
- The intercostal vessels form an arcade between the aorta and the internal mammary vessels and divide in 4 segments: vertebral, intercostal, intermuscular, and rectus segments (**FIG 3A**).[11,12]
- The ICAP flaps are classified as follows (**FIG 3B**):
  - The dorsal intercostal artery perforator (DICAP) flap. The flap is based on perforators originating from the vertebral segment of the intercostal vessels.
  - The lateral intercostal artery perforator (LICAP) flap, based on perforators arising from the intercostal segment.
  - The anterior intercostal artery perforator (AICAP) flap. The nutrient perforators of this flap arise from the muscular or rectal segment.
- The intercostal segment, which is the longest (12 cm), is very important because it gives 5 to 7 musculocutaneous perforators.[11]

- The LICAP, commonly used in breast surgery, originates from the costal segment of the intercostal vessels. The largest perforator is most frequently found in the 6th intercostal space, 0.8 to 3.5 cm from the anterior border of the LD muscle.[12] The pedicle has adequate length, allowing the rotation of the flap up to 180 degrees without tension and with no need to extend the dissection into the costal groove. An intercostal nerve may be included in the harvesting as an ICAP-sensate flap.
- For small defects, the LICAP is designed on the lateral aspect of the thorax. For moderate-large defects, the distal limit of the skin pad can reach the posterior thoracic region, planned in a fashion similar to the skin pad of an LD flap.[12]
- The AICAP flap is outlined over the upper abdomen, so that the final scar will be hidden under the brassiere strap. The donor site can be closed primarily if it is up to 6 cm wide (preoperative pinch test to be assured) or else in a reversed abdominoplasty fashion. The advantage of AICAP and SEAP flaps (see below) is that the patient is prepped in a supine position throughout the whole procedure. These flaps are mostly known for defects in the inferomedial quadrant of the breast.

SAAP Flap

- The SAAP flap is based on a connection between the thoracodorsal artery branch to the serratus anterior muscle and the intercostal perforators. It is not a constant perforator; 21% of cases there is a connection between the serratus anterior branch & the intercostal perforators.[12]
- When an appropriately sized perforator is identified in front of the anterior border of the LD, it can be followed back to the nutrient artery, which in this case is the serratus anterior branch, by dissecting the pedicle within the fascia and the fibers of the aforementioned muscle.

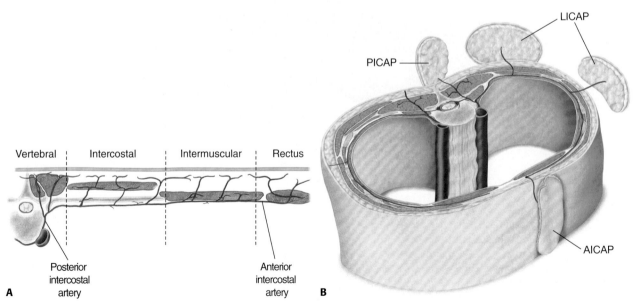

FIG 3 • The anatomy of the intercostal perforators. **A.** Four segments to the intercostal vessels: the vertebral, intercostal, intermuscular, and rectus segment. **B.** Intercostal perforator flap classification: PICAP, posterior intercostal artery perforator; LICAP, lateral intercostal artery perforator; AICAP, anterior intercostal artery perforator.

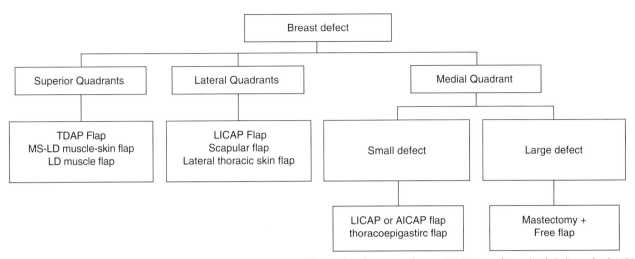

FIG 4 • Algorithm for using flaps for partial breast reconstruction. TDAP, thoracodorsal artery perforator; MS-LD, muscle-sparing latissimus dorsi; LICAP, lateral intercostal artery perforator; AICAP, anterior intercostal artery perforator.

SEAP Flap

- The SEAP flaps are based on perforators arising from either the superficial or the deep branch of the superior epigastric artery, and the perforator flaps are named SSEAP and DSEAP, respectively.[15]
- The SEAP flap has similar indications as the AICAP flap[15]; however, it has a longer pedicle that allows it to reach the defect with less tension.
- Pedicled SEAP flaps should be used only in selected cases, because it excludes the secondary use of abdominal tissue for autologous breast reconstruction (DIEAP, SIEAP, TRAM flaps) if completion mastectomy is later on indicated (**FIG 4**).

Preoperative Planning

- Perforator mapping with correct flap design is the keystone in these oncoplastic techniques.[3]
    - To localize the thoracodorsal perforators, a unidirectional Doppler (8 Hz) ultrasonography examination is performed for perforator mapping in the planned skin flap area. This device, although quite handy and less costly, has the disadvantage of generating false-negative and false-positive signals and provides less detailed anatomic vessel information.
    - This is due to the misleading background signal from the thoracodorsal vessels, which can be confusing and difficult to distinguish from the perforator signal. To avoid this, the patient is positioned, as in surgery, at a lateral position with 90 degrees of shoulder abduction and 90 degrees of elbow flexion.
    - Also, multidetector (MD) row CT scan can be used with accuracy to localize the perforator.[3]
- The patient is marked before surgery. The breast size, tumor size, and location as well as the final defect size are estimated.
- The incisions for the tumor resection are chosen from an oncological aspect but in the most aesthetically pleasing fashion.

- The TDAP (thoracodorsal artery perforator) flap planned for the partial breast reconstruction is designed to include the located perforators (one or more) at the proximal part if feasible, in the directions of relaxed skin lines, the brassiere line, or even horizontally according to the patient's preference.
- Skin laxity and fat excess in the lateral thorax and back area are estimated by the pinch test. The size of the flap is determined by the need for defect coverage and is an average of 20 × 8 cm.
- The skin drawings are applied at first with the patient in an upright position, and the anterior border of the LD muscle is palpated and marked also.
- Then the patient is placed in a lying position on her side, with the reconstruction side facing upward, as in surgery, for the perforator mapping and the flap design in the lateral thorax. The skin island is always extended over the anterior border of the LD to include the premuscular perforators if present.
- If the defect is more medially, the flap is designed more distally, further in the back. The same design is applied for the LICAP; however, the flap is placed more anteriorly, toward the breast. The AICAP or SEAP flaps are usually designed under the inframammary fold along the rib.

Positioning

- The patient is prepped and positioned in the supine position for the tumor excision. After the lumpectomy/quadrantectomy at clear margins, clips are placed in the wound bed and left there, in order to indicate the area for future radiation therapy.
- If the plan is to proceed with TDAP, LICAP, or SAAP flap, the patient is positioned and prepped again in the lateral position as in the typical LD musculocutaneous flap dissection.
- For AICAP/SEAP flap, the patient remains in the original position.

TECHNIQUES

■ Basics of Flap Harvesting

- The flap harvesting starts with skin incisions.
- A posterior approach is usually used in TDAP flap. The surgeon continues dissection down to the LD suprafascial plane while beveling in favor of the flap in order to gain as much of extra tissue as possible. Harvesting proceeds from the back to the axillary region. Further harvesting under loop magnification continues meticulously, until the perforator vessel is visualized. If the perforator is visibly pulsatile and adequate in caliber (greater than 0.5 mm for the whole bundle), the dissection continues along the perforator course up to the nutrient thoracodorsal pedicle. If a large pedicle length is required, the TD vessels can be dissected up to their subscapular vessel origin and included in the flap.
- If the perforators have an intramuscular course, dissection is performed in the direction of the muscle fibers, and any nerves that come across are carefully preserved. Within the muscle, all the perforator side branches are either ligated or coagulated. If two perforators are found along the same course, they can both be included within the flap, without sacrificing any muscle fibers.
- In case the perforators are inadequate in size, the flap harvesting is continued as muscle-sparing LD, preserving a small piece of muscle attached to the posterior wall of the perforators, sacrificing only minimum fibers and,

most important, salvaging the muscle innervation. This modification is also useful when the flap is intended for the medial breast area, because it protects the perforators from presumed tension.

- The flap harvesting carries on, with the skin incisions continued proximal to the axilla and lateral to the LD, and the dissection proceeds anteriorly, until the flap is freed from the donor-site tissues and left connected only to the vascular pedicle. The pedicle is carefully passed under a subcutaneous tunnel in the axilla–lateral thoracic area that has been previously prepared to the recipient breast area, avoiding any avulsion of the pedicle.
- The donor site is sutured in three anatomical layers with a drain in place, and the patient is returned again to the supine position.
- Before final closure of the defect, the flap can be partially or totally de-epithelialized (depending on the native skin reservations of the recipient site) and folded accordingly, to give extra projection to the reconstructed breast mount but always in a tension-free manner.
- In LICAP flap dissection, an anterior approach is performed from the breast side toward the anterior-free border of LD muscle. Perforator dissection is done within the serratus muscle until its origin from the costal grove. Further dissection is usually not needed.

■ TDAP Flap

Flap Design

- The patient is positioned in lateral decubitus with the shoulder in 90 degrees of abduction and the elbow in 90 degrees of flexion.
- In this position, the anterior border of the LD muscle is palpated through the skin and marked.
- A 5- to 8-MHz Doppler probe allows accurate location of the perforators in the posterior axillary line, 8 cm below the axillary crease and within 5 cm from the anterior border of the LD muscle.
  - More recently, CT scanning has been successfully used to preoperatively detect the best perforator and will certainly become a great tool for thoracodorsal perforator mapping in the future.
- Subsequently, the skin island is designed to include the audible perforators and can be oriented in different directions depending on the reconstructive needs and anticipated orientation of the scar (**TECH FIG 1**).
- The flap paddle is better oriented to fit into the skin lines and parallel to the rib direction, which provides the best inclusion of the angiosome territory.

Flap Harvesting

- The incision starts at the inferior anterior border of the flap, which allows for identification of the anterior

border of the LD muscle and eventual repositioning of the anterior border of the flap.

- The dissection proceeds from distal to proximal and from medial to lateral at the level just above the LD muscle fascia until a suitable perforator is identified (**TECH FIG 2**).
  - A perforator originating from the vertical branch is preferred because dissection is easier due to fewer connections with other vessels and a shorter intramuscular course.
  - If two perforators lie along the same line, both can be incorporated within the flap without cutting additional muscle.
  - A perforator should be visibly pulsatile and have a diameter suitable for microvascular anastomosis.
- Once a suitable perforator is identified, intramuscular dissection is rather straightforward.
  - The muscle is split longitudinally and the perforator dissected cranially.

Flap Placement and Completion

- The next step is to free the anterior border of the LD muscle and look underneath.
- Total pedicle length depends on the location of the perforator on the muscle, as the length of the intramuscular course adds up with the length of the oblique course on

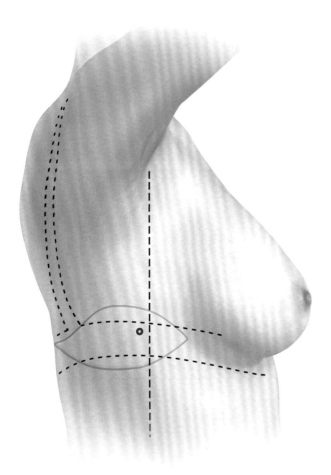

TECH FIG 1 • Surgical technique of TDAP flap harvesting. Flap design. The perforator is located using unidirectional Doppler and is usually found 6 to 8 cm from the posterior axillary fold. The flap is designed within the brassiere region (*dotted line*) and crosses the anterior border of the LD muscle (*dashed line*).

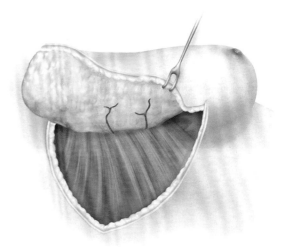

TECH FIG 2 • The flap is dissected from the LD muscle until the perforators are encountered.

top of the muscle and the length of the thoracodorsal pedicle itself (**TECH FIG 3A**).

- This usually yields a pedicle length of 7 to 12 cm.
- The motor nerves to the LD run on a deeper plane, which allows for complete freeing of the pedicle without injuring the nerves.
- Once the complete intramuscular trajectory has been dissected, harvesting the thoracodorsal pedicle proceeds.
- The skin paddle is carefully passed through the split muscle and subcutaneously into the defect through the axilla (**TECH FIG 3B**).
- At the end, closed suction drains are placed and donor site is closed primarily in three layers.
- The technique is illustrated in a clinical case (**TECH FIG 4**).

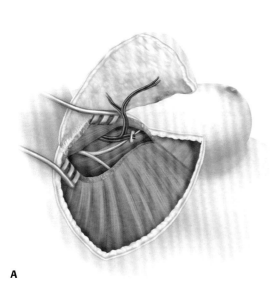

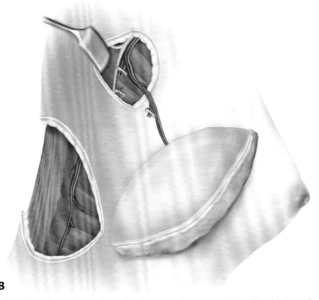

A   B

TECH FIG 3 • **A.** The LD muscle is split and the perforator dissected back to the main pedicle. The TD nerve is preserved. **B.** The flap is pulled through the axillary incision and into the breast defect.

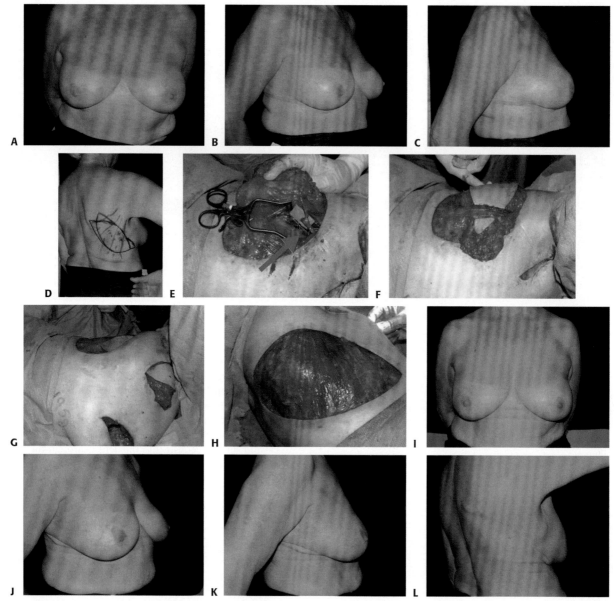

TECH FIG 4 • A patient undergoing a quadrantectomy for a tumor of the superolateral quadrant of the right breast. The quadrantectomy specimen weighed 195 g. Reconstruction is with a completely de-epithelialized TDAP flap based on one perforator. **A–C.** Preoperative views. **D.** The flap design with the marked perforators, located by Doppler. **E.** The dissection of the perforator through the split LD muscle. The TD nerve is preserved (*arrow*). **F,G.** The TDAP flap is passed through the split LD muscle and then through the axilla. **H.** The LD muscle is left intact. **I–K.** Postoperative views. **L.** Donor site.

PEARLS AND PITFALLS

Indications	▪ Any immediate partial reconstruction should be delayed if the surgeon is uncertain about the margins or tumor extension. ▪ A delayed reconstruction can still be performed within a few days after the definitive margin status is known.
Flap markings	▪ Using Doppler or CT scan imaging is essential to locate the perforators. ▪ Skin paddle should be extended anteriorly toward the inframammary fold.
Perforator flap harvesting	▪ Perforators must be pulsating and have a good diameter (more than 0.5 mm) if a flap is to be harvested.
Outcome	▪ Seroma incidence at the donor site after harvesting perforator flap is reduced to 0%. ▪ Long-term aesthetic result after pedicled flaps is very satisfactory despite the irradiation.

POSTOPERATIVE CARE

- Postoperatively, protocol perforator flap monitoring is implemented.
- Patients are administered VTE prophylaxis during the time of relative immobilization.
- Patients leave the hospital when the drains are removed, which is in average 3 to 5 days.
- The arm is hold in 45-degree abduction. Arm stretching is restricted for a week. Physiotherapy can be started afterward. Most of patients required between 9 and 14 sessions of shoulder physiotherapy.
- Patients treated for BCT with pedicled perforator flaps have a short rehabilitation course.[18]
- Adjuvant irradiation of the breast, if indicated, can be started at 6-week postreconstruction. Adjuvant chemotherapy can start 3 weeks postoperatively.

OUTCOME AND COMPLICATIONS

- Donor-site morbidity after harvesting locoregional pedicle perforator flaps for partial breast reconstruction is reduced to a minimum. Only a very limited rate of seroma formation has been observed and treated mainly conservatively. Wound dehiscence of the donor site usually when closed under tension is another infrequent event managed with local treatment.
- Data from a recent study show a seroma rate of 5.5% in MS-TDAP II flaps, compared to no seroma formation in perforator flaps. Other postoperative complications observed were wound dehiscence (4%), infection (2%), and hematoma (2%).[9]
- Partial or total flap losses are rare incidents and one must exclude coagulopathies or other medical diseases and conditions.
- Palpable (partial) fat necrosis of the flap has been observed and can be treated, if necessary, by excision and primary closure or reconstruction by a local flap. Or if necrosis is too extensive, a mastectomy with total breast reconstruction can be indicated.[9]
- Unpleasing scars, flap contractures, and volume loss are less rare sequelae and may need secondary surgical treatment.
- Flap reconstruction of breast defect may give a "plugged-in" appearance, which seems to slightly improve after radiation therapy. It is hard to predict the long-term outcomes of partial breast reconstruction with pedicled perforator flaps due to the indefinite impact of irradiation to the final result.
- Some patients who undergo partial breast reconstruction with a TDAP flap document an initial decrease in forward arm elevation and passive abduction, which recovers over time.[18]

Prognosis

- Many concerns have been raised about oncologic safety of oncoplastic surgery.
- A recent meta-analysis showed that oncoplastic surgery is an oncological safe procedure, with even lesser recurrence rates (4%) compared to breast conservative surgery (7%) alone.[19]
- After oncoplastic reduction mammoplasty, resection margins are more often negative, and if recurrences occur, they most often occur in the preoperative quadrant of the tumor and not the location after displacement techniques.[20]
- As stated earlier, if DCIS is present, oncoplastic techniques should be used cautiously.
- Local recurrence rates reported in the literature for oncoplastic surgery vary from 0% to 7% of the patients.[19–21]

Oncological Follow-Up

- Oncological follow-up after oncoplastic procedures remains important.
- Given the rearrangement of parenchymal tissues, scar tissue or fat necrosis is not uncommon and might be suspicious on several radiological imaging modalities.
- Biopsy with fine needle aspiration, core biopsy, or excisional biopsy can be necessary to rule out tumor recurrence (up to 25%).[21]
- The addition of breast remodeling procedures does not seem to affect mammographic sensitivity, and qualitative changes are similar to those found following BCT alone.[21]

REFERENCES

1. Losken A, Hamdi M. Partial breast reconstruction: current perspectives. *Plast Reconstr Surg.* 2009;124(3):722-736.
2. Honart JF, Reguesse AS, Struk S, et al. Indications and controversies in partial mastectomy defect reconstruction. *Clin Plast Surg.* 2018;45(1):33-45.
3. Hamdi M, Van Landuyt K, Van Hedent E, Duyck P. Advances in autogenous breast reconstruction: the role of preoperative perforator mapping. *Ann Plast Surg.* 2007;58(1):18-26.
4. Bostwick J III, Nahai F, Wallace JG, Vasconez LO. Sixty latissimus dorsi flaps. *Plast Reconstr Surg.* 1979;63(1):31-41.
5. Bartlett SP, May JW Jr, Yaremchuk MJ. The latissimus dorsi muscle: a fresh cadaver study of the primary neurovascular pedicle. *Plast Reconstr Surg.* 1981;67(5):631-636.
6. Blondeel PN, Van Landuyt K, Hamdi M, Monstrey SJ. Perforator flap terminology: update 2002. *Clin Plast Surg.* 2003;30(3):343-346.
7. Angrigiani C, Grilli D, Siebert J. Latissimus dorsi musculocutaneous flap without muscle. *Plast Reconstr Surg.* 1995;96(7):1608-1614.
8. Spinelli HM, Fink JK, Muzaffar A. The latissimus dorsi perforator-based fasciocutaneous flap. *Ann Plast Surg.* 1996;37:500-506.
9. Hamdi M, Van Landuyt K, Hijjawi JB, et al. Surgical technique in pedicled thoracodorsal artery perforator flaps: a clinical experience with 99 patients. *Plast Reconstr Surg.* 2008;121(5):1632-1641.
10. Hamdi M, Van Landuyt K, Monstrey S, Blondeel P. Pedicled perforator flaps in breast reconstruction: a new concept. *Br J Plast Surg.* 2004;57(6):531-539.
11. Hamdi M, Van Landuyt K, de Frene B, et al. The versatility of the inter-costal artery perforator (ICAP) flaps. *J Plast Reconstr Aesthet Surg.* 2006;59(6):644-652.
12. Hamdi M, Spano A, Van Landuyt K, et al. The lateral intercostal artery perforators: anatomical study and clinical application in breast surgery. *Plast Reconstr Surg.* 2008;121(2):389-396.
13. Losken A, Hamdi M. Partial breast reconstruction: current perspectives. *Plast Reconstr Surg.* 2009;124(3):722-736.
14. Munhoz AM, Montag E, Arruda E, et al. Immediate conservative breast surgery reconstruction with perforator flaps: new challenges in the era of partial mastectomy reconstruction? *Breast.* 2011;20(3):233-240.

15. Hamdi M, Van Landuyt K, Ulens S, et al. Clinical applications of the superior epigastric artery perforator (SEAP) flap: anatomical studies and preoperative perforator mapping with multidetector CT. *J Plast Reconstr Aesthet Surg.* 2009;62(9):1127-1134.

16. Hamdi M, Wolfli J, Van Landuyt K. Partial mastectomy reconstruction. *Clin Plast Surg.* 2007;34(1):51-62.

17. Hamdi M. Oncoplastic and reconstructive surgery of the breast. *Breast.* 2013;22(suppl 2):S100-S105.

18. Hamdi M, Decorte T, Demuynck M, et al. Shoulder function after harvesting a thoracodorsal artery perforator flap. *Plast Reconstr Surg.* 2008;122(4):1111-1117.

19. Losken A, Dugal C, Styblo T, Carlson G. A meta-analysis comparing breast conservation therapy alone to the oncoplastic technique. *Ann Plast Surg.* 2014;72(2):145-149.

20. Eaton B, Losken A, Okwan-Duodu D, et al. Local recurrence patterns in breast cancer patients treated with oncoplastic reduction mammoplasty and radiotherapy. *Ann Surg Oncol.* 2014;21:93-99.

21. Losken A, Schaefer TG, Newell M, Styblo TM. The impact of partial breast reconstruction using reduction techniques on postoperative cancer surveillance. *Plast Reconstr Surg.* 2009;124(1):9-17.

Section V: Prosthetic Breast Reconstruction

Delayed Tissue Expansion

Hana Farhang Khoee, Edward C. Ray, and Joseph J. Disa

13

CHAPTER

DEFINITION

- Delayed breast tissue expansion occurs after mastectomy skin has healed and after all adjuvant therapy has been completed.

ANATOMY

- Diagram of the chest wall (sagittal) showing tissue planes of the breast (**FIG 1**). From superficial to deep, layers include the skin, subcutaneous tissue, breast parenchyma, and *pectoralis major* muscle.
- The dissection involves creating a pocket deep to the *pectoralis major* muscle but above the *pectoralis minor* muscle.

PATIENT HISTORY AND PHYSICAL FINDINGS

History Taking

- Cancer history
- Previous adjuvant therapy, including radiation and chemotherapy
- Define the goals and expectations of the patient
- Psychosocial
- Overall fitness for surgery

Physical Exam

- Breast dimension: base width, height, projection, position, and symmetry of inframammary fold (IMF)
- Skin integrity
- Changes in skin due to prior irradiation
- Scars
- Contralateral breast
- Presence of a functioning ipsilateral *latissimus dorsi* muscle

IMAGING

- Imaging usually not necessary
- May consider ultrasound to assess thickness of skin flap

SURGICAL MANAGEMENT

- Delayed tissue expansion

Preoperative Planning

- Tissue expander (TE) selection
    - Size is determined by breast width of patient.
    - Most TE are anatomical and textured with integrated valves.

- Assessment of skin integrity and suitability for expansion
    - Irradiated skin or poor skin quality may suggest the need for *latissimus dorsi* myocutaneous flap.
- Markings
    - Should be done with patient in standing position prior to the operation
    - The most important is to identify the IMF.
        - Achieve symmetry with contralateral breast or, if bilateral, create a natural-appearing fold that is not too high.
    - Mark breast footprint.
        - Superior, medial (2 cm from midline), IMF, and anterior axillary fold (AAF)

Positioning

- Supine with arms either extended on arm boards (preferred) or tucked
- Ensure body and shoulders are centered on the table.

Approach

- One standard approach for delayed tissue expanders

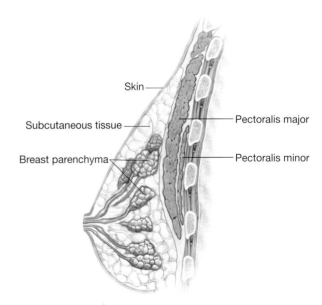

Skin

Subcutaneous tissue

Breast parenchyma

Pectoralis major

Pectoralis minor

FIG 1 • Relevant anatomy of the chest wall: Sagittal cross section: *Note skin, subcutaneous tissue, breast parenchyma, pectoralis major, and minor muscle on diagram.*

■ Creation of Submuscular Tissue Expander Pocket (TECH FIG 1)

- Excise mastectomy scar.
- Elevate mastectomy skin flaps.
- Expose *pectoralis major* muscle enough to allow entry of TE.
- Enter the submuscular layer either at the inferior or lateral border of the *pectoralis major* muscle or split the muscle in the direction of its fibers.

- Avoid elevation of *pectoralis minor* muscle.
- If needed, dissection of the *pectoralis major* muscle can be extended either to the subcutaneous plane inferiorly and laterally or into the submuscular/subfascial plane (ie, elevating *serratus anterior* muscle).
  - The decision is based on the quality of the mastectomy skin flaps.

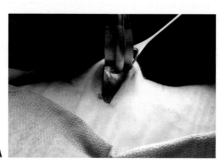 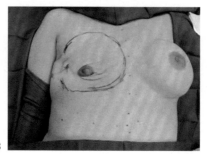

TECH FIG 1 • **A.** Creating the submuscular pocket using a lighted retractor. **B.** Showing the extent of submuscular pocket dissection. Solid line indicates the extent of dissection.

■ Release of Capsule Scar

- Must release any scar tissue that will restrict expansion of the mastectomy flaps
- Capsulotomy performed as needed (if there was a prior implant)
  - Typically, limited to a superior and medial capsulotomy
  - Care taken to avoid allowing the TE to migrate too far laterally
  - When lowering of IMF or greater lower pole expansion is desired, an inferior capsulotomy is performed.
- Capsulectomy as needed
  - Can facilitate better expansion

■ Insertion of Tissue Expander

- Expander is placed such that the zone of maximum expansion is located in the lower pole of the reconstructed breast.
- May insert some fluid in TE, depending on the amount of skin laxity.
- Ensure proper orientation of the TE (markings on TE can be helpful) (**TECH FIG 2**).
- When coverage of the expander by the muscle is insufficient, an engineered tissue substitute may be used.
  - The most common is acellular dermal matrix (ADM) such as AlloDerm. (LifeCell, Bridgewater, NJ).
  - These may be fenestrated to minimize the risk of undrained submuscular seromas and to optimize incorporation into the overlying subcutaneous tissue.

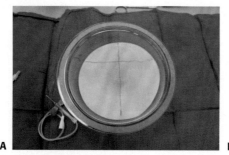 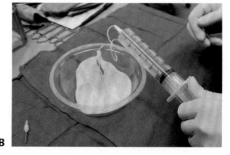

TECH FIG 2 • **A,B.** Show marking and filling of TE.

■ Closure of Wound

- Layered closure of the muscle and skin
- Use of drains is optional, depending on surgeon preference, expected fluid accumulation, or use of ADM.

PEARLS AND PITFALLS

Tissue expander selection	■ Based on breast width and volume
Tissue expander placement	■ Ideally, should establish IMF in the preoperative setting, with patient in a standing position
Skin quality	■ Thin or radiation-damaged skin may require *latissimus dorsi* myocutaneous flap to facilitate expansion.

POSTOPERATIVE CARE

■ If used, drains are kept in place until output drops below a given threshold.
  ■ Drains may be subcutaneous, submuscular, or both.
■ Postoperative antibiotics are used according to surgeon preference and patient risk factors.
■ The patient is placed in a loosely fit surgical brassiere.
  ■ The use of an underwire brassiere is avoided for several weeks after surgery.

OUTCOMES

■ Cochrane review identifies only one randomized control trial (RCT) assessing outcomes for immediate vs delayed breast reconstruction.[1]
  ■ This RCT was subject to high bias, and no conclusion could be made.
■ In general, immediate reconstruction provides better aesthetic outcomes due to preservation of the native skin envelope.[3]
  ■ This allows for a more rapid expansion to desired volume and better control of breast shape and ptosis.
■ Immediate reconstruction may also reduce the psychological burden of patients living with the disease, thus decreasing anxiety and depression while improving self-esteem.[2]
■ Delayed reconstruction allows for mastectomy skin flaps to heal before implant placement, thus decreasing the risk of infection and seroma formation.[3]
■ A recent retrospective study suggested that delayed reconstruction was associated with decreasing operative and non-operative complications relative to immediate reconstruction.[3]

COMPLICATIONS

Bleeding or Hematoma

■ Hematomas around the tissue expander increase the risk of infection and predispose to the development of capsular contracture.
■ If a hematoma of significant size is recognized, it should be promptly evacuated.
■ Drains do not prevent hematomas but may be useful indicators of excessive bleeding after surgery.

Infection

■ May present early or late and in the form of cellulitis or periprosthetic infection.
■ Uncomplicated mastectomy skin cellulitis can be treated with a trial of intravenous antibiotics or, occasionally, oral antibiotics.
■ If cellulitis fails to resolve with antibiotic therapy, or the infection worsens (eg, patient develops sepsis or skin breakdown), then the TE is removed, drains are placed, and the patient is given an appropriate course of antibiotics.
■ Signs of systemic illness related to a periprosthetic infection indicate the need for prompt implant removal.

Mastectomy Skin Necrosis

■ Superficial or partial-thickness flap necrosis is managed conservatively with local wound care.
■ Small areas of full-thickness necrosis may also be managed with local wound care if there is muscle or other vascularized tissue deep to the skin that will allow secondary healing.
  ■ When ADM becomes exposed, salvage becomes much more challenging.
■ Larger areas of mastectomy skin flap necrosis require resection of the necrotic skin with immediate wound closure.
  ■ Should consider removing fluid from the TE to allow for tension-free closure of the mastectomy skin.
  ■ If skin defect is too large, the device may require removal and possibly skin grafting over the *pectoralis major* muscle.
  ■ Secondary attempts at reconstruction may require autologous tissue flaps if the chest skin cannot be expanded.

REFERENCES

1. D'Souza N, Darmanin G, Fedorowicz Z. Immediate versus delayed reconstruction following surgery for breast cancer (Review). *Cochrane Database Syst Rev.* 2011;(7):CD008674.
2. Fernandez-Delgado J, Lopez-Pedraza MJ, Blasco JA, et al. Satisfaction with and psychological impact of immediate and deferred breast reconstruction. *Ann Oncol.* 2008;19(8):1430-1434.
3. Seth AK, Silver HR, Hirsch EM, et al. Comparison of delayed and immediate tissue expander breast reconstruction in the setting of postmastectomy radiation therapy. *Ann Plast Surg.* 2015;75(5):503-507.

14
CHAPTER

Tissue Expander With Acellular Dermal Matrix

Gabriel M. Kind

DEFINITION

- Two-stage tissue expander-to-implant reconstruction with prosthetic implants is the most common type of breast reconstruction in the United States.[1,2]
- The use of acellular dermal matrix (ADM), originally described for direct-to-implant reconstruction,[3,4] has become increasingly common in two-stage procedures as well.[5-7]
- The potential benefits of this technique include more precise recreation of the inframammary fold (IMF), control of the pectoralis major muscle, reduced risk of implant palpability, reduction in capsular contracture rates, and a larger initial expander volume (and consequently fewer office visits for tissue expansion), with less dissection of the chest wall musculature when compared to total muscle coverage of the tissue expander (TE).
  - All of these potential benefits would presumably improve aesthetic results and, at least for the latter benefit, result in less morbidity.
- Recently, there have been reports describing the placement of implants wrapped with dermal allograft in the prepectoral position.
  - This technique has the potential to decrease the incidence of some of the muscle-related complications associated with subpectoral placement, namely, pain associated with manipulation of the muscle at the initial surgery, discomfort associated with pectoralis major flexion postoperatively, and the animation deformity seen in some patients with flexion of the pectoralis major muscle.[8]

ANATOMY

- The pectoralis major muscle has sternocostal, costal, and abdominal origins and inserts on to the proximal humerus. It is a type V muscle, with a dominant arterial pedicle from the thoracoacromial trunk and multiple secondary arterial sources from parasternal perforators.

PATHOGENESIS

- Breast cancer occurs in approximately 12% of women in the United States. It is estimated that nearly 250 000 new cases of invasive breast cancer will be diagnosed in 2016, along with 61 000 cases of in situ disease.
- Although there are significant regional differences, mastectomy is performed in approximately 35% of those newly diagnosed, and approximately 35% of those women undergo breast reconstruction.
- The rate of breast reconstruction has risen steadily, from 11.6% in 1998 to 36.4% in 2011.[9]
- In 2014, of the 102 215 breast reconstructions performed in the United States, 74 694 (73%) used a TE and implant.[2]

PATIENT HISTORY AND PHYSICAL FINDINGS

- The use of dermal allograft for soft tissue support at the time of mastectomy is an intraoperative decision based on several factors, including the thickness of the mastectomy skin flaps, the anatomy of the pectoralis major muscle, and the desired initial volume of the TE.
- If ADM is not used, either a total submuscular pocket is created or partial muscle coverage of the expander is accepted.

IMAGING

- Not indicated or necessary

SURGICAL MANAGEMENT

Preoperative Planning

- The footprint of the breast is measured. The height and width of the breast are used to determine which TE to order. Usually two or three differently sized expanders are ordered for each case.
- If mastectomy has already been performed, the pectoralis major muscle function is assessed. Rarely, a paralytic or atretic muscle is identified preoperatively. In such cases, a larger piece of ADM may be necessary.

Positioning

- The patient is placed supine with both arms abducted and secured on well-padded arm boards or tucked depending upon surgeon preference.

Approach

- There are a number of different incisions used for mastectomy. TE insertion can be performed via any of the incisions used.
- In nipple-sparing procedures, care should be taken to avoid handling of the nipple to decrease the chance of contamination. Adhesive plastic drapes can be placed for this purpose.

■ Subpectoral Tissue Expander Placement With Dermal Allograft

Markings

- The footprint of the breast, including the IMF, is marked with the patient standing and again under anesthesia.
- Once the mastectomy is completed, hemostasis is confirmed.

Creation of Subpectoral Pocket

- The pectoralis major muscle is elevated to create a subpectoral pocket across the footprint of the breast (**TECH FIG 1**). The sternocostal origin is released as necessary.
  - There is significant variability in the location of the origin of the pectoralis major muscle.
  - Muscle attachments are preserved wherever possible. This will reduce the size of the ADM required.

Preparation and Suturing of Dermal Allograft

- A sheet of dermal allograft is prepared by irrigating it with normal saline followed by antibiotic solution. ADM is provided in various sizes.
  - Generally 4 to 8 cm × 14 to 18 cm sheets are used; more recently shaped pieces have become available.
  - Prefenestrated ADM is used, or fenestrations are cut into the ADM, to encourage revascularization.
  - The use of thick or thin ADM also depends upon the preference of the surgeon.
- Care is taken to place the dermal (shiny) side of the ADM facing the undersurface of the mastectomy flaps.
- The dermal allograft is sutured to the chest wall along the desired position of the IMF.
  - I prefer running absorbable barbed suture (2-0 PDO Quill) for this, although other suture types have been described, perhaps most commonly some type of an absorbable suture is used.

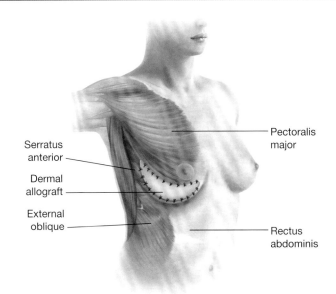

Serratus anterior —
Dermal allograft —
External oblique —
Pectoralis major
Rectus abdominis

TECH FIG 2 • The dermal allograft is secured to the IMF. The ADM is secured along the IMF to a point equal or superior to the vertical midpoint of the breast.

  - The lateral extent of the ADM-IMF suture line should be at least to a point equal to the vertical midpoint of the breast.
  - Patients with thin mastectomy flaps may benefit from continuing the ADM further superolaterally, but this may tether the pectoralis major and is generally not required (**TECH FIG 2**).

Preparation and Placement of Tissue Expander

- A TE is selected based on the width of the breast footprint, the weight of the mastectomy specimen, and the patient's desired size.

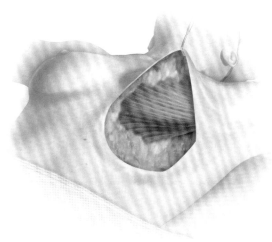

A

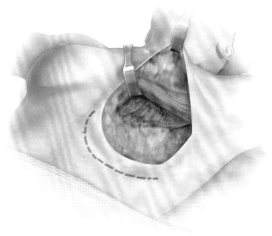

B

TECH FIG 1 • **A,B.** The pectoralis major muscle is elevated across the footprint of the breast.

- The TE is prepared by removing the air and inserting 50 to 100 mL of saline.
  - Some prefer methylene blue–tinted saline, whereas others prefer to fill the expander with air.
- The TE is placed in the wound and secured in place using 2-0 PDS suture if suture tabs are utilized. For expanders without tabs, precise pocket formation will limit movement of the expander.
- The ADM is trimmed to fit the defect in the inferolateral aspect of the subpectoral pocket.
- The upper border of the ADM is sutured to the lower border of the pectoralis major muscle (**TECH FIG 3**).
- Additional saline is injected into the TE.
  - In a total skin and nipple-sparing mastectomy, the expander is filled to approximately 50% of its capacity.
  - In non–nipple-sparing mastectomies, the final volume is determined by the limitation of the skin flaps.

Closure

- Closed suction drains are placed through stab incisions in the lateral chest wall.
  - For larger breasts and cases where axillary dissection is performed, two drains are used. For smaller breasts, one drain is used.

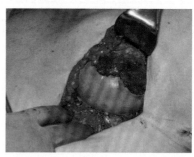

TECH FIG 3 • Typical appearance of ADM secured to the chest wall inferiorly and the pectoralis major muscle superiorly.

- The mastectomy flaps are debrided of nonviable skin and closed in layers.
  - Usually, 2-0 Vicryl is used in the deep tissues followed by 3-0 and 4-0 Monocryl in the skin.
  - The incision is dressed with dermal glue and a sterile dressing.
  - The chest is wrapped with an Ace wrap.

■ Prepectoral Tissue Expander Placement With Dermal Allograft

- As in the subpectoral technique, markings are made of the breast footprint and IMF, and following mastectomy, hemostasis is confirmed.
- The prepectoral technique is not recommended in patients with excessively thin or poorly vascularized flaps.
- A large sheet of dermal allograft (16 × 20 cm) is secured across the chest wall, several centimeters superior to the desired position of the IMF.
- The ADM is draped inferiorly and sutured to the chest wall slightly inferior to the desired position of the IMF.
- The TE is placed, and the ADM is folded over the tissue expander and then secured superiorly to the chest wall.
- The ADM is trimmed to the shape of the expander and then secured medially and laterally to the chest wall (**TECH FIG 4**).

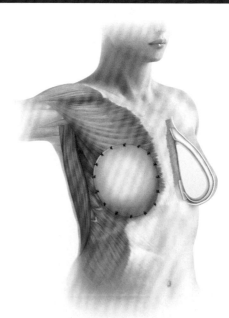

TECH FIG 4 • Dermal allograft secured to the chest wall with the implant in the prepectoral position.

PEARLS AND PITFALLS

Symmetry of the IMF	▪ Begins with symmetrical skin markings. In a bilateral case, leaving the first side open after placing the TE and ADM allows for visual confirmation of symmetrical placement of the TE and ADM along the IMF on the second side.
Symmetry of tissue expander placement	▪ The patient can be brought to a sitting position after inserting the TE(s) to confirm adequate symmetry.
Proper placement of the tissue expander	▪ Care must be taken to place the TE in the appropriate location and orientation. It is common to leave it too far superior and/or lateral on the chest wall.
Inset of the ADM	▪ The ADM should be trimmed so that there are no folds or corners. If there is a palpable fold, it should be excised and closed (similar to a "dog-ear" excision). Redundancy of the ADM should be minimized. This can sometimes be accomplished by filling the expander. If the muscle or skin does not permit enough filling to eliminate significant redundancy, the ADM needs to be trimmed further.
Seroma management	▪ Seromas can be safely aspirated superficial to the expander port. Tissue expansion can proceed as scheduled during seroma aspiration. Oral antibiotics should be considered if a seroma requires multiple aspirations.

POSTOPERATIVE CARE

- Oral antibiotics are continued until drains are removed.
- Drains are removed when the output is less than 30 mL/24 hours for 2 consecutive days.
- Tissue expansion is usually started 2 to 3 weeks postoperatively.
- Expansion volume can vary but typically ranges from 30 to 120 cc per fill.
- Overexpansion is avoided, as that can lead to a more redundant pocket and more visible rippling.

OUTCOMES

- Many of the benefits of ADM use in breast reconstruction are subjective and surgeon dependent. Several authors have reported favorable aesthetic outcomes.[3–6]
- With regard to more objective measures of outcomes, there are multiple retrospective series that report increased TE fill at the time of mastectomy plus TE/ADM and fewer postoperative visits for expansion.[4,10–14]
- There are several retrospective series that report diminished pain with ADM use.[4,5,15]
- There are several reports of an absence of capsular contracture in breasts reconstructed with ADM, with follow-up times ranging from 6.5 to 52 months.[3–5,16] This compares favorably with reported rates of capsular contracture as high as 14% in patients undergoing reconstruction without ADM.[17]
- There are also published data showing lower rates of capsular contracture in radiated breasts reconstructed with TE/ADM compared to historical controls.[13,18,19]
- Published reports describing prepectoral reconstruction with ADM are encouraging, but preliminary, as there is only short-term follow-up available at this time. A large series reports low complication rates at 6 to 26 months but gives no data regarding aesthetic results or pain compared to the subpectoral approach.[8]
- Questions remain regarding the role of fat grafting to mask rippling and the visibility of the upper pole of the implant, as well as the long-term complication rates using the prepectoral technique.

COMPLICATIONS

- Complications associated with ADM use in breast reconstruction are similar to those reconstructed without ADM. Published series comparing ADM use with TE reconstruction generally do not show statistically relevant differences in overall complication rates.
- The overall complication rates for reconstructions using ADM range from 3% to 49%.[20–23] Two studies show statistically significant higher incidences of seroma,[12,21] but several other studies do not show an increased rate of seroma with ADM use.[13,14,22,24] A recent review showed that the use of dermal allograft has a pooled relative risk of seroma of 1.85.[25]
- Mastectomy flap necrosis was shown in two reports to be higher in patients undergoing TE/ADM reconstruction.[14,21] However, in both series, there was a higher TE volume, which is known to cause a higher rate of mastectomy skin necrosis.
  - Caution should be taken when filling TEs at the time of mastectomy, as increased TE volume has been shown to correlate with mastectomy skin necrosis, with or without the use of ADM.
- There are multiple conflicting reports regarding the use of ADM and infection, with authors concluding both an increased risk and no increased risk of infection. Meta-analyses have shown increased relative risk of infection with ADM use in breast reconstruction of 2.47 and 2.7.[26,27]

REFERENCES

1. Albornoz CR, Bach PB, Mehrara BJ, et al. A paradigm shift in U.S. breast reconstruction: increasing implant rates. *Plast Reconstr Surg.* 2013;131:1,15-23.
2. American Society of Plastic Surgeons. *National Clearinghouse of Plastic Surgery Procedural Statistics.* 2014 Plastic Surgery Statistics Report. Available at http://www.plasticsurgery.org/Documents/news-resources/statistics/2014-statistics/plastic-surgery-statsitics-full-report.pdf
3. Breuing KH, Warren SM. Immediate bilateral breast reconstruction with implants and inferolateral AlloDerm slings. *Ann Plast Surg.* 2005;55:232-239.
4. Salzberg CA. Nonexpansive immediate breast reconstruction using human acellular tissue matrix graft (AlloDerm). *Ann Plast Surg.* 2006;57:1-5.

5. Bindingnavele V, Gaon M, Ota KS, et al. Use of acellular cadaveric dermis and tissue expansion in postmastectomy breast reconstruction. *J Plast Reconstr Aesthet Surg.* 2007;60(11):1214-1218.

6. Spear SL, Parikh PM, Reisin E, Menon NG. Acellular dermis-assisted breast reconstruction. *Aesthetic Plast Surg.* 2008;32(3):418-425.

7. Sbitany H, Serletti JM. Acellular dermis–assisted prosthetic breast reconstruction: a systematic and critical review of efficacy and associated morbidity. *Plast Reconstr Surg.* 2011;128(6):1162-1169.

8. Sigalove S, Maxwell GP, Sigalove NM, et al. Prepectoral implant-based breast reconstruction: rationale, indications, and preliminary results. *Plast Reconstr Surg.* 2017;139:287-294.

9. Kummerow KL, Du L, Penson DF, et al. Nationwide trends in mastectomy for early-stage breast cancer. *JAMA Surg.* 2015;150(1):9-16.

10. Sbitany H, Sandeen SN, Amalfi AN, et al. Acellular dermis assisted prosthetic breast reconstruction versus complete submuscular coverage: a head-to-head comparison of outcomes. *Plast Reconstr Surg.* 2009;124(6):735-1740.

11. Zienowicz RJ, Karacaoglu E. Implant-based breast reconstruction with allograft. *Plast Reconstr Surg.* 2007;120(2):373-381.

12. Parks JR, Hammond SE, Walsh WW, et al. Human acellular dermis (ACD) vs. No-ACD in tissue expansion breast reconstruction. *Plast Reconstr Surg.* 2012;130(4):739-746.

13. Seth AK, Hirsch EM, Fine NA, Kim JY. Utility of acellular dermis-assisted breast reconstruction in the setting of radiation: a comparative analysis. *Plast Reconstr Surg.* 2012;130(4):750-758.

14. Weichman KE, Wilson SC, Weinstein AL, et al. The use of acellular dermal matrix in immediate two-stage tissue expander breast reconstruction. *Plast Reconstr Surg.* 2012;129(5):1049-1058.

15. Namnoum JD. Expander/implant reconstruction with AlloDerm: recent experience. *Plast Reconstr Surg.* 2009;124(2):387-394.

16. Baxter RA. Intracapsular allogenic dermal grafts for breast implant-related problems. *Plast Reconstr Surg.* 2003;112(6):1692-1696.

17. Spear SL, Newman MK, Bedford MS, et al. A retrospective analysis of outcomes using three common methods for immediate breast reconstruction. *Plast Reconstr Surg.* 2008;122(2):340-347.

18. Spear SL, Seruya M, Rao SS, et al. Two-stage prosthetic breast reconstruction using AlloDerm including outcomes of different timings of radiotherapy. *Plast Reconstr Surg.* 2012;130(1):1-9.

19. Breuing KH, Colwell AS. Immediate breast tissue expander-implant reconstruction with inferolateral AlloDerm hammock and postoperative radiation: a preliminary report. *Eplasty.* 2009;9:e16.

20. Rawlani V, Buck DW II, Johnson SA, et al. Tissue expander breast reconstruction using prehydrated human acellular dermis. *Ann Plast Surg.* 2011;66(6):593-597.

21. Chun YS, Verma K, Rosen H, et al. Implant-based breast reconstruction using acellular dermal matrix and the risk of postoperative complications. *Plast Reconstr Surg.* 2010;125(2):429-436.

22. Antony AK, McCarthy CM, Cordeiro PG, et al. Acellular human dermis implantation in 153 immediate two-stage tissue expander breast reconstructions: determining the incidence and significant predictors of complications. *Plast Reconstr Surg.* 2010;125(6):1606-1614.

23. Losken A. Early results using sterilized acellular human dermis (Neoform) in post-mastectomy tissue expander breast reconstruction. *Plast Reconstr Surg.* 2009;123(6):1654-1658.

24. Vardanian AJ, Clayton JL, Roostaeian J, et al. Comparison of implant-based immediate breast reconstruction with and without acellular dermal matrix. *Plast Reconstr Surg.* 2011;128(5):403e-410e.

25. Jordan SW, Khavanin N, Kim JY. Seroma in prosthetic breast reconstruction. *Plast Reconstr Surg.* 2016;137(4):1104-1116.

26. Kim JYS, Davila AA, Persing S, et al. A meta-analysis of human acellular dermis and submuscular tissue expander breast reconstruction. *Plast Reconstr Surg.* 2012;129:1.

27. Ho G, Nguyen TJ, Shahabi A, et al. A systematic review and meta-analysis of complications associated with acellular dermal matrix-assisted breast reconstruction. *Ann Plast Surg.* 2012;68:4,346-356.

Immediate Tissue Expander

Eric G. Halvorson and Joseph J. Disa

DEFINITION

- Immediate tissue expander placement is performed following skin-sparing or nipple-sparing mastectomy as a prelude to either two-stage implant reconstruction or "delayed-immediate" autologous reconstruction.
- The advantages of expander placement (compared to immediate autologous reconstruction) include shorter operation, lack of donor site, shorter hospital stay, shorter recovery, ability to adjust final volume, and a "perkier" result.
- The disadvantages of expander placement include multiple postoperative office visits for expansions, discomfort associated with the expansion process, a second (albeit outpatient) surgery if proceeding with two-stage implant reconstruction, and the permanent risks of implants (capsular contracture, rupture, rotation, rippling, infection, malposition, and exposure).

PATIENT HISTORY AND PHYSICAL FINDINGS

- It is beneficial for the initial consultation to occur separate from multidisciplinary clinic visits focused on cancer care. Patients presenting to the plastic surgeon after such visits are often overloaded with information and overwhelmed by all the options and information related to reconstruction.
- It is critical to determine the patient's goals for reconstruction and to ascertain their preferences with respect to breast size, breast shape, willingness to accept surgical risk, willingness to accept donor-site morbidity, operative length, hospital stay, recovery process, postoperative follow-up protocol, secondary surgeries, and long-term complications.
- Having a physician extender well versed in reconstructive options to meet with patients and show them patient photographs is an incredibly helpful prelude to the physician-patient consultation.
- Physical examination of the breasts is performed to evaluate any masses and whether or not skin involvement or peau d'orange is present. The overall size and degree of ptosis are noted.
  - Patients with skin involvement or significant ptosis will typically require skin excision. If performed as an inverted "T" or Wise pattern, the risk of mastectomy flap necrosis is increased.
  - Alternatively, one can perform a generous horizontal, oblique, or vertical ellipse or two-stage Wise pattern excision with the vertical closure first and a horizontal excision at the inframammary fold (IMF) 3 to 6 months later.
- The breast width, height, and projection are measured in centimeters. These measurements are used for selecting a tissue expander (as described in the following text).

SURGICAL MANAGEMENT

- Ideal candidates for expander placement are thin nonsmokers undergoing bilateral mastectomy who have not, and will not, receive radiotherapy.
  - Smokers are prone to mastectomy flap necrosis and infection.
  - Radiotherapy increases the risk of infection, implant exposure, and capsular contracture.
  - Previously radiated skin will not expand well.
- Although obesity increases the risk of complication for any type of reconstruction, heavier patients tend to have better cosmetic results with autologous reconstruction than with implants, as it can be difficult to match the opposite breast after a unilateral mastectomy or give adequate volume/ptosis after a bilateral mastectomy.
- Patients with very large breasts who require skin removal during mastectomy are at risk for mastectomy flap necrosis and tend to require secondary procedures to address residual excess skin. These patients often have ample donor sites for autologous reconstruction, which may be a better option.
- Patients with small breasts who want them to be larger can achieve that goal through expansion.
- Patients who have minimal ptosis and want their breasts to be slightly smaller are candidates for single-stage implant reconstruction.
- Using a tissue expander as a bridge to autologous reconstruction, so-called delayed-immediate reconstruction, is considered when the patient is likely to receive postoperative radiation therapy, as radiating autologous flaps can result in fat necrosis, firmness, and shrinkage.
  - A minority of surgeons prefer to accept the risks of radiating an autologous flap when compared to the risks of performing delayed reconstruction in a radiated field.
  - Other reasons to consider delayed-immediate reconstruction are to gain control of the skin envelope, to expedite surgery and adjuvant therapy, and to modify risk factors (smoking, obesity) and when patients are undecided.

Preoperative Planning and Implant Selection

- Good communication with the breast surgeon is important to ensure oncologic goals are maintained and that reconstruction is appropriately staged.
- Patients with advanced disease, requirement for immediate postoperative adjuvant therapy, unstable social environment, and/or uncertainty regarding goals for reconstruction may be better served by delayed reconstruction.
- Prior to mastectomy, the patient must be marked in the standing position. The IMF is marked on each side, and the midline is drawn between the sternal notch and xiphoid process. The overall outline of the breasts is marked.

- Although a transverse ellipse around the nipple-areolar complex (NAC) is commonly used for the mastectomy incision, the authors' preference is an oblique ellipse parallel to the pectoralis major fibers (**FIG 1**). This renders the medial scar less visible in clothing, allows for better subincisional muscular coverage, and facilitates a stair-step approach during the exchange procedure (as described in the following chapter).

- Tissue expanders are selected preoperatively based on the width of the patient's breast. There are many different tissue expanders to choose from, but most are textured and anatomic, providing lower pole projection.
  - Some are taller than they are wide, some are wider than they are tall, and some are semicircular or crescentic and focus on lower pole expansion.
  - Some have tabs to secure the expander.
  - Most have integrated metal ports that are located with magnets, although a remote port is useful when placing the expander under a thick flap (such as a latissimus dorsi flap in an obese patient). In such patients, finding the port with a magnet can be difficult and a longer needle is required, placing the expander at risk for rupture.

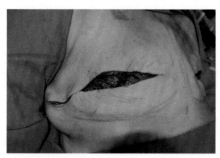

FIG 1 • An oblique mastectomy incision is used. (From: Halvorson EG. Two-stage implant breast reconstruction. In: Mulholland MW, ed. *Operative Techniques in Surgery*. Vol. 2. Philadelphia, PA: Wolters Kluwer, 2000.)

Positioning

- Patients are placed in the supine position under a general anesthetic with arms padded circumferentially and abducted at 80 to 90 degrees.
- Following mastectomy, the patient is positioned such that the sternum is parallel to the floor (via head elevation or reverse Trendelenburg).

■ Tissue Expander Placement

First Step—Wound Assessment

- Following mastectomy, the wounds are irrigated and hemostasis is obtained.
- The mastectomy flaps are evaluated by examining their thickness and assessing color and capillary refill.
- Areas where dermis is exposed internally should be carefully evaluated externally.
- Areas where the external skin is pale without capillary refill should be excised.
- Laser-assisted indocyanine green fluoroscopy has been promoted to assess mastectomy flap perfusion; however, guidelines for its use and interpretation have not been firmly established.[1]
- Use of tumescent solution by the extirpative surgeon makes assessment of mastectomy flaps difficult and has been shown in some studies to be associated with a higher rate of mastectomy flap necrosis.[2–4]
- When there is significant concern for mastectomy flap necrosis, or if debridement of questionable tissue will lead to closure under tension or an open wound, then aborting reconstruction is strongly advised.
- If necessary, the IMF can be recreated with interrupted suture; however, the position of the inferior edge of the expander will ultimately determine the IMF, which can be adjusted further during an exchange procedure if desired.
  - Some surgeons try to establish the native IMF during this initial procedure (which may make the exchange procedure simpler), whereas others intentionally place the expander lower than the IMF to increase lower pole expansion and projection (which requires recreation of the IMF with suture during the exchange procedure).

- The author's preference is to preserve the native IMF when performing single-stage implant reconstruction, when placing a significant initial fill volume in the expander, or when the IMF is already low.
- When performing delayed two-stage implant reconstruction or when placing minimal initial fill volume in the expander, placing the implant below the IMF will preferentially expand the lower pole and permit the surgeon to create minimal ptosis at the exchange procedure (as described in the following chapter).
- Another reason to consider placing the expander lower than the native IMF is when adjuvant radiotherapy is expected. Radiotherapy almost always causes fibrosis and contracture of the pectoralis major and soft tissue surrounding the implant, with superior migration of the expander.

Second Step—Creation of Implant Pocket

- The tissue expander cannot be covered by the mastectomy flaps alone, which are thin and offer poor soft tissue coverage. Ideally, the surgeon should provide complete musculofascial coverage with the pectoralis major and serratus anterior muscles (**TECH FIG 1A**) or use an acellular dermal allograft (ADM) or other product in addition to the pectoralis major muscle.
  - An emerging technique is to use complete acellular dermal matrix (ADM) coverage with adjuvant fat grafting at the time of implant exchange, which is beyond the scope of this chapter.
- The lateral edge of the pectoralis major muscle is pinched between the surgeon's index finger and thumb and pulled away from the chest, revealing a loose areolar plane between the pectoralis major and minor muscles. Dissection in this plane commences with Bovie cautery, but once the

subpectoral space is entered, much of the superior and medial implant pocket can be created via blunt digital dissection before using lighted retractors for direct visualization.

- A lighted retractor is quite helpful to finish medial dissection, as great care must be taken to ligate or cauterize the intercostal perforators (**TECH FIG 1B,C**).
- The medial boundary is defined externally by the preoperative markings that define the patient's native breast form. Internally, it is quite common to release the medial and inferomedial origins of the pectoralis major muscle. It is important not to release this area excessively, as symmastia can result and is difficult to correct.
- After the subpectoral plane is developed, the inferior insertion of the pectoralis major muscle is examined (**TECH FIG 1D**).

- If the patient's muscle reaches the IMF, then a submuscular pocket can be created down to the IMF with supple and adequate soft tissue coverage that will respond well to expansion (**TECH FIG 1E**).
- More commonly, however, the pectoralis major inserts above the IMF. In this scenario, to provide autologous implant coverage inferiorly, one must continue dissection past the pectoralis major insertion and under the anterior rectus sheath until just below the IMF.
- Transitioning from the subpectoral plane to underneath the anterior rectus sheath is sometimes technically difficult and may result in a few gaps in coverage that can be closed after the pocket is fully created. A lighted retractor is necessary for this portion of the procedure.

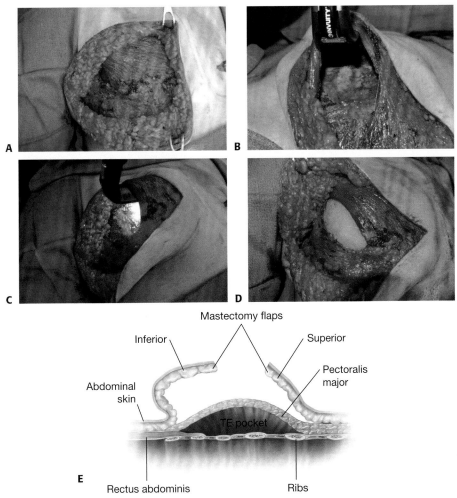

TECH FIG 1 • A. Following mastectomy, the pectoralis major and serratus anterior muscles are visualized as these are the muscles used for expander coverage. If these muscles have been affected by mastectomy, using an ADM in their place is considered. (From: Halvorson EG. Two-stage implant breast reconstruction. In: Mulholland MW, ed. *Operative Techniques in Surgery*. Vol. 2. Philadelphia, PA: Wolters Kluwer, 2000.) **B, C.** A lighted retractor is very helpful for both expander placement and the implant exchange procedure. Here, the lighted retractor is shown during creation of the subpectoral pocket superomedially, where dissection proceeds carefully so intercostal perforators can be visualized and carefully ligated if necessary. (From: Halvorson EG. Two-stage implant breast reconstruction. In: Mulholland MW, ed. *Operative Techniques in Surgery*. Vol. 2. Philadelphia, PA: Wolters Kluwer, 2000.) **D.** The relationship between the most caudal extent of the pectoralis major muscle and the IMF determines whether or not the anterior rectus sheath will be necessary to provide complete submusculofascial coverage of the expander. If the muscle originates at or below the IMF, as shown in this figure, then there is no need to elevate the anterior rectus sheath. (From: Halvorson EG. Two-stage implant breast reconstruction. In: Mulholland MW, ed. *Operative Techniques in Surgery*. Vol. 2. Philadelphia, PA: Wolters Kluwer, 2000.) **E.** Schematic diagram patient anatomy when the pectoralis major originates at or below the IMF. In this case, a submuscular pocket can be created down to the IMF that will be supple and respond well to expansion. TE, tissue expander. (From: Halvorson EG. Two-stage implant breast reconstruction. In: Mulholland MW, ed. *Operative Techniques in Surgery*. Vol. 2. Philadelphia, PA: Wolters Kluwer, 2000.)

TECHNIQUES

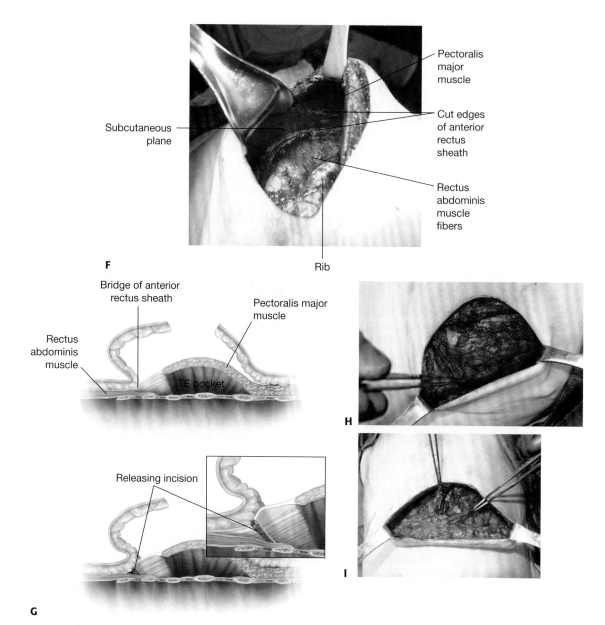

TECH FIG 1 (Continued) • **F.** At or just below the IMF, the anterior rectus sheath is divided horizontally to enter the subcutaneous plane. If this is not performed, lower pole expansion will be limited by the stiff anterior rectus sheath. (From: Halvorson EG. Two-stage implant breast reconstruction. In: Mulholland MW, ed. *Operative Techniques in Surgery*. Vol. 2. Philadelphia, PA: Wolters Kluwer, 2000.) **G.** Schematic diagram patient anatomy when the pectoralis major muscle originates above the IMF. In this case, the gap between the caudal border of the pectoralis and IMF must be bridged by elevating the anterior rectus sheath. At or just below the IMF, the sheath must be incised horizontally to enter the subcutaneous space; otherwise, the inferior pocket will not expand well. Alternatively, an ADM can be used to bridge this gap. TE, tissue expander. (From: Halvorson EG. Two-stage implant breast reconstruction. In: Mulholland MW, ed. *Operative Techniques in Surgery*. Vol. 2. Philadelphia, PA: Wolters Kluwer, 2000.) **H.** For lateral and inferolateral coverage, a partial-thickness serratus anterior muscle flap is elevated and shown in this photograph. If the fascia is robust and intact, that can be used alone; however, this is seldom the case. An incision in the muscle parallel to the inferolateral edge of the pectoralis major muscle is made and the flap is elevated laterally until the anterior axillary line or sufficiently to create the desired pocket width for the chosen expander. (From: Halvorson EG. Two-stage implant breast reconstruction. In: Mulholland MW, ed. *Operative Techniques in Surgery*. Vol. 2. Philadelphia, PA: Wolters Kluwer, 2000.) **I.** Following elevation of the serratus anterior muscle, the inferolateral aspect of the implant pocket will still be adherent to the chest wall. If retractors are placed under the pectoralis major and serratus anterior muscles, this area of adhesion will be exposed and inferolateral dissection will elevate the serratus anterior and external oblique muscles off the chest wall to complete implant pocket dissection. (From: Halvorson EG. Two-stage implant breast reconstruction. In: Mulholland MW, ed. *Operative Techniques in Surgery*. Vol. 2. Philadelphia, PA: Wolters Kluwer, 2000.)

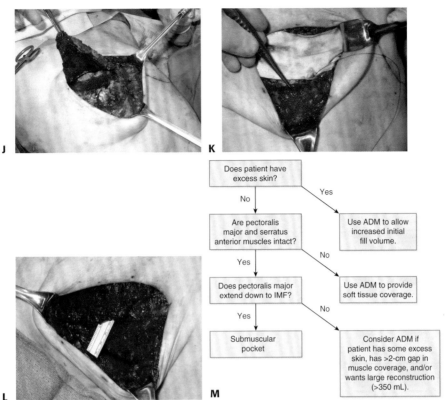

TECH FIG 1 (Continued) • **J.** If an ADM is used, the pectoralis major muscle is elevated from the chest wall by dividing its inferior and infero-medial origin. (From: Halvorson EG. Two-stage implant breast reconstruction. In: Mulholland MW, ed. *Operative Techniques in Surgery*. Vol. 2. Philadelphia, PA: Wolters Kluwer, 2000.) **K.** A piece of ADM is prepared appropriately, according to the manufacturer's recommendations, and is sewn in with the epidermis side facing the implant. A 6- × 16-cm piece is usually sufficient. The inferomedial and inferolateral corners of the ADM are trimmed to create a curved inferior border, and it is secured to the IMF and lateral pocket using a running 2-0 monofilament slowly absorbing suture. The transition from the IMF to the lateral pocket must be a gentle arc that mimics the opposite side. (From: Halvorson EG. Two-stage implant breast reconstruction. In: Mulholland MW, ed. *Operative Techniques in Surgery*. Vol. 2. Philadelphia, PA: Wolters Kluwer, 2000.) **L.** A ruler is used to measure the width of the surgically created pocket. The proper pocket width can be determined by either patient anatomy (eg, the anterior axillary line) or the dimensions of the expander desired. (From: Halvorson EG. Two-stage implant breast reconstruction. In: Mulholland MW, ed. *Operative Techniques in Surgery*. Vol. 2. Philadelphia, PA: Wolters Kluwer, 2000.) **M.** Algorithm to determine when to use ADM. IMF, inframammary fold. (From: Halvorson EG. Two-stage implant breast reconstruction. In: Mulholland MW, ed. *Operative Techniques in Surgery*. Vol. 2. Philadelphia, PA: Wolters Kluwer, 2000.)

- The anterior rectus sheath is quite stiff and will not expand well unless an incision is made transversely across the sheath just below the IMF, entering the subcutaneous plane (**TECH FIG 1F,G**).
  - If the anterior rectus sheath is released above the IMF, one would obviously enter the implant pocket. The goal is to provide complete and supple submusculofascial coverage without gap between the pectoralis major and the IMF.
  - Alternatively, the pectoralis major can be released from the chest wall and a piece of ADM (or other product) can be sewn to the IMF inferiorly using a running 2-0 absorbable braided suture.
- Following creation of a subpectoral pocket with or without elevation of the anterior rectus sheath, inferolateral coverage must be provided.
  - Autologous coverage is provided by elevating the serratus anterior fascia if robust, or more commonly a partial-thickness muscle flap if the fascia is thin or traumatized from the mastectomy.

- An incision in the serratus anterior is made at the level of, and parallel to, the inferolateral edge of the pectoralis major muscle, and a fascial or musculofascial flap is elevated to the anterior axillary line (**TECH FIG 1H**).
- Alternatively, one can determine the width of the implant pocket based on the width of the desired tissue expander and stop lateral dissection when a sufficient pocket width is achieved (usually 1 cm wider than tissue expander).
- At this point, the inferior and lateral dissections will be complete, but the inferior serratus and superolateral external oblique muscles will still be attached to the chest wall. By retracting inferiorly and laterally, this plane is exposed and the muscles can be elevated off the chest wall to open the inferolateral pocket (**TECH FIG 1I**).
- If an ADM is used, the origin of the pectoralis major is taken down starting inferolaterally and extending medially and then superiorly along the sternal origin to approximately the 4th rib (**TECH FIG 1J**).

- The ADM will provide inferolateral implant coverage, and there is no need to elevate the serratus anterior. In this case, the IMF and anterior axillary line are marked internally and the ADM is sutured along a line that transitions in an arc from the IMF to the anterior axillary line using a running 2-0 absorbable braided suture (**TECH FIG 1K**).
- Alternatively, one can mark the lateral mammary fold based on the width of the desired tissue expander and suture the ADM to this line (**TECH FIG 1L**).
- One can tailor the surgically created IMF to match the contralateral native IMF during unilateral reconstruction. If performing bilateral reconstruction, then it is imperative to create symmetric IMFs.
- The advantages of using an ADM are that it avoids any morbidity associated with elevation of the rectus sheath and serratus anterior, it allows for a greater initial fill volume (and thus fewer postoperative expansions), it allows precise control of the IMF, it may reduce operative time, and it may preserve lower pole fullness.
- Disadvantages include cost and an increased incidence of seroma, infection, and reconstructive failure in patients with risk factors such as obesity, smoking, and/or radiation.[5]
- Although some surgeons use an ADM routinely and others do not, the author's preference is to use ADM selectively (**TECH FIG 1M**).
- If the pectoralis major muscle extends to the IMF and the patient does not desire a large breast reconstruction, then complete submusculofascial coverage is performed. In most other cases, ADM is utilized unless the patient has significant risk factors (obesity, radiation, tobacco use).

Third Step—Preparation of Tissue Expander

- Intraoperatively, a ruler is used to measure the width of the surgically created implant pocket, which ultimately determines the expander to be used. Alternatively, one can create a pocket wide enough to accommodate the desired expander.
- The authors' preference is to measure the surgically created pocket based on native patient anatomy and choose an expander that is 1 cm narrower in width (the expander is always wider than its base when expanded).
- Tissue expanders come with air in them to prevent the inner shell from sticking to itself. There are usually markings for orientation, but it is helpful to draw a vertical line on the expander with a marking pen to assist with positioning the expander in the pocket.
- A needle (usually 23 gauge) is inserted into the port, and all air is removed.
  - The most commonly used tissue expanders are anatomic (creating lower pole expansion), and thus, they are textured (to prevent rotation). There is typically more shell inferiorly, and while deflating the expander, it is important to fold excess shell inward as opposed to folding it upward and on to itself, where it might cover the port and get punctured (**TECH FIG 2**).
- The authors' preference is to place 60 to 180 mL of sterile saline in the tissue expander prior to placement, which allows the anterior shell to move away from the rigid backing. It is important to control positioning of this backing as it is what determines final expander position.

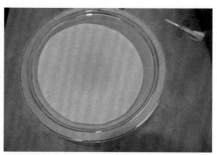

TECH FIG 2 • The tissue expander is marked with a vertical line for orientation. All air is removed with the excess inferior implant folded inward as shown to avoid puncturing the inferior implant while placing needles for expansion in clinic postoperatively. A minimum of 60 mL of saline is instilled. (From: Halvorson EG. Two-stage implant breast reconstruction. In: Mulholland MW, ed. *Operative Techniques in Surgery*. Vol. 2. Philadelphia, PA: Wolters Kluwer, 2000.)

- It can be helpful to put 1 mL of methylene blue in 1 L of injectable saline and use this for the initial expander fluid. If the expander is punctured during closure, it will be evident due to the dye. Additionally, during expansions in clinic, the blue dye will confirm when the port is accessed.

Fourth Step—Placement of Tissue Expander and Closure

- The pectoralis is retracted away from the chest wall and the expander is placed into the pocket taking great care to orient it correctly.
  - It is important to note the rigid backing of the expander and place the caudal edge at the IMF or below if desired. Be sure to unfold all edges of the expander and ensure it is as medial as desired.
  - If performing bilateral reconstruction, symmetry in expander placement should be confirmed by palpating the expander ports on each side and ensuring symmetric horizontal and vertical positioning.
  - If an expander requires adjustment in positioning, it is critical to grasp the rigid backing of the implant and then adjust the position. If only the ports or anterior shell are adjusted, this usually has no effect on the position of the backing, which determines implant position once fully inflated.
- The inferolateral edge of the pectoralis major muscle is sutured to the anteromedial edge of the serratus anterior muscle with running absorbable 2-0 braided suture, closing the pocket. A small opening is left superolaterally to allow egress of fluid.
  - Alternatively, if an ADM is used, the pectoralis major muscle is sewn to the ADM with interrupted figure-of-8 braided absorbable 2-0 suture (**TECH FIG 3A**).
- The author's preference is to inflate the tissue expander with sterile saline as much as the soft tissue (muscle/skin) will allow without creating tension. This is typically 120 to 240 mL.
  - It is important to do this prior to skin closure, as placing the needle through the muscle will occasionally cause bleeding, which can be controlled directly. Otherwise, a hematoma could expand in the subcutaneous space without notice until the patient is out of surgery.

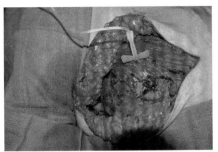
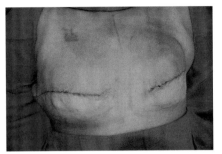

TECH FIG 3 • A. The inferolateral edge of the pectoralis major is sewn to the superomedial edge of the serratus anterior with a running 2-0 absorbable polyfilament suture to cover the implant. The expander can then be subsequently filled further depending upon the tolerance of the submuscular pocket and the mastectomy skin flaps. (From: Halvorson EG. Two-stage implant breast reconstruction. In: Mulholland MW, ed. *Operative Techniques in Surgery*. Vol. 2. Philadelphia, PA: Wolters Kluwer, 2000.) **B.** The patient is shown following placement of tissue expanders and closure over closed suction drains. Internal absorbable sutures are used, with skin glue as the only dressing. No bra is applied, which might apply pressure to tenuous mastectomy flaps. (From: Halvorson EG. Two-stage implant breast reconstruction. In: Mulholland MW, ed. *Operative Techniques in Surgery*. Vol. 2. Philadelphia, PA: Wolters Kluwer, 2000.)

- In cases where there is significant concern regarding the cutaneous circulation, then only 0 to 60 mL of inflation is advisable.
- Two closed suction drains are placed in the subcutaneous space. One is oriented superiorly and the other inferiorly.
  - In low-risk patients with smaller breasts, a single drain may be placed via the axilla and extending inferiorly along the lateral border and then across the IMF toward the midline.
- The skin is closed with interrupted 3-0 absorbable monofilament suture for the dermis and a running 4-0 absorbable monofilament suture for subcuticular closure (**TECH FIG 3B**).
  - The authors' preference is to use skin glue alone as a dressing, without placement of a surgical bra, which applies pressure to the tenuous mastectomy flaps and is an impediment to physical examination.

- Antibiotics are continued parenterally for at least 24 hours postoperatively.
  - Although some studies support the use of postoperative prophylactic antibiotics until the drains are removed[6], others have shown no difference between this regimen and 24 hours alone.[7]
- Drains are removed when output is less than 30 mL per 24 hours and expansion is begun typically 2 weeks postoperatively. Expansion can continue on a weekly basis, adding as much fluid as the patient will tolerate without discomfort (usually 60 to 120 mL).
- Once expansion is complete according to patient preference and surgeon's satisfaction, the author's preference is to perform one additional overexpansion, which can provide some additional tissue to create minimal ptosis at the exchange procedure at least 1 month later (as described in the following chapter).

PEARLS AND PITFALLS

Indications	▪ Patients with a history of radiation are poor candidates for implant reconstruction. ▪ Risk factors for infection and wound healing complications include smoking, radiation, and obesity.
Incision placement	▪ An oblique incision parallel to the pectoralis muscle fibers provides the best appearance and easiest approach for the exchange procedure. ▪ Excess skin can be excised through a linear incision only, as additional incisions will compromise circulation and risk mastectomy flap necrosis. Secondary procedures are frequently necessary in patients with excess skin.
Expander selection	▪ Expanders are selected based on breast width, not volume.
Expander placement	▪ Marking the expander assists in correct orientation. ▪ Remove all air and place saline dyed with methylene blue to allow detection of implant rupture as well as confirmation of port access for staff performing expansions. ▪ Provide 24 hours of postoperative antibiotics.

POSTOPERATIVE CARE

- Following the mastectomy and tissue expander placement, the patient is maintained on antibiotics for at least 24 hours.
- Drains remain in place at least 3 days and then are removed when output is less than 30 mL/d.
  - Only one drain from each side should be removed at a time, as sometimes the output of the second drain will increase after the first drain is removed.
  - The author's preference is to allow patients to shower with drains in place.
- The patient should be seen within 1 week to evaluate for postoperative infection and/or mastectomy flap necrosis and to remove drains if appropriate.
- Range of motion is limited to 90 degrees of shoulder abduction for 2 weeks, and then full range of motion is permitted. Heavy lifting (greater than 10 lb) is avoided for 1 month.
- Expansion is begun 2 weeks after surgery and continued on a weekly basis thereafter until the patient and surgeon are happy with the final volume.
- One additional "overexpansion" is performed, and the exchange procedure is scheduled at least 1 month later to allow the tissues to soften.

OUTCOMES

- Please see the chapter on implant exchange for a discussion of the outcomes of implant reconstruction in general.
- Although patients are typically happy to have "something there" following mastectomy, expanders are often uncomfortable, and the process of tissue expansion can cause discomfort, especially after each expansion.
- Many patients will describe the expander as a "rock under my arm," and it is important to reassure them that this improves dramatically following the exchange procedure.

- The overall success rate of expander reconstruction is roughly 95% to 98%, with a 2% to 5% risk of implant loss due to necrosis and infection.

COMPLICATIONS

- Bleeding
- Infection
- Injury to surrounding structures (eg, cutaneous nerves)
- Mastectomy flap necrosis
- Seroma
- Asymmetry, imperfect cosmetic result

REFERENCES

1. Moyer HR, Losken A. Predicting mastectomy skin flap necrosis with indocyanine green angiography: the gray area defined. *Plast Reconstr Surg.* 2012;129(5):1043-1048.
2. Abbott AM, Miller BT, Tuttle TM. Outcomes after tumescence technique versus electrocautery mastectomy. *Ann Surg Oncol.* 2012;19(8):2607-2611.
3. Seth AK, Hirsch EM, Fine NA, et al. Additive risk of tumescent technique in patients undergoing mastectomy with immediate reconstruction. *Ann Surg Oncol.* 2011;18(11):3041-3046.
4. Chun YS, Verma K, Rosen H, et al. Use of tumescent mastectomy technique as a risk factor for native breast skin flap necrosis following immediate breast reconstruction. *Am J Surg.* 2011;201(2):160-165.
5. Ho G, Nguyen TJ, Shahabi A, et al. A systematic review and meta-analysis of complications associated with acellular dermal matrix-assisted breast reconstruction. *Ann Plast Surg.* 2012;68(4):346-356.
6. Clayton JL, Bazakas A, Lee CN, et al. Once is not enough: withholding postoperative prophylactic antibiotics in prosthetic breast reconstruction is associated with an increased risk of infection. *Plast Reconstr Surg.* 2012;130(3):495-502.
7. Phillips BT, et al. Are prophylactic postoperative antibiotics necessary for immediate breast reconstruction? Results of a prospective randomized clinical trial. *J Am Coll Surg.* 2016;222(6):1116-1124.

Replacement of Expander With Permanent Implant

Eric G. Halvorson and Joseph J. Disa

DEFINITION

- Exchange of an expander for a permanent implant is performed as the second stage in two-stage implant breast reconstruction, following mastectomy and tissue expander placement (covered in previous chapter).
- The advantages of two-stage implant reconstruction (compared to autologous reconstruction) include shorter operation, lack of donor site, shorter hospital stay, shorter recovery, patient control over final volume, and a "perkier" result.
- The disadvantages of two-stage implant reconstruction include multiple postoperative office visits for expansions, discomfort associated with the expansion process, a second (albeit outpatient) surgery, and the permanent risks of implants (capsular contracture, rupture, rippling, infection, malposition, and exposure).

PATIENT HISTORY AND PHYSICAL FINDINGS

- The initial consultation will have taken place prior to mastectomy and tissue expander placement; however, it is important to review the patient's interim medical history prior to the exchange procedure, as interim changes are not uncommon as a patient progresses through breast cancer treatment, and their medical problems to assess risk factors for wound healing complications, for example, diabetes, radiation therapy, obesity, and smoking.
  - If patients have had radiotherapy, then waiting 3 to 6 months before performing the exchange procedure is advised.
- Physical examination of the breasts is performed to evaluate expander size and position as well as the soft tissue envelope.
  - Implants often require position adjustment using capsulotomy and/or capsulorrhaphy.
  - Radiation changes are noted (if applicable), and if the skin and soft tissue surrounding the mastectomy scar are very thin, then an IMF approach to the exchange procedure should strongly be considered. Cutaneous recurrence should always be excluded.
- Areas of soft tissue deficiency are evaluated for possible autologous fat grafting. This is fairly common in the upper pole.
- Donor sites are also assessed. The medial thighs and hips are good donor sites. The abdomen should be spared as a possible future donor site for autologous reconstruction, if appropriate.
- Expander size and volume is reviewed and determines implant selection (covered in the following text).

SURGICAL MANAGEMENT

- Ideal candidates for two-stage implant reconstruction are thin, nonsmokers undergoing bilateral mastectomy who have not, and will not, receive radiotherapy.
  - Smokers are prone to wound healing complications and infection.
  - Radiotherapy increases the risk of infection, implant exposure, and capsular contracture.
- Although obesity increases the risk of complications for most procedures, unless other risk factors are present, the exchange procedure on obese patients is very safe. Most of their risk will have occurred during the mastectomy and expander placement.
- The exchange procedure can be an opportunity to modify implant position and also address some excess skin via lenticular excision.

Preoperative Planning and Implant Selection

- Good communication with the breast surgeon and medical oncologist ensures oncologic goals are maintained and that reconstruction is appropriately staged.
- The exchange procedure is typically delayed until one month following chemotherapy.
  - If radiotherapy is planned, the exchange procedure can be performed between chemotherapy and radiation, or 3 to 6 months following radiation. This is often determined by the preferences of the medical oncologist and radiation oncologist.
  - Patients on extended adjuvant therapy can safely undergo the exchange procedure; however, the specific agent must be assessed for risk of wound healing complications and/ or thromboembolic events, and a discussion with the medical oncologist is advised.
- Prior to the exchange procedure, the patient must be marked in the standing position.
  - The IMF is marked on each side and the midline is drawn between the sternal notch and xiphoid process.
  - A horizontal line is drawn from the lowest point of the IMF on each side to the midline, which helps identify vertical asymmetries in expander position.
  - The medial silhouette of each expander is marked, which helps identify horizontal asymmetries in expander position.
  - The ideal contour for the final implants is marked, revealing areas where capsulotomy will need to be performed to adjust the implant pocket.
- If applicable, areas of soft tissue deficiency are outlined for autologous fat grafting, and the donor sites are marked.

- Final implants are selected primarily based on volume, although width should be taken into consideration. A full discussion of implant types is beyond the scope of this chapter.
  - The majority of surgeons use smooth, round, high-profile silicone implants for reconstructive purposes, although textured anatomic silicone implants are also available.
  - Patients with very wide chests may require a moderate-profile implant that will have a larger base diameter for a given volume (although less projection).
- A comparison of saline vs silicone implants is also beyond the scope of this chapter, but suffice it to say that the issue is controversial. The authors' preference is to offer both types to patients noting the following advantages and disadvantages for each implant type:
  - Saline
    - Advantages: Implant rupture is immediately detected; removal/replacement of a ruptured implant is simple and quick.
    - Disadvantages: Re-expansion may be required if implant ruptures and is not replaced expeditiously;

firmer than silicone, although this difference is negligible when good soft tissue coverage is present; higher potential for rippling if underfilled.
  - Silicone
    - Advantages: Softer, more "natural" feel
    - Disadvantages: Rupture is often clinically silent until capsular contracture and/or extracapsular rupture occurs, removal of a ruptured implant is a difficult operation that can involve removal of native tissue thus compromising subsequent reconstruction, and monitoring for silent implant rupture using magnetic resonance imaging (MRI) is not proven and has a definite risk of false positives and unnecessary surgeries.

Positioning

- Patients are placed in the supine position under a general anesthetic with arms padded circumferentially and abducted at 80 to 90 degrees. The patient is positioned such that the sternum is parallel to the floor via head elevation or reverse Trendelenburg.

TECHNIQUES

■ Implant Exchange

First Step—Removal of Tissue Expander

- As noted earlier, the patient is marked in the standing position. Asymmetries are noted, and the ideal contour for the final implants is marked.
- If performing fat grafting, the donor sites should be injected with tumescent solution at the beginning of the case to allow the epinephrine to take effect.
- The mastectomy scars have often widened during expansion and these can be excised.
- A stair-step approach to the implant pocket is usually performed, so any wound breakdown in one layer does not expose the suture line of the other layer.
  - If the scar is oriented obliquely (**TECH FIG 1A**), 2 to 4 cm of superomedial skin elevation will expose the pectoralis major, which can be incised parallel to the muscle fibers.

- If a transverse approach was used, then superolateral and inferomedial skin elevation is required to expose the pectoralis major and allow for an incision parallel to the muscle fibers.
- The implant pocket is entered and the capsule is bluntly separated from the expander, which is removed. If the expander is too large, it can be ruptured with a needle or scalpel to assist in removal. If there was any doubt about the final expander volume, it can be measured at this point (**TECH FIG 1B**).

Second Step—Creation of Implant Pocket

- Ideally, the expanders can be removed and the permanent implants placed without further intervention; however, this is rarely the case. Superior and superomedial capsulotomy is often required to soften the transition from the chest wall to the implant (**TECH FIG 2A,B**).

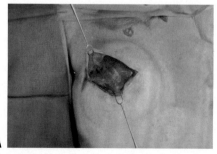 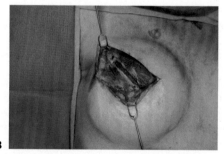

A   B

TECH FIG 1 • A. If the oblique incision is used for mastectomy, it is easy at the exchange procedure to elevate a superomedial flap exposing the pectoralis major muscle where it tends to be thicker. This will allow a "stair-step" approach to the implant pocket. Any wound healing issue at one level will not expose the suture line at the other level. (From Halvorson EG. Two-stage implant breast reconstruction. In: Mulholland MW, ed. *Operative Techniques in Surgery*. Vol 2. Philadelphia, PA: Wolters Kluwer; 2014.) **B.** A muscular incision is made parallel to the pectoralis major muscle fibers to access the implant pocket. The capsule is also incised with cautery, and the expander is bluntly separated from the capsule. (From Halvorson EG. Two-stage implant breast reconstruction. In: Mulholland MW, ed. *Operative Techniques in Surgery*. Vol 2. Philadelphia, PA: Wolters Kluwer; 2014.)

- The pocket may need to be medialized, lateralized, elevated, or displaced inferiorly. These can all be accomplished through capsulotomy.
- If the final implant is roughly the same width as the expander, then a corresponding capsulorrhaphy at the opposite side of the pocket is necessary using figure-of-eight interrupted 0 suture.
- If the implant is wider than the expander, this may not be necessary as the capsulotomy will increase pocket diameter.
- If the expander was placed below the IMF, or if the IMF needs to be elevated, this is accomplished with figure-of-eight interrupted 0 suture.
  - The patient is sat upright (**TECH FIG 2C,D**) and the inferior mastectomy flap is lifted away from the chest wall.
  - Usually, the old IMF can be visualized and marked; otherwise, the desired IMF can be marked.
  - The needle is passed through the capsule and the IMF marking externally is visualized. The needle tip should just catch the deep dermis, resulting in a small indentation when tied. These indentations will resolve in several weeks.
  - After passing the needle through the capsule/dermis, tension can be adjusted by examining the fold externally and elevating it as desired.
  - Internal inspection with the suture still under tension will indicate where the corresponding suture throw in the chest wall must be made. Suturing into the rib should be avoided, as this results in pain.
  - The first suture is placed at the center of the IMF and then one to two sutures are placed medially and laterally until an adequate fold is created (**TECH FIG 2E**).

- Some surgeons prefer to establish the IMF at the initial operation, potentially with an acellular dermal matrix (ADM), which has the added benefit of permitting a higher initial fill volume. A greater initial fill volume has the potential to better preserve lower pole fullness.
- No time is spent reconstructing the IMF at the exchange procedure. Although this may be a simpler approach, it may result in a blunted IMF.
  - The authors' preference is to treat each case individually and surgically create a crisp IMF at the exchange procedure if necessary. For example, patients undergoing delayed reconstruction will benefit from significant lower pole expansion and thus the expander is placed inferior to the desired IMF and the IMF is reconstructed at the exchange procedure.
  - A patient with minimal excess skin and ptosis undergoing immediate reconstruction may benefit from an ADM to maximize the initial fill volume (preserve lower pole fullness), establish the IMF, and avoid inferior capsulorrhaphy at the exchange procedure.
- To further expand the lower pole and create minimal ptosis, capsulotomy of the inferior pocket is then performed. A horizontal capsulotomy half way up the inferior mastectomy flap, at least 4 cm off the chest wall, will expand the lower pole of the pocket. Additional radial capsulotomies can be added for further lower pole expansion or elsewhere to create symmetric pockets.
- During pocket creation, it is helpful to have a temporary sizer inflated (with air or saline) to roughly the desired implant volume, which can be placed into the implant pocket to assess position, shape, and volume. This is

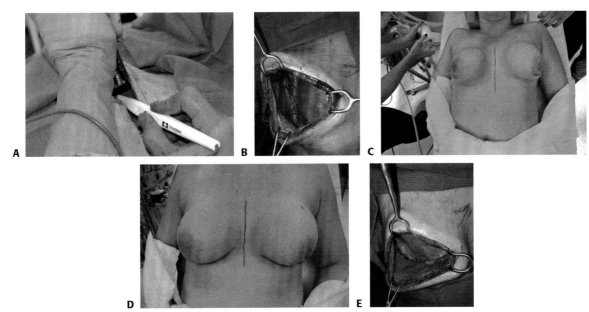

TECH FIG 2 • A,B. A superomedial and superior capsulotomy is made just above the chest wall using a lighted retractor. This will soften the transition from chest wall to implant and allow for more implant mobility within the pocket. (From Halvorson EG. Two-stage implant breast reconstruction. In: Mulholland MW, ed. *Operative Techniques in Surgery*. Vol 2. Philadelphia, PA: Wolters Kluwer; 2014.) **C,D.** The patient is positioned upright with both upper extremities well padded and secured to the operating room table or arm boards. **E.** Inframammary fold and/or lateral mammary fold sutures are place to define the fold and adjust pocket dimensions as needed. (From Halvorson EG. Two-stage implant breast reconstruction. In: Mulholland MW, ed. *Operative Techniques in Surgery*. Vol 2. Philadelphia, PA: Wolters Kluwer; 2014.)

TECHNIQUES

particularly important in bilateral reconstructions, where two sizers are required to confirm pocket symmetry.

- If the sizer is loose and slips laterally, lateral capsulorrhaphy sutures should be placed.
- If autologous fat grafting is to be performed, the authors' preference is to do it while the temporary sizers are in place to avoid inadvertent rupture of the permanent implants.
    - Fat grafts are harvested, processed, and injected into the subcutaneous, intramuscular, and submuscular planes via the incision or small stab incisions as determined by preoperative examination and markings.
    - The sizers are removed, and the implant pocket is once again irrigated to remove any possible fat grafts that have been placed into the implant pocket. A full description of fat grafting techniques is beyond the scope of this chapter.

Third Step—Implant Selection and Closure

- When ordering implants for the exchange procedure, it is wise to order implants that are one size smaller and one size larger than the implant size determined by the patient's final expansion volume (prior to final overexpansion). As mentioned earlier, temporary sizers are usually used and can be adjusted to determine an acceptable final implant volume.
    - Inflating the sizer beyond the final expander volume usually results in excessive upper pole fullness, a noticeable step-off between the chest and implant, and tight closure. The chest should transition to the implant smoothly, and the breast mound should have slight ptosis.
- When placing saline implants, choose an implant that has the desired volume as the upper end of its volume range. For example, if 380 mL is the desired implant volume, use an implant with a volume range of 360 to 390 mL.
    - This avoids rippling at the expense of making the implant slightly firmer. Some surgeons will in fact overfill the implant by 10% to avoid rippling.
- Disposable sizers can be used prior to final implant placement (**TECH FIG 3A**).

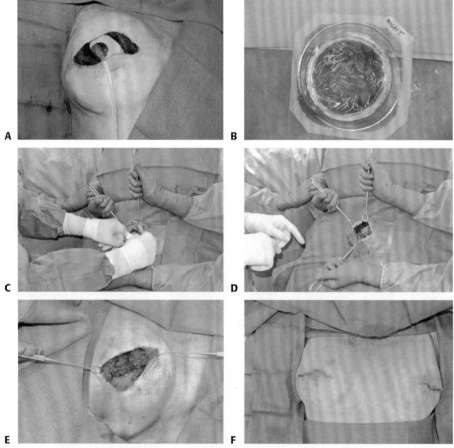

TECH FIG 3 • **A.** Disposable sizers are used to determine the optimal implant. The patient is viewed in the upright position. (From Halvorson EG. Two-stage implant breast reconstruction. In: Mulholland MW, ed. *Operative Techniques in Surgery*. Vol 2. Philadelphia, PA: Wolters Kluwer; 2014.) **B–D.** Next, the permanent implant is selected. The field is surrounded by clean sterile drapes and clean gloves are used to place the implant. Care is taken to avoid implant contact with the skin. (Credit: Halvorson EG. Two-stage implant breast reconstruction. In: Mulholland MW, ed. *Operative Techniques in Surgery*. Vol 2. Philadelphia, PA: Wolters Kluwer, 2014.) **E,F.** The pectoralis is reapproximated with an absorbable suture, and the wound is closed in layers. (From Halvorson EG. Two-stage implant breast reconstruction. In: Mulholland MW, ed. *Operative Techniques in Surgery*. Vol 2. Philadelphia, PA: Wolters Kluwer; 2014.)

- The pockets are irrigated, hemostasis is obtained, and the final implants are opened.
  - Although many surgeons will reprep the patient, place new drapes, dip retractors in prep solution, and handle the implants with fresh gloves, there is no data to support these practices. The authors do not take any special precautions, as the procedure is a clean, sterile procedure (**TECH FIG 3B–D**).
- The implants are placed and the muscular closure is performed with a running 2-0 braided absorbable suture.

The capsule is not included in this closure if possible, thus creating an anterior capsulotomy (made upon initial approach to the implant pocket).

- No drains are placed. The skin is closed with interrupted deep dermal 3-0 monofilament absorbable suture and a running 4-0 subcuticular absorbable suture (**TECH FIG 3E,F**). A skin glue is applied, and a brassiere is only used if supporting the implant in a particular position is desired.

PEARLS AND PITFALLS

Implant selection	▪ Implants are selected based on volume primarily, taking breast width into consideration. High-profile implants are typically used, except in patients with wide chests who benefit from moderate-profile, wider implants.
Adjunct procedures	▪ Consider fat grafting to address contour deformities, improve the soft tissue, and soften the contours of the implant.
Patient expectation	▪ Two-stage implant breast reconstruction is typically a year-long process. ▪ Symmetry in the nude is always the goal but is seldom achieved. Symmetry in clothing is the most reasonable expectation.

POSTOPERATIVE CARE

- Following the exchange procedure, patients may shower after 48 hours. The exchange procedure is sterile, and the mastectomy flaps have been delayed and have robust perfusion. No postoperative antibiotics are given. Range of motion is limited to 90 degrees of shoulder abduction for 2 weeks, and then full range of motion is permitted. Heavy lifting (greater than 10 lb) is avoided for 1 month.

OUTCOMES

- Patient satisfaction with implant breast reconstruction is high, provided the preoperative consultation appropriately identified the patient's priorities, goals, and preferences with respect to reconstructive options, and realistic expectations were discussed.
  - Although some studies have indicated that patients undergoing prosthetic reconstruction are less satisfied than are those undergoing autologous tissue reconstruction,[1,2] other studies have shown significant improvements in psychosocial outcomes regardless of the type of reconstruction.[3]
- It is common to tell patients undergoing implant reconstruction that, on average, they will require some form of surgery every 10 years. These could be procedures for symmetry, infection, rupture, or capsular contracture. Although some surgeons exchange silicone implants every 10 years to avoid extracapsular ruptures, most only offer surgery if a problem is identified.
- One study evaluated long-term outcomes of autologous vs implant reconstruction and noted stable survival of 90% of autologous reconstructions vs a gradual decline to 70% survival of implant reconstructions.[4] In general, autologous

reconstructions improve or remain stable with time, whereas implant reconstructions tend to worsen slightly over time.

- There is no increased risk of breast cancer recurrence in patients undergoing therapeutic mastectomy and implant reconstruction. Detection of recurrence and outcome when recurrence is detected are not affected by the presence of an implant reconstruction.[5]

COMPLICATIONS

- Bleeding
- Infection
- Long-term risks of implants: capsular contracture, rupture, rippling, infection, malposition, and exposure
- Asymmetry, imperfect cosmetic result

REFERENCES

1. Alderman AK, Wilkins EG, Lowery JC, et al. Determinants of patient satisfaction in postmastectomy breast reconstruction. *Plast Reconstr Surg.* 2000;106:769-776.
2. Christensen BO, Overgaard J, Kettner LO, et al. Long-term evaluation of postmastectomy breast reconstruction. *Acta Oncol.* 2011;50(7): 1053-1061.
3. Wilkins EG, Cederna PS, Lowery JC, et al. Prospective analysis of psychosocial outcomes in breast reconstruction: one-year postoperative results from the Michigan Breast Reconstruction Outcome Study. *Plast Reconstr Surg.* 2000;106(5):1014-1025.
4. Rusby JE, Waters RA, Nightingale PG, et al. Immediate breast reconstruction after mastectomy: what are the long-term prospects? *Ann R Coll Surg Engl.* 2010;92(3):193-197.
5. McCarthy CM, Pusic AL, Sclafani L, et al. Breast cancer recurrence following prosthetic, postmastectomy reconstruction: incidence, detection, and treatment. *Plast Reconstr Surg.* 2008;121(2):381-388.

17

CHAPTER

Direct-to-Implant Breast Reconstruction

Amy S. Colwell and Eric J. Wright

DEFINITION

- Following mastectomy, the reconstructive goal is to recreate a natural-appearing breast, which may improve quality of life and body image.
- Direct-to-implant (DTI) reconstruction involves placement of the permanent implant at the time of mastectomy in one stage.
- DTI reconstruction is a cost-effective, low complication rate procedure with outcomes similar to two-stage tissue expander/implant reconstruction in experienced centers.[1]
- Alternatives to DTI include no reconstruction, two-stage tissue expander/implant reconstruction and autologous reconstruction with flaps or fat.
- In comparison with tissue expander reconstruction, there are fewer office visits and one less surgical procedure. Compared to autologous reconstruction, there is no donor site morbidity.

ANATOMY

- The breast skin is preserved or reduced to accommodate an appropriate-size implant.
- Skin-sparing or nipple-sparing mastectomy keeps the native breast skin envelope intact by crafting a natural shape with immediate round or shaped implant insertion. In nipple-sparing procedures, the nipple ducts are removed with the mastectomy and the outer epidermis and dermis are retained with the rest of the breast skin.
- Ideal candidates for nipple-sparing mastectomy have grade 1 to grade 2 nipple ptosis.
- Patients with grade 3 ptosis may be better candidates for skin-sparing mastectomy or mastopexy prior to mastectomy.
- The implant has total, partial, or no muscle coverage under the breast skin.
- The pectoralis major muscle most commonly covers the implant superiorly. Inferiorly, acellular dermal matrix (ADM) or mesh serves as an extension of the pectoralis major muscle to cover the implant inferiorly.

PATIENT HISTORY AND PHYSICAL FINDINGS

- DTI reconstruction can be performed in unilateral or bilateral mastectomies and in reconstruction for cancer or prophylaxis.
- Ideal candidates for DTI reconstruction are otherwise healthy patients, with moderate size breasts, who desire to retain approximately the same breast size.

- Patients who desire a significantly larger size are more safely treated with tissue expander/implant reconstruction.
- Relative contraindications to DTI include active smoking, uncontrolled diabetes, and immunosuppressive medications.
- Planned postoperative radiation, obesity, prior breast scars, and previous lumpectomy/radiation may increase the risk of complications, but they are not absolute contraindications to performing DTI reconstruction.
- The breasts are assessed for volume, symmetry, nipple position, inframammary fold (IMF) position, and breast base width.
- Patients with very small (less than 100 g) or very large (greater than 900 g) breasts are typically better candidates for tissue expander/implant reconstruction.
- If a patient has asymmetry, a better cosmetic outcome may be achieved in two stages for bilateral reconstructions.

IMAGING

- Preoperative mammogram or MRI can determine the oncologic safety of proceeding with a nipple-sparing vs skin-sparing mastectomy based upon the proximity of the cancer to the nipple.

SURGICAL MANAGEMENT

- Surgical management requires either a team approach with the surgical oncologist and plastic surgeon or an oncoplastic surgeon experienced in both mastectomy and reconstruction.
- During the preoperative visit, patients are to be counseled on the possibility of a two-stage tissue expander/implant reconstruction or delayed reconstruction depending on the intraoperative mastectomy skin viability.
- Though saline implants can be used, silicone implants are used more commonly to create a more nature look and feel.
- Smooth round implants are softer than are anatomic implants and typically provide more superior pole fullness.
- Textured anatomic implants are firmer than round implants and typically have reduced risk of rippling. These implants may better match a contralateral breast in unilateral reconstructions and may have less contracture after postmastectomy radiation.
- Partial pectoralis muscle coverage of the implant is the most common technique with an inferior sling of ADM or synthetic mesh.
- Compared to total muscle coverage, partial muscle coverage gives more natural breast shape and can accommodate a larger size implant.

- Compared to no muscle coverage, partial muscle coverage has better soft tissue coverage in the upper pole, and it is less expensive.
- Human ADM is the most common material used to provide an inferior sling.[2] Alternative materials include porcine skin, bovine skin, and synthetic meshes made from silk, Vicryl, and titanium. These products provide precise control of the lateral and inframammary pocket borders along with the lower pole projection. They also support the implant and help keep the pectoralis muscle on stretch.
- The authors describe their preferred technique using partial muscle coverage with an inferior pole sling of human ADM.

Preoperative Planning

- A paravertebral block can be performed for perioperative and postoperative analgesia.
- Reference markings are placed including the IMF bilaterally and planned lateral border of the breasts.
- For skin-sparing procedures, the incision is placed around the areola, with or without small medial and lateral extensions.
- For nipple-sparing procedures, an inferolateral IMF incision optimizes mastectomy, lymph node sampling, and reconstruction.
- Alternative incisions in NSM include lateral radial, vertical, or extension of a nonradiated scar (**FIG 1**).
  - A full-thickness periareolar incision is typically avoided to decrease risk of nipple and skin loss.
- Circumvertical mastopexy or Wise pattern mastopexy procedures at the time of mastectomy are associated with a higher risk of complications and are typically avoided.
- The goal is for placement of an appropriate-sized implant within the pocket for uneventful wound healing and centralization of the nipple if preserved.

Positioning

- The patient is placed in the supine position with arms extended, secured on arm boards, and angled to the side.

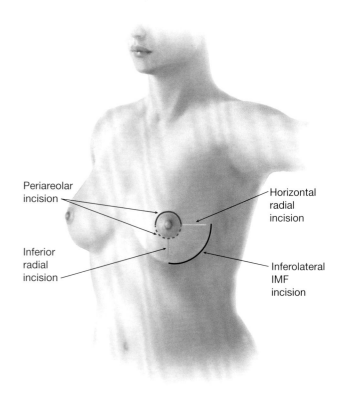

Periareolar incision

Horizontal radial incision

Inferior radial incision

Inferolateral IMF incision

FIG 1 • Depending on tumor location and surgeon preference, these are the possible incision locations for nipple-sparing mastectomy.

- Intraoperatively, the patient will be placed in the sitting position to assess size and symmetry before permanent implant placement.

Approach

- Implant placement can be performed through any access incision used for the mastectomy.
- For NSM, an inferolateral IMF incision is most commonly used and has excellent appearance.[3]

■ Direct-to-Implant Reconstruction with Partial Muscle Coverage and Acellular Dermal Matrix (Video)

Pocket Creation

- Intravenous antibiotics are administered prior to the surgical incision (**TECH FIG 1A**).
- The patient is reprepped with chlorhexidine, and new drapes are placed over existing drapes after completion of the mastectomy.
- The mastectomy skin flaps are assessed for perfusion based upon appearance/color, thickness of skin flaps/visibility of the dermis, and capillary refill (**TECH FIG 1B**).
  - Concern for ischemia necessitates two-stage or delayed reconstruction. If available, perfusion devices can be used to help assess relative skin ischemia and perfusion.

- Ideal mastectomy skin flaps have a relatively even layer of subcutaneous fat with no exposed dermis and no red or blue discoloration.
- Mastectomy specimens are weighed to assess the volume removed.
- The patient is paralyzed for easier subpectoral dissection and pocket closure once the implant is placed.
- The pectoralis major muscle is elevated from the lateral border to create a subpectoral pocket. The inferior insertion of the pectoralis major muscle is released to approximately the 4 or 8 o'clock position (**TECH FIG 1C,D**).
  - Care is taken to not violate the IMF with muscle release if intact. Hemostasis is confirmed throughout the pocket.

TECHNIQUES

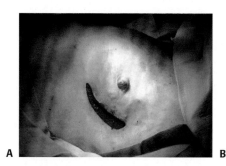 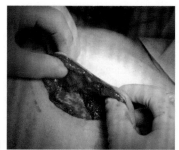 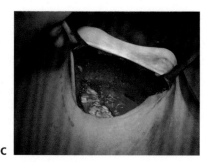

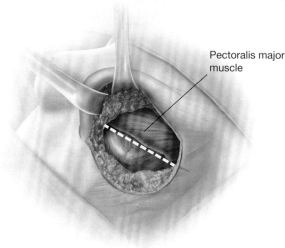

Pectoralis major muscle

TECH FIG 1 • **A.** The inferolateral inframammary fold incision is commonly used to perform the nipple-sparing mastectomy and reconstruction. This incision gives access to perform the sentinel lymph node biopsy. **B.** Mastectomy flaps are inspected at the start of the case. Ideal flaps will have an even layer of subcutaneous fat with no skin discoloration. **C,D.** The pectoralis muscle is released along the sternum from 4 o'clock to 8 o'clock along the inferior border. (**D** from Colwell AS. Direct-to-implant breast reconstruction. In: Mulholland MW, ed. *Operative Techniques in Surgery*. Vol 2. Philadelphia, PA: Wolters Kluwer Health; 2015:1471-1475.)

- Based upon the natural breast diameter and volume/diameter of the expected implant, the lateral border of the pocket is marked by extending over the serratus muscle.
  - This marking is placed 1 cm less than the expected diameter of the implant to compensate for the stretch of human ADM. If a stiffer material is used, this marking can be adjusted.

ADM and Implant Placement and Closure

- Rectangular or contoured ADM is sutured to the released border of the pectoralis muscle and IMF loosely medially to accommodate medial implant placement (**TECH FIG 2A**).
  - The ADM is sewn to the chest wall in the inferior and lateral position to help prevent bottoming out and lateral malposition. The authors prefer braided permanent sutures for the chest wall stitches, although absorbable sutures are also commonly used.
- Silicone or saline sizers are used to confirm implant size and pocket dimensions.
- Temporary tacking sutures secure the pectoralis muscle to the ADM, and the patient is placed in the upright position.

- After symmetry and appropriate pocket appearance are confirmed, the permanent implant is chosen based primarily on the volume and breast base width.
- New gloves are used when handling the implant.
  - Triple antibiotic solution with cefazolin, gentamicin, and bacitracin is used for pocket irrigation.
- Two no. 15 Bard drains are placed lateral to the incision and secured.
  - One drain is placed internally along the IMF, and the other is placed laterally toward the axilla and extending over the pectoralis muscle.
- After implant insertion, the pectoralis muscle is secured to the ADM using a braided absorbable suture (**TECH FIG 2B,C**).
  - The tension is adjusted and ADM trimmed as necessary to create a tight pocket around the implant that helps to avoid lateral and inferior malposition.
- The incision is de-epithelialized 2 to 3 mm, and a three-layered closure is performed with absorbable sutures followed by skin glue.
  - An occlusive dressing is applied over the incision and Biopatches are placed around the drains.
- Elastic foam tape and Tegaderm are often used to help stabilize the implant and nipple position (**TECH FIG 2D**).

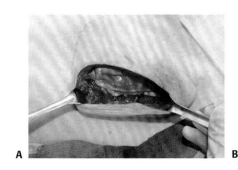
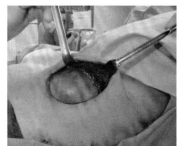

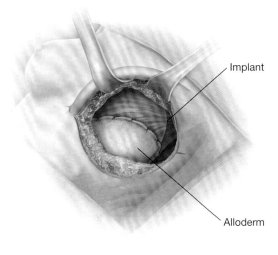

Implant

Alloderm

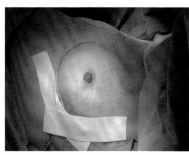

TECH FIG 2 • A. The acellular dermal matrix is sutured with permanent suture to the chest wall and pectoralis muscle. **B,C.** After implant placement, the acellular dermal matrix is sutured to the released inferior border of pectoralis muscle. **D.** After closure, final dressing with elastic foam is placed to help with position. (**C** from Colwell AS. Direct-to-implant breast reconstruction. In: Mulholland MW, ed. *Operative Techniques in Surgery.* Vol 2. Philadelphia, PA: Wolters Kluwer Health; 2015:1471-1475.)

PEARLS AND PITFALLS

Preoperative assessment	▪ Appropriate patient selection improves outcomes.
Intraoperative assessment	▪ Before committing to a direct-to-implant reconstruction, the mastectomy skin flaps must be viable without injury. The patient should always be consented for possible tissue expander placement.
Technique	▪ Suture the ADM loose medially and tight laterally to avoid lateral displacement. Use of a sizer will help determine appropriate pocket dimensions for proper implant selection.
	▪ For skin-sparing mastectomy, choose higher profile implants if possible to help overcome the flattening effect of losing the nipple.
	▪ For NSM, choose the width of implant to centralize the nipple. A lower profile implant may be necessary to avoid shifting the nipple laterally, which can be seen when the implant is too narrow.

POSTOPERATIVE CARE

▪ Patients are typically hospitalized overnight but may stay 2 days postoperatively.
▪ On postoperative day 1, a supportive surgical brassiere is placed avoiding excess constriction that can decrease perfusion.
▪ Patients are allowed to shower following the surgery.
▪ Patients are discharged home on oral antibiotics until the drains are removed.

▪ Drains are removed in follow-up clinic once the output has decreased to less than 30 cc per 24 hours. Typically, one drain per side is removed 1 week after surgery and the other is removed the second week after surgery. Drains are not kept longer than 4 weeks.
▪ Strenuous activity is limited for 8 to 12 weeks following the procedure.
▪ For smooth round implants, massage begins 1 month after the procedure.

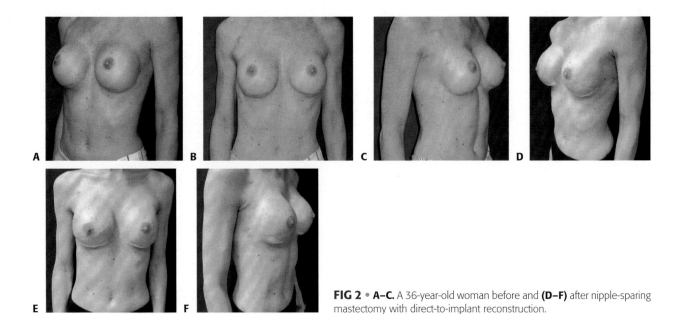

FIG 2 • A–C. A 36-year-old woman before and **(D–F)** after nipple-sparing mastectomy with direct-to-implant reconstruction.

- Pathology of the nipple specimen is reviewed. If positive, the nipple is excised with a 2- to 3-mm margin of areolar skin.
- The immediate postoperative appearance may have contour irregularities due to the unevenness of the mastectomy skin flaps and ADM-muscle interface. This resolves over the course of a few weeks once the suction drains are removed and the skin begins its recovery.

OUTCOMES

- A single-institution, three-surgeon study found DTI reconstruction with ADM had similar low rates of complications and explantations compared to traditional tissue expander/

implant reconstruction[1] (**FIGS 2** and **3**). This cohort was followed for an average of 5 years and was found to have similar revision rates for malposition, size, fat grafting, and capsular contracture between DTI and tissue expander reconstruction.[4]

- In a review of 500 nipple-sparing mastectomies with immediate reconstruction performed at one center, DTI reconstruction was performed in 59% vs 41% for two-stage expander/implant reconstruction. The rate of implant loss was 1.9% with no significant difference between DTI and two-stage tissue expander reconstructions.[4]
- An 8-year experience with DTI reconstructions using ADM in 466 reconstructed breast had an overall complication rate

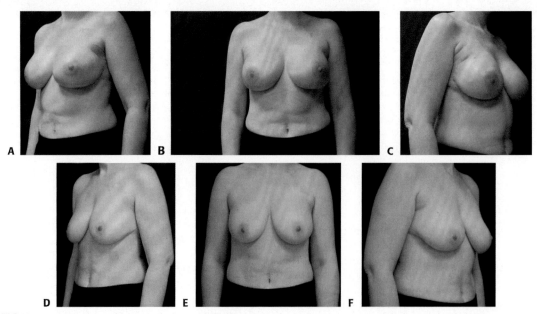

FIG 3 • A–C. A 40-year-old woman before and **(D–F)** after nipple-sparing mastectomy with direct-to-implant reconstruction.

of 3.9% and overall revision rate of 9.4%, similar to two-stage reconstructions.[5]

- A 5-year experience with 682 reconstructions found no difference in the revision rate between DTI and two-stage expander reconstructions.[6]

COMPLICATIONS

- Skin/nipple necrosis: Skin necrosis requires aggressive management to prevent infection or exposure of the implant. Small areas can be debrided and closed in the clinic setting. Larger areas require return to the OR for excision and possible downsize of the implant or placement of a tissue expander.
- Infection: Erythema, fever, drainage, pain, and swelling are signs of a cellulitis or periprosthetic infection. If symptoms are mild, oral antibiotics can be administered. If severe, the patient is admitted to the hospital for intravenous antibiotics. If the symptoms do not improve, the patient is returned to the operating room for washout and removal or replacement of the implant.
- Hematoma, seroma, and asymmetry are other potential complications.
- Long-term complications include implant rippling, capsular contracture, implant rupture, malposition, and contour irregularities.

REFERENCES

1. Colwell AS, Damjanovic B, Zahedi B, et al. Retrospective review of 331 consecutive immediate single-stage implant reconstructions with acellular dermal matrix: indications, complications, trends, and costs. *Plast Reconstr Surg.* 2011;128:1170-1178.
2. Scheflan M, Colwell AS. Tissue reinforcement in implant-based breast reconstruction. *Plast Reconstr Surg Glob Open.* 2014;2:e192.
3. Colwell AS, Gadd M, Smith BL, et al. An inferolateral approach to nipple-sparing mastectomy: optimizing mastectomy and reconstruction. *Ann Plast Surg.* 2010;65:140-143.
4. Colwell AS, Tessler O, Lin AM, et al. Breast reconstruction following nipple-sparing mastectomy: predictors of complications, reconstruction outcomes, and 5-year trends. *Plast Reconstr Surg.* 2014; 133:496-506.
5. Salzberg CA, Ashikari AY, Koch RM, et al. An 8-year experience of direct-to-implant immediate breast reconstruction using human acellular dermal matrix (AlloDerm). *Plast Reconstr Surg.* 2011;127:514-524.
6. Clarke-Pearson EM, Lin AM, Hertl C, et al. Revisions in implant-based breast reconstruction: how does direct-to-implant measure up? *Plast Reconstr Surg.* 2016;137:1690-1699.

Section VI: Latissimus Flap Breast Reconstruction

Latissimus Flap

Peter Henderson and Joseph J. Disa

DEFINITION

- The principal reason to undergo a latissimus dorsi (LD) myocutaneous flap for breast reconstruction is to recruit healthy skin to replace lost breast skin. The volume of subcutaneous tissue is often insufficient to adequately replace the breast mound. In this case, the most common approach is to place tissue expanders (TEs) at the time of the LD flap, followed by expansion and ultimately exchange for permanent implants at a later date (but in the appropriately selected patient, breast reconstruction can be performed in a single stage, with the permanent implants placed at the time of the LD flap).[1]
- LD flap breast reconstruction without placement of any sort of prosthetic device (TEs or permanent implants) would be done in one of three scenarios:
  - First, if the patient's build is so thin that minimal breast mound is needed in order to provide the desired breast projection
  - Second, if the patient is obese and has a large amount of fat in the four fat compartments of the back, as described for the low transverse extended LD flap concept by Bailey et al. (parascapular fold, lumbothoracic fold, lumbar fold, or suprailiac ford).
  - Third, if the decision has been made that there will be no attempt to recreate any appreciable breast mound at the current time (if the patient's preferences change in the future change, a prosthetic device could be placed at a subsequent operation). In the case of this reason, the LD flap would be best thought of as a means of providing soft tissue coverage for chest wounds and not of actual "breast reconstruction," per se.

ANATOMY

- The LD is a Mathes-Nahai type V muscle. The dominant pedicle is the thoracodorsal artery and vein (off the subscapular artery and vein), and multiple secondary pedicles arise from the lumbar vessels (**FIG 1**).
- The origins of the muscle are the spinous processes of T7-T12, the thoracolumbar fascia, the iliac crest, the inferior angle of the scapula, and ribs 9 to 12.
- The insertion is the floor of the intertubercular or bicipital groove of the humerus.
- The innervation is the thoracodorsal nerve (off the posterior cord of the brachial plexus).
- The function of the LD is to adduct, extend, and internally rotate the ipsilateral arm.

PATHOGENESIS

- The indication for the LD myocutaneous flap is most commonly breast skin loss due to ischemia (particularly following skin-sparing or nipple-sparing mastectomy) and/or radiation-induced injury.

PATIENT HISTORY AND PHYSICAL FINDINGS

- The patient's breast history (prior procedures as well as adjuvant or neoadjuvant therapy) should be elicited to understand the timing and expected progression of the sequelae.
- If TEs are in place, it is important to understand if tissue expansion is complete or if it is still under way.
- Physical examination should focus on assessing the surface area of skin needed, and the volume of breast mound needed.
- The back should be examined for thickness/volume of the skin and subcutaneous tissue, as well as any prior incisions.

IMAGING

- No imaging is necessary for preoperative planning.
- If necessary, appropriate surveillance for breast disease (mammography, MRI, etc.) should be performed.

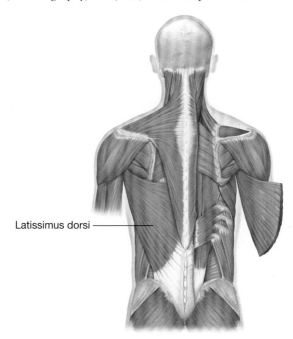

Latissimus dorsi ——————

FIG 1 • Latissimus dorsi anatomy.

NONOPERATIVE MANAGEMENT

- If TE is in place and skin necrosis has occurred in the absence of infection or exposure of the TE, one approach is to continue expansion—in fact overexpansion—in order to excise and perform primary closure at the time of exchange, which obviates the need for recruitment of additional skin.

SURGICAL MANAGEMENT

Preoperative Planning

- If breast TE will be used, it is chosen based on base diameter and then desired projection.
- If permanent implants are to be used, they must be chosen prior to the procedure. Important variables are fill substance, size, shape, and texture. This should be a joint decision-making process between the patient and the reconstructive surgeon.
- The fill substance can be either saline or silicone (the outer shell is made of silicone in both cases). Saline has a less "natural" feel, but no surveillance is recommended; if rupture were to occur, it would be readily apparent, and saline is assuredly medically inert. Silicone has a more "natural" feel, though it is recommended to have a regular MRI surveillance imaging to evaluate for the possibility of rupture.
- The most important variable in choosing the size of the implant is the base diameter (there is a decreasing emphasis on the volume, as it is a variable that can change based on the shape of the device).
- The shape can be either round or anatomic ("form stable" or "gummy bear"). Anatomic implants were designed, in theory, to give more of a natural appearance. Round implants have greater upper pole projection and may not look as "natural" and instead have an "augmented" look, which may be desirable to some patients.
- All anatomic implants have a textured surface, whereas round implants can be either textured or smooth.[2,3]

Positioning

- Positioning is one of the greatest challenges of performing the LD flap.
- If bilateral LD flaps will be performed, then prone positioning is mandated for harvest of the flaps.
- If a unilateral LD flap will be performed, then flap harvest can be performed either prone or in the lateral decubitus position.
- If the patient had been prone for harvest, then inset is best performed after the patient is flipped supine. If the patient had been in the lateral decubitus position for harvest, then options include repositioning supine or else releasing the devices used to hold in the lateral decubitus position in order to place the patient in a "near-supine" position.

Approach

- The optimal orientation of the skin paddle has been debated. Some advocate for a skin paddle that will be closed in a roughly horizontal orientation, thereby making it easily hidden in the "bra line." Others advocate for orienting the skin paddle obliquely, with the medial aspect being more cranial and the lateral aspect being more caudal. An orientation of 90 degrees from that orientation has been done but commonly leads to a widened scar and is therefore usually avoided.

■ Latissimus Dorsi Myocutaneous Flap

- If the mastectomy was not performed on the same day, the mastectomy defect must be recreated, and decisions need to be made about the excision of any amount of skin.
- Position the patient in the prone or lateral decubitus position; ensure that appropriate padding of all sensitive areas (axilla, face, genitals, limbs, etc.) is performed with a deflatable beanbag, pillows, and foam.
- Incise the epidermis and dermis of the skin paddle (full thickness).
- Divide the subcutaneous tissue down to the LD fascia. Some surgeons prefer to divide straight down to the fascia, whereas others bevel away from the skin paddle to increase volume and/or capture additional perforators (**TECH FIG 1A**). Commonly, this beveling is performed particularly in the fat deep to the Scarpa fascia.
- Some advocate for suturing the skin paddle to the fascia to reduce the chance of injury (or even avulsion) of the skin paddle.
- Raise the skin flaps in the plane either just superficial to the LD fascia or deep to the LD fascia directly on the muscle. Borders of the dissection plane include the superior (free) margin of the LD, nearly to the midline, the thoracolumbar fascia near the iliac crest, and the lateral (free) margin of the LD. Of note, the inferior aspect of the trapezius muscle will be encountered at the superomedial aspect of the LD, and the plane of dissection must remain deep to the trapezius. Additionally, the serratus muscle can be difficult to distinguish from the LD at the lateral margin.
- Elevate the LD off the underlying fascia (**TECH FIG 1B**). Two approaches are possible: create the plane deep to the muscle first and then divide the nonfree margins (medial and inferior) or else divide the nonfree margins first, and then peel the LD muscle off the underlying fascia. Either way, be careful not to raise the serratus muscle with the LD; this can be best protected against by mobilizing in a medial-to-lateral direction at the superior aspect.
- As dissection continues superolaterally toward the thoracodorsal pedicle, care must be taken to avoid injury to the artery and vein that run in the plane immediately deep to the muscle (**TECH FIG 1C**).
- If arc of rotation is not sufficient to reach the recipient site on the anterior chest wall, a number of maneuvers can be used to increase the arc of rotation. First, one can mobilize the latissimus all the way up to the tendinous insertion on the humerus; this will require skeletonization of the thoracodorsal vessels. Second,

TECHNIQUES

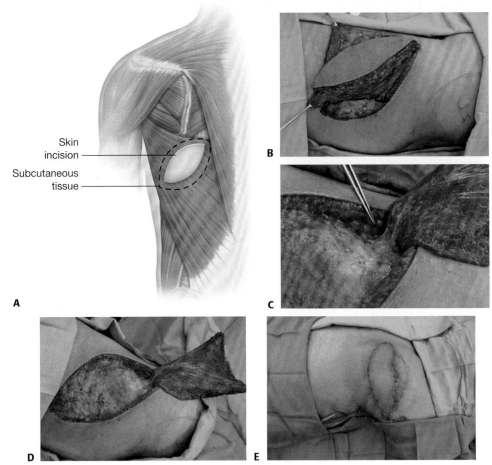

TECH FIG 1 • A. Diagram of beveling. **B.** Raising latissimus dorsi muscle flap. **C.** Thoracodorsal pedicle. **D.** Elevated flap. **E.** Inset of flap.

one can divide the serratus branch of the thoracodorsal pedicle. Third, one can divide the proximal tendinous insertion of the LD, partially, 90%, or completely; doing so enhances the arc of rotation, but increases the likelihood of stretch injury to and/or avulsion of the pedicle (**TECH FIG 1D**).[4]

- Create the subcutaneous tunnel from the back to the anterior mastectomy wound. The tunnel should be 3 to 4 fingerbreadths wide, and the tunnel should be made as far superior as possible in order to preserve the inframammary fold and to prevent an unsightly bulge that is not obscured in the axilla.
- Pass the flap through the tunnel into the anterior mastectomy pocket. While doing so, ensure that there is no unnecessary torque or twisting of the pedicle.
- Place closed-suction drains in the donor site.
- Irrigate and ensure hemostasis and close the back wound in layers.
- Dress the back wound.
- Turn the patient to the supine position for inset. If the patient was prone, this will require reprepping. If the patient was in the lateral decubitus position, it is possible to release the beanbag and ease the patient into a nearly supine position (otherwise, the patient should be positioned and reprepped as if she had been prone).

- Complete delivery of the flap through the subcutaneous tunnel.
- Inset the LD muscle to the chest wall, taking care to recreate the inframammary fold and affixing medial enough to generate medial fullness and avoid excess lateral/axillary fullness.
- If TEs will be placed, do so in the pocket created by the LD muscle, prior to completion of inset.
- If permanent implants will be placed, most surgeons recommend using a removable sizer intraoperatively in order to choose the most appropriate size and shape of implant and then place the appropriately sized permanent implant into the pocket.
- Though unequivocal evidence is lacking, many surgeons choose to employ a combination of Betadine, topical antibiotics, and the "no touch" technique in order to reduce the risk of infection and capsular contracture. Most surgeons will place 100 to 150 mL of saline in each expander at the time of placement and then begin serial expansions as an outpatient in about 2 weeks.
- Place at least one closed-suction drain in the mastectomy pocket.
- The native breast skin is closed to the LD skin paddle with sutures in the deep dermal and the subcuticular positions (**TECH FIG 1E**).[5–7]

PEARLS AND PITFALLS

Technique
- Some surgeons advocate for transection of the thoracodorsal nerve. This has the advantage of reducing animation, but increases the likelihood of vascular pedicle injury and may lead to increased muscle atrophy.
- Keeping the tunnel as superior as possible (near the axilla) will preserve the inframammary fold and prevent an unsightly bulge on the inferior, lateral chest wall.
- Hematoma and seroma are common complications at the back donor site. Ensure meticulous hemostasis, place drains, and consider "quilting sutures" to reduce the amount of dead space.

POSTOPERATIVE CARE

- The anterior (breast) drains may be removed relatively early, though the posterior (back) drains should be left longer (at least 7 days) to minimize the incidence of seroma.
- If breast TEs were placed, then serial percutaneous expansions usually begin approximately 2 weeks postoperatively and continue with weekly or biweekly expansions of approximately 50 mL/session until the desired size is achieved.
- Patients can expect to resume full activities by 6 weeks.

OUTCOMES

- Functional deficiency as a result of loss of one (or even both) LD muscles is minimal, except in individuals who would otherwise participate in strenuous physical activity that emphasizes the upper body (swimming, rock climbing, etc).[8]

COMPLICATIONS

- Seroma at the donor (back) site is not uncommon and can be protected against by leaving drains for at least 7 days and performing intraoperative measures that reduce the dead space.
- Transient venous congestion of the skin paddle can be observed, though tissue loss is uncommon.
- Fat necrosis is uncommon, because of the limited amount of subcutaneous tissue in the LD flap (compared to the abdomen-based flaps).
- Exposure of the breast device can occur. If it is a TE and if there are no signs of infection, it is possible to complete expansion and then exchange for permanent implant. If the exposed device is a permanent implant, or if signs of infection are present, the device almost always must be removed (and can be replaced immediately in only limited circumstances).

REFERENCES

1. Bailey SH. The low transverse extended latissimus dorsi flap based on fat compartments of the back for breast reconstruction. *Plast Reconstr Surg.* 2011;128:382-394.
2. Feng J, Pardoe CI, Mota AM, et al. Two-stage latissimus dorsi flap with implant for unilateral breast reconstruction: getting the size right. *Arch Plast Surg.* 2016;43(2):197-203.
3. Hammond DC. Latissimus dorsi flap breast reconstruction. *Plast Reconstr Surg.* 2009;124:1055-1063.
4. Hwang MJ, Sterne G. Thoracodorsal nerve division in latissimus dorsi breast reconstruction to avoid unwanted breast animation: a safe and simple technique to ensure division of all branches. *J Plast Reconstr Aesthet Surg.* 2015;68(2):e43-e44.
5. Moore HG Jr, Harkins HN. The use of a latissimus dorsi pedicle flap graft in radical mastectomy. *Surg Gynecol Obstet.* 1953;96(4):430-432.
6. Sternberg EG, Perdikis G, McLaughlin SA, et al. Latissimus dorsi flap remains an excellent choice for breast reconstruction. *Ann Plast Surg.* 2006;56(1):31-35.
7. van Huizum MA, Hage JJ, Rutgers EJ. Immediate breast reconstruction with a myocutaneous latissimus dorsi flap and implant following skin-sparing salvage mastectomy after irradiation as part of breast-conserving therapy. *J Plast Resconstr Aesthet Surg.* 2016;69:1080-1086.
8. Yang JD, Huh JS, Min Yes, et al. Physical and functional ability recovery patterns and quality of life after immediate autologous latissimus dorsi breast reconstruction: a 1-year prospective observational study. *Plast Reconstr Surg.* 2015;136(6):1146-1154.

19

CHAPTER

Section VII: Abdominal Flap Breast Reconstruction

TRAM

Peter Henderson, Jeffrey A. Ascherman, and Joseph J. Disa

DEFINITION

- The pedicle transverse rectus abdominis myocutaneous (TRAM) flap for breast reconstruction was first described by Hartrampf et al. in 1982, and it heralded the onset of a new era of abdomen-based autologous breast reconstruction. This procedure has been modified and improved upon, such that today free perforator flaps from the abdomen (as well as other sites such as the buttocks and thighs) have become the most modern, cutting-edge procedures available. But it is indisputable that the pedicle TRAM is a procedure that every reconstructive surgeon must have available in his or her armamentarium, to use as both a form of primary breast reconstruction as well as a salvage procedure in the case of failure of device-based reconstruction or other non–abdomen-based autologous reconstruction.[1,2]

ANATOMY

- The rectus abdominis (RA) is a Mathes-Nahai type III muscle. The two dominant pedicles are the superior epigastric vessels (off the internal mammary artery and vein) and the deep inferior epigastric vessels (off of the external iliac artery and vein). The superior epigastric vessels approach the RA from the cranial direction on the central portion of the deep surface of the RA. The deep inferior epigastric vessels approach the RA from the lateral aspect of the caudal portion of the RA, on the deep surface (**FIG 1**).[3]
- The origins of the RA are the sternum and the 5th-7th ribs.
- The insertion is the pubic symphysis.
- Innervation is from multiple branches of the intercostal nerves, which penetrate the lateral aspect of the posterior rectus sheath and enter the RA muscle on its deep surface.
- The function of the paired RA is to flex the trunk at the waist.
- The rectus sheath is composed of the aponeuroses of the external oblique, internal oblique, and transversus abdominis muscles (**FIG 2**). Cranial to the arcuate line (aka "arcuate line of Douglas" and "linea semicircularis"), the anterior rectus sheath is composed of the aponeuroses of the external oblique and the anterior leaflet of the internal oblique, and the posterior rectus sheath is composed of the aponeuroses of the posterior leaflet of the internal oblique

and the transversus abdominis (as well as the transversalis fascia). Caudal to the arcuate line, the anterior rectus sheath is composed of the aponeuroses of the external oblique, internal oblique, and transversus abdominis muscles, and the posterior rectus sheath is composed of only the transversalis fascia.

PATHOGENESIS

- The pedicle TRAM procedure is indicated for breast reconstruction when skin and/or subcutaneous tissue is needed, and the patient has sufficient excess abdominal skin and fat to serve as donor tissue.

PATIENT HISTORY AND PHYSICAL FINDINGS

- The patient's breast history (prior procedures as well as adjuvant or neoadjuvant therapy) should be elicited to understand the timing and expected progression of the sequelae.
- Nicotine use is highly deleterious to the outcomes of this operation and should be avoided at all costs. Tumor resection must occur in a timely fashion, but reconstruction can be delayed until the patient has stopped smoking.

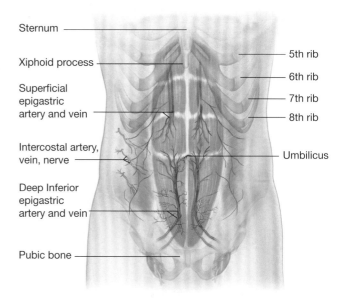

FIG 1 • Rectus abdominis anatomy.

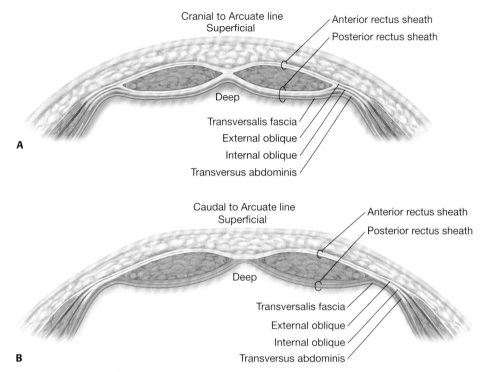

FIG 2 • Contributions to rectus sheath cranial and caudal to arcuate line.

- In patients who will undergo radiation therapy, the surgeon and patient may choose to delay the reconstruction until the radiation is completed.
- Surgical history should focus on prior abdominal operations, breast operations, and cardiac procedures (to determine if the internal mammary artery has been used as a cardiac bypass or has potentially been damaged during rewiring of a sternotomy; this is the source vessel for the superior epigastric artery).
- Physical exam of the chest should focus on assessing the surface area of skin needed, and the volume of breast mound needed.
- The abdomen should be examined for amount of subcutaneous tissue and excess skin and estimated laxity (in terms of defect that can be closed without undue tension). Prior abdominal scars should be noted (midline scars usually render the tissue contralateral to the pedicle unable to be included in the flap). Any hernias (umbilical, incisional, etc.) should be noted.
- An acoustic (handheld) Doppler can be used to identify perforators (especially if a fascia-sparing approach is to be used)

IMAGING

- CT angiography can be performed if there is any question about the patency of the superior epigastric vessels, as well as for identification of abdominal wall perforators.

NONOPERATIVE MANAGEMENT

- Breast reconstruction is never mandatory and can be deferred if the patient's wishes or comorbidities preclude it from happening.

SURGICAL MANAGEMENT
Preoperative Planning

- Decision must be made as to whether the amount of skin and subcutaneous tissue that is needed at the recipient (breast) site can be reliably met with a unipedicle TRAM. Smoking, prior abdominal incisions, and large breasts can decrease the likelihood that a unipedicle TRAM is suitable. Near-infrared fluorescent angiography can provide valuable semiquantitative data to assist in clinical decision-making.
- If concern that a single pedicle will not suffice, available measures to increase the surface area and volume that can be safely carried with the flap include performing a bipedicle TRAM (using both superior epigastric pedicles) and performing surgical delay (2 weeks prior to the reconstruction).[4,5]

Positioning

- Supine
- Ideally, arms are tucked (but sometimes that is not possible if breast surgeons are performing axillary sentinel lymph node biopsy or full axillary dissection; in that case, the arms can be tucked after the breast surgeons complete their portion of the operation).
- The patient's waist should be positioned at the appropriate break in the bed so that a flexed (semi-Fowler) position can be utilized to assist with closure of the abdomen.

■ TRAM Flap for Breast Reconstruction

Preparation

- Preoperatively, the patient is marked in the standing position (**TECH FIG 1**).
- Prep the patient, including the entire bilateral breasts and abdomen to the groin. Make sure to clean the umbilicus.
- If necessary, perform surgical delay of the TRAM flap prior to definitive reconstruction.
  - This can take the form of either dividing the skin and subcutaneous tissue but not otherwise raising the flap, or dividing the deep inferior epigastric pedicle alone.
- At the time of definitive reconstruction, inspect the mastectomy defect, or else recreate the mastectomy defect (in the plane immediately superficial to the pectoralis major muscle) if the reconstruction is delayed relative to the mastectomy.
- If the procedure will be performed as a unipedicle TRAM, the surgeon must decide which superior epigastric pedicle will be used (left or right); some surgeons advocate for using the pedicle ipsilateral to the breast defect, whereas others advocate for using the contralateral pedicle.
  - The ipsilateral pedicle will often allow the surgeon to create more ptosis in the reconstructed breast, whereas the contralateral pedicle may initially allow the pedicle to appear flatter as it crosses the upper abdomen.
  - It is also possible to use a bipedicle TRAM to maximize the amount of tissue that can be harvested. The surgeon can either split the flap in the midline or leave it intact, depending on the needs of the defect.

Dissection and Flap Elevation

- Incise the skin and subcutaneous tissue down to the external oblique fascia (laterally) and the anterior rectus sheath (medially).
  - If direction of dissection bevels outward, the volume of recruited tissue is greater, and the likelihood of capturing important perforators increases.
  - Also incise the skin and subcutaneous tissue surrounding the umbilicus down to the anterior rectus sheath.
- Elevate the "abdominoplasty" flap off of the anterior rectus sheath, using the costal margin and the xiphoid as the limits of dissection (**TECH FIG 2B**).

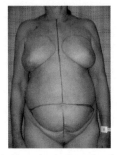

TECH FIG 1 • Markings for ipsilateral unipedicle TRAM breast reconstruction.

- At the level of the external oblique fascia, separate the skin and fat flap from the underlying fascia in a lateral-to-medial direction; one can move quickly until the lateral edge of the rectus sheath (linea semicircularis) (**TECH FIG 2C**).
- Depending on the amount of fascia intended to be taken as part of the flap, one can either incise anterior rectus sheath at the lateral edge or carefully continue dissecting the flap off of the anterior rectus sheath until the lateral row perforators are found (**TECH FIG 2D**).
  - In this case, a maximal amount of anterior rectus sheath can be spared, and the likelihood of postoperative incisional hernia decreases.
- If unilateral breast reconstruction and unipedicle TRAM will be used, the flap on the side contralateral to the pedicle is completely raised.
  - If bipedicle TRAM will be used, or if bilateral TRAM flaps are being raised, the tissue connection between the flap and the underlying fascia will be maintained overlying both the left and the right pedicles.
- Moving in a direction away from the flap, elevate the anterior rectus sheath off of the rectus abdominis (RA) muscles (this dissection must continue cranial to the costal margin).
  - Separating the fascia and the muscle will be difficult at the tendinous insertions; at these points, err on the side of fascia to avoid injury to the superior epigastric pedicle, which can be very superficial at the level of the inscriptions.
- Determine how much RA muscle will be included in the flap.
  - Most surgeons will use the entire width of the muscle, but it is possible to preserve a lateral strip (the intercostal neurovascular pedicle enters the muscle from the deep surface of the lateral aspect).
- Isolate and divide the deep inferior epigastric vessels; do so as far caudally as possible to preserve length in case the flap would benefit from "supercharging" (anastomosing the deep inferior epigastric vein to augment venous outflow) because of venous congestion.
- Moving in a caudal-to-cranial direction, raise the flap (skin, subcutaneous tissue, fascia, and muscle) off of the posterior rectus sheath (**TECH FIG 2E**).
  - Ensure that the vascular pedicle is included in the flap (and minimize the risk of injury to the pedicle) by dissecting precisely at the superficial surface of the posterior rectus sheath (ie, all areolar tissue is included in the flap).

Passing and Insetting the Flap

- Create a subcutaneous tunnel between the mastectomy space and the abdomen that is at least four fingerbreadths wide.
  - Most surgeons advocate for the tunnel being as far medial as possible, but that may increase the likelihood of an unsightly bulge near the midline.
- Pass the flap through the tunnel, ensuring that no problematic twisting, or kinking, of the pedicle has occurred.
- Inset the flap to the chest wall and the overlying skin.

T E C H N I Q U E S

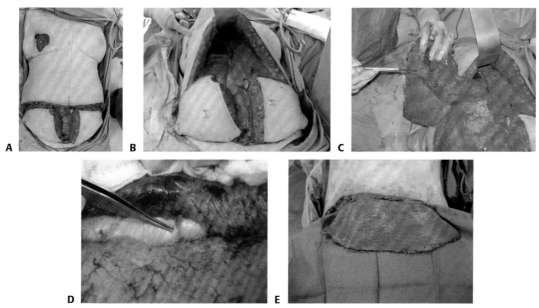

TECH FIG 2 • A. Right mastectomy defect and skin incisions done bilaterally for unipedicle TRAM. (Only a hemiflap was needed in this case.) **B.** Abdominal skin flap elevated and anterior rectus sheath elevated off the muscle. **C.** Deep inferior epigastric pedicle has been divided, and the flap is raised off the posterior rectus sheath in preparation for delivery in to the mastectomy space. **D.** Lateral row perforator exiting the muscle and entering the skin paddle. **E.** Pedicled TRAM in situ completely de-epithelialized in a different patient.

- If nipple-sparing mastectomy was performed, it is possible to have a flap with no cutaneous portion, but even in that case some surgeons would advocate for including a skin paddle to use as an indicator (this can easily be excised under local anesthesia after the viability of the flap has been ensured).
  - Place closed suction drains.
- Some surgeons close the anterior rectus sheath with non-absorbable sutures, whereas others may use long-lasting absorbable sutures (**TECH FIG 3A**).
- Ensure that all layers of anterior rectus sheath are included (caudally, the external oblique and internal oblique aponeuroses tend to separate) (**TECH FIG 3B**).

- If the wound cannot be primarily closed, mesh should be used (**TECH FIG 3C**). Even if it can be primarily closed, some surgeons choose to reinforce the fascial closure with mesh.
- Place closed suction drains.
- Flex the patient at the waist to reduce tension, and then close the abdominal defect by suturing the Scarpa fascia, the deep dermis, and the skin.
- Mature the umbilicus by incising the skin at the point overlying the umbilical stalk. There is no consensus on the best shape for the skin excision, but most would advocate for some noncircular shape (as an uninterrupted circle is prone to contracture/stenosis in the long term).

TECH FIG 3 • A. Primary closure of the rectus sheath with permanent sutures. **B.** Contralateral plication of the abdominal wall to centralize the umbilicus. **C.** Mesh reinforcement of the primary rectus sheath repair.

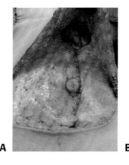
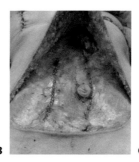
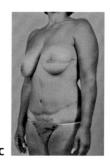

PEARLS AND PITFALLS

Dissection of rectus abdominis	■ It is advisable to dissect the rectus abdominis muscle to a point cranial to the costal margin; doing so maximizes the arc of rotation. Remember that the superior epigastric pedicle pierces the posterior rectus sheath at a point caudal to the costal margin; thus, the superior aspect of the muscle can be disinserted from the cranial attachments to the ribs and xiphoid to further increase arc of rotation as long as it is done very carefully *cranial* to the costal margin.
Dissection of umbilicus	■ A previously unidentified umbilical hernia is not uncommon and must be watched for during the umbilical dissection. If identified, it should be reduced and repaired.
Dissection of anterior rectus sheath	■ The locations at which the pedicle is most at risk during the dissection of the anterior rectus sheath off of the rectus abdominis muscle are at the tendinous inscriptions (the muscle is very thin and fused with the overlying aponeurosis; the underlying pedicle is in close proximity). Risk can be minimized by erring on the side of the rectus sheath, instead of dissecting into the muscle.
Equipment	■ Have hospital bed available at end of operation (instead of stretcher); this will reduce the number of transfers between beds and thereby reduce the likelihood of undue tension being placed on the patient's abdominal closure

POSTOPERATIVE CARE

- Ensure that patient remains in semi-Fowler ("beach chair") position for the early postoperative period (staying flexed at the waist reduces tension at the abdominal closure).
  - This should be maintained both while in bed and when walking.
  - Restrictions can usually be relaxed in 1 to 2 weeks.
- Avoid strenuous activity for 6 weeks to reduce likelihood of developing hernia at fascial closure site(s).

OUTCOMES

- In case of unipedicle TRAM, functional deficit is minimal (**FIG 3**).
- If bipedicle TRAM has been performed, or bilateral TRAMs have been raised (and therefore both RA muscles have been rendered nonfunctional), some weakness in flexing the waist (ie, sit-ups) may occur.

COMPLICATIONS

- Complete flap loss is extremely rare. Partial flap loss can occur and is more commonly due to venous congestion than to arterial insufficiency. Use of near-infrared laser angiography to assess for flap perfusion can help in operative decision-making.
- Wound healing complications at the breast site can occur due to flap ischemia or native breast skin damage (such as due to radiation or ischemia due to excessive thinning of the mastectomy flaps). Wound healing complications at the abdominal closure site can occur due to excess tension or systemic vasoconstriction (such as caused by nicotine use).
- Infection is relatively uncommon, though of greater significance when prosthetic mesh was used in the abdominal closure.
- Hernia development at the fascial closure site can occur due to poor technique (most notably excess suture tension

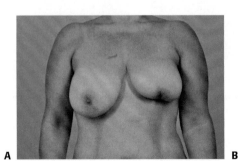
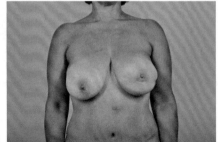
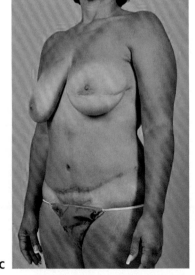

FIG 3 • Preoperative **(A)** and postoperative **(B,C)** appearance of a patient who underwent partial breast reconstruction with a ipsilateral pedicle TRAM flap.

leading to fascial ischemia) and can be decreased by avoiding strenuous activity for 6 weeks after the operation. Including mesh in the abdominal closure may further minimize the chance of hernia and bulge development.

REFERENCES

1. Hartrampf CR, Scheflan M, Black PW. Breast reconstruction with a transverse abdominal island flap. *Plast Reconstr Surg.* 1982; 69(2):216-225.

2. Jones G. The pedicled TRAM flap in breast reconstruction. *Clin Plast Surg.* 2007;34(1):83-104.

3. Moon HK, Taylor GI. The vascular anatomy of rectus abdominis musculocutaneous flaps based on the deep superior epigastric system. *Plast Reconstr Sur.* 1988;82(5):815-832.

4. Nahabedian MY, Patel K. Autologous flap breast reconstruction: surgical algorithm and patient selection. *J Surg Oncol.* 2016;113(8): 865-874.

5. Wagner DS, Michelow BJ, Hartrampf CR Jr. Double-pedicle TRAM flap for unilateral breast reconstruction. *Plast Reconstr Surg.* 1991;88(6):987-997.

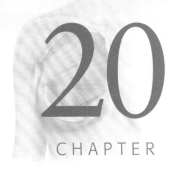

Free TRAM

CHAPTER **20**

Jennifer A. Klok and Toni Zhong

DEFINITION

- The free transverse rectus abdominis myocutaneous (TRAM) flap is composed of lower abdominal skin, subcutaneous fat, anterior rectus fascia, and a segment of the rectus abdominis muscle. The pedicle for this flap is the deep inferior epigastric artery (DIEA).
- The variations in free abdominal flaps based off the DIEA have been classified according to the inclusion and width of the rectus abdominis muscle used. The muscle-sparing (MS) free TRAM flaps spare either the lateral muscle (MS-1) or the medial and lateral muscle segments (MS-2). At either extreme are the free TRAM flap (MS-0), which includes the entire width and partial length of the muscle, and the MS-3 or deep inferior epigastric perforator (DIEP) flap, which preserves the entire muscle.[1]
- For the purposes of this chapter, the free TRAM (MS-0) flap will be discussed. This flap was first described by Holstrom in 1979.[2]
- The free TRAM flap has typically been used for the purpose of breast reconstruction. However, other uses include chest wall, upper extremity, lower extremity, and head and neck reconstruction.

ANATOMY

- The rectus muscle has a dual blood supply that coalesces in choke vessels at the umbilicus where the deep superior epigastric and deep inferior epigastric systems meet.[3]
- The free TRAM flap is based off the deep inferior epigastric vessels. The pedicle originates from the external iliac artery and then travels cephalad to enter the lateral and deep surface of the rectus abdominis muscle a few centimeters below the arcuate line. Just above the level of the arcuate line, the vessels typically divide into a medial and lateral row and

continue superiorly, sending perforating branches through the muscle to supply the overlying skin and fat (**FIG 1A,B**).[3,4]
- Three variations in DIEA branching patterns have been described, the type II variation with medial and lateral row branching being the most common at 57% to 84%. Type I vessels continue cephalad with the muscle as a single artery (27% to 29%), whereas type III vessels divide into three branches and are least common (14% to 16%).[3–5]
- On average, five to six perforators originate from the DIEA.[4] In a free TRAM flap, all or most of these perforators are preserved.
- The nerve supply to the rectus abdominis muscle originates from the lower six thoracic intercostal nerves. The nerves travel in the fascia of the transversus abdominis muscle and enter posteriorly at the junction between the lateral and middle third of the muscle.[3]
- Functionally, the rectus abdominis muscle acts to flex the torso, originating at the pubic symphysis and inserting onto the fifth to seventh rib cartilages.

PATIENT HISTORY AND PHYSICAL FINDINGS

- Discussing patient goals and expectations for breast reconstruction is one of the most important aspects of the initial consultation for surgery.
- It is essential to conduct a thorough review of past medical history, surgical history, medications, allergies, smoking history, personal or family history of clotting disorders, and detailed breast cancer history.
- Of particular importance on surgical history are number and type of abdominal surgeries to assess adequacy of the donor site.
- It is important to understand the details of the patient's breast cancer history. All neoadjuvant and expected adjuvant therapies need to be discussed and documented.

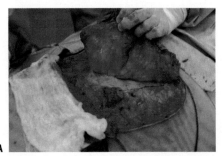
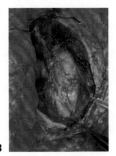

FIG 1 • **A.** Photo showing the most superior perforators from the medial and lateral rows near the level of the umbilicus. **B.** The course of the DIEA with its two venae comitantes is seen here through a long window in the rectus abdominis muscle (top of photo is cephalad). The forceps at the bottom of the image is lifting the transversalis fascia. This layer is elevated to expose the pedicle in proximity to the vessel origin.

- If the patient is expected to have postoperative radiation, it is still our typical practice to delay autologous reconstruction until 12 months after completion of radiation.
  - Tamoxifen is stopped for 2 weeks prior to and after surgery.
- Any questionable clotting disorder history warrants consultation with a hematologist.
- We will not operate on patients who are smokers. They are required to quit smoking a minimum of 6 weeks prior to surgery. This includes being off nicotine patches. Nicotine urine tests are performed on recent ex-smokers.
- On physical exam, assess the patient's overall body habitus, BMI, and brassiere cup size.
- Examine breasts for scars, skin quality (including radiation changes), palpable masses, symmetry, ptosis, and perform standard breast measurements.
- Examine abdomen for scars, skin quality, and amount of excess skin and subcutaneous tissue (pinch test), and palpate for hernias.

IMAGING

- At our center, all patients have computed tomography angiography (CTA) of the abdomen prior to their surgery.
- The CTA assists with surgical planning in identification of dominant perforators as well as their intramuscular course from the pedicle.[5,6]
- Having this preoperative understanding of the vessel anatomy for each individual patient can help to guide the decision between doing an MS-3 perforator flap (**FIG 2A**), which is our preference, and flap that includes muscle to incorporate additional perforators (**FIG 2B**).
- Alternative imaging techniques include color Doppler (duplex) ultrasound, handheld Doppler, and magnetic resonance angiography.[6]

SURGICAL MANAGEMENT

- Broad indications for choosing autologous reconstruction over implant-based reconstruction include the following: patient goals and expectations, adequate donor site tissue, longevity of reconstruction, resistance to undergo multiple future surgeries, amount of ptosis of the contralateral native breast, importance that the patient places on natural look and feel of

the reconstruction, and history of chest or breast radiation.[7]
- Although we perform free TRAM flaps, we aim for DIEP and MS-TRAM flaps in the majority of our breast reconstructions. Sometimes, a full free TRAM is needed; however, this is rarely the case. Maximum preservation of rectus fascia and muscle whenever possible to limit abdominal morbidity should be the goal in reconstruction.
- Indications for choosing a full free TRAM over a MS-TRAM or DIEP flap are few but relate to a need for increased flap perfusion and can be divided into patient and intraoperative factors.[1]
- Patient factors include recent history of smoking, prior abdominal liposuction, abdominoplasty or multiple abdominal surgeries with extensive scarring in the rectus abdominis muscle, and large flap volume (greater than 1000 g) required in patients with aforementioned risk factors.[1,8-10]
- Intraoperative factors include the number and size of perforators located during flap elevation. The presence of a dominant perforator at least 1.5 mm in diameter would indicate suitability for a perforator flap. If no single dominant perforator is located or the reliability of selected perforator(s) for supply of the flap becomes questionable after temporary occlusion of other identified perforators, then an MS-TRAM or free TRAM is indicated.[1]
  - If the medial and lateral row perforators are found to be so widely separated that they come off the extreme edges of the muscle and are so small in caliber to the extent that at MS-TRAM off one row would be inadequate, then the whole width of the muscle would need to be harvested in a full TRAM.
- An additional intraoperative scenario that might steer the surgeon to convert to a free TRAM includes encountering a severely scarred or attenuated rectus abdominis muscle where the musculocutaneous perforators are encased in scar and unidentifiable.

Preoperative Planning

- Optimize the patient for surgery with appropriate consultations to anesthesia, medicine, and/or hematology as needed.
- Carefully review the CTA to understand the size, location, and intramuscular course of the perforators.

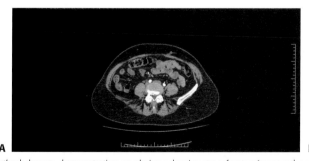
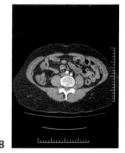

FIG 2 • **A.** CTA of a patient's abdomen demonstrating an obvious dominant perforator (greater than 1.5 mm in size) coming from the medial branch of the left DIEA. This patient will likely be a good candidate for a DIEP flap. **B.** The largest perforator seen on the right hemiabdomen is shown here and is quite small in size (less than 1.5 mm). Intraoperatively, it may be determined not to be reliable enough to support the flap. More perforators may be required, and in this case, a free TRAM or MS-TRAM would be considered.

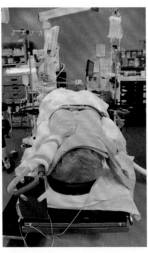

FIG 3 • Demonstrates positioning of the patient. The bed is turned 180 degrees so that the anesthetic machine is at the foot of the bed. The patient's arms are tucked, the face is protected, and all bony prominences are well padded.

- Prior to surgery administer heparin 5000 U subcutaneously and apply thromboembolism deterrent stockings (TEDs) and sequential compression devices (SCDs).
- Give intravenous antibiotics (usually cefazolin) prior to incision.

Positioning

- Position the patient supine with the arms tucked and the surgical table turned 180 degrees (**FIG 3**). This creates more space for surgeons and assistants as well as room for the microscope in the field.

Approach

- **Retrograde approach:** Start distally by lifting the lateral edge of muscle to identify the pedicle and elevate flap from caudal to cephalad.
- **Anterograde approach:** Transect superior edge of muscle just above the most superior perforators and elevate flap from cephalad to caudad.
- **Fascial sparing approach:** Always try to spare as much muscle fascia as possible by closely hugging the medial and lateral perforator rows during dissection.

■ Markings

- Markings are done preoperatively with the patient standing.
- Start with the breast markings and mark the sternal notch, sternal midline, inframammary folds (IMF), and breast borders.
  - We use one of three mastectomy incisions in immediate reconstruction cases. These include circumareolar, circumvertical pattern with skin reduction, or circumareolar with straight vertical incision (**TECH FIG 1A–C**).

- In delayed reconstruction, the mastectomy incision is marked for excision. A superolateral back-cut or pleat is drawn on the superior mastectomy skin to avoid the pinched appearance of the flap just below the mastectomy scar. The lower mastectomy skin borders are marked for eventual excision (**TECH FIG 1D**).
- The abdominal incision is marked superiorly above the umbilicus and inferiorly along the suprapubic crease. The incision lines are checked using a pinch test. The height of the abdominal flap should match the width of the breast (**TECH FIG 1E**).

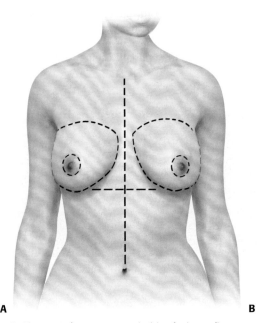

A

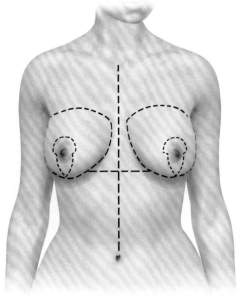

B

TECH FIG 1 • A. Circumareolar mastectomy incision for immediate reconstruction. **B.** Circumvertical mastectomy incisions resulting in mosque pattern with vertical scar used in immediate reconstruction for patients with skin laxity and ptosis.

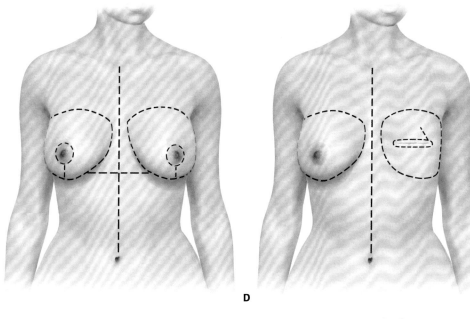

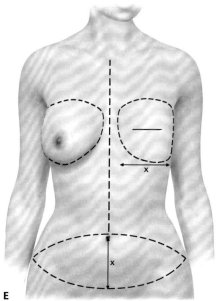

TECH FIG 1 (Continued) • **C.** Circumareolar mastectomy incision with vertical extension for immediate reconstruction in patients with a tight skin envelope to aid in exposure of the recipient vessels without over-retraction on the mastectomy flaps. **D.** Markings for delayed breast reconstruction illustrating excision of the mastectomy scar and back-cut incision on the upper lateral mastectomy flap to improve final flap contour. The shaded lower mastectomy skin will eventually be removed and the flap inset on top. **E.** Abdominal flap markings demonstrating the height of the flap midline equaling the width of the breast.

◾ Perforator Identification

- Confirm preoperative markings with patient on the operative table.
- Use a handheld Doppler to identify perforators based on CTA mapping and mark with suture.
- Isolate the umbilicus, leaving a cuff of fat around the stalk but taking care not to dissect too widely and inadvertently injure the periumbilical perforators.
- Make superior abdominal incision and dissect down to rectus fascia, beveling superiorly.
- Create inferior incision, taking care to first identify and dissect approximately 5 cm of the superficial inferior epigastric vein (SIEV) before completing the incision down to the fascia (**TECH FIG 2A**).
- Ensure that patient is fully paralyzed before proceeding.

- Start elevating skin flap from lateral to medial in suprafascial plane using electrocautery. Proceed carefully upon reaching the lateral border of the rectus abdominis muscle and begin to identify the lateral row perforators. At this point, lower the cautery settings.
- In a bilateral case, split the flap along the midline and elevate flap from medial to lateral to reveal the medial row perforators. In a unilateral case, the flap often crosses midline to incorporate a portion of the contralateral side depending on size requirements for the reconstruction. Once the size of the flap is determined, divide the flap and elevate from medial to lateral to identify the medial row perforators.
- In the free TRAM flap, all identified perforators in both the medial and lateral rows are preserved (**TECH FIG 2B,C**).

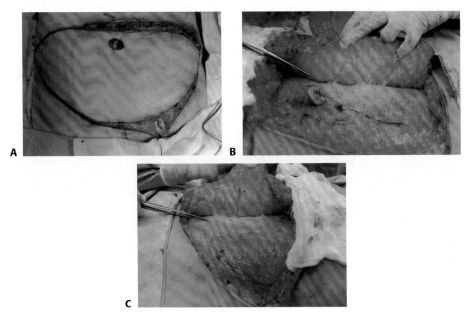

TECH FIG 2 • **A.** The superficial inferior epigastric vein (SIEV) is shown at the bottom right of the photo. Its location is superficial to the Scarpa fascia at this level and approximately one-third of the distance between midline and the anterior superior iliac spine (ASIS). This vein is spared whenever possible in our dissection to provide a backup for venous outflow. **B,C.** Exposure of the medial and lateral row of perforators originating from the deep inferior epigastric system. All of these perforators will be preserved and included in the free TRAM flap.

■ Fascial Dissection

- Mark fascia closely around selected perforators with methylene blue to spare as much fascia as possible (**TECH FIG 3A–C**).
- Use forceps and a scalpel to make the first incisions through fascia immediately around the perforators. The forceps are used to lift the fascia upward prior to incision to avoid injury to vessels directly beneath fascia.

- Once dissection around the perforators is done, complete the fascial incision with cautery on the cutting setting along a line to the lateral and inferior end of the muscle where the pedicle is expected.
- Once the incisions are complete, use forceps and electrocautery to elevate the fascia off the rectus abdominis muscle medially and laterally.
- Reflect fascia back on itself and staple for retraction (**TECH FIG 3D**).

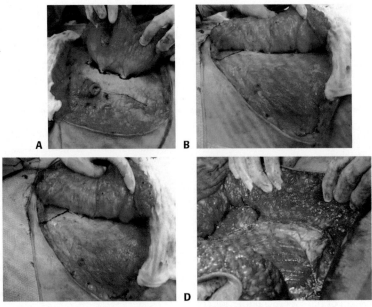

TECH FIG 3 • **A,B.** Fascial sparing technique is used during flap dissection. The methylene blue is used to mark out the fascial incision, ensuring that it is tight to exposed perforators. **C.** View of the lateral row in **(B)** shows the oblique inferolateral extension made to complete the fascial incision down to the level of the pedicle. **D.** After the fascia has been incised and elevated off the rectus abdominis muscle, it is stapled back to provide optimal exposure for the intramuscular dissection.

■ Intramuscular Dissection

- We typically perform the intramuscular dissection in a retrograde approach. Perform this part systematically and carefully. Dissect layer by layer to avoid diving into the muscle and injuring the pedicle or perforators.
- First, elevate the inferolateral edge of the rectus abdominis muscle to find the pedicle as it begins to travel beneath the muscle (**TECH FIG 4A**). Dissect through transversalis fascia to visualize its location and note its course as it travels superiorly under the muscle.
- Then dissect a long window through the muscle directly over the pedicle in a retrograde direction. Use tenotomy dissecting scissors and bipolar cautery to make this opening in the muscle down to the pedicle (**TECH FIG 4B**). Ligate larger branches with clips to prevent thermal damage to the main vessels.
- As the inferior perforators from the medial and lateral row are approached, transect the muscle transversely to its medial and lateral edge. Perform this one layer at a time keeping in mind that some perforators have a tortuous course through the muscle.

- Once the inferior edge of the muscle is divided, transect the superior edge of muscle just above the upper periumbilical perforators. Take care to identify the superior epigastric vessels at this level and ligate with clips.
- Once the muscle has been released inferiorly and superiorly, gently lift the flap and use bipolar cautery to divide any further attachments to the pedicle or muscle on its posterior surface.
- Caudally, use deep retractors to find the origin of the main vessels in the pelvis. The free TRAM flap requires a longer pedicle than does the perforator flap. We prefer to dissect a pedicle of at least 7 cm in length in situ on mild stretch (**TECH FIG 4C**).
- Temporarily staple the flap in place on the abdomen until the recipient vessels have been prepared (see below).
- When ready to do microsurgery, mark the anterior surface of the vessels for orientation, ligate the deep inferior epigastric artery and vein(s) with two vascular clips on each vessel, and start ischemia time.

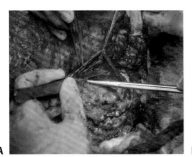 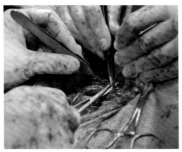 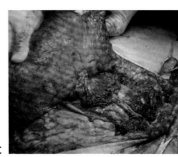

A   B   C

TECH FIG 4 • **A.** Photo showing the inferolateral edge of the rectus abdominis muscle being elevated to identify the deep inferior epigastric vessels entering the undersurface of the muscle. **B.** Demonstrating layer-by-layer dissection through the muscle using tenotomy scissors and bipolar cautery. This approach reduces risk of injury to perforators and pedicle. It also allows for precise hemostasis, keeping the operative field unstained. **C.** Photo demonstrating the fully dissected TRAM flap prior to ligation of the pedicle. Note that the length of the pedicle is at least 7 cm in the free TRAM flap.

■ Recipient Vessel Dissection—Internal Mammary Vessels

- This step is performed after completion of the mastectomy in an immediate reconstruction or after creation of a subcutaneous breast pocket under the superior mastectomy flap in a delayed reconstruction. It is done simultaneously during the abdominal flap harvest.
- The third rib is identified via palpation and using sternal notch and angle landmarks.
- Electrocautery is used to split the pectoralis major muscle directly over the rib cartilage. Use clips for ligating perforators seen along the medial pectoralis border. This reduces the risk of any thermal damage transmitted to the recipient vessels below.
- Split the rib perichondrium longitudinally over the rib from the sternum to about 3 cm lateral using cautery or a scalpel. Make vertical incisions at each end of the cut to create an H-type incision.
- Use a periosteal elevator to strip the perichondrium off the rib cartilage, taking care to hug the surface of the rib as the posterior perichondrium is released.

- Remove the rib cartilage with a rongeur (**TECH FIG 5A**).
- Use bipolar cautery and tenotomy scissors to remove the perichondrium overlying the internal mammary vessels, which are typically about 1 cm lateral to the sternum. Start about 1 to 2 cm lateral to where the vessels are expected and elevate perichondrium from lateral to medial.
- Proceed cautiously when removing the perichondrium from directly above the recipient vessels. Take care to first visualize any branches and ligate with clips as these tear and bleed quite easy.
- If further length on the vessels is desired, remove intercostal muscle above the vessels.
- A medial and lateral vein may be seen on either side of the artery. Often, there is only a medial vein present (**TECH FIG 5B,C**).
- Clear the vessels of surrounding tissue beneath the perichondrial layer under the microscope in preparation for the microsurgical anastomosis.
- The thoracodorsal artery and vein are an alternative option for recipient vessels. For some surgeons, these are preferential in the immediate reconstruction setting as they are often exposed following mastectomy and axillary dissection.

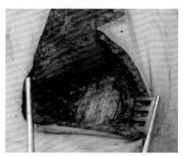 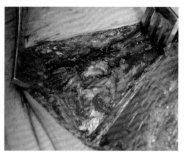 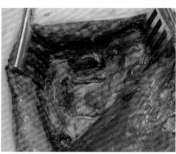

TECH FIG 5 • A. View of the perichondrium after removal of the third rib cartilage. The posterior perichondrium overlies the recipient vessels and will subsequently be removed. **B.** The perichondrium has been removed and the medial and lateral internal mammary veins as well as the internal mammary artery in between are seen in this photo. **C.** The vessels have been completely cleared under the microscope and are ready for microsurgical anastomosis.

Microsurgery and Flap Inset

- Typically, the contralateral abdominal flap is used for reconstruction of the breast when the internal mammary vessels are used as recipients. In this way the flap is positioned vertically to better match the contour of a natural breast shape.[7]
- Rotate the flap 90 degrees such that the pedicle lies medially on the chest and the umbilical incision is positioned laterally toward the axilla. In a right breast reconstruction, the flap is rotated 90 degrees counterclockwise, and in a left breast reconstruction, the flap rotates 90 degrees clockwise.

- Note that if the ipsilateral abdominal flap is used, then the umbilical incision will rotate to lie at the inferomedial aspect of the reconstructed breast.
- Wrap the flap in a saline-soaked sponge and staple to the chest to prevent shifting of flap and eliminate tension on the pedicle during microsurgery.
- Use self-retaining retractor and fishhook retractors for optimal exposure. We also use a pediatric size drain applied to suction and stapled into place at our anastomosis site to minimize pooling of fluid during the microsurgery (**TECH FIG 6A**).

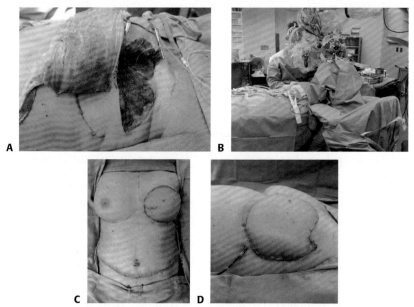

TECH FIG 6 • A. Demonstrates a standard setup in preparation for microsurgery. A single self-retaining retractor and fishhook retractor provide excellent exposure of the recipient vessels as well as adequate space for the anastomosis. A pediatric size drain attached to suction (upper left side of the photo) is stapled into place just above the recipient vessels. This keeps the field dry for better visualization during the microsurgery. A moist saline gauze is wrapped around the flap and secured into place with staples. The pedicle is draped into the chest to meet the recipient vessels without being under any tension. **B.** Both surgeons are comfortably seated for microsurgery. The microscope easily fits into the space at the head of the bed, the hassle of maneuvering around the anesthetic machine having been eliminated by turning the bed at the beginning of the case. **C,D.** Flap inset in delayed breast reconstruction. An oblique back-cut dart was made in the superolateral mastectomy skin to improve upper pole contour and prevent a pin cushioned appearance. In this patient, the ipsilateral abdominal flap was harvested, and the repaired umbilical opening is seen on the medial aspect of the breast. If the contralateral flap had been used, the umbilical incision would be positioned laterally on the reconstructed breast.

- Clear the flap vessels and separate the artery from the vein(s) to provide enough length for comfortable anastomosis to the recipient vessels. Flush the artery with heparinized saline until clear fluid is seen coming out of the vein.
- The surgeons are seated comfortably throughout the microsurgery procedure (**TECH FIG 6B**).
- The microanastomosis is performed, first of the vein and then of the artery. A coupler device is used for the vein. The artery is sutured with 8-0 or 9-0 nylon suture.
- Once the microsurgery is complete, the flap is inset. Often, the medial aspect of the flap is sutured to the medial pectoralis in two to three places to reduce traction on the pedicle.

- The flap is de-epithelialized in all areas that will lie under the mastectomy flaps, and the flap is trimmed conservatively as needed for the desired breast size. Observe the color and amount of bleeding during de-epithelialization as indication of the patency of the anastomoses.
  - In immediate reconstruction, the skin paddle on the flap becomes a circle in place of the nipple-areola complex.
  - In delayed reconstruction, the mastectomy scar is completely excised and sent to pathology. The mastectomy skin below the scar is removed after the microsurgery is complete and the flap is inset in its place. The TRAM flap is only de-epithelialized superiorly where it will lie under the upper mastectomy flap (**TECH FIG 6C,D**).

■ Abdominal Closure

- Close the abdomen with the bed partly flexed during the microsurgery for better efficiency.
- We do minimal undermining of the superior abdominal flap as we have found this to lower overall seroma rates (**TECH FIG 7**).
- Repair the anterior rectus sheath fascia with no. 1 Prolene suture. Use a Prolene inlay mesh if the fascial closure is too tight.
- Insert two Jackson-Pratt drains under the abdominal flaps.
- Mark the umbilical position.
- Close the abdominal incision in three layers, starting with the Scarpa fascia and then the deep dermal and skin layers.
- Create an incision (we use a chevron style) for the umbilicus and inset.

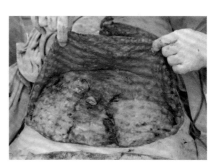

TECH FIG 7 • Demonstrates minimal undermining of the upper abdominal flap. This reduces seroma formation and maintains vascularity to the skin.

PEARLS AND PITFALLS

Muscle relaxation	■ Ensure full muscle relaxation during flap elevation. ■ Communicate with anesthetist before and during surgery.
Fascia	■ Always try to spare as much rectus fascia as possible to avoid tension with closure.
Pedicle dissection	■ Dissect pedicle in retrograde fashion. ■ Create long muscle window to have better visualization of vessels.
Pedicle length	■ Longer pedicle length is required in free TRAM compared to perforator flap.
Recipient vessel	■ Ensure ample length on IMA exposure so as avoid working in a deep hole during microsurgery.
Abdominal flap	■ Minimize undermining of upper flap to decrease seroma formation.

POSTOPERATIVE CARE

- Each patient receives a standardized care routine postoperatively with experienced nursing care on the ward.
  - Hourly flap monitoring (color, capillary refill, temperature, turgor, and Doppler) for first 24 hours in step-down unit or ICU
  - Bed rest for the first night, up to chair the next day, and walking on postoperative day (POD) 2
  - NPO the first night with progression of diet the next day if no flap concerns

  - Enoxaparin 40 mg SC daily while in hospital, started POD 0
  - Aspirin 81 mg daily for the first 6 weeks, started POD 1
  - Abdominal binder applied for 6 weeks
- The typical discharge date is POD 3 for unilateral reconstructions and POD 4 for bilateral or immediate reconstructions.

OUTCOMES

- Several studies have reported abdominal donor site morbidity, including bulge or hernia and functional weakness, to be higher in free TRAM vs DIEP patients.[11,12]

- However, a recent multicenter, patient-reported outcomes study found no significant difference in BREAST-Q scores for physical well-being of the abdomen between free TRAM and DIEP flap reconstruction.[11]
- With regard to other outcomes, the literature has shown that the risk of fat necrosis is lower in free TRAM flaps when compared to DIEP flaps.[12]

COMPLICATIONS

- Early complications
  - Hematoma or seroma (donor site or flap site)
  - Venous congestion
  - Flap loss (partial or total)
  - DVT/PE
  - Infection
  - Mastectomy flap necrosis
  - Abdominal skin or umbilical necrosis
- Late complications
  - Fat necrosis (flap)
  - Delayed wound healing
  - Abdominal bulge or hernia
  - Aesthetic (asymmetry, malposition)

REFERENCES

1. Nahabedian MY, Momen B, Galdino G, Manson PN. Breast reconstruction with the free TRAM or DIEP flap: patient selection, choice of flap, and outcome. *Plast Reconstr Surg.* 2002;110(2): 466-475.
2. Holmström H. The free abdominoplasty flap and its use in breast reconstruction. An experimental study and clinical case report. *Scand J Plast Reconstr Surg.* 1979;13(3):423-427.
3. Moon HK, Taylor GI. The vascular anatomy of rectus abdominis musculocutaneous flaps based on the deep superior epigastric system. *Plast Reconstr Surg.* 1988;82(5):815-832.
4. Ireton JE, Lakhiani C, Saint-Cyr M. Vascular anatomy of the deep inferior epigastric artery perforator flap: a systematic review. *Plast Reconstr Surg.* 2014;134(5):810e-821e.
5. Rozen WM, Palmer KP, Suami H, et al. The DIEA branching pattern and its relationship to perforators: the importance of preoperative computed tomographic angiography for DIEA perforator flaps. *Plast Reconstr Surg.* 2008;121:367-373.
6. Mathes DW, Neligan PC. Current techniques in preoperative imaging for abdomen-based perforator flap microsurgical breast reconstruction. *J Reconstr Microsurg.* 2010;26(1):3-10.
7. Serletti JM. Breast reconstruction with the TRAM flap: pedicled and free. *J Surg Oncol.* 2006;94(6):532-537.
8. Chang DW, Reece GP, Wang B, et al. Effect of smoking on complications in patients undergoing free TRAM flap breast reconstruction. *Plast Reconstr Surg.* 2000;105(7):2374-2380.
9. Karanas YL, Santoro TD, Da Lio AL, Shaw WW. Free TRAM flap breast reconstruction after abdominal liposuction. *Plast Reconstr Surg.* 2003;112(7):1851-1854.
10. Jandali S, Nelson JA, Wu LC, Serletti JM. Free transverse rectus abdominis myocutaneous flap for breast reconstruction in patients with prior abdominal contouring procedures. *J Reconstr Microsurg.* 2010;26(9):607-614.
11. Macadam SA, Zhong T, Weichman K, et al. Quality of life and patient-reported outcomes in breast cancer survivors: a multicenter comparison of four abdominally based autologous reconstruction methods. *Plast Reconstr Surg.* 2016;137(3):758-771.
12. Man LX, Selber JC, Serletti JM. Abdominal wall following free TRAM or DIEP flap reconstruction: a meta-analysis and critical review. *Plast Reconstr Surg.* 2009;124:752-764.

Muscle-Sparing Free Transverse Rectus Abdominis Myocutaneous (TRAM) Flap

Arash Momeni and Liza C. Wu

DEFINITION

- Acquired amastia following mastectomy is associated with significant psychological distress.[1]
- Breast reconstruction following prophylactic mastectomy or mastectomy for breast cancer has been demonstrated to improve health-related quality of life and patient-reported outcomes.[2]
- Favorable long-term patient satisfaction is particularly associated with autologous breast reconstruction using abdominal tissue.[3-5]
- In contrast to the traditional free TRAM flap in which the entire width of the rectus abdominis muscle is harvested, the muscle-sparing free TRAM flap only incorporates a small amount of rectus abdominis muscle along with overlying anterior rectus sheath, thus, reducing donor-site morbidity.

ANATOMY

- The rectus abdominis muscles are flat muscles located on either side of the midline that originate from the 6th to 8th costal cartilages and the xiphoid process and insert on the pubic symphysis.
- Each rectus abdominis muscle rests within a fascial sheath (ie, rectus sheath) that is formed by the confluence of the aponeuroses of the oblique (external and internal) and transversus abdominis muscles.
  - Above the arcuate line, the aponeurosis of the internal oblique splits, thus contributing to the anterior and posterior rectus sheath by joining with the external oblique aponeurosis and transversus abdominis aponeurosis, respectively.
  - Below the arcuate line, all three aponeuroses form the anterior rectus sheath.
- The rectus abdominis muscle has a dual blood supply via the superior and deep inferior epigastric vascular arcade.
  - These vessels originate from the external iliac vessels.
  - Perforating vessels from these arcades pierce the rectus abdominis muscle to perfuse the overlying skin and soft tissues.
  - The blood supply to the lower anterior abdominal skin via the superior epigastric artery is indirect and relies on "choke" vessels located in the midabdomen.
  - In contrast, perforators emanating from the deep inferior epigastric artery represent a more direct source of blood supply to the lower anterior abdominal skin.
    - This represents the anatomic basis for the more robust blood supply of the free muscle-sparing (MS) TRAM flap compared to the pedicled TRAM flap.

PATIENT HISTORY AND PHYSICAL FINDINGS

- The preoperative evaluation for patients presenting for autologous breast reconstruction using an MS-TRAM flap includes a detailed history and focused physical examination.
- History
  - Preoperative smoking cessation is strongly encouraged in order to decrease the risk of wound infection, mastectomy skin necrosis, and abdominal flap necrosis.[6]
  - Pre-existing medical conditions, such as diabetes mellitus, hypertension, etc., need to be optimized preoperatively.
  - Obesity is a specific consideration that may lend itself to increased intraoperative and postoperative complications such as increased blood loss, wound healing issues, and hernia formation.[7]
- Physical examination
  - The abdomen is inspected for pre-existing scars that may preclude MS-TRAM flap harvest.
    - Although appendectomy and Pfannenstiel scars do not pose clinical problems (unless the deep inferior epigastric vessels were previously ligated), subcostal incisions can be associated with a higher rate of delayed wound healing due to compromised perfusion to the watershed area of the abdominal flap.
    - Midline scars are not necessarily problematic, particularly in bilateral reconstructions.
      - Merely unilateral reconstructions in patients with large breasts in whom more than two perfusion zones are required may occasionally necessitate raising the MS-TRAM flap as a bipedicled flap.
      - Previous liposuction is not a contraindication; however, a true abdominoplasty is.[8]
  - Palpation of the abdomen is performed to document the presence of ventral and/or umbilical hernias.
    - Repair of an umbilical hernia at the time of autologous breast reconstruction risks the development of umbilical necrosis.
  - The height of the MS-TRAM flap is determined preoperatively and should correspond to breast width.
    - It may be helpful to determine the degree of abdominal tissue laxity by having the patient flex at the waist, as this gives a reasonable estimate of how much tissue can be harvested without subjecting the closure line to undue tension.
  - Breast examination/palpation is important to assess preoperative beast volume as this can necessitate modification of flap design to optimize a volume match.

IMAGING

- Preoperative imaging is not routinely required prior to MS-TRAM flap harvest.
  - Only in select patients, ie, patients with previous abdominal procedures in which the deep inferior epigastric vessels or its perforators were at risk for injury, is a CT angiography obtained to confirm the presence of suitable vessels.

SURGICAL MANAGEMENT

- Parameters to consider include the following:
  - Timing of reconstruction
    - Immediate vs delayed reconstruction
- Immediate reconstruction has several advantages. These include the ability to reconstruct a breast mound in a single procedure as well as ease of obtaining an aesthetically appealing result due to the presence of the breast skin envelope.
- Delayed reconstruction can be offered at anytime after mastectomy and adjuvant chemotherapy. In cases of postmastectomy radiotherapy, we recommend waiting 6 months after the end of radiation to allow for the recovery of the soft tissues from radiation injury. Furthermore, scarred or irradiated skin that prevents adequate ptosis should be excised and replaced with abdominal skin.
  - Need for adjuvant radiotherapy
    - Radiotherapy after MS-TRAM flap-based reconstruction can result in volume loss, skin contracture, fat necrosis, and poor appearance.[9]
    - Options to remedy the detrimental radiation-induced effects include a "delayed-immediate" approach, in which a tissue expander is placed immediately and eventually replaced with autologous tissue following completion of radiotherapy, or immediate reconstruction with an MS-TRAM flap that is designed approximately 10% to 15% larger than the contralateral breast to account for the anticipated volume loss.
  - Recipient vessels
    - The decision as to whether the ipsilateral or contralateral MS-TRAM flap is used is predominantly determined by the choice of the recipient vessels (see Techniques).

Preoperative Planning

- Preoperative patient assessment should reveal the presence of adequate amount of lower abdominal soft tissue for the purpose of breast reconstruction.
- Clinical examination should rule out pre-existing abdominal scars that would preclude the harvest of an MS-TRAM flap.
- Preoperative landmarks include the umbilicus, anterior superior iliac spines (ASIS), and the suprapubic crease.
  - The elliptical skin island of the MS-TRAM flap includes the areas between the upper border of the umbilicus and the suprapubic crease and the ASIS bilaterally.

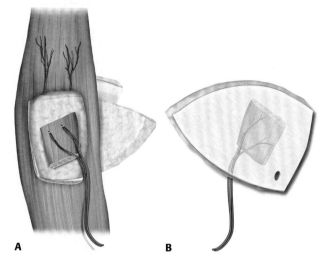

FIG 1 • **A,B.** Illustration of a free MS-TRAM flap based on the deep inferior epigastric vessels with limited rectus abdominis muscle attached to the skin island. (Courtesy of D.W. Low, MD.)

Positioning

- The patient is positioned supine on the operating table with bilateral upper extremities abducted.
- The operating table should allow hip flexion to decrease tension during donor-site closure.

Approach

- The lower abdominal skin can be harvested in a variety of different ways based on the amount of rectus muscle included as well as its vascular pedicle.
  - Options include
    - Pedicled TRAM flap (see Chapter 19)
    - Free TRAM flap—Full width of rectus abdominis muscle is harvested (see Chapter 20)
    - Free MS-TRAM flap—Part of the rectus abdominis muscle is harvested (**FIGS 1** and **2**)
    - Free deep inferior epigastric perforator (DIEP) flap—No rectus abdominis muscle is harvested (see Chapter 22)
    - Free superficial inferior epigastric artery (SIEA) flap—The anterior rectus sheath is not violated and the abdominal flap is raised based on the superficial epigastric vessels (see Chapter 23)

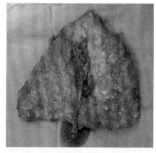

FIG 2 • Clinical image of a free MS-TRAM flap. Note the small segment of rectus abdominis muscle harvested with the flap.

■ Free MS-TRAM Flap Harvest

- Landmarks: Umbilicus, anterior superior iliac spines (ASIS), suprapubic crease
- Skin incision is made along the upper border of the flap.
- Dissection is carried down to the abdominal wall fascia followed by undermining of the upper abdominal skin and soft tissues to the level of the xiphoid and costal margin.
  - It is critical to spare perforating vessel in the subcostal region to maximize perfusion to the abdominal skin flap.
- The patient is temporarily sat up and the superior abdominal skin is draped over the MS-TRAM flap island to confirm the ability to obtain donor-site closure at the completion of the procedure.
- The lower border of the MS-TRAM flap is incised followed by identification of the superficial inferior epigastric (SIE) vessels.
  - The SIE vein (SIEV) is found approximately 4 to 5 cm lateral to the midline. The SIEA is approximately 2 to 3 cm lateral to the SIEV.
  - At this point, the surgeon should determine if the SIE vessels are suitable to apply a SIEA flap.
  - If the SIEA is of inappropriate caliber (less than 1.5 mm) or not present, the SIEV is dissected over the course of 4 to 5 cm and ligated. This provides for an additional outflow vein or a source of vein graft.
- Next, flap dissection proceeds from lateral to medial until the lateral row of perforators emanating from the anterior rectus sheath is visualized.
  - In unilateral breast reconstruction, the skin island opposite the vascular pedicle is dissected off of the abdominal wall, across the midline, and up to the medial row of perforators.
  - In bilateral breast reconstruction, the skin island is transected in the midline followed by medial-to-lateral dissection until the medial row of perforators is identified.

- Once the decision is made on which perforators to include, the anterior rectus sheath is incised below to the inferior-most perforator. The anterior rectus sheath is divided inferolaterally toward the vascular pedicle of the flap.
- The deep inferior epigastric vessels are identified along the lateral edge of the rectus abdominis muscle and followed all the way to their origin, ie, the external iliac vessels.
- Superiorly, the anterior rectus sheath incision is extended to incorporate the chosen perforators. It is critical to keep the amount of fascial harvest to a minimum.
- The amount of muscle divided in a MS-TRAM flap is dependent on the topography of perforators.
  - The lateral- and medial-most perforators determine the width of rectus abdominis muscle that is divided.
  - The rectus abdominis muscle is split along its fibers at the level of the lateral-most perforator and the medial-most perforator, respectively.
    - It is important to confirm that the main vascular pedicle is located within the harvested segment of rectus abdominis muscle.
    - Small vascular branches traveling away from the perforator-carrying central muscle segment are carefully ligated and divided.
    - In order to reduce the width of rectus abdominis muscle that is sacrificed, it is critical to stay close to the perforators and to follow their intramuscular course (**TECH FIG 1**).
- After recipient vessel dissection and confirmation of adequate recipient vessels, the deep inferior epigastric vessels are ligated close to their origin, followed by transection of the central rectus abdominis muscle segment inferiorly and superiorly.

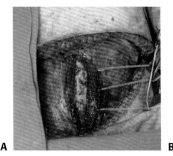 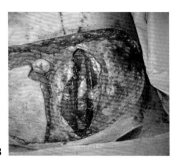

TECH FIG 1 • A. Donor-site defect following MS-TRAM flap harvest. **B.** Donor-site defect following MS-TRAM flap harvest. Note, preservation of rectus abdominis muscle medially and laterally. **A**　　**B**

■ Recipient Vessel Dissection

- The most common recipient vessels are the internal mammary artery (IMA) and vein (IMV) (**TECH FIG 2**).
- The pectoralis major muscle is divided along its fibers at the level of the 3rd rib.
- After identification of the 3rd rib, the intercostal space between the 3rd and 4th rib is assessed for the possibility of a rib-sparing approach to the IM vessels.
  - If the intercostal space is adequately wide (greater than 2 cm), a rib-sparing approach is chosen.

- The pectoralis major muscle is divided along its fibers between the 3rd and 4th rib.
  - The intercostal muscles are divided lateral to the level of the IM vessels vertically beginning inferolaterally at the level of the cartilaginous and bony junction. Next, in a lateral to medial direction, the intercostal muscle cuff is excised at the level of the pleura until the IM vessels are visualized encased in adipose tissue.

- Completion IM vessel dissection follows after removal of the adipose tissue and lymphatics surrounding the IMA and V in the space between the 3rd and 4th rib.
- If a rib-sparing approach is not possible, the cartilage of the 3rd rib is most commonly removed for the purpose of IM vessel dissection.
  - The perichondrium of the 3rd rib is incised transversely on its anterior surface from its junction with the sternum to approximately 1 cm medial to the costochondral junction.
  - Subperichondrial dissection follows anteriorly, superiorly, and inferiorly. Complete posterior dissection is not mandatory.
  - The costal cartilage is then removed with a rongeur.
  - The posterior perichondrium is incised vertically lateral to the IM vessels followed by lateral-to-medial dissection.
    - Meticulous dissection with ligation of small intercostal branches is critical to maintain a bloodless field.

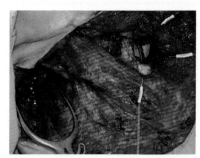

TECH FIG 2 • Recipient vessel dissection: The pectoralis major muscle is split and the right internal mammary vessels are dissected.

- After identification of the IM vessels, the soft tissues between the superior border of the 4th rib and the inferior border of the 2nd rib are excised, thus, providing for a long vascular segment that facilitates microsurgical anastomosis.
- Other possible recipient vessels include the thoracodorsal vessels, the circumflex scapular vessels, the thoracoacromial vessels, and the axillary artery and vein.

■ Abdominal Donor-Site Closure

- Meticulous donor-site closure is critical if abdominal hernias and bulges are to be avoided.
- Inferiorly primarily fascial closure is performed with figure-of-eight polypropylene sutures with buried knots.
- Fascial closure is routinely reinforced with polypropylene mesh.
- The polypropylene mesh is placed between the rectus abdominis muscle and the anterior rectus sheath.
  - It is critical to ensure that the mesh is positioned inferiorly within the rectus sheath so as to buttress the fascial repair site.
  - Size 0 polypropylene sutures are used to secure the mesh.
  - The mesh is secured with buried mattress sutures: first, inferiorly; then superiorly and medially; and, finally, laterally.
- In cases on minimal fascial excision with MS-TRAM flap harvest, primary fascial closure is performed. However, in

cases of moderate (greater than 2–3 cm) fascial excision, a bridging mesh technique of anterior rectus sheath closure is preferred to minimize postoperative abdominal discomfort secondary to an overly tight fascial closure.
- Next, the patient is raised to facilitate skin closure.
- The superior abdominal skin flap is temporarily stapled into place and the site of the umbilical transposition is marked.
  - An opening in the abdominal skin flap is created, followed by removal of a core of subcutaneous tissue.
  - The umbilicus is sutured into place with interrupted deep dermal 4-0 absorbable monofilament sutures followed by a subcuticular closure with a 5-0 absorbable monofilament suture.
- Two suction drains are placed exiting the abdominal wound laterally.
- Layered closure is performed with approximation of Scarpa fascia followed by deep dermal and subcuticular closure.
- Sterile dressings are applied.

■ MS-TRAM Flap Inset

- Whenever the internal mammary vessels are chosen as recipient vessels, the contralateral MS-TRAM flap is used for reconstruction.
  - The MS-TRAM flap is rotated 90 degrees with the umbilicus positioned inferolaterally (**TECH FIG 3**).
- The ipsilateral MS-TRAM flap is used whenever the thoracodorsal vessels are chosen as recipient vessels.
  - Here, the umbilicus is positioned inferomedially after rotating the flap 90 degrees.
- After performing microsurgical anastomoses, the flap is secured in place with 2-0 absorbable sutures.

- The flap is secured medially at the level of the 3rd rib as well as along the superomedial, superior, and superolateral borders of the breast footprint.
- A suction drain is placed and wound closure performed with interrupted absorbable sutures for deep dermal closure following by subcuticular closure.
- Finally, Doppler examination is performed and the site with an audible Doppler signal is marked with a 5-0 polypropylene suture.
- **TECH FIG 4** displays a case example of bilateral immediate breast reconstruction with free MS-TRAM flaps.

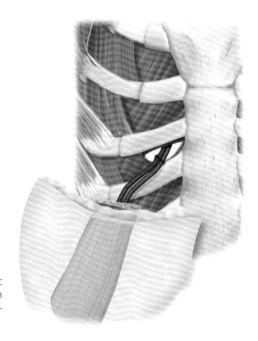

TECH FIG 3 • Illustration demonstrating anastomosis of the deep inferior epigastric vessels to the internal mammary vessels. Note that the left MS-TRAM flap has been transferred to the right chest with the flap being rotated 90 degrees so that the umbilicus is positioned inferolaterally. (Courtesy of D.W. Low, MD.)

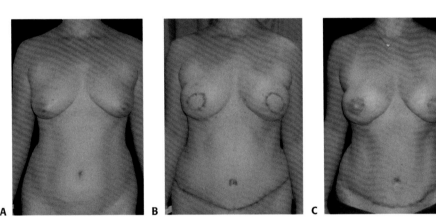

A   B   C

TECH FIG 4 • Preoperative **(A)**, early postoperative (prior to nipple-areola reconstruction) **(B)** and late postoperative (after nipple-areola reconstruction) **(C)** images of a patient who underwent bilateral immediate breast reconstruction with free MS-TRAM flaps.

PEARLS AND PITFALLS

Indications	▪ Patients with adequate amount of lower abdominal soft tissue for the purpose of breast reconstruction. ▪ Absence of abdominal scars precluding MS-TRAM flap harvest.
Imaging	▪ Routine use of preoperative imaging is not indicated. ▪ Merely in cases in which prior abdominal surgery places the deep inferior epigastric vessels or its perforators at risk is preoperative CT angiography warranted.
Flap dissection	▪ Minimize abdominal wall morbidity by having the lateral- and medial-most perforators determine the width of rectus abdominis muscle that is divided. ▪ Minimize fascial excision. ▪ Preserve the SIEV as an additional drainage source or potential vein graft.
Donor-site closure	▪ Meticulous fascial closure is paramount to minimize the risk of abdominal hernia or bulge formation. ▪ Routinely use polypropylene mesh in donor-site closure, even if primary fascial closure is performed. ▪ Avoid an overly tight fascial closure; use bridging mesh in cases of moderate fascial excision (>2–3 cm).
Flap inset	▪ The contralateral MS-TRAM flap is used whenever the IM vessels are chosen as recipient vessels. ▪ The ipsilateral MS-TRAM flap is used in cases in which the thoracodorsal vessels are used as recipients.

POSTOPERATIVE CARE

- Following extubation and transfer to the PACU, the patient is admitted to a step-down unit.
- Flap checks are performed via a combination of clinical and Doppler examination hourly for the first 48 hours, followed by every 4 hours until discharge.
- The patient is kept NPO until the morning of postoperative day (POD) 1 and is then started on a clear liquid diet. Diet is advanced to a regular diet on POD 2.
- Activity restrictions include out of bed to chair on POD 1 followed by ambulation on POD 2.
- No specific anticoagulation is indicated. Patients merely receive heparin 5000 U subcutaneously every 8 hours for the duration of the hospitalization.
- The patient is typically discharged home on POD 3 to 4. Instructions are provided regarding incision and drain care.

OUTCOMES

- The issue of donor-site morbidity associated with MS-TRAM flap harvest was investigated in a matched-pair analysis of a total of 104 patients.[10]
  - Fifty-two MS-TRAM flap patients were matched with 52 abdominoplasty patients.
  - Postoperative complication rate, including the rate hernia and abdominal bulge formation were similar in both groups.
  - A higher degree of patient satisfaction with the appearance of the abdominal scar was noted among TRAM flap patients.[10]
- Using the BREAST-Q, Macadam et al. performed a multicenter study including 1790 patients and did not detect any significant difference in patient-reported outcomes between patients undergoing reconstruction with DIEP flaps vs MS-TRAM flaps.[11]

COMPLICATIONS

- Wound-related complications can be as high as 30% to 50%[9] and include
  - Simple infections
  - Seromas
  - Hematomas
  - Skin flap necrosis
  - Delayed wound healing

- Additional complications include
  - Fat necrosis
  - Flap loss (approximately 1%)[12]
  - Abdominal bulge/hernia formation

REFERENCES

1. Gomez-Campelo P, Bragado-Alvarez C, Hernandez-Lloreda MJ. Psychological distress in women with breast and gynecological cancer treated with radical surgery. *Psychooncology.* 2014;23(4):459-466.
2. Koslow S, Pharmer LA, Scott AM, et al. Long-term patient-reported satisfaction after contralateral prophylactic mastectomy and implant reconstruction. *Ann Surg Oncol.* 2013;20(11):3422-3429.
3. Hu ES, Pusic AL, Waljee JF, et al. Patient-reported aesthetic satisfaction with breast reconstruction during the long-term survivorship Period. *Plast Reconstr Surg.* 2009;124(1):1-8.
4. Liu C, Zhuang Y, Momeni A, et al. Quality of life and patient satisfaction after microsurgical abdominal flap vs staged expander/implant breast reconstruction: a critical study of unilateral immediate breast reconstruction using patient-reported outcomes instrument BREAST-Q. *Breast Cancer Res Treat.* 2014;146(1):117-126.
5. Atisha DM, Rushing CN, Samsa GP, et al. A national snapshot of satisfaction with breast cancer procedures. *Ann Surg Oncol.* 2015;22(2):361-369.
6. Selber JC, Kurichi JE, Vega SJ, et al. Risk factors and complications in free TRAM flap breast reconstruction. *Ann Plast Surg.* 2006;56(5):492-497.
7. Fischer JP, Nelson JA, Sieber B, et al. Free tissue transfer in the obese patient: an outcome and cost analysis in 1258 consecutive abdominally based reconstructions. *Plast Reconstr Surg.* 2013;131(5):681e-692e.
8. Jandali S, Nelson JA, Wu LC, Serletti JM. Free transverse rectus abdominis myocutaneous flap for breast reconstruction in patients with prior abdominal contouring procedures. *J Reconstr Microsurg.* 2010;26(9):607-614.
9. Serletti JM, Fosnot J, Nelson JA, et al. Breast reconstruction after breast cancer. *Plast Reconstr Surg.* 2011;127(6):124e-135e.
10. Momeni A, Kim RY, Heier M, et al. Abdominal wall strength: a matched-pair analysis comparing muscle-sparing TRAM flap donor-site morbidity with the effects of abdominoplasty. *Plast Reconstr Surg.* 2010;126(5):1454-1459.
11. Macadam SA, Zhong T, Weichman K, et al. Quality of life and patient-reported outcomes in breast cancer survivors: a multicenter comparison of four abdominally based autologous reconstruction methods. *Plast Reconstr Surg.* 2016;137(3):758-771.
12. Pannucci CJ, Basta MN, Kovach SJ, et al. Loupes-only microsurgery is a safe alternative to the operating microscope: an analysis of 1,649 consecutive free flap breast reconstructions. *J Reconstr Microsurg.* 2015;31(9):636-642.

DIEP Flap Breast Reconstruction

Pierre M. Chevray

DEFINITION

- Breast reconstruction following mastectomy can be accomplished with prosthetic breast implants, autologous tissue flaps, or a combination of the two.
- Autologous tissue flaps from the lower abdomen are capable of creating the most natural, lasting, and maintenance-free reconstructed breasts with the highest long-term patient satisfaction when compared to other methods of breast reconstruction.[1]
- Autologous tissue flaps have donor-site morbidity and require longer and more complex surgery, with a longer recovery period, compared to implant-based breast reconstruction.
- Techniques to harvest lower abdominal flaps of skin and subcutaneous tissue for breast reconstruction have evolved from the pedicled TRAM flap, to the free TRAM flap, to the muscle-sparing free TRAM flap, to the DIEP flap, to the SIEA flap, in order to minimize donor-site morbidity.[2]
- The DIEP (Deep Inferior Epigastric Perforator) flap has become the most popular lower abdominal free flap used for breast reconstruction because of its balance of sparing rectus abdominis muscle function while still providing a well-vascularized and reliable flap of skin and subcutaneous tissue.[3-5]

ANATOMY

- The vascular pedicle of the DIEP flap is the deep inferior epigastric (DIE) artery and veins, and their branches which perforate through the rectus abdominis muscle (perforators), into the subcutaneous fat of the anterior abdominal wall.
- The DIE vessels originate from the external iliac vessels in the pelvis, course anteriorly and superiorly, in the retroperitoneal plane, to the inferolateral border of the rectus abdominis muscle. The DIE vessels continue superiorly, within the rectus sheath, on the deep surface of the rectus abdominis muscle, from which branches to the muscle and perforators into the overlying flap tissue originate. Terminal branches of the DIE vessels coalesce with the terminal branches of the deep superior epigastric vessels (**FIG 1**).
- The single most common branching pattern of the DIE artery is that it bifurcates into two parallel branches that course superiorly on the underside of the rectus abdominis muscle. One branch runs along the medial side of the muscle, giving rise to the "medial row" of perforators, and the other runs along the lateral side of the muscle, giving rise to the "lateral row" of perforators. However, this branching pattern is variable.
- Generally, lateral row perforators pierce the muscle perpendicular to the plane of the flat, straplike, rectus abdominis muscle and are easier to dissect compared to medial row perforators, which tend to travel obliquely, from medial

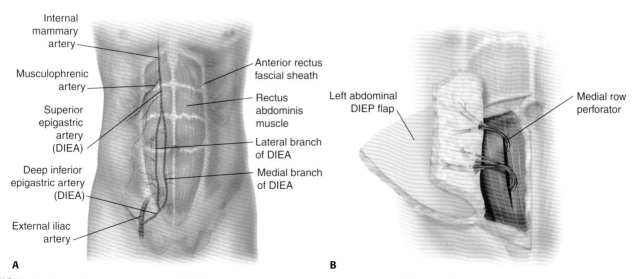

Internal mammary artery

Musculophrenic artery

Superior epigastric artery (DIEA)

Deep inferior epigastric artery (DIEA)

External iliac artery

Anterior rectus fascial sheath

Rectus abdominis muscle

Lateral branch of DIEA

Medial branch of DIEA

Left abdominal DIEP flap

Medial row perforator

A

B

FIG 1 • **A.** Deep inferior epigastric artery (DIEP) flap anatomy showing a right hemiabdominal DIEP flap skin paddle overlying the right rectus abdominis muscle containing the medial and lateral branches of the deep inferior epigastric (DIE) artery, which gives off the medial and lateral row of perforators. **B.** The left hemiabdominal DIEP flap is reflected laterally, as it would be during exposure of the medial row of perforators.

to lateral, and superior to inferior, through the muscle and require dissection along greater distances within the muscle when compared to lateral row perforators.

- The limits of the DIEP flap skin paddle are several centimeters superior to the superior edge of the umbilicus, inferiorly to the level of the pubic bone, and laterally to the anterior axillary line. It is possible, usually in younger and thinner patients, to transfer this entire lower abdominal flap based on the perforators from one DIE vascular pedicle.

- The skin paddle of lower abdominal flaps has been divided into zones.[6] Zone 1 is the paramedian region of the flap skin paddle overlying the rectus abdominis muscle and is the best perfused area of the flap. Zone 2 is lateral to Zone 1. Zone 3 is the mirror image of Zone 1, on the opposite side of the vertical midline. Zone 4, lateral to Zone 3, is the furthest from the perforators and thus the least well-perfused zone and most likely to suffer fat necrosis.

- Selecting which perforators to keep, and which are not necessary and can be sacrificed, is one of the critical decisions during this operation and requires the most experience and judgment.

- Generally, the single largest perforator will perfuse Zone 1 of a DIEP flap. However, in most breast reconstructions, Zones 1 and 2 are necessary to reconstruct a large enough breast.

- Zones 1, 2, and 3, and sometimes Zone 4, can be perfused by including more perforators.

- The rectus abdominis muscle is segmentally innervated, and the skin paddle of the DIEP flap receives sensory innervation from the thoracoabdominal branches of the intercostal nerves T7-T11, which run between the internal oblique and transversus abdominis muscles and then enter the lateral border of the anterior rectus sheath.

- These thoracoabdominal nerves run roughly transversely, just deep, and within the rectus abdominis muscle along with the accompanying vascular branches of the intercostal arteries and veins to anastomose with the DIE vessels, which run roughly vertically.

- The sensory nerve fibers run with the perforators through the rectus abdominis muscle and anterior rectus sheath, into the overlying subcutaneous tissue of the DIEP flap, to innervate the skin. The motor fibers branch into the substance of the rectus abdominis muscle to innervate it.

- These motor and sensory nerves run superficial to the DIE vessels, and for all practical purposes, must be divided to harvest and transfer the DIEP flap. Some surgeons repair the nerves that are divided.

PATHOGENESIS

- The DIEP flap is most commonly used for breast reconstruction following mastectomy for treatment of breast cancer, or risk reduction in patients with a genetic increased risk of breast cancer such as BRCA 1 or 2 gene mutations.

NATURAL HISTORY

- Rates of breast reconstruction have been slowly rising over the past 40 years. However, in the United States, less than half of patients who are treated with mastectomy have breast reconstruction,[7,8] and rates of breast reconstruction are substantially lower elsewhere in the world.

PATIENT HISTORY AND PHYSICAL FINDINGS

- The DIEP flap can be used for total, or partial, breast reconstruction in patients who have had a mastectomy or partial mastectomy (lumpectomy, segmental mastectomy), respectively.

IMAGING

- CT and MR angiography is used by some surgeons to visualize the DIE vascular pedicle and perforators preoperatively. Some believe this can decrease operative times; however, the author does not use preoperative imaging of any kind.

NONOPERATIVE MANAGEMENT

- Breast reconstruction has been shown to improve the quality of life of patients who have had a mastectomy.

- The Women's Health and Cancer Rights Act of 1998, a federal law in the United States, mandates commercial health insurance companies to cover breast reconstruction after a mastectomy, surgery on the opposite breast to improve breast symmetry, and breast prostheses. Despite this law, less than half of patients who have a mastectomy in the United States have breast reconstruction.

- Nonsurgical treatment would include using an external breast prosthesis, which fits into a brassiere cup or is part of a custom-made brassiere.

SURGICAL MANAGEMENT

Preoperative Planning

- The objective of the operation is to improve the quality of life of the mastectomy patient by reconstructing a breast mound that is as similar to a natural breast as possible.

- Absolute contraindications for this operation are prior full abdominoplasty or uncorrectable hypercoagulable state.

- Relative contraindications are a body mass index greater than 40 kg/m², hypercoagulable state, previous abdominal liposuction, and prior abdominal surgery that may compromise the flap or abdominal wall.

- The risks of the surgery to be discussed with the patient include the risks of surgery in general (infection, bleeding, pain, scarring, hematoma, seroma, and delayed healing) and the specific risks of this surgery, which are abdominal hernia, bulge, weakness, and partial or total flap loss.

- For immediate breast reconstruction, the incisions for the mastectomy are discussed with the breast surgeon. A common issue is, should a patient with ptotic breasts who would like smaller or more lifted reconstructed breasts have a nipple-sparing mastectomy (NSM), even if it is oncologically acceptable? If yes, how long after the NSM and DIEP flap reconstruction will you perform a mastopexy that involves a periareolar incision?
  - Anecdotally, the author likes to wait at least 6 months.
  - Alternatively, the patient may be treated with a lumpectomy and oncoplastic mastopexy and complete any adjuvant treatments and then undergo NSM and DIEP flap breast reconstruction.
  - A third option, in patients without breast cancer such as patients with BRCA mutations, is to have a mastopexy or breast reduction first and then, 6 or more months later, undergo NSM and DIEP flap reconstruction.

Preoperative Markings

- Preoperatively, with the patient standing upright, mark the anterior midline from the sternal notch down to the pubis. Mark both inframammary folds (IMFs). Then draw a horizontal line from the most inferior point of each IMF across the midline to the opposite IMF to determine if one side is lower or higher than the other side (**FIG 2**).
- Also with the patient standing, mark the superior flap incision line. This is typically about 2 cm superior to the superior border of the umbilicus but can vary from the level of the superior border of the umbilicus, up to about 5 cm above this.
  - This transverse line curves inferiorly as it is extended laterally in both directions, and generally ends several centimeters lateral and superior to the anterior superior iliac spine (ASIS).
  - The lower this incision is made, the lower and more easily concealed, the longer the transverse abdominal donor-site scar will be, but the less flap skin surface area and less flap subcutaneous fat volume that is harvested (see **FIG 2**; **FIG 3**).
- The lower transverse abdominal incision is also marked preoperatively with the patient standing. This is typically drawn in the natural suprapubic crease and extends

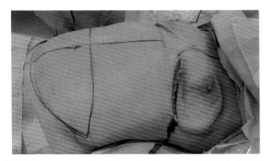

FIG 2 • Patient prepared and draped with arms abducted at 90 degrees on arm boards. The vertical midline, bilateral inframammary folds (IMF), horizontal extension of the nadir of both IMF, and the proposed DIEP flap skin paddles have been marked preoperatively with the patient standing. Bilateral nipple-sparing mastectomies via IMF incisions have been completed.

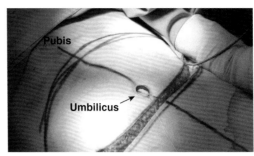

FIG 3 • Initial DIEP flap harvest with patient supine. (Note that in all intraoperative photos, the patient's head is to the right.) The umbilicus has been cored out from the DIEP flaps, and the upper abdominal incision has been made. The umbilicus has been tagged at its 12 o'clock position with a suture, which will be used later to find the umbilicus and bring it out for insetting once the abdominal donor site has been closed. Note that the initial, more superior, upper and lower abdominal incision markings, which were made preoperatively, have both been lowered by about 2 cm based on an intraoperative pinch/grab evaluation of the abdominal donor site with the patient's head and back raised to 45 degrees.

laterally, curving gently upward to meet the superior incision line several centimeters superior and lateral to the ASIS (see **FIGS 2** and **3**).

Positioning

- The patient is positioned supine with the arms abducted 90 degrees on arm boards. Alternatively, if no axillary lymph node surgery is planned, the arms may be tucked. This allows for easier positioning of a dual head operating microscope for two surgeons, but care must be taken not to injure the patient's hands and arms when raising the patient's head and back to close the abdominal donor site.
- The operating table may be reversed (turned 180 degrees) underneath the patient, in what is sometimes called a "C-arm position." This allows the head and back to be raised nearly to 90 degrees upright, which some surgeons desire for evaluating insetting and shaping of the DIEP flap.

- In immediate breast reconstruction, DIEP flap harvest can begin at the abdomen at the same time the breast surgeon is performing the mastectomy at the chest. Alternatively, the DIEP flap surgery can begin after the breast surgeon is finished.
- Typically, the patient cannot be paralyzed until the breast surgeon has completed any axillary lymph node surgery, and this may make dissection of perforators at the abdomen difficult due to the contraction of the rectus abdominis muscle when stimulating the motor nerves with the electrocautery.
- In a unilateral breast reconstruction, assess if a hemi-DIEP flap will provide sufficient volume and skin surface for the reconstruction or if tissue across the midline needs to be harvested.

- Once the patient is under general anesthesia, raise the head and back of the patient to about 45 degrees, or more, and perform a pinch/grab test to assess if the abdominal donor site can be closed after flap harvest along the marked incision lines. Raise or lower the upper abdominal incision line to adjust.
- The upper abdominal incision is commonly at the level of the superior border of the umbilicus or up to several centimeters superior to this. Return the patient to the supine position. **FIG 3** shows an example where the initially marked upper and lower abdominal incision lines were both lowered intraoperatively by about 2 cm after the pinch/grab test of the donor site.

TECHNIQUES

■ DIEP Flap Harvest

Incision and Flap Elevation

- The abdominal incisions are made. The superior incision is beveled superiorly to capture more subcutaneous tissue volume with the flap and to decrease the thickness of the cut edge of the upper abdominal donor-site flap. This creates a better thickness match between the upper and lower cut edges of the abdominal donor-site incision at closure.
- The upper abdominal donor-site flap of skin and subcutaneous tissue is elevated off the anterior rectus fascia for 5 to 10 cm to allow closure of the donor site. Raising this abdominal skin flap superiorly to the xiphoid process usually does not substantially increase mobility of the skin flap and will decrease vascularity of the midline upper abdominal tissue.
- The lower abdominal incision is made just barely through the dermis and into the subcutaneous fat, in order to identify, and not injure, the superficial inferior epigastric and/or the superficial circumflex iliac vessels. If there is a large enough superficial artery, harvest of a superficial inferior epigastric artery (SIEA) flap may be considered (see SIEA flap chapter). If there is a large vein, it is dissected free inferiorly for 4 to 8 cm, ligated, and divided. This is done to provide additional venous drainage or to be used as a vein graft, if needed, in the case of venous congestion of the DIEP flap.
- The umbilicus is cored out from the surrounding DIEP flap tissue and tagged with a suture. Leave some fat around the stalk of the umbilicus to minimize the risk of devascularization. Minimize the diameter or the umbilicus because a smaller diameter umbilicus will draw surrounding upper abdominal skin inward and deeply, resulting in a less visible circumferential scar (see **FIG 3**).
- For bilateral DIEP flap reconstructions, or unilateral cases where a hemiflap is sufficient, the vertical midline incision separating the right and left DIEP flaps is made.

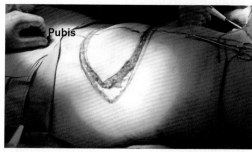

TECH FIG 1 • Left lateral view of patient just before beginning elevation of the left abdominal DIEP flap to expose and dissect vascular perforators. Note that the surgical oncologist is performing the right mastectomy. Note also that in this patient, the right IMF is about 2 cm lower than the left IMF. This is indicated by the markings extending medially from the nadir of each IMF, which were drawn preoperatively while the patient was standing. This IMF asymmetry will be corrected with sutures.

- The DIEP flaps are elevated off the abdominal muscle fascia using electrocautery at a low setting of 20 in the coagulation mode. The edge of the flap tissue is grasped and is retracted and reflected at a greater than 90-degree angle away from the abdominal wall in order to spread the plane between the subcutaneous fat of the flap and the anterior rectus fascia so that vascular perforators can be visualized (**TECH FIG 2A**).

Perforator Location and Selection

- The DIEP flaps are raised from lateral to medial (**TECH FIGS 1** and **2A,B**) to expose the lateral row of perforators, from medial to lateral to expose the medial row of perforators, and from superior to inferior, and inferior to superior.
- Rarely are perforators located superior to the umbilicus used because they are located at one corner of the flap and thus are less likely to perfuse a large area of the flap,

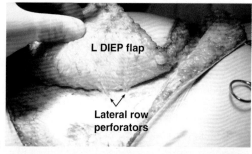

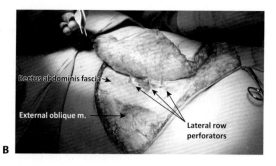

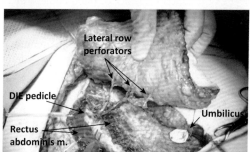

TECH FIG 2 • **A.** Left abdominal DIEP flap elevation showing identification of two lateral row perforators. **B.** Left abdominal DIEP flap elevation showing three lateral row perforators. The anterior rectus abdominis muscle fascia between the perforators has been divided, and perforator dissection through the muscle is about to begin. **C.** The left abdominal DIEP flap has been raised on three lateral row perforators. The DIE pedicle is visible and about to be dissected.

and they require incision and dissection through more rectus abdominis muscle.

- Perforators located more than 10 cm inferior to the umbilicus are rarely used because they tether the pedicle to the underside of the flap and shorten the effective length of the pedicle.
- The largest perforator is most commonly in the medial row, located within several cm of the umbilicus. However, sometimes the largest perforator is in the lateral row. When harvesting a hemiabdominal DIEP flap, the one largest perforator is often sufficient to perfuse the flap. This can be tested by occluding the other perforators with Acland clamps for 5 to 10 minutes and evaluating the color of the flap and arterial bleeding at the edges of the flap.
- Two or three perforators may be necessary to adequately perfuse the flap.
- It is advantageous to select perforators within the same medial or lateral row as this minimizes the amount of rectus abdominis muscle fibers that are divided during flap harvest (**TECH FIG 2C**).

Perforator Dissection

- The selected perforators are dissected free from the anterior rectus fascia. There is an opening in the fascia that each perforator passes through. The edge of this hole in the fascia is exposed with the cautery, grasped with toothed forceps, elevated to allow the underlying perforator to fall away, and divided with the cutting cautery to enlarge the opening. These enlarged openings around the selected perforators in the fascia are connected by incising the fascia between them (see **TECH FIG 2B**).
- The perforators are carefully dissected free from the rectus abdominis muscle using bipolar cautery on a low setting, such as 20. It is important to retract the muscle fibers away from the perforator vessels using "fish-hook" or Weitlaner retractors and directly grasp the muscle fibers immediately adjacent to the perforator vessels, pulling them away and dividing them with bipolar cautery (see **TECH FIG 2C**).
- Much of the muscle can be bluntly dissected (pushed) away from the perforator vessels until a small vascular branch of the perforator into the muscle is encountered. The smallest of these branches are divided using the bipolar cautery. Others are clipped with small vascular clips and divided with scissors.
- Dissection of the selected perforators continues until they are freed from the rectus abdominis muscle, and the junction with the DIE vascular pedicle is reached (see **TECH FIG 2C**).
- The DIE vessels are sometimes within the rectus abdominis muscle and have to be dissected free from the muscle

fibers like the perforators. Further inferiorly, the DIE vessels will always be in a fatty or loose areolar plane deep to the rectus abdominis muscle, between the muscle and the posterior rectus sheath.

DIE Vessel Dissection

- There are segmental intercostal neurovascular bundles entering the lateral border of the rectus sheath. These run in a superolateral to inferomedial direction and anastomose with the DIE vessels. The intercostal vessels must be divided.
- These intercostal nerves within these intercostal neurovascular bundles continue over (superficial to) the DIE vessels and branch into the rectus abdominis muscle to innervate the muscle and follow the perforator branches of the DIE vessels through the muscle and into the flap to provide sensory innervation to the abdominal flap skin. These intercostal nerves are divided where they cross over the DIE vessels. If desired, these nerves can be repaired, after transposing the ends deep to the DIE vessels.
- Continue to dissect the DIE vessels inferiorly toward their origin from the external iliac vessels. Deep to the inferior quarter of the rectus abdominis muscle, the DIE vessels diverge from the underside of the muscle and run in a deep and lateral direction through the preperitoneal fat to meet the external iliac vessels (**TECH FIG 3**).
- The pedicle vessels are dissected to within a few cm of their origin from the external iliac vessels to ensure adequate pedicle length to reach the internal mammary or thoracodorsal recipient vessels at the chest.
- De-epithelialize as much of the flap skin as possible while the flap is still in situ at the abdomen (see section below on Insetting the DIEP Flap).

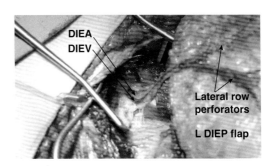

TECH FIG 3 • Dissection of the left abdominal DIEP flap pedicle continues to within 1 to 2 cm of its origin from the external iliac vessels. Two Weitlaner retractors are used for exposure. DIEA, deep inferior epigastric artery. DIEV, deep inferior epigastric vein.

◼ Exposure and Preparation of Internal Mammary Recipient Vessels

- The breast surgeon will typically have completed the unilateral or bilateral mastectomy surgery by the time the DIEP flap dissection is completed, and dissection of the recipient vessels can begin.
- The internal mammary recipient vessels are preferred over the thoracodorsal vessels as the arteries are larger in caliber and a better size match to the DIE pedicle vessels

and are more superficially and centrally located making microsurgical vascular anastomosis technically easier and allowing improved flap positioning.

- The mastectomy skin flaps must be retracted sufficiently to expose the third intercostal space adjacent to the sternum and to allow the operating microscope a line of sight to this area perpendicular to the chest wall. The mastectomy incision may have to be lengthened to achieve this exposure. A combination of Weitlaner retractors and fishhook elastic retractors or retaining sutures are used for this exposure (**TECH FIG 4A**). The tension, pressure, and time of retraction of the mastectomy skin flaps should be minimized to minimize the risk of mastectomy skin flap necrosis.

- A small 3 × 5 cm trapezoidal flap of pectoralis major muscle is elevated off the underlying third intercostal space and reflected laterally (**TECH FIG 4B**). It is important to divide the origins of the pectoralis major muscle of this small flap far enough medially to expose the lateral border of the sternum at the third intercostal space.
- The perichondrium of the medial-most 2.5 cm of the third rib costochondral cartilage is incised in the shape of an "H" and opened like window shutters off of the cartilage using a freer elevator.
- A rongeur is used to remove the medial-most 2.5 cm of the third costochondral cartilage, being careful not

to enter, tear, or avulse any of the underlying posterior perichondrium.

- Once the rib cartilage has been removed (**TECH FIG 4C**), the posterior perichondrium is incised at the lateral end of the exposure and divided from lateral to medial carefully avoiding injuring the internal mammary vessels, which are immediately deep to the posterior perichondrium.
- The internal mammary vein is medial to the internal mammary artery when there is only one vein (**TECH FIG 4D**).
- The posterior perichondrium and the third intercostal space soft tissue are excised and discarded.
- The internal mammary artery and vein are dissected free from each other, and the surrounding soft tissue from the second intercostal space (just superior to the excised third rib cartilage and perichondrium) inferiorly to the superior border of the 4th rib (see **TECH FIG 4D**).

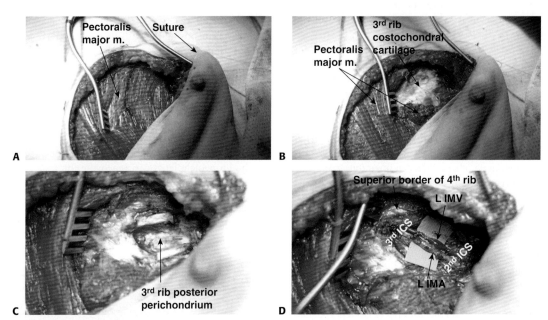

TECH FIG 4 • A. Exposure for left internal mammary recipient vessel preparation following nipple-sparing mastectomy via an inframammary incision. A Weitlaner retractor and suture are used for this exposure. The incisions along the lines of the muscle fibers to raise a laterally based flap of pectoralis major muscle are marked. **B.** Left internal mammary recipient vessel preparation. The trapezoidal flap of pectoralis major muscle overlying the third costochondral cartilage has been reflected laterally. **C.** Left internal mammary recipient vessel preparation. The left third costochondral cartilage has been removed with a rongeur, leaving the perichondrium. **D.** Left internal mammary recipient vessel preparation. The third rib perichondrium and portions of the second and third intercostal muscles have been removed. The left internal mammary artery and vein are exposed and dissected free circumferentially from the second intercostal space (ICS) down to the superior border of the fourth rib. IMA, internal mammary artery. IMV, internal mammary vein. ICS, intercostal space.

■ Control of the Footprint of the Reconstructed Breast

- Two 15 French fluted closed suction drains are exited from the chest wall lateral to the lower lateral border of the breast. One drain is placed along the inframammary fold (IMF) of the reconstructed breast, and the second drain is placed superficial to the pectoralis major muscle in the upper breast.
- The IMF is fixed in the desired position using three to four simple interrupted 2-0 PDS sutures placed through the pectoralis major muscle fascia and into rib periosteum.

- In delayed breast reconstructions, the skin and subcutaneous tissue lateral to the breast is dissected free from the underlying chest wall and axillary contents. In immediate reconstructions, this dissection will have been done by the breast surgeon performing the mastectomy.
- This lateral breast and subaxillary lateral chest wall skin and subcutaneous tissue is advanced anteriorly (in the anatomic position) and sutured into position using several simple interrupted 2-0 PDS sutures. If this is not done, this tissue tends to fall posteriorly and inferiorly, creating a roll of excess tissue, and/or the DIEP flap can migrate laterally into this space.

- The skin of the DIEP flap that is not needed is de-epithelialized while the flap is still in situ at the abdomen. This way, the flap does not need to be removed from within the mastectomy skin envelope once it is placed there.
- For immediate reconstructions with a nipple-sparing mastectomy, a small elliptical segment of skin paddle measuring 1.5 × 6 cm is kept to be brought out along the IMF (**TECH FIG 5**). For immediate reconstructions with a skin-sparing mastectomy, a 9-cm-diameter circular skin paddle in the middle of the DIEP flap is kept initially. Later, once the flap is transferred, a 5-cm-diameter skin paddle is made for future nipple reconstruction. For delayed breast reconstructions, only the lateral-most few cm of the DIEP flap is de-epithelialized while the flap is still in situ at the abdomen.

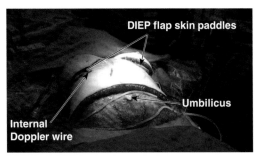

TECH FIG 5 • Abdominal donor site and flap insetting. The anterior rectus fascia is closed primarily, and two drains are placed at the abdominal donor site.

■ Harvest, Transfer, and Revascularization of the DIEP Flap

- The operating microscope is prepared, brought into position over the internal mammary recipient vessels, and adjusted (**TECH FIG 6**). Note that some surgeons use loupes only and do not use an operating microscope.
- The DIEP flap is harvested by ligating the DIE artery and vein(s) with metal clips and dividing them with scissors.
- The DIE artery and vein(s) are flushed with 2 cc each of 100 mg/mL heparinized saline.
- The flap is transferred to the chest wall and secured with two or three simple interrupted 3-0 Vicryl sutures to the chest wall skin if needed.
- The internal mammary vein (IMV) is ligated with a metal clip and divided with scissors. The microvenous anastomosis is created using a flow-coupler device. Most commonly, 2.5 or 3.0 mm diameter couplers are used for the larger right IMV, and 2.0 or 2.5 mm couplers are used for the smaller left IMV.
- The arterial anastomosis is completed after the venous microanastomosis. The IMA is ligated with a metal clip and divided with scissors. The IMA and DIEP flap artery are placed in a double approximating Acland clamp and the anastomosis completed with typically eight simple interrupted 9-0 nylon sutures.

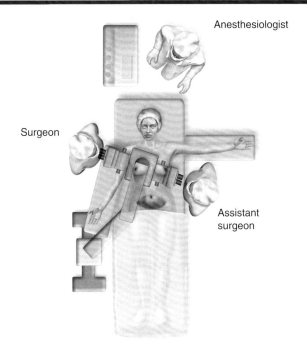

TECH FIG 6 • Setup of the surgeon, assistant surgeon, and microscope for DIEP flap revascularization to the internal mammary recipient vessels at the chest. The ipsilateral patient arm is lowered so the surgeon can stand by the ipsilateral patient shoulder. The assistant surgeon stands below the contralateral abducted patient arm. This allows both surgeons to stand close enough to the microsurgical field and be 180 degrees apart to be able to simultaneously use a dual head operating microscope.

■ Insetting the DIEP Flap and Shaping a Breast

- It is important that the flap volume matches the footprint of the reconstructed breast and mastectomy skin flap volume. If the DIEP flap is not wide enough, or not large enough in volume to fill out the mastectomy skin envelope, it will leave a depression or hollow at the superomedial reconstructed breast. Suspending the flap to the superomedial mastectomy pocket with sutures will result in flattening of the flap and loss of projection of the reconstructed breast. Therefore, if the flap volume is

inadequate to fill out the mastectomy pocket, it is best to reduce the perimeter of the reconstructed breast by elevating the IMF and closing down the lateral mastectomy pocket with 2-0 PDS sutures. See Section "Control of the footprint of the reconstructed breast" above.
- The thickest part of the flap, which is usually the vertical midline cut edge, is placed along the IMF. In other words, a right abdominal DIEP flap is turned 90 degrees clockwise to inset, whereas a left abdominal DIEP flap is turned 90 degrees counterclockwise to inset, for either the left or right breast. The DIEP flap is placed within the mastectomy skin envelope.

TECHNIQUES

- The vascular pedicle, anastomoses, internal mammary vessels, and flow-coupler wire are examined by retracting the DIEP flap and carefully arranged to avoid kinks or twists.
- In immediate reconstruction with a nipple-sparing mastectomy, I leave a small skin paddle within the mastectomy incision. For an inframammary incision, I leave a 1.5 × 6 cm fusiform-shaped ellipse of skin within this incision (see **TECH FIG 5**). For a vertical infra-areolar incision, I leave a smaller, 1.5 × 3 cm fusiform-shaped ellipse of DIEP flap skin. Both of these small narrow skin paddles are usually excised at the revision/touch-up surgery done 3 or more months after the DIEP flap breast reconstruction.

- In immediate reconstruction with a skin-sparing mastectomy, I usually leave a 4.5 to 5 cm circular DIEP flap skin paddle to replace the excised nipple-areolar complex. This diameter allows future nipple reconstruction with a C-V flap entirely within the flap skin paddle, which will eventually be tattooed.
- The dermal edges of the DIEP flap are sutured to the mastectomy skin envelope with a single layer of inverted dermal 3-0 Monocryl and dressed with antibacterial ointment and Xeroform gauze. No brassiere or other dressings, or support, are used.

■ Closure of the Abdominal Donor Site

- The anterior rectus fascia is closed with buried interrupted figure-of-eight 0 PDS sutures. The rectus abdominis muscle is not sutured (see **TECH FIG 5**).
- The upper abdominal skin and subcutaneous tissue flap is elevated off the fascia for several cm superiorly. It is not necessary to elevate this all the way to the xiphoid process.
- Fluted 15-Fench round drains are brought out from each end of the abdominal donor-site incision and secured with 2-0 nylon sutures. The left drain is placed transversely along the lower donor site, and the right sided drain is placed transversely across the upper donor site, superior to the umbilicus (see **TECH FIG 5**).
- The head and back of the patient are raised sufficiently to be able to close the donor site without excessive tension.

With the patient flexed at the hips, the bed is placed in Trendelenburg to bring the back of the patient parallel to the floor.
- The upper and lower abdominal skin flaps are closed with multiple simple interrupted 2-0 clear PDS sutures to reapproximate the superficial fascia and subcutaneous fat. The skin is closed with a running subcuticular 2-0 Monoderm Quill suture.
- A 20 × 8 mm ellipse of skin and underlying cylindrical core of fat are excised from the upper abdominal skin flap overlying the umbilicus. The umbilicus is brought out through this hole, and inset using multiple inverted dermal 4-0 Monocryl sutures.
- The umbilicus and abdominal donor-site incision are dressed with antibiotic ointment, Xeroform gauze, dry sterile gauze, and tape.

PEARLS AND PITFALLS

Perforator selection	■ Lateral row perforators, in general, have a more direct course through the rectus abdominis muscle to the DIE pedicle and are easier to dissect, compared to medial row perforators, which often run diagonally through greater amounts of the rectus abdominis muscle. The largest perforators are more commonly in the medial row, but medial row perforators are not required, unless a DIEP flap including tissue across the midline is being harvested.
Congested flap during harvest	■ Occasionally, a DIEP flap will become venous congested during flap harvest, while still in situ at the abdomen. If this is mild, it will often resolve over 1–2 hours as venous interconnections within the flap "open up" and venous outflow redistributes.
Venous insufficiency	■ Venous insufficiency, manifest by venous congestion of the DIEP flap, is more common and more difficult to detect than arterial insufficiency. I recommend using an internal venous Doppler probe, especially one where the Doppler probe is integrated into a venous anastomotic coupling device. You cannot leave the operating room if the flap skin paddle is at all blue in hue and has less than 1-second capillary refill. This is venous congestion and must be addressed. On the other hand, a free flap can appear very pale, and without detectable capillary refill, as long as there is an arterial Doppler flow signal present.
Insetting	■ Set the perimeter/footprint of the reconstructed breast, and de-epithelialize the DIEP flap before transfer, so that the flap is placed within the mastectomy skin envelope only once, and does not have to be removed for de-epithelializing the periphery or adjusting the perimeter of the mastectomy pocket. This will avoid the risks of taking the flap in and out of the mastectomy skin envelope, and it will save time.
Flap orientation	■ A typical DIEP flap pedicle is long enough to allow the ipsilateral or contralateral flap to be used to reconstruct a breast. All else being equal, it is advantageous to use an ipsilateral flap, especially in delayed breast reconstruction, because this places the least well-perfused tissue, and most likely portion to suffer partial flap loss or fat necrosis, at the lateral and inferior region of the reconstructed breast.
Postoperative	■ No postoperative anticoagulation regimen has been proven more effective than others. I give patients 325 mg of aspirin daily while they are inpatients starting as soon as the patient is awake enough to swallow. I also give patients 40 mg of low molecular weight heparin subcutaneously daily while they are inpatients, starting at 5 PM on the 1st postoperative day.

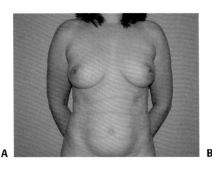 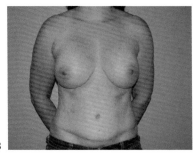

FIG 4 • A. Preoperative frontal view of patient shown in **FIG 2** and **TECH FIG 6**. **B.** Postoperative frontal view of patient shown in **FIG 2** and **TECH FIG 6**, 8 months after bilateral nipple-sparing mastectomies, and bilateral immediate breast reconstruction with DIEP flaps. Bilateral 190-cc smooth silicone implants were added to augment the reconstructed breast volume.

A　　　　　　　　　　　　　　　**B**

POSTOPERATIVE CARE

- Patients have perfusion of the DIEP flap monitored hourly for the first 24 hours and then every 2 hours for the next 48 hours by the nurses.
- Patients are not allowed to eat or drink, except for ice chips to moisten their mouths, until viability of the DIEP flap is confirmed on the morning of the 1st postoperative day, at which time a regular diet is allowed.
- Patients are given aspirin 325 mg orally daily starting immediately postoperatively and as long as they are inpatients.
- Patients are given 40 mg of low molecular weight heparin subcutaneously daily starting at 24 hours after completion of the surgery.
- On the morning of the 1st postoperative day, patients transfer with assistance from their bed into a chair for 15 minutes to 3 hours.
- On the 2nd postoperative day, patients ambulate with assistance outside of their hospital room at least once.
- On the 3rd postoperative day, intravenous fluids and the Foley catheter are discontinued in the morning, and patients are asked to ambulate with assistance outside of their hospital room at least three times.
- Starting of the 3rd postoperative day, patients are asked to shower and wash all surgical sites with soap and water daily.
- Some patients are discharged home in the afternoon of the 3rd postoperative day. Most patients are discharged home on the 4th postoperative day.
- Patients are asked not to wear a brassiere, not to sleep prone or on their sides, and not to raise their elbows higher than their shoulders for the first 2 weeks after surgery.
- Patients are asked not to submerge any surgical wound underwater (so no bathtub, hot tub, or swimming) and not to perform any activity which causes impact, or jarring of their body, for 4 to 5 weeks postoperatively.
- Patients are given prophylactic intravenous antibiotics as long as they have an I.V. in the hospital, and then Bactrim DS twice daily until removal of the last drain.
- Drains are removed once the output has fallen to less than, or equal to, 30 mL/d, for 2 consecutive days. Occasionally, one or two drains are removed before discharge from the hospital. Typically, some of the drains are removed at the first office visit 5 to 10 days after discharge from the hospital, and the remaining drains are removed at the second postoperative office visit 1 week later.
- An outpatient surgery to improve reconstructed breast shape and symmetry, repair abdominal donor-site dog-ears, and for nipple reconstruction is typically done, at the earliest, 3 months after the initial DIEP flap reconstruction surgery.

OUTCOMES

- Autologous tissue flaps from the lower abdomen are capable of producing the best, long-lasting, and most maintenance-free reconstructed breasts of any method of breast reconstruction.[1]
- A reconstructed breast, which looks and feels like a natural breast, can be achieved with a DIEP flap and nipple-sparing mastectomy done via an inframammary incision (**FIG 4**).

COMPLICATIONS

- With experience, the DIEP free flap loss rate, and emergent take-back rate, should be at or below 1% and 5%, respectively.
- Partial flap loss and fat necrosis are more common in obese patients and patients who smoke. Both of these are usually managed nonoperatively.
- A true hernia at the abdominal donor site is exceedingly rare, with a frequency of a fraction of a percent of patients.
- A lower abdominal bulge, to some degree, occurs in about 5% of patients. Abdominal bulges are not a health risk and are repaired if the patient desires by plication and polypropylene mesh overlay.
- The most common reasons for emergent take back are venous insufficiency/congestion of the DIEP flap and hematoma at the reconstructed breast. Venous congestion can cause a hematoma secondarily and can be mistaken for a hematoma by the inexperienced surgeon. A breast hematoma does not cause venous occlusion of the DIEP flap pedicle or anastomosis, but can result from venous congestion.

REFERENCES

1. Hu ES, Pusic AL, Waljee JF, et al. Patient-reported aesthetic satisfaction with breast reconstruction during the long-term survivorship period. *Plast Reconstr Surg.* 2009;124:1-8.
2. Chevray PM. Breast reconstruction with superficial inferior epigastric artery flaps: a prospective comparison with TRAM and DIEP flaps. *Plast Reconstr Surg.* 2004;114:1077-1083.
3. Koshima I, Soeda S. Inferior epigastric artery skin flaps without rectus abdominis muscle. *Br J Plast Surg.* 1989;42:645-648
4. Allen RJ, Treece P. Deep inferior epigastric perforator flap for breast reconstruction. *Ann Plast Surg.* 1994;32:32-38.
5. Chevray PM. Update on breast reconstruction using free TRAM, DIEP, and SIEA flaps. *Semin Plast Surg.* 2004;18:97-104.
6. Holm C, Mayr M, Hofter E, Ninkovic M. Perfusion zones of the DIEP flap revisited: a clinical study. *Plast Reconstr Surg.* 2006;117:37-43.
7. Jagsi R, Jiang J, Momoh AO, et al. Trends and variation in use of breast reconstruction in patients with breast cancer undergoing mastectomy in the United States. *J Clin Oncol.* 2014;32:919-926.
8. Howard-McNatt MM. Patients opting for breast reconstruction following mastectomy: an analysis of uptake rates and benefit. *Breast Cancer.* 2013;5:9-15.

23
CHAPTER

Abdominal Breast Reconstruction Using a SIEA Flap Approach

Adrian S. H. Ooi, Deana Shenaq, Julie E. Park, and David H. Song

DEFINITION

- Abdominal-based flaps for breast reconstruction can be divided into pedicled and free flaps based on their arterial supply.
  - Pedicled
    - Transverse rectus abdominis myocutaneous (TRAM) flap
  - Free
    - TRAM flap
    - Muscle-sparing TRAM (MS-TRAM) flap
    - Deep inferior epigastric perforator (DIEP) flap
    - Superficial inferior epigastric artery (SIEA) flap
- The free TRAM, MS-TRAM, and the DIEP flaps are based on a deep inferior epigastric vascular pedicle arising directly from the external iliac vessels.
  - In the free TRAM flap, the entire width of rectus muscle is taken to capture all the perforators within that segment.
  - In the MS-TRAM flap, a cuff of rectus muscle is harvested to capture multiple perforators from the deep inferior epigastric pedicle.
  - In the DIEP flap, only the perforating vessels to the subcutaneous fat and skin are harvested and the rectus muscle is not sacrificed.

- The SIEA flap is based on the subcutaneous superficial inferior epigastric vascular pedicle arising from the femoral vessels in the femoral triangle. Harvest of the flap does not involve any rectus muscle or fascia.

ANATOMY

- The SIEA flap is a Mathes and Nahai fasciocutaneous type A flap, harvested from the lower abdomen.
  - The skin island for the SIEA flap extends laterally to the anterior superior iliac spine (ASIS), medially to the midline or just past it, and from the level of the umbilicus superiorly to the pubic tubercle inferiorly.
- Vascular anatomy
  - Arterial
    - The SIEA is a branch of the femoral artery and arises from the femoral artery 2 to 3 cm below the inguinal ligament (**FIG 1**).
    - It is present in 49% to 91% of patients.[1,2]
    - The average size of the SIEA is 1.2 to 1.6 mm and average length 4 to 6 cm.[3]
    - It is present in both groins in 58% of patients.[4]

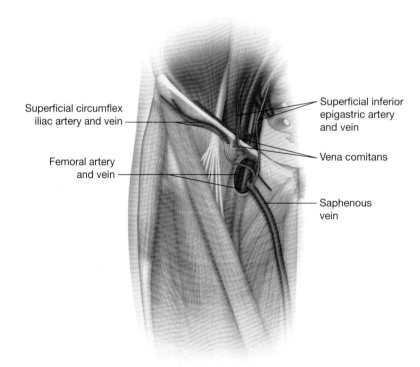

Superficial circumflex iliac artery and vein

Femoral artery and vein

Superficial inferior epigastric artery and vein

Vena comitans

Saphenous vein

FIG 1 • Vascular anatomy of the superficial inferior epigastric system.

- In about 75% of cases, it arises from a common origin with the superior circumflex iliac artery (SCIA).[5]
- The course of the artery is variable in relation to the superficial inferior epigastric vein (SIEV), usually arising up to 3 cm lateral to the SIEV and deep to the Scarpa fascia.
- After piercing the cribriform fascia, the SIEA courses inferolaterally for a short distance immediately above the deep fascia.
- It runs in a superolateral direction before crossing the inguinal ligament at roughly the midpoint between the pubic tubercle and the ASIS.
- The SIEA then pierces the Scarpa fascia to run in the superficial fatty later of the abdomen before arborizing with the periumbilical perforators of the deep inferior epigastric artery.
- Venous drainage
  - The venous drainage of the flap is through up to two venae comitantes of the epigastric artery and/or the SIEV (see **FIG 1**).
  - Diameter: 1.3 to 4 mm[1]
  - The surface marking of the SIEV is one-third of the way between the pubic symphysis and the ASIS.
  - The SIEV directly drains the subcutaneous plexus and is usually located superficial and medial to the SIEA in the superficial fatty layer of the abdomen.
  - The venae comitantes of the SIEA typically drain into SIEV.[6]
  - Occasionally, the superficial circumflex iliac vein (SCIV) and SIEV join into a common branch before draining into the femoral vein and if taken together can be used to enhance venous drainage of the flap (**FIG 2**).
- Flap vascular territory
  - The literature consists of varying reports using different measurement parameters stating flap perfusion can range from the hemiabdomen to 100% of the entire abdominal flap.[1,2,6]
  - We have found harvesting of the tissue across the midline to be unreliable, and would not advocate going past the hemiabdomen without testing perfusion either clinically with clamping off all other vascular input on the contralateral side or utilizing intraoperative fluorescence imaging.
- The flap receives sensory innervation via the segmental intercostal nerves T10-T12.

PATHOGENESIS

- Breast defects requiring SIEA flap reconstruction can be partial or total mastectomy defects and can arise from a variety of pathologies including:
  - Postcancer resection

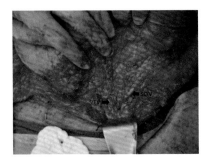

FIG 2 • The left superficial inferior epigastric (SIEV) and superficial circumflex iliac veins (SCIV) draining into a common branch.

- Prophylactic resection
- Failed implants
- A single large mastectomy defect may require a complete abdominal flap for coverage. An SIEA flap can be used together with the contralateral SIEA, DIEP, or MS-TRAM flap.
- The SIEA flap has been used for coverage of other defects including:
  - Head and neck
  - Upper extremity and hand
  - Lower extremity

NATURAL HISTORY

- Holmström reported the first use of a free abdominoplasty flap based on the deep inferior epigastric vessels in 1979.[7]
- Hartrampf pioneered the use of the pedicled TRAM flap for breast reconstruction in 1982.[8]
- While sacrificing rectus muscle, the free TRAM gained increasing popularity for breast reconstruction due to the use of the dominant blood supply to the rectus muscle, the deep inferior epigastric pedicle, to perfuse the abdominal tissue. It also allowed for more freedom in insetting and shaping the breast.[9]
- To minimize donor-site morbidity from harvest of the rectus muscle, the free MS-TRAM and DIEP flaps were developed following improvements in microsurgical knowledge and technique. Varying amounts of rectus muscle are left behind after harvest to maintain abdominal wall integrity and strength.
- Further evolution of the abdominal tissue flaps led to the development of the SIEA flap. The flap, first used by Antia and Buch for facial reconstruction in 1971 and further elucidated by Taylor and Daniel in their cadaveric studies of 1975, is based on a subcutaneous pedicle and completely spares the rectus fascia and muscle. Grotting first reported on its use in breast reconstruction in 1991, and owing to its obvious donor-site benefits has rapidly gained popularity ever since.[10–12]

PATIENT HISTORY AND PHYSICAL FINDINGS

- A focused history and examination relevant to any form of free flap reconstruction should be performed. In particular, the following should be elucidated and corrected if possible:
  - History of tobacco use
  - Obesity
  - Previous irradiation
  - Prothrombotic conditions
  - Anticoagulant use
- Similar criteria are applied to the SIEA flap as when determining the suitability of a patient for a free DIEP, MS-TRAM, or TRAM.
  - Sufficient redundant lower abdominal skin and fat
    - Approximates final desired breast volume
    - Allows for primary donor-site closure analogous to an abdominoplasty
  - Abdominal scars
    - Transverse lower abdominal scars such as in a Pfannenstiel incision may preclude the use of the SIEA or even deep inferior epigastric pedicles.
    - Midline laparotomy scars limit the abdominal tissue use to a single hemiabdomen as the perfusion across the midline is no longer reliable.

IMAGING

- Though not essential, several preoperative investigative techniques can be used to elucidate the vascular anatomy of the abdominal flap.
    - Doppler ultrasound
        - Can be used pre- and intraoperatively to locate perforators and pedicle position.
        - Used postoperatively for flap monitoring
    - CT-angiogram and MR-angiogram
        - Used preoperatively to elucidate location of abdominal perforators and the route of the source vessels
        - Can be used to select cases where the SIEA is suitable for use
    - Fluorescence imaging
        - Intraoperative administration of ICG via a peripheral vein after the hemiabdominal flap has been isolated on its pedicle and imaging with an infrared camera can help to assess the flap vascular territory.

DIFFERENTIAL DIAGNOSIS

- Reconstructive options for breast defects include but are not limited to:
    - Implant-based reconstruction +/− acellular dermal matrix
        - Immediate implant
        - Primary expander with implant exchange
        - Expander-implant
    - Pedicled flaps
        - Latissimus dorsi (LD)
        - TRAM
    - Free flaps
        - LD
        - TRAM
        - MS-TRAM
        - DIEP
        - SIEA
        - Superior gluteal artery perforator (SGAP) flap
        - Inferior gluteal artery perforator (IGAP) flap
        - Gracilis muscle–based flaps
        - Anterolateral thigh
        - Pudendal artery perforator (PAP) flap
        - Lateral thigh perforator (LTP) flap

SURGICAL MANAGEMENT

- Options of breast reconstruction should be tailored to each individual patient based on her disease process, adjuvant treatment, body habitus, and personal preference.
- Although implant-based breast reconstruction provides an expeditious reconstructive option, it is associated with implant-related complications as well as aesthetic outcomes which can be below expectations, especially in the setting of postoperative radiotherapy.
- We consider implant-based reconstruction in these scenarios:
    - The patient refuses autologous tissue use or has no autologous options.
    - Bilateral mastectomies
    - No postreconstructive radiation planned
    - Patient is unable to tolerate prolonged surgery.
- Abdominal tissue-based breast reconstruction has been the standard for the past few decades. Whether used in an immediate or delayed setting, it is associated with better aesthetic outcomes and higher rates of patient satisfaction.[13]
- The TRAM, MS-TRAM, and DIEP have been described in detail in other chapters, and owing to the variability of the SIEA remains the workhorse of abdominal tissue transfer options.
- However, in the instances when an SIEA flap can be used, there is decreased donor-site morbidity, an expedited harvesting, and similar aesthetic outcomes.

Preoperative Planning

- Indications
    - Patients desiring breast reconstruction with autologous tissue and having sufficient abdominal skin and fat without limiting abdominal scars.
- Flap selection
    - If the internal mammary (IM) vessels are used as recipients, a contralateral SIEA flap is used. This allows the short pedicle to be positioned at the internal IM vessels once the flap is placed in the breast pocket. If anastomosis to the thoracodorsal (TD) system is planned, an ipsilateral SIEA flap is used (**FIG 3**).

Internal mammary vessels

Thoracodorsal vessels

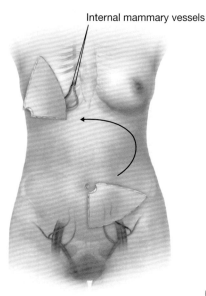
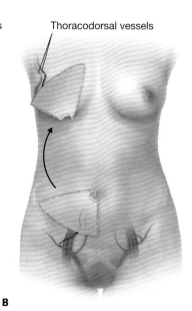

A   B

FIG 3 • A. If anastomosis to the internal mammary vessels is planned, a contralateral SIEA flap is used. **B.** If anastomosis to the thoracodorsal system is planned, an ipsilateral SIEA flap is used.

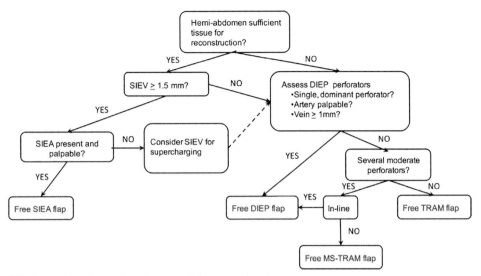

FIG 4 • Our decision-making algorithm for free abdominal flap breast reconstruction.

- We base our selection of SIEA flap reconstruction based on a simple intraoperative algorithm (**FIG 4**).
  - Assess the SIEV
    - If the SIEV is present and ≥1.5 cm, then the SIEA is assessed.
  - Assess the SIEA
    - If the SIEA pulsation is palpable and a hemiabdomen is sufficient for reconstruction, then a SIEA flap is used.
    - If the SIEA is not present or palpable, then a DIEP or MS-TRAM is performed.
- Many authors have used the caliber of the SIEA to as a criterion of suitability for the SIEA flap. In our experience, if the SIEA is palpable at the incision and the SIEV is ≥1.5 cm, the SIEA flap can be used even if the SIEA artery is less than 1 mm. In our consecutive series of 500 abdominal-based flaps, we have found the SIEA to be of use in 123 cases (29%).[14]
- We do not advocate the routine use of preoperative imaging for SIEA flap reconstruction.
- Marking
  - Patient marking is similar to that of the DIEP and free TRAM, with the lateral borders of the abdominal ellipse ending at the right and left ASIS (**FIG 5**).
  - The superior transverse incision of the abdominal ellipse is designed to include the periumbilical perforators.

- The major difference is the location of the inferior incision of the transverse ellipse. To encounter the SIEA at a larger caliber and optimize it as an option, it is recommended to lower the inferior incision, and we frequently mark this 5 cm above the mons pubis.

Positioning

- Positioning is similar to the free DIEP and TRAM.
- The patient is placed supine with hips positioned at the flex point of the operating table to enable a "jack-knife" position which aids in the closure of the abdominal incision.
- Calf compression pumps are placed for mechanical DVT prophylaxis.

Approach

- Intravenous antibiotics are given 30 minutes before skin incision.
- Whenever possible, the procedure is done by two teams, with one team harvesting the flap and the other preparing the recipient pocket and vessels.
- The IM vessels are the first choice for SIEA flap reconstruction. Use of the TD system leads to difficult microsurgical anastomosis and in cases where the SIEA pedicle is of insufficient length may necessitate vein grafts which increase the complexity of the procedure.

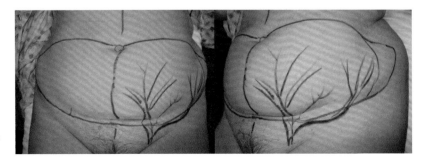

FIG 5 • Superficial inferior epigastric artery flap marking.

■ SIEA Flap

Incision and Exposure

- The lower incision is sharply incised, and careful dissection proceeds as the SIEA and SIEV are in the superficial fat layer of the flap. The SIEV in particular can be very superficial and lie just beneath the dermis (**TECH FIG 1**).
- The SIEV is located at approximately a point one-third between the pubic tubercle and the ASIS.
- The SIEA lies in an area up to 3 cm lateral to the SIEV and can be found deeper in the superficial fat compartment.
- The SIEV and SIEA are exposed and suitability determined as previously described. If suitable, the procedure proceeds with pedicle dissection.

Dissection

- Anterior dissection of the pedicle proceeds initially without circumferential isolation. This protects the artery from traction injury and prevents spasm.
- Gentle cephalad retraction of the flap coupled with vertical retraction of the lower groin skin will give clear access to anterior dissection of the pedicle (**TECH FIG 2A**).
- The route of the SIEV is straightforward and it can be easily dissected caudally toward the femoral vein.
  - When the SCIV is identified at the lower lateral edge of the flap and can be traced to a common origin with the SIEV at the femoral vein, the common branch is taken. This helps to improve venous drainage of the flap (see **FIG 2**).
  - If more than one superficial vein is found draining the flap and entering into separate source veins, these should be dissected out and clamped prior to pedicle ligation to determine dominancy.

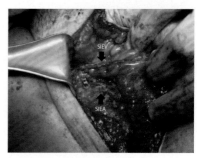

TECH FIG 1 • Exposure of the SIEV and SIEA.

- The path of the SIEA from the flap to its origin at the femoral artery is more complex.[6]
  - The SIEA initially travels caudally from the flap.
  - Prior to entering the femoral sheath, the SIEA sharply turns superomedially.
  - To increase the length and caliber of the artery, the cribriform fascia should be fully opened and the vessel traced all the way to its origin at the common femoral artery. This increases SIEA length by 1 to 2 cm and yields a larger diameter vessel (**TECH FIG 2B–D**, Video 1).
  - Any branches close to the origin from the femoral artery are clipped long for potential use as a point at which to spatulate the artery to address size mismatch.
  - Caution should be taken in cases where the SCIA merges with the SIEA to form a common pedicle at the take-off from the femoral artery. In these cases, both the SCIA and SIEA can be taken together with the flap.

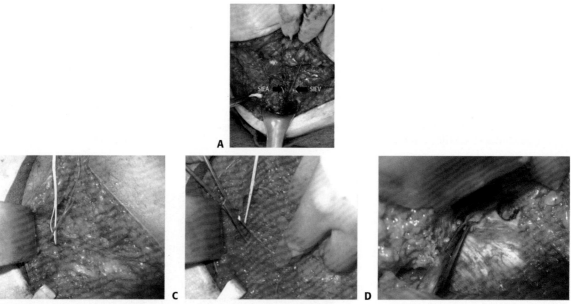

TECH FIG 2 • **A.** Dissection of the right SIEV and SIEA with cephalad retraction of the flap and vertical retraction of the lower groin skin. **B.** Dissection of the right superficial inferior epigastric artery (SIEA) to the cribriform fascia. **C.** Opening of the cribriform fascia to maximize exposure of the origin of the SIEA. **D.** Close up of the cribriform fascia outlined in *blue ink*.

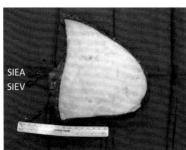
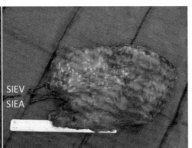
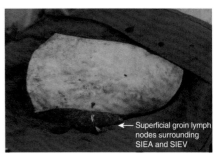

E

F

TECH FIG 2 (Continued) • **E.** Completion of harvest a right sided SIEA flap. **F.** Harvest of the superficial groin lymph nodes lateral to the SIEV (*yellow microvascular clamp*) together with a left-sided SIEA (*green microvascular clamp*) flap.

- Once the anterior dissection is complete along the full length of the vessel, posterior dissection of the pedicle can proceed. This is done carefully to avoid traction on the vessels (**TECH FIG 2E**).
- Concomitant vascularized lymph node transfer (VLNT).
  - The superficial groin lymph nodes lie lateral to the SIEV and can be harvested together with the pedicle (**TECH FIG 2F**). To avoid harvesting the deeper lymph nodes, which can lead to lower limb lymphedema, we recommend the use of reverse lymphatic mapping with radioisotope to identify the sentinel lymph node.[15]

Completion of Flap Harvest

- Once pedicle dissection is completed, harvest of the abdominal tissue proceeds.
- The superior incision is completed sparing the umbilicus, and the flap is dissected off the abdominal muscular fascia in the avascular plane.
  - Any intercostal perforators encountered along the way are carefully ligated.
- When dissection reaches the borders of the rectus muscle at the semilunaris, care must be taken to identify the DIEP perforators.
- If there is any question of SIEA perfusion of the flap, microvascular clamps can be applied to the DIEP perforators to assess the perfusion based upon the superficial system.
- Once it is determined that the flap can survive on the SIEA alone, the DIEP perforators are securely ligated.
- Because the SIEA has a short pedicle, we recommend de-epithelializing the majority of the flap in situ on the abdomen to avoid injuring the microanastomosis once the flap has been delivered to the mastectomy defect. This is especially important for larger flaps with the small aperture of a skin-sparing mastectomy.

Recipient Vessels and Microanastomosis

- Our order of choice of recipient vessels are:
  - Pulsatile IM artery (IMA) perforator with adequate IM vein (IMV) perforator
  - IMA and IMV—the rib can usually be spared with an intercostal space of 3 cm. We typically target the 2nd or 3rd intercostal space.
  - If lymph nodes are required in the axilla, or on the rare occasion where the internal mammary vessels are not available, the thoracodorsal system is used.

- If the flap pedicle is too short, vein grafts have to be used to prevent tension on the anastomosis.
- When there is significant vessel size mismatch between the IMA and the SIEA, manipulation via back cuts or spatulation can be performed. The back-cut on the antimesenteric side of the vessel allows for a technically easier anastomosis. Alternatively, if there are any distal branches, the pedicle could be spatulated at a branch point to increase vessel diameter.[14] Finally, end-to-side anastomosis between the SIEA and the IMA has been described.
- The SIEV is usually of sufficient size and there is rarely any mismatch with the IMV. Use of a venous coupler usually facilitates any venous anastomosis size mismatch and short pedicle. We hand sew the vein if the SIEV is greater than 4 mm in diameter as use of a coupler can cause redundancy of the thick SIEV within the lumen and cause occlusion.
- Overall, the SIEA is particularly prone to spasm and careful dissection, as well as minimizing the amount of anastomotic revisions, is paramount to successful execution of this flap.

Flap Inset

- The main issue when insetting the SIEA flap is the short pedicle length. Care must be taken not to cause traction on the vessels, especially in the setting of an immediate reconstruction with a skin-sparing mastectomy and small aperture.
- As mentioned previously, we perform the majority of flap de-epithelialization with the flap in situ in the abdomen before ligation of the pedicle and transfer. Any de-epithelialization performed with the flap in the chest must be undertaken with the utmost care. Remember the superficial nature of the SIEV when de-epithelizing, insetting, and securing the flap.
- Insetting the flap in the superomedial direction first takes the tension off the pedicle. The remainder of the mastectomy skin can then be carefully draped around the flap.
- The mastectomy skin envelope to flap relationship must be evaluated. If the flap is relatively small within a large skin envelope:
  - Reduce the skin envelope
  - Consider a contralateral breast reduction
  - Place anchoring sutures from the flap to the chest wall

T E C H N I Q U E S

- Use external support such as a surgical brassiere that is fitted carefully to prevent compression while giving inferior and lateral support.
- A closed suction drain is placed exiting at the lateral IMF and draining the superior portion of the flap, ending just away from the microanastomoses site.

Donor Site Closure

- Donor-site closure is similar to that of the free DIEP and TRAM, except that the abdominal muscular fascia remains untouched and no closure of this is required.
- The upper abdominal flap is undermined to the border of the ribs laterally and the xiphoid process superiorly, being careful to ligate any significant perforators along the way.

- Once the microanastomosis is complete and de-epithelialization is complete and the flap has been secured in position in the breast defect, the operating table can be adjusted into a "jack-knife" position with the patient's hips flexed to allow tension-free abdominal closure.
- Skin staples are used to temporarily approximate the skin edges, usually requiring some adjustment from lateral to medial.
- Key to donor-site closure is approximating the Scarpa fascia from the upper and lower abdominal flaps with absorbable 2-0 polyfilament sutures. Once this is done, skin closure can be done with technique of choice. Abdominal closed suction drains should be used.

PEARLS AND PITFALLS

Preoperative preparation	■ Caution in patients who are heavy, active smokers for increased risk of vasospasm
Exposure	■ Lower the abdominal incision to encounter the SIEA at a larger caliber.
Pedicle dissection	■ Perform anterior rather than circumferential dissection of the artery first to minimize vasospasm. ■ Dissect the artery completely to the femoral artery. ■ Avoiding unnecessary periarterial lymph node harvest increases pedicle length.
Raising the flap	■ De-epithelialize the flap in situ on the abdomen.
Microanastomosis	■ Maximize recipient vessel length. ■ Back-cut or spatulate the SIEA for cases where there is vessel mismatch. ■ Intraoperative papavarine is useful to address any arterial spasm.
Inset	■ Careful support of the flap to prevent ptosis
Postoperative care	■ Keep the patient warm and reduce pain and anxiety to prevent vasospasm.

POSTOPERATIVE CARE

- General care for the SIEA flap is similar to the postoperative care for other free tissue reconstruction of the breast. At our institution:
  - A near infrared (NIRS) tissue spectroscopy monitor is placed on the flap and the patient is sent to the postoperative care unit for a period of monitoring.
  - Once the patient is stable, she is sent to the floor. The flap is monitored clinically for color, temperature, capillary refill, turgor, and handheld Doppler signal as well as continuous tissue oximetry.
  - Incentive spirometry as well as chemical and mechanical DVT prophylaxis is started.
  - Patients are kept NPO for the approximately the first 24 hours. If the patient and flap are doing well by the first postoperative day (POD) morning, the diet is advanced after evaluation on morning rounds. The urinary catheter is removed and the patient is advised to sit out of bed in a chair and encouraged to ambulate later in the day. Intravenous antibiotics are converted to oral antibiotics after the first 24 hours.
  - POD 2 and 3 are spent with continuation of ambulation and converting all pain control to oral medications. Patients are usually discharged on POD 3.

- Specific considerations regarding the postoperative care of the SIEA flap center around arterial spasm, which can happen up to more than 48 hours postoperatively.
  - This can manifest in a variety of ways:
    - A clinically cool, pale flap
    - Absent Doppler signal
    - Steady drop in NIRS tissue spectroscopy of 15 to 20 points and leveling off
  - Arterial spasm can result from any combination of factors including:
    - Ptosis of the flap placing stretch on the vascular anastomosis
    - Patient pain and anxiety
    - Dehydration
    - Reduced patient core temperature
  - Maneuvers to alleviate arterial spasm include the following:
    - A surgical brassiere can be placed to give support.
    - Adequate treatment of pain, warming, and antianxiolytics can be administered as necessary.
  - If the spasm does not resolve after these measures, operative exploration is warranted.

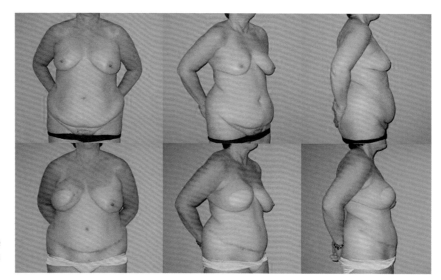

FIG 6 • Preoperative (*above*) and postoperative (*below*) photos of a right breast reconstructed with a left abdominal SIEA flap.

OUTCOMES

- The SIEA flap has similar aesthetic outcomes to the other abdominal-based flaps (**FIG 6**).
- There is a steep learning curve associated with the flap and high conversion rate to another free flap.[16]
- There are no risks of hernia or bulge because the rectus fascia and motor nerves to the rectus muscles are not disturbed.
- In our series of 145 free abdominal flaps based on the superficial system, overall success rates were 95%.[14]

COMPLICATIONS

- Vascular thrombosis and flap loss
  - An analysis of 99 SIEA flaps performed in 82 patients showed an overall arterial thrombosis rate of 6.1%, venous congestion rate of 2%, partial flap loss of 5.1%, and total flap loss of 5.1%.[17]
  - In an analysis of 69 SIEA flaps, the rate of venous or arterial thrombosis was 17.4%, with 2.9% total flap loss, significantly greater numbers than in a comparative DIEP flap group.[18]
  - Another study of outcomes of 44 SIEA flaps against 125 DIEP flaps showed significantly higher re-exploration rates in the SIEA group (20%) vs the DIEP group (7%). A subset analysis showed arterial problems to be significantly higher among SIEA flaps (14%) vs DIEP flaps (1%). None of the arterial thrombosis were salvageable.[19]
  - In our series, there were nine cases of re-exploration for vascular problems (6.2%), three with purely venous thrombosis and six with arterial thromboses. Two of the flaps with venous thromboses were salvaged, whereas none of the flaps with arterial thromboses were salvaged. Eighty percent of the flaps with arterial thromboses lost had arterial revisions at the initial operation. SIEA spatulation did not correlate with increased thromboses rate.[14]
- Fat necrosis
  - In a large series of 99 free SIEA flaps, fat necrosis rates were found to be 1%. These authors routinely used tissue across the midline, discarding zone IV of the flap and any tissue assessed to have poor perfusion intraoperatively.[17]
  - In a case series of 228 patients, it was found that the fat necrosis rates for free SIEA, DIEP, and MS-TRAM flaps were 14%, 25%, and 5%, respectively.[20]

- A further systemic review of fat necrosis rates in abdominal free flaps reinforced this and showed the SIEA to have a mean fat necrosis rate of 8.1% (range 5.7% to 13.5%). This was lower than the free DIEP flap and slightly higher than the free MS-TRAM. Risk factors for necrosis included obesity, pre-existing abdominal scars, pre- and postoperative irradiation, and smoking.[21]
- In a more recent study of a single center's experience of SIEA flaps vs DIEP flaps, the flap necrosis requiring debridement in the SIEA group was 14% (6/44 patients) vs 3% (4/125 patients) in the DIEP group.[19]
- An analysis of our series of 145 free flaps based on the superficial system, the fat necrosis rate was 10.3%.[14]

REFERENCES

1. Chevray PM. Breast reconstruction with superficial inferior epigastric artery flaps: a prospective comparison with TRAM and DIEP Flaps. *Plast Reconstr Surg.* 2004;114(5):1077-1083.
2. Ulusal BG, Cheng MH, Wei FC, et al. Breast reconstruction using the entire transverse abdominal adipocutaneous flap based on unilateral superficial or deep inferior epigastric vessels. *Plast Reconstr Surg.* 2006;117(5):1395-1403.
3. Kim BJ, Choi JH, Kim TH, et al. The superficial inferior epigastric artery flap and its relevant vascular anatomy in Korean women. *Arch Plast Surg.* 2014;41(6):702-708.
4. Rizzuto RP, Allen RJ. Reconstruction of a partial mastectomy defect with the superficial inferior epigastric artery (SIEA) flap. *J Reconstr Microsurg.* 2004;20(6):441-445.
5. Arnez ZM, Smith RW, Eder E, et al. Breast reconstruction by the free lower transverse rectus abdominis musculocutaneous flap. *Br J Plast Surg.* 1988;41(5):500-505.
6. Dorafshar A, Januszyk M, Song D. Anatomical and technical tips for use of the superficial inferior epigastric artery (SIEA) flap in breast reconstructive surgery. *J Reconstr Microsurg.* 2010;26(06):381-389.
7. Holmström H. The free abdominoplasty flap and its use in breast reconstruction: an experimental study and clinical case report. *Scand J Plast Reconstr Surg.* 1979;13(3):423-427.
8. Hartrampf CR, Scheflan M, Black PW. Breast reconstruction with a transverse abdominal island flap. *Plast Reconstr Surg.* 1982;69(2):216-224.
9. Friedman RJ, Argenta LC, Anderson R. Deep inferior epigastric free flap for breast reconstruction after radical mastectomy. *Plast Reconstr Surg.* 1985;76(3):455-458.
10. Antia NH, Buch VI. Transfer of an abdominal dermo-fat graft by direct anastomosis of blood vessels. *Br J Plast Surg.* 1971;24:15-19.
11. Grotting JC. The free abdominoplasty flap for immediate breast reconstruction. *Ann Plast Surg.* 1991;27(4):351-354.

12. Taylor GI, Daniel RK. The anatomy of several free flap donor sites. *Plast Reconstr Surg.* 1975;56(3):243-253.

13. Chang DW. Breast reconstruction with microvascular MS-TRAM and DIEP flaps. *Arch Plast Surg.* 2012;39(1):3-10.

14. Park JE, Shenaq DS, Silva AK, et al. Breast reconstruction with SIEA flaps. *Plast Reconstr Surg.* 2016;137(6):1682-1689.

15. Dayan JH, Dayan E, Smith ML. Reverse lymphatic mapping. *Plast Reconstr Surg.* 2015;135(1):277-285.

16. Thoma A, Jansen L, Sprague S, Stat EDP. A comparison of the superficial inferior epigastric artery flap and deep inferior epigastric perforator flap in postmastectomy reconstruction: a cost-effectiveness analysis. *Can J Plast Surg.* 2008;16(2):77-84.

17. Spiegel AJ, Khan FN. An intraoperative algorithm for use of the SIEA flap for breast reconstruction. *Plast Reconstr Surg.* 2007;120(6):1450-1459.

18. Selber JC, Samra F, Bristol M, et al. A head-to-head comparison between the muscle-sparing free TRAM and the SIEA flaps: is the rate of flap loss worth the gain in abdominal wall function? *Plast Reconstr Surg.* 2008;122(2):348-355.

19. Coroneos CJ, Heller AM, Voineskos SH, Avram R. SIEA versus DIEP arterial complications: a cohort study. *Plast Reconstr Surg.* 2015;135(5):802e-807e.

20. Baumann DP, Lin HY, Chevray PM. Perforator number predicts fat necrosis in a prospective analysis of breast reconstruction with free TRAM, DIEP, and SIEA flaps. *Plast Reconstr Surg.* 2010;125(5):1335-1341.

21. Khansa I, Momoh AO, Patel PP, et al. Fat necrosis in autologous abdomen-based breast reconstruction: a systematic review. *Plast Reconstr Surg.* 2013;131(3):443-452.

Recipient Vessel Exposure—Internal Mammary and Thoracodorsal

Theodore A. Kung and Adeyiza O. Momoh

CHAPTER 24

DEFINITION

- Recipient vessels for microsurgical breast reconstruction are required to re-establish perfusion in transferred free flaps.
- Perfusion through these vessels is most critical early on after free tissue transfers, when flaps are entirely dependent on the recipient vessels for inflow and outflow. Over time, collateral perfusion is typically established from the surrounding soft tissue bed.
- The primary recipient vessels for breast reconstruction are the internal mammary and thoracodorsal vessels.

ANATOMY

Internal Mammary Vessels

- The internal mammary artery (IMA) is a paired artery on both sides of the sternum that arises from the subclavian artery. It transitions into the superior epigastric vessels at about the sixth intercostal space.
- The internal mammary vein (IMV) is also paired, runs parallel to the IMA, arising from the superior epigastric vein and ending in the brachiocephalic vein.
- The vessels are 1 to 2 cm lateral to the sternum and run deep to the intercostal muscles and ribs.
- Both vessels give off intercostal branches laterally that run inferior to the first six ribs. Perforators to the overlying breast and skin are also given off by the IMA and IMV in the first 5 to 6 intercostal spaces.
- The right and left IMAs are of similar diameter (1.9–2.1 mm) at 3rd and 4th intercostal spaces where they are typically used.[1,2] At the level of the 3rd intercostal space, the IMA lies lateral to the IMV or between two IMVs.
- The left IMV bifurcates at a higher level than does the right IMV (3rd rib on the left vs 4th rib on the right). At the level of the 3rd ICS, the left IMV is on average smaller than the right (2.5 mm vs 3 mm).[3]

Thoracodorsal Vessels

- The thoracodorsal artery (TDA) and the circumflex scapular artery are the two main branches of the subscapular artery, which arises from the third division of the axillary artery (**FIG 1**).
- The TDA travels along the lateral thoracic wall before diving into the latissimus dorsi muscle about 9 from its origin. Prior to its entry into the muscle, the TDA consistently (99%) gives off a branch to the serratus anterior muscle.[4]
- The TD vessels are commonly divided for microvascular anastomosis just proximal to the serratus branch where the diameter of the artery is approximately 3 mm.[5] Preservation of the serratus branch also allows for the use of a pedicled

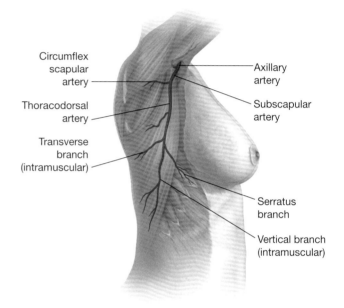

FIG 1 • Illustration of the thoracodorsal vessels arising from the subscapular system.

latissimus dorsi flap and an implant for breast reconstruction in case free tissue transfer is unsuccessful.

- Proximally, there are often two veins that unify into a single TD vein. The TD vein travels with the TD artery and has an average diameter of 3.4 mm at its origin and 1.6 mm where it enters the latissimus dorsi muscle.[6]
- The TD nerve enters the axilla deep to the axillary vein at a point several centimeters medial to the origin of the subscapular vessels. The nerve then continues toward the subscapular system and eventually travels parallel with the TD vessels along the lateral thoracic wall (**FIG 2**).

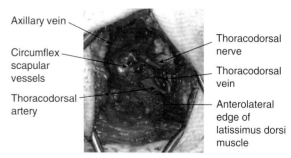

FIG 2 • Exposure of the thoracodorsal artery, vein, and nerve prior to their entry into the latissimus dorsi muscle. The nerve should be dissected free to prevent any kinking of the vessels after anastomosis.

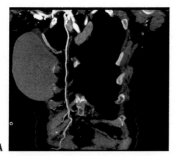 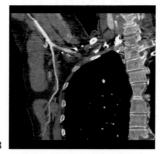 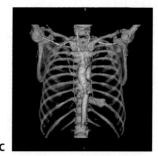

A **B** **C**

FIG 3 • **A.** A CT angiogram of the chest with sagittal slices showing continuity of the IM. **B.** TD arteries. **C.** Additional 3D reconstruction provides an overall view of the thoracic vessel anatomy.

PATIENT HISTORY AND PHYSICAL FINDINGS

- A thorough history of prior thoracic and breast procedures including axillary lymph node dissections and prior chest wall radiation are important to determine possible compromise to the IM or TD vessels.
- The continuity of IM vessels is seldom affected by oncologic breast procedures; however, a history of radical chest wall tumor resections or coronary bypass procedures may prevent use of the IM vessels as recipients.
- Thoracodorsal vessels are at greater risk of injury during axillary lymph node dissections and should be approached with caution in the setting of delayed reconstruction in such patients.
- A history of radiation should prompt an anticipation of friable recipient vessels. IM vessel friability introduces technical challenges with exposure and anastomosis but can be consistently overcome with careful vessel handling.

IMAGING

- There is limited value to routine preoperative imaging of IM or TD vessels in the absence of a history that suggests potential compromise.
- If a patient has had a preoperative breast MRI, that status of the mammary vessels may be evident.
- When needed, CT angiography provides detailed information on the vascular anatomy for surgical planning (**FIG 3**).

SURGICAL MANAGEMENT

- The decision on which recipient vessel is to be used is made preoperatively. The internal mammary vessels are the authors' preferred option for immediate and delayed microsurgical breast reconstruction with the TD vessels serving as a backup option.
- If immediate reconstruction following mastectomy and axillary lymph node dissection is performed, the TD vessels are often already partially exposed and may be considered for anastomosis. However, the vessels must be carefully inspected for any injury or spasm resulting from the extirpation surgery. Additionally, the flap pedicle must be of sufficient length to reach the TD vessels for anastomosis.
- In contrast, with delayed breast reconstruction and especially following radiation therapy, significant scarring can be expected within the axilla. Dissection of the thoracodorsal vessels in this setting is usually more time-consuming and has a higher risk of vessel injury.

Preoperative Planning

- The risks and benefits of costal cartilage resection with IM vessel exposure should be discussed in addition to the rare potential for a pneumothorax during vessel exposure.

Positioning

- When the IM vessels are selected for anastomosis, the patient is positioned supine with arms either tucked at the sides or abducted at 90 degrees.
- When the TD vessels are used, the ipsilateral arm should be prepped to allow for adjustments in position during the operation. The arm boards should be kept under sterile drapes in order to adjust arm abduction during the operation. It is most ergonomic for the surgeon to be positioned above the arm board on the side of the anastomosis while the assistant is positioned below the contralateral arm board (**FIG 4**).

Approach

- IM vessels are either exposed with costal cartilage resection or in the intercostal space through a rib-sparing approach. The former is the authors' preferred approach.

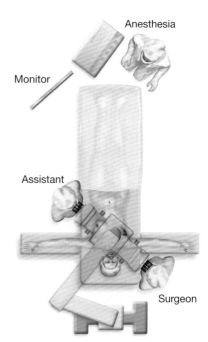

FIG 4 • Ergonomic surgeon and assistant positioning with use of the TD vessels as recipients.

- TD vessels may be accessed through the mastectomy incision. From this approach, adequate exposure is often difficult and requires retraction of the lateral border of the pectoralis major muscle or the use of additional instruments.[7] Alternatively, the authors favor a separate incision in the axilla. In many breast cancer patients, a previous scar from sentinel lymph node biopsy may already be present. Slight abduction of the arm and the use of self-retaining retractors facilitate microsurgical anastomosis even in overweight patients.[8]

T
E
C
H
N
I
Q
U
E
S

■ Internal Mammary Vessel Exposure

- In the setting of an immediate reconstruction following a skin-sparing mastectomy, the breast pocket is first irrigated and hemostasis achieved with electrocautery as needed.
- An Army-Navy retractor is temporarily introduced to retract medial mastectomy skin for visualization of the medial anterior chest wall.
- The cartilaginous portion of the 3rd rib is palpated through the pectoralis major muscle. The muscle fibers over this medial aspect of the rib are split along the fibers with electrocautery and a Weitlaner retractor is introduced between the muscle fibers (handles lateral) to provide exposure of the underlying rib. The muscle split is performed from the lateral edge of the sternum to a point approximately 6 cm lateral to the sternum.
- The anterior costal perichondrium is scored along its length with the electrocautery and also perpendicular to the lengthwise incision at the medial and lateral extents of the exposed cartilage.
- A Freer elevator is then used to elevate the perichondrium off the underlying cartilage on its superficial surface, around the superior and inferior borders of the rib (**TECH FIG 1A**).
- The lateral cartilage is then excised with a rongeur down to the posterior perichondrium, taking care not to violate this posterior plane at this time.
- A second Weitlaner retractor is introduced perpendicular to the first (handles cephalad), anchored laterally at the cut edge of the rib, and used to retract the medial mastectomy skin out of the field. At this point, the Army-Navy retractor is no longer needed. In patients with large skin flaps, a few skin hooks might be necessary to adequately retract redundant mastectomy skin.
- Excision of the remainder of the cartilage proceeds from lateral to medial to expose the posterior perichondrium. The IMA and vein are sometimes visible through the posterior perichondrium at this point.
- An incision parallel to the cut edge of the rib is made laterally through the posterior perichondrium with a scalpel. A Freer is then introduced underneath the perichondrium and used to push all soft tissue and vessel downward, proceeding toward the sternum.
- The posterior perichondrium is then split with a tenotomy scissor from lateral to medial exposing the underlying IMA and IMV.
- The posterior perichondrium is bluntly dissected off the underlying vessels with a Freer.
- Small vessel branches from the IMA and IMV are identified, ligated with microsurgical clips, and cut.
- The posterior perichondrium is then excised completely with a cautery at low settings to provide optimal exposure of the recipient vessels.
- If additional length is desired, the intercostal muscles cephalad and caudal to the vessels can be excised. To gain size in the exposed vessels, the intercostal muscles cephalad to the vessels can be excised.
- The IMA and IMV are dissected circumferentially with a Freer elevator. All side branches are ligated with microsurgical clips and cut with tenotomy scissors.
- A background mat with attached suction (authors' preference) is then placed beneath both vessels (**TECH FIG 1B**).
- Papaverine is applied, and a warm moist gauze is placed over the vessels until they are ready to be used.

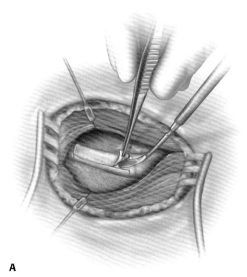

A

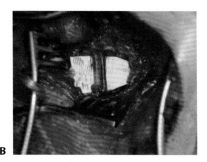

B

TECH FIG 1 • **A.** The 3rd rib exposed deep to the pectoralis major muscle (fibers retracted with a Weitlaner retractor). Elevation of perichondrium over medial segment of the rib with a Freer. **B.** Exposure of the internal mammary vessels with a background in place.

TECHNIQUES

Thoracodorsal Vessel Exposure

- A 6-cm curvilinear incision is made within the axillary fossa just inferior to the axillary crease. The incision should not extend anteriorly beyond the anterior axillary fold. If present, a previous scar from sentinel lymph node biopsy should be incorporated into the incision.
- Dissection is performed through the subcutaneous fat using the electrocautery until the axillary fat is reached. The axillary fat pad is more yellow in color than the subcutaneous fat.
- Two Weitlaner retractors are positioned within the incision to spread the axillary fat pad apart.
- Branches of the intercostobrachial nerve are encountered within the axillary fat pad and should be preserved if possible.
- At this point, nontoothed forceps and bipolar cautery should be used.
- The TD vessels can be found by two approaches:
  - Locating the anterolateral edge of the latissimus dorsi first and then performing dissection along its deep surface to identify the TD neurovascular bundle
  - Locating the axillary vein first and then exposing the takeoff of the subscapular vessels. Dissection is then carried distally to identify the TD vessels.
- With the first method, the lateral edge of the latissimus dorsi muscle can be found by gentle tapping of the electrocautery tip to bring about muscle contractions. The point at which the neurovascular hilum enters the undersurface of the muscle is approximately 2 to 3 cm away from its anterolateral edge. The TD vessels are identified, separated from the TD nerve, and followed proximally.
- With the second method, blunt dissection with a finger through the axillary fat pad is performed in the direction of the axillary vessels. The pulsations of the axillary artery can easily be appreciated by palpation, and this can guide the direction of dissection. The axillary vein is anterior to the axillary artery; when it is encountered, meticulous dissection should proceed along its length to identify branches traveling inferiorly. Once the subscapular artery and vein are identified, they are dissected distally to locate the branch point of the circumflex scapular vessels and their continuation as the TD vessels.
- Often, the circumflex scapular branch needs to be ligated to achieve adequate pedicle length and to prevent kinking of the pedicle.
- The branch to the serratus anterior muscle should be identified and preserved. The TD vessels are usually divided just proximal to the serratus anterior branch point.
- When sufficient pedicle length has been obtained, a McCabe dissector is used to separate the TD artery, vein, and nerve. Once divided, the TD vessels should be positioned superficial to the nerve to prevent a "clotheslining effect" of the nerve on the pedicle.
- Particularly in larger patients, performing the anastomosis deep within the axilla can be quite difficult. To ameliorate this problem, a moist gauze is packed into the axilla and the divided TD vessels may subsequently be positioned more superficially.

PEARLS AND PITFALLS

Technique	■ IMA and IMV size at the level of the 3rd rib are consistently well matched with the commonly utilized deep inferior epigastric vessels; as often as possible, this is the ideal site for recipient vessel.
	■ The 4th rib in some cases is in a central location within mastectomy defects and might be easier to access than the 3rd rib. The IMVs on the left are appreciably smaller at the level of the 4th rib; plan to dissect proximal through the intercostal muscles to improve on IMV size.
	■ Plan for additional length of the IM vessels with possible proximal and distal dissection extending to the ribs above and below in cases with a traditionally short flap pedicle or in morbidly obese patients with very large flaps.
	■ To avoid injury to the IM vessels, it is critical to begin rib resection and elevation of the posterior perichondrium lateral to the vessel location. Dissect from lateral to medial.
	■ Keep vessel handling and cleaning of the adventitia to a minimum in radiated fields to avoid vessel injury.
	■ In some patients, exposed to radiation or with a low BMI, there may be very little adipose tissue between the posterior perichondrium and the pleura. Careful blunt dissection is needed to avoid an injury to the pleura.
Pleural injury	■ During exposure of the IM vessels, small tears in the parietal pleura may occur. These rents may either be left unrepaired or carefully closed with fine absorbable suture.
	■ To evaluate for a pneumothorax, a positive pressure test may be performed. The rent is completely submerged in normal saline and the anesthesiologist delivers a breath of positive pressure ventilation. When the injury is limited to the parietal pleura, a positive pressure test will not result in air escape.
Pneumothorax	■ A pneumothorax results when the injury extends through the parietal pleura, through the visceral pleura, and into the lung parenchyma.
	■ A positive pressure test will result in bubbles appearing from the injury.
	■ When this is detected in the operating room, the air within the pleural space must be evacuated and an airtight closure of the parietal pleura should be performed. A small red rubber catheter on suction is placed into the pleural space and a purse-string suture is thrown around the pleural rent but left untied. As the anesthesiologist delivers a breath of positive pressure ventilation, the catheter is removed and the purse string is tied securely. The positive pressure test is repeated to check for air escape. Postoperatively, a chest x-ray is performed. Any significant lung collapse warrants a chest tube.

POSTOPERATIVE CARE

- Based primarily on postoperative flap care or protocol

OUTCOMES

- Flap complication and survival rates with use of the internal mammary or thoracodorsal vessels are similar.[9,10]
- Conversions from TD vessels to IM vessels tend to be more common in radiated patients with previous axillary lymph node dissections.[11]
- Occasional contour deformities and temporary discomfort at the site of rib resection are experienced by patients with IM vessel exposure. When present, contour deformities are easily addressed with autologous fat grafting, and chest wall discomfort resolves with time.

COMPLICATIONS

- Hematomas in the early postoperative period can be experienced with potential rapid enlargement of the breast mound with an arterial bleed. Large hematomas place pressure on the vascular pedicle and increase the risk of vascular compromise. Clinically significant hematomas are taken back to the operating room for evacuation and hemostasis.
- The axillary artery and vein are in close approximation to the brachial plexus. Careful dissection using bipolar cautery will prevent iatrogenic nerve injury.
- Arms should be well padded to avoid pressure-related complications.
- Neuropraxia due to prolonged arm abduction may be treated expectantly, but prevention is the best strategy.

REFERENCES

1. Rozen WM, Ye X, Guio-Aguilar PL, et al. Autologous microsurgical breast reconstruction and coronary artery bypass grafting: an anatomical study and clinical implications. *Breast Cancer Res Treat*. 2012; 134(1):181-198.
2. Tan O, Yuce I, Aydin OE, Kantarci M. A radioanatomic study of the internal mammary artery and its perforators using multidetector computed tomography angiography. *Microsurgery*. 2014;34(4):277-282.
3. Clark CP III, Rohrich RJ, Copit S, et al. An anatomic study of the internal mammary veins: clinical implications for free-tissue-transfer breast reconstruction. *Plast Reconstr Surg*. 1997;99(2):400-404.
4. Rowsell AR, Davies DM, Eisenberg N, Taylor GI. The anatomy of the subscapular-thoracodorsal arterial system: study of 100 cadaver dissections. *Br J Plast Surg*. 1984;37(4):574-576.
5. Robb GL. Thoracodorsal vessels as a recipient site. *Clin Plast Surg*. 1998;25(2):207.
6. Bartlett SP, May JW Jr, Yaremchuk MJ. The latissimus dorsi muscle: a fresh cadaver study of the primary neurovascular pedicle. *Plast Reconstr Surg*. 1981;67(5):631-636.
7. Mehrara BJ, Santoro T, Smith A, et al. Improving recipient vessel exposure during microvascular breast reconstruction. *Ann Plast Surg*. 2003;51(4):361.
8. Gravvanis A, Caulfield RH, Ramakrishnan V, Niranjan N. Recipient vessel exposure in the axilla during microvascular breast reconstruction. *J Reconstr Microsurg*. 2008;24(8):595-598.
9. Moran SL, Nava G, Benham AB, Serletti JM. An outcome analysis comparing the thoracodorsal and internal mammary vessels as recipient sites for microvascular breast reconstruction: a prospective study of 100 patients. *Plast Reconstr Surg*. 2003;111:1876-1882.
10. Temple CL, Strom EA, Youssef A, Langstein HN. Choice of recipient vessels in delayed TRAM flap breast reconstruction after radiotherapy. *Plast Reconstr Surg*. 2005;115:105-113.
11. Saint-Cyr M, Youssef A, Bae HW, et al. Changing trends in recipient vessel selection for microvascular autologous breast reconstruction: an analysis of 1483 consecutive cases. *Plast Reconstr Surg*. 2007;119:1993-2000.

25

CHAPTER

Inferior Gluteal Artery Perforator Flap Breast Reconstruction

Katie E. Weichman

DEFINITION

- Fujino et al. first popularized the gluteal donor site for breast reconstruction in 1975 as a free myocutaneous flap, and Shaw further refined it in 1983.[1,2] Additional modification of this myocutaneous flap by Paletta and Le-Quang et al. to use the inferior gluteal vessels as donor vessels was also described. However, despite initial success, it was abandoned secondary to technical difficulty and postoperative morbidity to the sciatic nerve.
- After the popularization of perforator flaps by Koshima, both the inferior and superior gluteal artery perforator flaps were described and gained popularity in reconstructive surgery.
- The inferior gluteal artery perforator (IGAP) flap was first described as a pedicled flap for ischial pressure sores by Blondeel in 2002.
- Allen further expanded the IGAP flap for breast reconstruction in 2004.[3] He further advanced this perforator flap, with a widely accepted in-crease technique. This technique uses skin and tissue in the buttock area based on the IGAPs and minimizes the scar in the gluteal crease.[4]
- Though abdominally based free flaps remain the most common choice for breast reconstruction secondary to sufficient skin and soft tissue, patients may require alternative donor sites for various reasons. These reasons include lack of abdominal donor sites secondary to prior abdominoplasty, inadequate volume in the abdomen, and patient preference. Approximately 20% of patients are not candidate for abdominally based free flaps.[2]
- Advantages of IGAP flaps include the ability to harvest as a sensate flap (posterior cutaneous nerve of the thigh), hidden donor site, lack of risk of abdominal hernia/bulge, and increased breast projection based on the consistency of the buttock fat. Additionally, IGAP has a slightly longer pedicle when compared to SGAP, and the risks of aesthetic donor-site morbidity with increased beveling of adjacent fat are decreased.
- Disadvantages include difficult patient positioning in bilateral cases, tedious dissection with a long oblique intramuscular course, potential injury to sciatic or posterior femoral cutaneous nerves, and significant arterial and venous mismatch of the pedicle.

ANATOMY

- The inferior gluteal artery originates from the internal iliac artery and is the smaller of its terminal branches. It exits the pelvis through the greater sciatic foramen and accompanies the greater sciatic nerve, internal pudendal artery and vein, and the posterior femoral cutaneous nerve.
  - Anatomically, after perforating the sacral fascia, the inferior gluteal vessels exit below (caudal) to the piriformis muscle and above (cranial) to the coccyx (**FIG 1**).
  - Once it exists below the piriformis, it divides into several perforators, usually more than the SGAP flap, and then travels in an intramuscular fashion to supply the inferior portion of the buttock.
  - The length of the perforator depends on the area of the buttock supplied. Inferomedial perforators tend to be shorter with less intramuscular course (3–5 cm), whereas superolateral perforators tend to have a longer intramuscular course (4–6 cm). Therefore, lateral perforators are preferentially chosen for longer pedicle length.
  - In 91% of patients, the inferior gluteal vessels travel with the posterior femoral cutaneous nerve (S1-S2) to the posterior thigh.[5] Therefore, if desired, a neurosensory flap is possible if nerves are preserved.
- The inferior gluteal vein is associated with the inferior gluteal artery; however, it receives multiple tributaries in the subsacral fascia fibroconnective tissue. These vessels are prone to bleeding at the level of the pelvis and are quite large and friable. These vessels are routinely larger than superior gluteal veins.
- The perforating vessels, which are all musculocutaneous, are located inferior to the exit point below the piriformis muscle.
- Several studies have looked at these perforating vessels and found IGAP flaps have a mean number of 7 perforators (range 4–10), with an average intramuscular length of 8.7 cm (range 6–14 cm) and a mean total pedicle length of 13.4 cm (range 10–17 cm). Additionally, the mean main vessel diameter was found to be 5 mm (range 4–7 mm) for the inferior gluteal artery and 7.7 mm (range 6–10 mm) for the inferior gluteal vein.[6]
- Understanding the course of the sciatic nerve and the posterior femoral cutaneous nerve is paramount to this flap

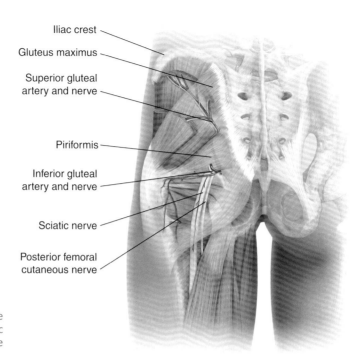

Iliac crest

Gluteus maximus

Superior gluteal
artery and nerve

Piriformis

Inferior gluteal
artery and nerve

Sciatic nerve

Posterior femoral
cutaneous nerve

FIG 1 • Location of the inferior gluteal artery in relation to the piriformis muscle, posterior femoral cutaneous nerve, and sciatic nerve as it penetrates the sacral fascia, the space behind the gluteus maximus muscle.

dissection. These nerves often run together with the inferior gluteal artery as it emerges from the sciatic foramen below the piriformis muscle. The posterior cutaneous nerve is generally more medial in relation to both the inferior gluteal artery and sciatic nerve. Both nerves run posterior to the gluteus maximus muscle.

- Sciatic nerve
  - The nerve is generally visualized during the submuscular dissection below the sacral fascia, as it exits the sciatic foramen below the piriformis muscle and travels posterior to the gluteus maximus muscle and anterior to the inferior gemellus muscle.
    - Provides motor and sensory control to almost the entire posterior leg and foot
    - Derived from spinal nerves L4-S3 and is the largest, widest, single nerve in the body
- Posterior femoral cutaneous nerve (S1-S2)
  - Can be observed at two points during the dissection
    - First, along the inferior incision of the skin paddle, in the gluteal crease, in the subfascial plane, where the investing muscular fascia of the gluteus maximus muscle and fascia lata coalesce
    - Second, during submusclar/subfascial dissection proximally with the inferior gluteal artery pedicle and sciatic nerve
      ○ Provides sensation to the posterior thigh, leg, and perineum
      ○ Derived from the sacral plexus and has three main branches:
        ■ Inferior cluneal nerves (most likely encountered on inferior skin paddle incision)
          • Three of four in number
          • Turn upward around the lower border of the gluteus maximus

- Provide sensibility to the skin covering the lower lateral portion of the gluteus maximus
  ■ Perineal branches
    • Supply the skin covering the perineum
  ■ Main continuation in the posterior thigh
    • Travels posterior to fascia lata anterior to long head of biceps femoris
    • In mid leg, pierces fascia and travels with the lesser saphenous vein in the subcutaneous plane
    • Provides sensation to posterior and medial thigh, popliteal fossa, and superior leg
- There are several muscles that are highlighted for IGAP dissection in the posterior gluteal area.
  - Gluteus maximus
    - Origin: Gluteal surface of the ilium, lumbar fascia, sacrum, and sacrotuberous ligament
    - Insertion: Gluteal tuberosity of the femur and iliotibial tract
    - Action: External rotation and extension of the hip joint
    - Arterial supply: Superior and inferior gluteal arteries
    - Innervation: Inferior gluteal nerve (L5, S1, and S2)
  - Gluteus medius (deep to the gluteus maximus)
    - Origin: Gluteal surface of the ilium
    - Insertion: Greater trochanter of the femur forming the iliotibial tract
    - Action: Abduction of the hip, preventing adduction of the hip, and medial rotation of the thigh
  - Piriformis (deep to the gluteus maximus)
    - Origin: Anterior portion of the sacrum
    - Insertion: Greater trochanter of the femur forming the iliotibial tract
    - Action: External rotator of the thigh

- Arterial supply: Interior gluteal artery, superior gluteal artery, and lateral sacral artery
- Innervation: Nerve to the piriformis (L5, S1, and S2)
- Gluteus minimus (deep to gluteus maximus and gluteus medius)
  - Origin: ilium under the gluteus minimus
  - Insertion: greater trochanter of the femur forming the iliotibial tract
  - Action—works in concert with gluteus medius: abduction of the hip, preventing adduction of the hip, and medial rotation of the thigh
  - Arterial supply: superior gluteal artery
  - Innervation: superior gluteal nerve (L4, L5, S1)

PATIENT HISTORY AND PHYSICAL FINDINGS

- This includes patients with a history of breast cancer, patients undergoing prophylactic mastectomy, patients with congenital abnormalities, and transgender patients.
- Physical examination includes examination of the abdomen, medial thighs, and buttock to assess availability of excess tissue.
- Patients who are candidates for IGAP flap are generally nulliparous, with inadequate abdominal soft tissue, prior abdominoplasty, prior abdominal flap harvest, or prior abdominal liposuction.
- Patients should have estimated mastectomy specimen weights of no more than 350 to 400 g and cup size no greater than C cup.
- Timing of reconstruction should be planned in patients with prior history of breast irradiation. The authors prefer to wait 6 months after the completion of radiation therapy prior to completing delayed reconstruction.
- Smoking status is assessed also.
- Additionally, tamoxifen should be withheld 3 weeks prior to surgery.

IMAGING

- Patients considering IGAP flap reconstruction should undergo preoperative imaging with either computed tomography angiogram (CTA) or magnetic resonance angiography (MRA) of the pelvis and lower extremity.
- Imaging is performed in the prone position and coordinating with the radiologist for appropriate evaluation of images.
- Perforators should be described as they exit the deep muscular fascia and described based on location in an x-y axis. The gluteal fold will be set as zero on the y-axis, and the midline will be set as zero on the x-axis. Important bony landmarks that should be noted including the coccyx, the summit of the posterosuperior iliac crest, and the most lateral point of the greater trochanter[7] (**FIG 2**).
- The description of the perforator should include the size of perforator as it exits the fascia and length of course to the

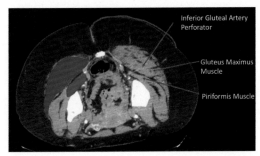

FIG 2 • Locations of IGAP perforator on axial CT scan including the gluteus maximus muscle and piriformis muscle.

inferior gluteal artery as it travels through the gluteus maximus and inferior to the piriformis back to the origin on the internal iliac artery. This should be described in relation to the coccyx, posterior superior iliac crest, and the most lateral point of the greater trochanter.

SURGICAL MANAGEMENT

- The authors perform IGAP flaps on patients either undergoing immediate or delayed breast reconstruction.
- Additionally, this procedure can be performed on patients who required multiple flaps secondary to volume and skin deficit and require reconstruction in a stacked fashion.[8] This includes both patients having immediate stacked reconstruction and patients who have autologous reconstruction that requires secondary augmentation in a delayed fashion.
  - Unilateral breast reconstruction with bilateral IGAP flaps has been described.[9]
- Flap weights have been seen between 148 and 833 g.[4]
- The operation requires loupe magnification for perforator dissection and microsurgical instruments.
- Although the microsurgical anastomosis can be performed under loupe magnification, the authors prefer the use of the operative microscope.

POSITIONING

- Patient is positioned in the lateral decubitus position for unilateral flaps and in the prone position for bilateral flaps.
- The perforator location should be double checked with the patient in the lateral decubitus position.

APPROACH

- A two-team approach can be used for IGAP flap harvest.
  - After intubation, the patient is placed in lateral decubitus position, and ipsilateral chest wall, buttock, arm, and leg are prepped into the field.
  - The second microsurgeon prepares the recipient site and vessels.
  - The primary microsurgeon will start with flap harvest.

Flap Design and Markings

- Patients are marked in the standing position.[10]
- The flap is designed as a horizontal ellipse with the axis centered over the gluteal fold.
- The inferior border of the flap is marked in the gluteal fold (**TECH FIG 1A**).
- Based on preoperative images, using a handheld 5- to 8-MHz Doppler, the main perforators are marked clearly on the skin.
- Dissection can be performed in a clockwise or counterclockwise fashion to determine the best perforators.
  - No more than two perforators should be chosen.

- The superior aspect of the skin island ellipse is marked to capture these perforators, and the direction that parallels the gluteal crease is determined by the pinch test.
- Flap dimensions have been described as large as 8 × 18 cm but can be as long as 25 cm. The desired width of the flap is based on judgment to avoid excessive tension on the closure.
- Additional fat to be captured in the flap harvest should also be noted during marking (**TECH FIG 1B**).

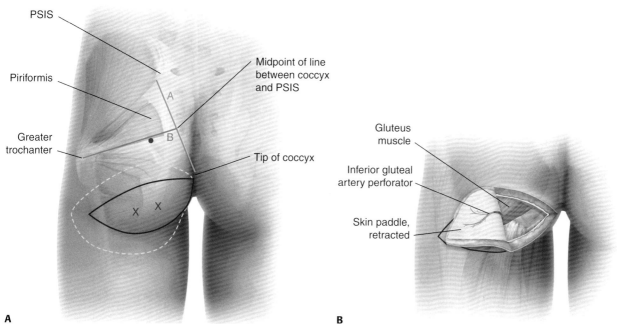

TECH FIG 1 • A. Inferior gluteal artery perforator flap markings in relation to the greater trochanter, *red line* represents the inferior border of the piriformis muscle (midpoint of the line connecting posterosuperior iliac spine and coccyx to the apex of the greater trochanter). Inferior incision lies within the gluteal fold and superior incision incorporates perforators. **B.** Inferior gluteal artery perforator flap marked on patient noting incorporation of surrounding fat to increase bulk of flap.

Flap Harvest

- Harvest of the flap should be done under loupe magnification.
- Incision of the skin ellipse is made inferiorly and medially first.
- Posterior cutaneous nerve of the thigh is identified and preserved along the inferior border of the incision.
- Superior and lateral incisions are then made and superior and inferior beveling to include the maximum amount of fat and soft tissue.
- Lateral fat can also be captured additionally to include the saddlebags.

- Care should be taken to preserve medial fat over the ischium to prevent pain and pressure in the postoperative period. The fat in this area is notable with lighter color and larger globule ration overlying the iliotibial tract.
- Flap elevation begins in a lateral to medial fashion and gluteal fascia is incised early (**TECH FIG 2A**).
- Subfascial dissection proceeds until perforators are identified.
- Once the chosen perforator has been identified, dissection proceeds with the use of bipolar cautery through the gluteus maximus muscle using standard perforator dissection techniques.

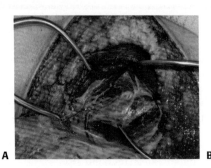 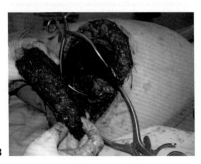

A   **B**

TECH FIG 2 • A. Elevation of IGAP flap in a lateral to medial fashion in subfascial plane over the gluteus maximus muscle. Inferior gluteal artery perforator is present and seen coming through the muscle to the flap. **B.** Intraoperative photo of dissection of inferior gluteal artery perforator and vena comitans with splitting of gluteus maximus muscle in the direction of the fibers.

- It is important to split the gluteus maximus muscle in the direction of the fiber along the septum to avoid technical error (**TECH FIG 2B**).
- Unlike the SGAP flap, it is often unnecessary to open the sacral fascia to dissect in the submuscular or subgluteal flap plane for increased pedicle length.
  - This is secondary to the risk of intraoperative damage to the sciatic nerve and posterior cutaneous nerve of the thigh.
  - However, as compared to SGAP flaps, the submuscular/subsacral fascia dissection and venous confluence are easier with less variability.

- Significant mismatch of the inferior gluteal artery and vein is seen under the sacral fascia. There are multiple communications and branches that require ligation near the pedicle.
- Flaps are then harvested with either tie or double clip in the pelvis and placed on ice on the back table.
- Closure of the donor site proceeds in layers and over closed suction drains. Care is taken to avoid raising the gluteal fold by more than 1 cm.
- Patient is then repositioned into the supine position for microsurgical anastomosis.

▪ Recipient Vessel Exposure

- Exposure of the recipient vessels proceeds in the standard technique.

- Both rib-sparing and rib-sacrificing techniques have been described.[11]

PEARLS AND PITFALLS

Physical findings	▪ This flap is really a tertiary flap choice; therefore, abdomen and thigh donor sites should be used preferentially based on high incidence of flap failure and technical difficulty associate with IGAP flaps.
	▪ Scar position in the gluteal crease should be marked preoperatively in the standing position.
Technique	▪ Two-surgeon approach is helpful when harvesting the flap and preparing the recipient site.
	▪ Choice of number of perforators and perforators selected should be aided by imaging and difficulty of intramuscular dissection. More than 2 perforators should not be selected.
	▪ Beveling superiorly, inferiorly, and laterally can help add additional tissue to the flap and is imperative for increasing flap volume. However, light-colored medial fat must be spared to prevent donor-site discomfort when sitting secondary to pressure over the ischium.
	▪ As the inferior gluteal artery perforator dissection moves proximally, the sciatic nerve is palpated to avoid injury. When the perforator enters the main trunk of the descending inferior gluteal artery, the sciatic nerve is separated and not visualized.
	▪ Dissection of the submuscular/subfascial pedicle is not always required and can prevent injury to posterior cutaneous nerve of the thigh and sciatic nerve.
	▪ Venous thrombotic complications are most common and size mismatch is possible. Therefore, avoiding kinking during inset is imperative.
Postoperative	▪ Compression garment should be worn for 1 month postoperatively.
Complications	▪ Postoperative donor-site problems remain the most common complication.
	▪ If venous thrombosis occurs, vein graft will likely be required for salvage, and possible vein donor sites include the dorsal foot, hand, and turn down from proximal cephalic vein.

POSTOPERATIVE CARE

- Patients routinely stay in the hospital for 3 to 4 days postoperatively.
- Pain control can be augmented with intraoperative subcutaneous bupivacaine (Exparel) administration in addition to scheduled ibuprofen/Toradol.
- Patients have routine transcutaneous Doppler checks, and monitoring can be further augmented by ViOptix technology. The authors prefer flap checks q 15 minutes × 2 hours, q 30 minutes × 1 hour, q 1 hour × 24 hours, and q 4 hours until discharge.
- Postoperatively, sitting can be initiated on POD no. 1 and ambulation on POD no. 2.
- Patients routinely stay in the hospital for 3 days and then are discharged home on postoperative aspirin × 30 days.
- Drains remain in place until less than 30 mL × 24 hours.

OUTCOMES

- IGAP flap for breast reconstruction provides an adequate reconstruction. The buttock fat is less pliable with a greater skin to fat ratio as compared to a natural breast due to a developed reticular system. This flap gives increased projection of the breast secondary to this quality.
- The IGAP flap offers a successful reconstruction in 90% to 96% of patients.
- Secondary revision with fat grafting to the breast and local tissue rearrangement to the donor site is common.
- Should be used as a tertiary flap in breast reconstruction, with abdominal and thigh donor site preferred (**FIG 3**)

COMPLICATIONS

- Donor-site complications remain the most common complications associated with IGAP flap dissection. These complications include:

- Seroma is common and reported in as many as 25% of patients.
- Hematoma
- Wound healing problems (including dehiscence and wound infection)
  - Avoid tension across the incision with minimal skin paddle height and focus on undermining superiorly, inferiorly, and laterally to gain additional fatty tissue.
- Total flap loss is a dreaded complication of breast reconstruction with IGAP flap. Based on available series, the failure rate is likely between 2.5% and 6.5%.[12]
  - These complications can be associated with arterial or venous thrombosis or difficulty with perforator dissection but most commonly associated with venous thrombosis in a delayed fashion with that being observed in up to 13% of flaps.
  - This can be attributed to kinking of the vein and significantly size mismatch. Prompt take back to the operating room is required for either revision of arterial anastomosis or venous anastomosis in the cases of arterial or venous insufficiency. Vein grafts are often necessary for salvage.
  - These complications often present in the first 24 to 48 hours.
- Fat necrosis in fasciocutaneous flaps for breast reconstruction is commonplace. However, the fat necrosis rate in IGAP flaps has been seen to be between 3.5% and 10%. Treatment of fat necrosis is variable and can include revision with direct excision or liposuction.
- Sciatic nerve injury is possible; however, reapproximation to the gluteus maximus muscle helps to avoid significant sequelae.
- Persistent sensory disturbances greater than 3 months can be seen in 19% of patients in their posterior leg. This complication is associated with injury or sacrifice of the posterior cutaneous nerve of the thigh, due to intimate association with the pedicle.[13] However, most of these complications diminish over time.

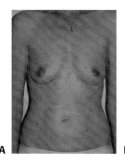
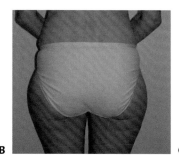
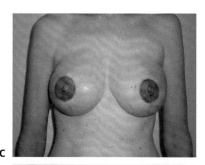
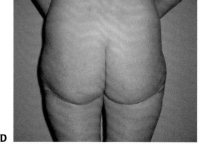

FIG 3 • Preoperative and postoperative results. **A.** Preoperative AP view of a 42-year-old female with history of right breast DCIS and size 34A breasts. **B.** Preoperative PA view of patient. **C.** Postoperative AP view of patient after bilateral mastectomy and immediate IGAP reconstruction. **D.** Postoperative PA view of patient after bilateral IGAP harvest.

REFERENCES

1. Fujino T, Harasina T, Aoyagi F. Reconstruction for aplasia of the breast and pectoral region by microvascular transfer of a free flap from the buttock. *Plast Reconstr Surg.* 1975;56(2):178-181.
2. Shaw WW. Breast reconstruction by superior gluteal microvascular free flaps without silicone implants. *Plast Reconstr Surg.* 1983;72(4):490-501.
3. Guerra AB, Metzinger SE, Bidros RS, et al. Breast reconstruction with gluteal artery perforator (GAP) flaps: a critical analysis of 142 cases. *Ann Plast Surg.* 2004;52(2):118-125.
4. Allen RJ, Levine JL, Granzow JW. The in-the-crease inferior gluteal artery perforator flap for breast reconstruction. *Plast Reconstr Surg.* 2006;118(2):333-339.
5. Boustred MA. Inferior gluteal free flap breast reconstruction. *Clin Plast Surg.* 1998;25:275.
6. Georgantopoulou A, Papadodima S, Vlachodimitropoulos D, et al. The microvascular anatomy of superior and inferior gluteal artery perforator (SGAP and IGAP) flaps: a fresh cadaveric study and clinical implications. *Aesthetic Plast Surg.* 2014;38(6):1156-1163.
7. Fade G, Gobel F, Pele E, et al. Anatomical basis of the lateral superior gluteal artery perforator (LSGAP) flap and role in bilateral breast reconstruction. *J Plast Reconstr Aesthet Surg.* 2013;66(6):756-762.
8. Blum CA, Frank D, Scott S, et al. Composite superior gluteal artery perforator flaps for unilateral breast reconstruction: a case report. *J Reconstr Microsurg.* 2015;31(7):541-543.
9. Satake T, Muto M, Ogawa M, et al. Unilateral breast reconstruction using bilateral inferior gluteal artery perforator flaps. *Plast Reconstr Surg Glob Open.* 2015;3(3):e314.
10. LoTempio MM, Allen RJ. Breast reconstruction with SGAP and IGAP flaps. *Plast Reconstr Surg.* 2010;126(2):393-401.
11. Haddock NT, Teotia SS. Five steps to internal mammary vessel preparation in less than 15 minutes. *Plast Reconstr Surg.* 2017;140(5):884-886.
12. Mirzabeigi MN, Au A, Jandali S, et al. Trials and tribulations with the inferior gluteal artery perforator flap in autologous breast reconstruction. *Plast Reconstr Surg.* 2011;128(6):614e-624e.
13. Windhofer C, Brenner E, Moriggl B, Papp C. Relationship between the descending branch of the inferior gluteal artery and the posterior femoral cutaneous nerve applicable to flap surgery. *Surg Radiol Anat.* 2002;24(5):253-257.

Superior Gluteal Artery Perforator Flap Breast Reconstruction

Katie E. Weichman

DEFINITION

- The superior gluteal artery perforator (SGAP) flap is a variation of the gluteal artery myocutaneous flap initially described by Shaw and further modified by Codner and Nahai for use in breast reconstruction.[1,2] This perforator flap was first described as a pedicled flap by Koshima and used for repair of sacral pressure sores[3] and further expanded for use as a free flap in breast reconstruction when described by Allen and Tucker in 1995.[4] This perforator flap uses skin and tissue in the buttock area based on the SGAPs. The flap has been further modified by Blondeel in 1999 for use in breast reconstruction as a sensate flap.[5]
- While abdominally based free flaps remain the most common choice for breast reconstruction secondary to sufficient skin and soft tissue, patients may require alternative donor sites for various reasons. These reasons include lack of abdominal donor sites secondary to prior abdominoplasty, inadequate volume in the abdomen, and patient preference.

ANATOMY

- The superior gluteal artery originates from the internal iliac artery and is its largest branch. It runs backward between the lumbosacral trunk and the first sacral nerve and exits the pelvis through the sciatic foramen just above the upper border of the piriformis muscle and inferior to the gluteus medius.
  - Anatomically, this exit point between the piriformis and the gluteus medius has been shown to be about 6 cm from the PSIS and 4.5 cm lateral to the midline of the sacrum or at the junction of the proximal and middle thirds of a line connecting the PSIS to the apex of the greater trochanter of the femur (**FIG 1**).
  - Once it passes out of the pelvis, it immediately divides into a superficial and deep branch.
  - The superficial branch enters the deep surface of the gluteus maximus muscle and divides into several branches that perforate through the gluteus maximus muscle onto the skin. These are the perforating vessels that will be followed in SGAP dissection.
- The superior gluteal vein is associated with the superior gluteal artery; however, it receives multiple tributaries as it enters the pelvis that requires ligation during harvest.
- The perforating vessels are located inferior to and lateral to the anatomical exit point of the superior gluteal artery. Several studies have looked at these perforating vessels and found SGAP flaps have a mean number of 7.2 perforators (range 5–10), with an average intramuscular length of 5.33 cm (range 3–11 cm) and a mean total pedicle length of 9.8 cm (range 6.0–15.5 cm).[6]

- There are several muscles that are highlighted for SGAP dissection in the posterior gluteal area (**FIG 2**).
  - Gluteus maximus
    - Origin: Gluteal surface of the ilium, lumbar fascia, sacrum, and sacrotuberous ligament
    - Insertion: Gluteal tuberosity of the femur and iliotibial tract
    - Action: External rotation and extension of the hip joint
    - Arterial supply: Superior and inferior gluteal arteries
    - Innervation: Inferior gluteal nerve (L5, S1, and S2)
  - Gluteus medius (deep to the gluteus maximus)
    - Origin: Gluteal surface of the ilium
    - Insertion: Greater trochanter of the femur forming the iliotibial tract
    - Action: Abduction of the hip, preventing adduction of the hip, and medial rotation of the thigh
  - Piriformis (deep to the gluteus maximus)
    - Origin: Anterior portion of the sacrum

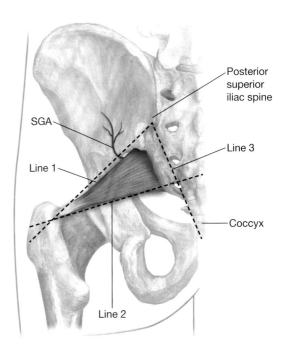

FIG 1 • Anatomical relationships of superior gluteal artery. *Line 1* connects posterior iliac spine to apex of greater trochanter. Superior gluteal artery is located at the junction between the proximal and middle third of this line. *Line 2* connects the midpoint of the gluteal crease to the superior greater trochanter. *Line 3* connects the posterior iliac spine to the coccyx. *Line 2* represents the inferior border of the piriformis muscle.

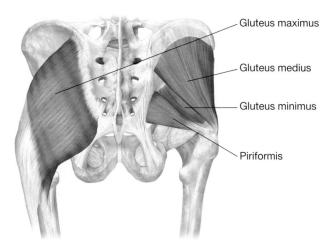

FIG 2 • Important musculature of the posterior trunk involved in SGAP dissection.

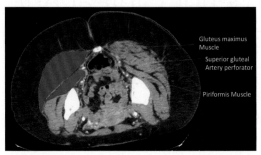

FIG 3 • Locations of SGAP perforator on axial CT scan including the gluteus maximus muscle and piriformis muscle.

- Insertion: Greater trochanter of the femur forming the iliotibial tract
- Action: External rotator of the thigh
- Arterial supply: Interior gluteal artery, superior gluteal artery, and lateral sacral artery
- Innervation: Nerve to the piriformis (L5, S1, and S2)
■ Gluteus minimus (deep to gluteus maximus and gluteus medius)
  - Origin: Ilium under the gluteus minimus
  - Insertion: Greater trochanter of the femur forming the iliotibial tract
  - Action: Works in concert with gluteus medius: abduction of the hip, preventing adduction of the hip, and medial rotation of the thigh
  - Arterial supply: Superior gluteal artery
  - Innervation: Superior gluteal nerve (L4, L5, S1)

PATIENT HISTORY AND PHYSICAL FINDINGS

- This includes patients with a history of breast cancer, patients undergoing prophylactic mastectomy, patients with congenital abnormalities, and transgender patients.
- Physical examination includes examination of the abdomen, medial thighs, and buttock to assess availability of excess tissue.
- Timing of reconstruction should be planned in patients with prior history of breast irradiation. The authors prefer to wait 6 months after the completion of radiation therapy prior to completing delayed reconstruction.
- Smoking status is also assessed.
- Additionally, tamoxifen should be held 3 weeks prior to surgery.

IMAGING

- Patients considering SGAP flap reconstruction should undergo preoperative imaging with either computed tomography angiogram (CTA) or magnetic resonance angiography (MRA) of the pelvis and lower extremity.
- Imaging is performed in the prone position and coordinating with the radiologist for appropriate evaluation of images.
- Perforators should be described as they exit the deep muscular fascia and described based on location in an x-y axis. The gluteal fold will be set as zero on the y-axis, and the midline will be set as zero on the x-axis. Important bony landmarks

that should be noted include the coccyx, the summit of the posterosuperior iliac crest, and the most lateral point of the greater trochanter[7] (**FIG 3**).
- The description of the perforator should include the size of perforator as it exits the fascia and length of course to the superior gluteal artery as it travels through the gluteus maximus and superior to the piriformis back to the origin on the internal iliac artery. This should be described in relation to the coccyx, posterosuperior iliac crest, and the most lateral point of the greater trochanter.

SURGICAL MANAGEMENT

- The authors perform SGAP flap on patients either undergoing immediate or delayed breast reconstruction.
- Additionally, this procedure can be performed on patients who required multiple flaps secondary to volume and skin deficit and require reconstruction in a stacked fashion.[8] This includes both patients having immediate stacked reconstruction and patients who have autologous reconstruction that requires secondary augmentation in a delayed fashion.
  ■ Unilateral stacked SGAP flaps have been described.[8]
  ■ PAP and augmenting prior SGAP flap have also been described. [9]
- Flap weights have been seen between 210 and 820 g.[4]
- The operation requires loupe magnification for perforator dissection and microsurgical instruments.
- While the microsurgical anastomosis can be performed under loupe magnification, the authors prefer the use of the operative microscope.

Preoperative Planning

- Patients are marked in the standing or sitting position.
- The superior gluteal artery is identified and marked as noted above at the junction of the proximal and middle thirds of a line connecting the posterior iliac crest to the lateral most portion of the greater trochanter of the femur. The perforators are most likely found in a 3-cm radius of the point.
- A second line is drawn from the PSIS to the coccyx.
- A third line is drawn to represent the piriformis muscle from the midpoint of the line between the PSIS and coccyx to the superior edge of the greater trochanter.
- Based on preoperative images, using a handheld 5- to 8-MHz Doppler, the main perforators are marked clearly on the skin.
- The flap is then designed and should be centered over the perforators. The skin island should be oriented parallel to

the bikini line and medially should be marked in a fishtail to avoid a dog-ear at the gluteal crease. In general, the flap should be at a 45-degree slant cranially from medial to lateral.

- The apex of the flap is marked beginning two to three fingerbreaths below the gluteal crease in the midline extending laterally and superiorly.
- Flap dimensions have been described as large as 30 cm × 13 cm; however, generally, it can be between 6 and 13 m wide and 20 and 25 cm in length.[5] The desired width of the flap is based on judgment to avoid excessive tension on the closure.
- Additional fat that you would like to capture in the flap harvest should also be noted during marking (**FIG 4**).

Positioning

- The patient is positioned in the lateral decubitus position for unilateral flaps and in the prone position for bilateral flaps. If bilateral reconstruction, this will have to start in the supine position for either mastectomy in immediate reconstruction or preparation of site in delayed reconstruction and vessel harvest. This supine position will be followed by prone positioning and finally supine positioning again.

Approach

- A two-team approach can be used for SGAP flap harvest. The first team is utilized for site preparation and vessel exposure and the second team for flap harvest. Alternatively, for bilateral cases, flap harvest can be performed synchronously.

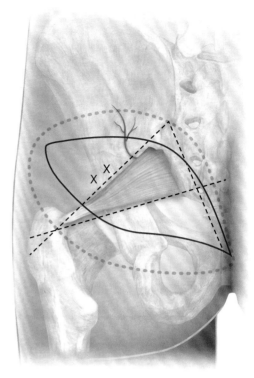

FIG 4 • Flap markings in relation to *Line 1* (from posterior iliac spine to apex of greater trochanter), *Line 2* (from the midpoint of the gluteal crease [*Line 3*] to the superior greater trochanter), and *Line 3* (postero-superior iliac spine to coccyx).

■ Superior Gluteal Artery Perforator Flap

- Markings: See above
- Harvest of the flap should be done under loupe magnification.
- Incision of the skin ellipse is made laterally with both superior and inferior incisions being opened (**TECH FIG 1A**).
- If additional fat is desired, beveling is necessary to capture the fat.
- Above the muscular fascia, the superior cluneal nerves can be identified at the superior border of the flap. These can be included if large enough to allow a sensate flap. The superior cluneal nerves are the terminal ends of the lateral rami of the posterior rami of lumbar spinal nerves L1, L2, and L3.
- Suprafascial dissection proceeds above the gluteus maximus muscle in the direction of the fibers until the area around SGAP perforator is encountered.
- The gluteal fascia is then incised and elevated in a lateral to medial fashion above the muscle.
- Once the chosen perforator has been identified, dissection proceeds with the use of bipolar cautery through the gluteus maximus muscle using standard perforator dissection techniques.
- It is important to split the gluteus maximus muscle in the direction of the fiber along the septum to avoid technical error (**TECH FIG 1B**).

- At the deepest point of dissection through the gluteus maximus, the posterior fascia is encountered, and it must be opened.
- Once opened, the subgluteal fat pad is exposed, there is a dangerous intricate vascular network, and the veins in this area tend to be fragile.
- At this point, Gelpi retractors in the piriformis and gluteus medius are required to get adequate exposure of the vessel at its origin (**TECH FIG 1C**).
- If pedicle length is adequate prior to dissection in the subgluteal fat pad, then dissection can stop prior to entry.
- Additional 2 to 3 cm of length can be gained in the subgluteal flat plane.
- Once the dissection of the perforator back toward the superior gluteal artery as it emerges between the piriformis and the gluteus medius has been completed, the remainder of the skin incisions can be made (inferiorly and medially).
- The skin paddle is then lifted from the muscle and the flap is isolated on the perforators.
- Flaps are then harvested with either tie or double clip in the pelvis and placed on ice on the back table.
- Closure of the donor site proceeds in layers and over closed suction drains. Care is taken to avoid undermining over the iliac crest and greater trochanter to avoid disruption of periosteal skin ligaments.
- The patient is then repositioned into the supine position for microsurgical anastomosis.

TECHNIQUES

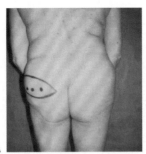 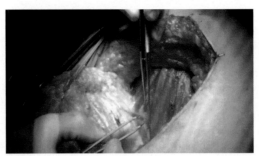 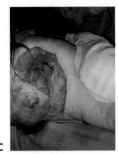

TECH FIG 1 • Intraoperative dissection. **A.** Intraoperative markings. **B.** Split of gluteus maximus muscle during perforator dissection. **C.** Dissection in the subgluteal fat plane.

■ **Recipient Vessel Exposure**

■ Exposure of the recipient vessels proceeds in the standard technique.

■ Rib-sparing and rib-sacrificing techniques have been described and can be utilized with this flap. [10]

PEARLS AND PITFALLS

Physical findings	■ Preoperative imaging and marking remain the most important part of the preoperative workup. When marking the skin paddle, make sure the paddle is centered over the perforators and is oriented in a 45-degree angle with the dog-ear run out into the gluteal crease.
Technique	■ Mark skin paddle without tension to avoid donor-site deformity and step-offs. ■ Make only superior and lateral incisions first. ■ Dissect in the suprafascial plane until the periperforator area, and then make fascial incision in the direction of the gluteus maximus muscle to avoid increased incidence of seroma. ■ Must split the muscle, after fascial incision is made, in the direction of the fibers to allow careful dissection. ■ When ligating large venous branches in the subgluteal fat plane, leave minimal length on the branch from the pedicle for risk of predisposition to venous thrombosis. ■ When closing donor site, close in layers and avoid undermining superiorly and laterally resulting in contour abnormalities and functional abnormalities.
Postoperative	■ Patient should be maintained in compression garment 1 month postoperatively.
Complications	■ High flap loss rates are possible, and donor-site complications remain the most difficult to handle and can require revision surgery with scar revision and fat grafting occasionally.

POSTOPERATIVE CARE

■ Patients routinely stay in the hospital for 3 to 4 days postoperatively.
■ Pain control can be augmented with intraoperative subcutaneous bupivacaine (Exparel) administration in addition to scheduled ibuprofen/Toradol.
■ Patients have routine transcutaneous Doppler checks, and monitoring can be further augmented by ViOptix technology. The authors prefer flap checks q 15 minutes × 2 hours, q 30 minutes × 1 hour, q 1 hour × 48 -hours, and q 2 hours until discharge.
■ Postoperatively, sitting can be initiated in patients on POD no. 1 and ambulation on POD no. 1 or POD no. 2 depending on the patient.

■ Foley is removed on POD no. 2.
■ Patients routinely stay in the hospital for 3 days and then are discharged home on postoperative aspirin × 30 days.
■ Drains remain in place until less than 30 mL × 24 hours.

OUTCOMES

■ SGAP flap for breast reconstruction provides an adequate reconstruction; however, the buttock fat is less pliable as compared to a natural breast due to a developed reticular system. The flap allows for increased projection of the breast secondary to this quality (**FIG 5**).
■ The SGAP flap offers a successful reconstruction in 93% to 97% of patients.[11,12]

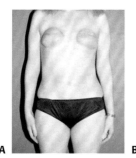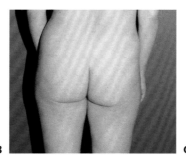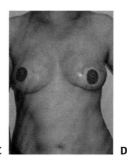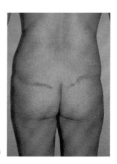

A   B   C   D

FIG 5 • A–D. Clinical case example.

COMPLICATIONS

- Donor-site complications remain the most common complications associated with SGAP flap dissection. These complications include the following:
  - Seroma of which the incidence can be decreased if suprafascial dissection is undertaken. The incidence of seroma has been seen in as many as 13.5% of patients.
  - Hematoma can be seen in as many as 1% to 3% of patients.
  - Wound healing problems (including dehiscence and wound infection) can be seen in as many as 4% to 6% of patients.
- Total flap loss is a dreaded complication of breast reconstruction with SGAP flap. There are no large series of SGAP for breast reconstruction in the literature; however, failure rates are likely between 5% and 8% secondary to the short pedicle and tedious perforator dissection. These complications can be associated with arterial or venous thrombosis or difficulty with perforator dissection. In the largest series describing SGAP, arterial thrombosis occurred in 3.7% of patients, venous thrombosis occurred in 3.7% of patients, and both arterial and venous thrombosis occurred in 3.7% of patients.[11] Prompt take back to the operating room is required for either revision of arterial anastomosis or venous anastomosis in the cases of arterial or venous insufficiency. These complications routinely present in the first 24 to 48 hours.
- Fat necrosis in fasciocutaneous flaps for breast reconstruction is commonplace. However, the fat necrosis rate in SGAP flaps is unknown secondary to the lack of large series. However, it has been seen in as many as 3% to 6% of patients, which is similar to other fasciocutaneous flaps.[11] Treatment of fat necrosis is variable and can include revision with direct excision or liposuction with fat grafting as an augmentation.

REFERENCES

1. Codner MA, Nahai F. The gluteal free flap breast reconstruction. Making it work. *Clin Plast Surg.* 1994;21(2):289-296.
2. Shaw WW. Superior gluteal free flap breast reconstruction. *Clin Plast Surg.* 1998;25(2):267-274.
3. Koshima I, Moriguchi T, Soeda S, et al. The gluteal perforator-based flap for repair of sacral pressure sores. *Plast Reconstr Surg.* 1993;91(4):678-683.
4. Allen RJ, Tucker C Jr. Superior gluteal artery perforator free flap for breast reconstruction. *Plast Reconstr Surg.* 1995;95(7):1207-1212.
5. Blondeel PN. The sensate free superior gluteal artery perforator (S-GAP) flap: a valuable alternative in autologous breast reconstruction. *Br J Plast Surg.* 1999;52(3):185-193.
6. Georgantopoulou A, Papadodima S, Vlachodimitropoulos D, et al. The microvascular anatomy of superior and inferior gluteal artery perforator (SGAP and IGAP) flaps: a fresh cadaveric study and clinical implications. *Aesthetic Plast Surg.* 2014;38(6):1156-1163.
7. Fade G, Gobel F, Pele E, et al. Anatomical basis of the lateral superior gluteal artery perforator (LSGAP) flap and role in bilateral breast reconstruction. *J Plast Reconstr Aesthet Surg.* 2013;66(6):756-762.
8. Blum CA, Frank D, Scott S, et al. Composite superior gluteal artery perforator flaps for unilateral breast reconstruction: a case report. *J Reconstr Microsurg.* 2015;31(7):541-543.
9. Haddock N, Nagarkar P, Teotia SS. Versatility of the profunda artery perforator flap: creative uses in breast reconstruction. *Plast Reconstr Surg.* 2017;139(3):606e-612e.
10. Haddock NT, Teotia SS. Five steps to internal mammary vessel preparation in less than 15 minutes. *Plast Reconstr Surg.* 2017;140(5):884-886.
11. Baumeister S, Werdin F, Peek A. The sGAP flap: rare exception or second choice in autologous breast reconstruction? *J Reconstr Microsurg.* 2010;26(4):251-258.
12. Guerra AB, Metzinger SE, Bidros RS, et al. Breast reconstruction with gluteal artery perforator (GAP) flaps: a critical analysis of 142 cases. *Ann Plast Surg.* 2004;52(2):118-125.

Section VIII: Other Free Flaps

Profunda Artery Perforator Flap for Breast Reconstruction

Katie E. Weichman and Nicholas Haddock

DEFINITION

- The profunda artery perforator (PAP) flap is a variation of the posterior thigh myocutaneous flap, which was initially described by Hurwitz[1] and further popularized for reconstruction of burn contractures, pressure sores, and extremity wounds.[2,3] Since its description by Allen et al. in 2010, it has been recently popularized for use in breast reconstruction.[4]
- Although abdominally based free flaps remain the most common choice for breast reconstruction secondary to sufficient skin and soft tissue, patients may require alternative donor sites for various reasons. These reasons include lack of abdominal donor site secondary to prior abdominal surgery or abdominoplasty, inadequate volume in the abdomen, and patient preference.

ANATOMY

- The profunda femoris artery originates from the common femoral artery. It runs deep in the thigh and between the pectineus and the adductor longus and on the posterior side of the adductor longus.
- The profunda femoris artery gives off several branches including lateral circumflex femoral artery, medial circumflex femoral artery, and several perforating branches that perforate the adductor magnus muscles to the posterior and medial compartments of the thigh.
- There are typically three to four perforating arteries originating from the profunda femoris.
  - First perforating artery passes posteriorly between the pectineus and adductor brevis and then pierces the adductor magnus close to the linea aspera.
  - Second perforating artery larger than the first pierces the tendons of the adductor brevis and adductor magnus and divides into anterior and posterior branches.
  - Third perforating artery is given off below the adductor brevis, and it pierces the adductor magnus and divides into branches that supply posterior femoral muscles.
- The perforating vessels used in the PAP flap have been evaluated in imaging studies based on both size and location and perfusion.
  - The perforator is consistently found in the upper medial thigh posterior to the gracilis. The most common location of the perforator in the medial thigh is exiting the fascia in the vicinity of the adductor magnus about 3.8 cm from the midline and 5.0 cm below the gluteal fold. The second most common perforator location is in the vicinity of the biceps femoris and vastus lateralis at 12 cm from the midline and 5.0 cm below the gluteal fold[5] (**FIG 1**).
- The thigh has three compartments: anterior compartment, medial compartment, and posterior compartment. The medial and posterior compartments are highlighted for profunda artery flap dissection (**FIG 2**).
- The medial compartment includes the obturator externus muscle, gracilis muscle, adductor longus muscle, adductor brevis, and adductor magnus.
  - Gracilis muscle
    - Origin: The line on the external surfaces of the body of the pubis, inferior pubis ramus, and the ramus of the ischium
    - Insertion: Medial surface of proximal shaft of the tibia
    - Action: Adducts the thigh at the hip and flexes the knee
    - Arterial supply: Medial femoral circumflex
    - Innervation: Obturator nerve
  - Adductor longus
    - Origin: External surface of the body of the pubis (triangular depression inferior to pubic crest and lateral to pubic symphysis
    - Insertion: Linea aspera to middle one-third of the shaft of the femur
    - Action: Adducts and medial rotates the thigh at the hip
    - Arterial supply: Profunda femoris
    - Innervation: Obturator nerve
  - Adductor magnus
    - Origin: Ischiopubic ramus
    - Insertion: Posterior surface of the proximal femur, linea aspera, and medial supracondylar line

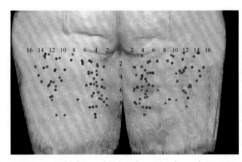

FIG 1 • Posterior thigh perforator location based on CT scanning. Described as location from the gluteal fold and from the midline.

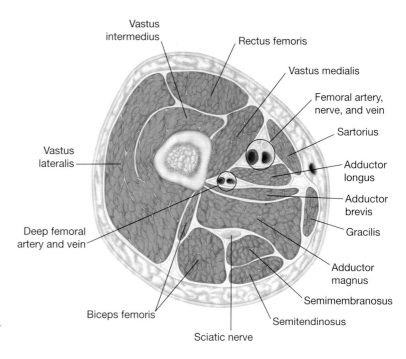

FIG 2 • Cross section of the thigh at the level of the profunda artery perforators.

- Action: Adducts and medially rotates the thigh at hip joint
- Arterial supply: Profunda femoris
- Innervation: Obturator nerve
- The posterior compartment has three muscles: biceps femoris, semitendinosus, and semimembranosus.
  - Biceps femoris
    - Origin—long head: Ischial tuberosity
    - Origin—short head: Linea aspera on posterior surface of the femur
    - Insertion: Both insert onto the head of the fibula as a single tendon.
    - Action: Flexion at the knee and extends the hip
    - Arterial supply: Profunda femoris artery and perforators of profunda femoris artery
    - Innervation: Sciatic nerve
  - Semitendinosus
    - Origin: Ischial tuberosity of the pelvis
    - Insertion: Medial surface of the tibia (pes anserinus)
    - Action: Flexes the leg at the knee joint and extension of the hip
    - Arterial supply: Inferior gluteal artery and perforating arteries from the profunda femoris
    - Innervation: Sciatic nerve (tibial portion)
  - Semimembranosus
    - Origin: Ischial tuberosity
    - Insertion: Medial tibial condyle
    - Action: Flexion of the leg at the knee joint and extension of the hip
    - Arterial supply: Profunda femoris and gluteal arteries
    - Innervation: Sciatic nerve (tibial portion)

PATIENT HISTORY AND PHYSICAL FINDINGS

- Patients present for evaluation for either delayed or immediate breast reconstruction.
  - This includes patients with a history of breast cancer, patients undergoing prophylactic mastectomy, patients with congenital abnormalities, and transgender patients.
- Physical examination includes examination of the abdomen and posteromedial thighs to assess availability of excess tissue.
- Timing of reconstruction should be planned in patients with prior history of breast irradiation. The authors prefer to wait 6 months after the completion of radiation therapy prior to completing delayed reconstruction.
- Smoking status is also assessed.
- Additionally, tamoxifen should be held 2 weeks prior to surgery and 2 weeks after surgery.

IMAGING

- Patients considering PAP flap reconstruction should undergo preoperative imaging with either computed tomography angiogram (CTA) or magnetic resonance angiography (MRA) of the pelvis and lower extremity.
- Imaging is performed in the supine position and coordinated with the radiologist for appropriate evaluation of images.
- Perforators should be described as they exit the deep muscular fascia and described based on location in an x-y axis. The gluteal fold will be set as zero on the y-axis, and the posterior border of the gracilis will be set as zero on the x-axis (**FIG 3**).

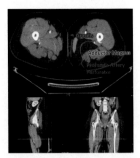

FIG 3 • CTA of the lower extremity identifying the location of the profunda artery perforator behind the gracilis traversing the adductor magnus toward the profunda femoris artery.

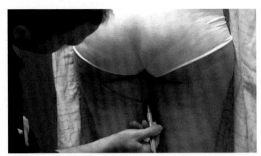

FIG 4 • Preoperative markings of profunda artery perforator flap. An elliptical incision starting medially at the adductor longus and laterally to the lateral edge of the gluteal crease. The flap measures 6 to 7 cm in width, and the perforators are identified with a handheld Doppler and based on the distance from the gluteal crease and the distance from midline.

- The description of the perforator should include the size of perforator as it exits the fascia, length of course to the profunda femoris, distance from midline, and distance from gluteal crease. Additional information includes location of the perforator in relation to gracilis, adductor longus, adductor magnus, and semimembranosus.

SURGICAL MANAGEMENT

- The authors perform PAP flap on patients either undergoing immediate or delayed breast reconstruction.
- Additionally, this procedure can be performed on patients who required multiple flaps secondary to volume and skin deficit and require reconstruction in a stacked fashion.[6,7] This includes both patients having immediate stacked reconstruction and patients who have autologous reconstruction that require secondary augmentation in a delayed fashion.
  - Unilateral stacked PAP flaps have been described.[8]
  - Bilateral stacked deep inferior epigastric artery perforator (DIEP) and PAP flaps have been described.[6]
  - PAP and augmenting prior superior gluteal artery perforator flap has also been described.[7]
- The technique has been shown effective on patients with body mass index between 18.2 kg/m^2 and 38.7 kg/m^2, and flap weights have been shown between 172 and 695 g.[4,7,9]
- The operation requires loupe magnification for perforator dissection and microsurgical instruments.
- Though the microsurgical anastomosis can be performed under loupe magnification, the authors prefer the use of the operative microscope.

Preoperative Planning

- Some surgeons prefer to mark the patients in the office on the day prior to surgery as the marking process is time-consuming.
- Patients are marked in the standing position (**FIG 4**).
- Based on preoperative images, a handheld Doppler can identify the main perforators. If marked in the standing position,

these perforator markings may shift once positioned in the operating room. Therefore, similar to other perforator flap elevations, this step may be unnecessary.
- The superior margin is marked at or approximately 1 cm below the gluteal crease.
- The inferior margin is marked 6 to 7 cm below the superior margin depending on perforator location and skin pinch.
- The horizontal markings are started laterally and carried medially in an ellipse to capture the perforators and traditionally extend 25 to 35 cm.
  - The medial border is the medial border of the adductor longus.
  - The lateral border is the lateral border of the gluteal crease.
- Additional fat that you would like to capture in the flap harvest should also be noted during marking.

Positioning

- Patient is positioned in the frog-leg position.
  - When initially described, patients underwent PAP harvest in the prone position and then flipped to the supine position, but authors have moved toward harvest in the supine position based on experience.
  - The entire leg is prepped and sterile sequential compression devices (SCDs) are routinely placed. This allows manipulation of the leg throughout the procedure.

Approach

- Routinely, a two-team approach is required.
  - One team performs recipient artery exposure, internal mammary artery and vein, thoracodorsal artery and vein, or serratus branches.
  - The second team performs flap harvest. This can be done either ipsilateral or contralateral depending on comfort.

■ Profunda Artery Perforator Flap

Team 1

- Harvest of the flap proceeds in a medial to lateral fashion.
- The incision at the medial tip of the flap is made first. This is overlying the adductor longus muscle. The flap is raised going laterally in subcutaneous plane until the gracilis muscle is encountered. Gracilis perforators are often encountered and if so they should be transected. If large, they can be maintained until the PAP perforator is identified.
- The muscular fascia overlying the gracilis is incised vertically (in the direction of the muscle's fibers) at the lateral/posterior border of the gracilis and subfascial dissection continues (**TECH FIG 1**).
- The gracilis is then retracted anteriorly, and the fascia overlying the adductor magnus is identified and also incised.
- Dissection proceeds in a subfascial plane going laterally/posteriorly until the perforator is identified.
- Once the perforator is identified, intramuscular (adductor magnus) perforator dissection continues in a standard fashion.
- Dissection stops at the origin on the profunda femoral artery. Occasionally, dissection may be stopped earlier

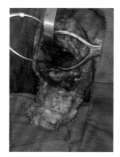

TECH FIG 1 • Profunda artery perforator intramuscular dissection with staggered approach to maintain adductor magnus viability and function. This dissection was performed to the vessel origin.

when the loose areolar plane at the end of the adductor magnus muscle is encountered. Here, the length and caliber of the vessels are usually adequate; however, you may dissect the perforator back to the origin on the profunda femoral artery if inadequate.[10]

Team 2

- Exposure of the recipient vessels proceeds in the standard technique.
  - Rib-sparing and rib-sacrificing techniques have been described.[11]

PEARLS AND PITFALLS

Physical findings	▪ Preoperative imaging and marking remains the most important part of the preoperative workup. Be careful with the height of the markings as this could create tension on the closure. Additionally, avoid extending the incision outside of the gluteal fold to maintain a well-hidden scar.
Technique	▪ Be prepared for the dominant perforator to be caudal within the adductor magnus. ▪ Pedicle dissection is often performed within a tunnel, and therefore, great care must be taken to identify and control posterior branches. ▪ If the perforator is deep in the adductor magnus, then a stair-step dissection can be performed from posterior and then a second dissection point anterior to the adductor magnus.
Postoperative	▪ Patients are maintained in a compression garment for the first month following surgery.
Complications	▪ Postoperative donor-site problems remain the most common complication.

POSTOPERATIVE CARE

- Patients routinely stay in the hospital for 3 to 4 days postoperatively.
- Patients are monitored in a flap unit for the first 48 hours with q 1 hour vascular checks.
- Patients have routine transcutaneous Doppler checks, and monitoring can be further augmented by other technologies based on surgeon preference.
- Postoperatively, sitting is initiated on POD no. 1 in a beach-chaired position.
- Patients are discharged home on postoperative aspirin for 30 days.

OUTCOMES

- Outcomes of breast reconstruction with PAP flap are superior. The flap allows for great coning of the breast as well as a soft contour on the chest. Patients who have an abundant posterior thigh tissue and small breasts are the best candidates for this type of reconstruction. The mean flap weights for this type of reconstruction are in the mid-400 g (**FIGS 5** and **6**).
- The new breast has the shape and feel of a natural breast.
- The PAP flap offers a successful reconstruction in 97.1% to 99.4% of patients.

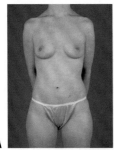 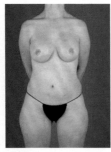 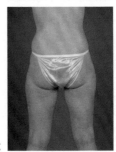 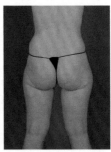

A **B** **C** **D**

FIG 5 • A 39-year-old female with history of left breast cancer who underwent bilateral mastectomy and bilateral profunda artery perforator flap followed by nipple reconstruction and tattooing. **A.** Preoperative AP photo. **B.** Postoperative AP photo. **C.** Preoperative posterior view. **D.** Postoperative posterior view.

COMPLICATIONS

- Hematomas can occur in either the thigh donor site or the breast. They occur in 1% to 2% of patients.[7,9] If a hematoma occurs in the breast, concern for venous congestion of the flap should be raised. Patients require reoperations for hematomas in both the breast and the thigh donor site due to concern for infection and direct pressure necrosis of the skin.
- Total flap loss is a dreaded complication of breast reconstruction with PAP flap. Fortunately, the reported incidences of total flap losses have been seen between 0.6% and 2.9% of flaps.[7,9] These complications can be associated with arterial or venous thrombosis or difficulty with perforator dissection. Prompt take back to the operating room is required for either revision of arterial anastomosis or venous anastomosis in the cases of arterial or venous insufficiency. These complications usually present in the first 24 to 48 hours.
- Fat necrosis in fasciocutaneous flaps for breast reconstruction is commonplace. In PAP flap reconstruction, the incidence has been reported between 1.3% and 7.0%.[7,9] Treatment of fat necrosis is variable and can include revision with direct excision or liposuction.

- The most common complication associated with PAP flap breast reconstruction remains donor-site complications. Dehiscence of the closure as well as infection can occur at the donor site and occurs between 3.6% and 8.2% of donor sites. Treatment of these complications ranges from healing by secondary intention to revision of donor-site scar closure in a secondary procedure.

REFERENCES

1. Hurwitz DJ, Walton RL. Closure of chronic wounds of the perineal and sacral regions using the gluteal thigh flap. *Ann Plast Surg.* 1982;8(5):375-386.
2. Angrigiani C, Grilli D, Siebert J, Thorne C. A new musculocutaneous island flap from the distal thigh for recurrent ischial and perineal pressure sores. *Plast Reconstr Surg.* 1995;96(4):935-940.
3. Song YG, Chen GZ, Song YL. The free thigh flap: a new free flap concept based on the septocutaneous artery. *Br J Plast Surg.* 1984;37(2):149-159.
4. Allen RJ, Haddock NT, Ahn CY, Sadeghi A. Breast reconstruction with the profunda artery perforator flap. *Plast Reconstr Surg.* 2012;129(1):16e-23e.
5. Haddock NT, Greaney P, Otterburn D, et al. Predicting perforator location on preoperative imaging for the profunda artery perforator flap. *Microsurgery.* 2012;32(7):507-511.
6. Mayo JL, Allen RJ, Sadeghi A. Four-flap breast reconstruction: bilateral stacked DIEP and PAP flaps. *Plast Reconstr Surg Glob Open.* 2015;3(5):e383.
7. Haddock N, Nagarkar P, Teotia SS. Versatility of the profunda artery perforator flap: creative uses in breast reconstruction. *Plast Reconstr Surg.* 2017;139(3):606e-612e.
8. Blechman KM, Broer PN, Tanna N, et al. Stacked profunda artery perforator flaps for unilateral breast reconstruction: a case report. *J Reconstr Microsurg.* 2013;29(9):631-634.
9. Allen RJ Jr, Lee ZH, Mayo JL, et al. The profunda artery perforator flap experience for breast reconstruction. *Plast Reconstr Surg.* 2016;138(5):968-975.
10. Haddock NT, Gassman A, Cho MJ, Teotia SS. 101 Consecutive profunda artery perforator flaps in breast reconstruction: lessons learned with our early experience. *Plast Reconstr Surg.* 2017;140(2):229-239.
11. Haddock NT, Teotia SS. Five steps to internal mammary vessel preparation in less than 15 minutes. *Plast Reconstr Surg.* 2017; 140(5):884-886.

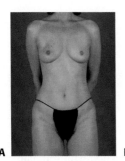 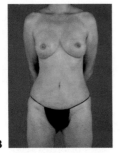

A **B**

FIG 6 • A 44-year-old female with history of right breast cancer s/p bilateral nipple-sparing mastectomy and immediate reconstruction with profunda artery perforator flap. **A.** Preoperative AP view. **B.** Postoperative AP view.

Transverse Upper Gracilis Flap for Breast Reconstruction

Adeyiza O. Momoh

DEFINITION

- The transverse upper gracilis (TUG) flap is a medial thigh–based musculocutaneous flap option for breast reconstruction.
- It serves as a second- or third-line autologous flap option in patients who lack abdominal donor tissue necessary for breast reconstruction (**FIG 1**).
- The TUG flap is typically used to reconstruct small to moderate-sized breasts based on limitations of medial thigh soft tissue volume.

ANATOMY

- The flap is based on the medial circumflex femoral vessels, which branch off the profunda femoris vessels.
- The ascending branch of medial circumflex femoral reliably perfuses the gracilis muscle and skin/adipose tissue of the upper medial thigh, extending from just medial to the femoral neurovascular bundle to the midline of the posterior infragluteal region.
- The flap pedicle is located at the anterior border of the gracilis and can be found approximately 8.5 cm inferior to the pubis.[1]
- The pedicle length is relatively short averaging 6.7 cm, with an average arterial diameter of 2.2 mm and average venous diameter of 2.3 mm.

- Anterior to the gracilis muscle, the pedicle runs deep to the adductor longus muscle and comes off the profunda femoris just anterior to the adductor longus.
- A transverse skin paddle measuring 30 × 10 cm is possible[2]; a vertical skin paddle extension positioned directly over the central aspect of the gracilis can be included to gain additional volume[1] (**FIG 2**).

PATIENT HISTORY AND PHYSICAL FINDINGS

- A detailed medical history is necessary given that there is a potential for a lengthy operation under general anesthesia.
- The surgeon should be aware of all medications that might have an impact on the operation and recovery such as anticoagulants, tamoxifen, and chemotherapeutic medications; also important to assess is the patient's smoking history and the presence of hypercoagulable conditions.
- The history should then focus on details of the patient's breast pathology and reasons for mastectomy. This should also include information on neoadjuvant or planned adjuvant treatment following mastectomy in the setting of immediate reconstruction.
- Prior treatments to the breast and chest wall including radiation therapy and the time from the last treatment should be discussed in cases of delayed breast reconstruction.

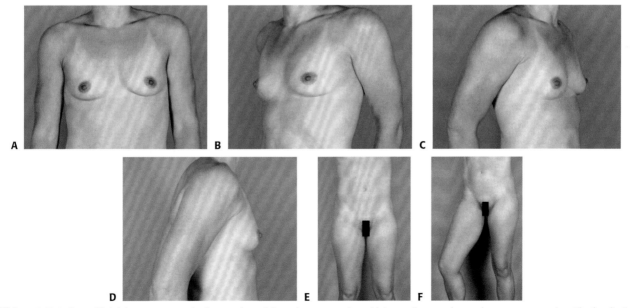

FIG 1 • A–F. Patient with left breast cancer who is to undergo bilateral mastectomies with immediate autologous breast reconstruction. She has limited tissue for an abdominal-based flap reconstruction. Her thigh soft tissue is a good option for small-sized breast reconstructions.

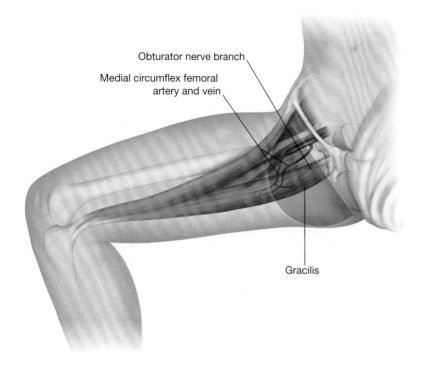

Obturator nerve branch

Medial circumflex femoral artery and vein

Gracilis

FIG 2 • Illustration demonstrating the flap skin paddle design and vascular anatomy.

■ Information on prior operations to the chest or breast and the potential donor sites (in this case the thighs) should be elicited.

■ In addition to the breast examination assessing breast size, degree of ptosis, and base width, the patient should be asked about her desired breast size postreconstruction.

■ With an appreciation of the patient's desired size, the medial thighs/posterior thigh can be assessed, palpating and gently pinching to determine the possibility of achieving the desired volume.

IMAGING

■ There is limited value to routine preoperative imaging of recipient vessels or the flap vasculature in the absence of a history that suggests potential compromise. CT angiography is currently the imaging modality of choice for recipient or donor-site vascular studies.

SURGICAL MANAGEMENT

■ The author performs immediate breast reconstruction with two teams, the oncologic and reconstructive team, working simultaneously. Flap harvest is performed while the mastectomies are performed.

■ The goal of the first operation is the free tissue transfer to establish the breast mound. In cases of unilateral breast reconstruction, contralateral procedures for symmetry are performed in a subsequent procedure.

Preoperative Planning

■ Appropriate referrals and consultations should be made for clearance and patient optimization prior to surgery based on the history and physical.

■ The risks and benefits of breast reconstruction using tissue from the medial thighs should be discussed, including the risk for flap loss, medial thigh scars that drift low onto the thighs and that could widen.

■ Preoperative markings of the breasts and thighs are performed prior to returning to the operating room.

■ Markings of breast landmarks including the midline and inframammary folds and the planned incisions for mastectomy are performed with the patient sitting.

■ The thighs are marked with the patient standing to visualize the inguinal and gluteal crease. The patient also externally rotates the thigh to aid with the markings. The upper marking is approximately 1 cm inferior to the inguinal and gluteal crease. A pinch test is performed just posterior to the gracilis to determine how far inferior the lower marking can be made over the medial thigh. This marking extends anterior and posterior, tapering to end medial to the femoral neurovascular bundle (anteriorly) and the midline of the posterior thigh.

Positioning

■ The entire procedure is performed with the patient in supine position. The arms are extended and secured to arm boards.

■ To aid with space for the two-team approach, the operating table is turned 180 degrees such that the patient's head is furthest from the anesthesiologist.

Approach

■ Flap harvest is performed from an anterior to posterior approach, and the hips are flexed and externally rotated (frog legged) for portions of the case as needed (**FIG 3**).

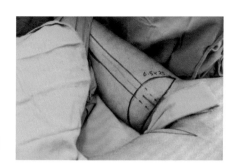

FIG 3 • Positioning of the hip in flexion and external rotation to provide exposure of the medial thigh for flap harvest.

■ Flap Harvest

Dissection

- An incision is made along the anterior half of the superior skin paddle markings.
- Bovie electrocautery is then used to dissect through the dermis and subcutaneous tissue down to the muscles of the medial thigh. The gracilis muscle and the adductor longus (just anterior to the gracilis) are identified.
- Once the gracilis is identified, dissect inferiorly along its anterior border to identify the circumflex femoral vessels (**TECH FIG 1A**).
- With identification of the vascular pedicle, the inferior skin paddle incision for the anterior half of the flap is completed with a scalpel. A Bovie is then used to dissect down to the muscle fascia inferiorly.
- The flap is then elevated from anterior to posterior in the suprafascial plane until the saphenous vein is encountered. The saphenous vein is preserved and the dissection plane deepened posterior to the vein and over the adductor longus muscle.
- At the anterior border of the gracilis, the adductor longus muscle is retracted anteriorly with Army-Navy retractors, and dissection of the vascular pedicle identified earlier is performed.
- Vessel branches from the pedicle to the underside of the adductor longus are isolated, ligated with clips, and divided (**TECH FIG 1B**).
- Additional dissection of the flap pedicle is performed from the anterior border of the adductor longus, exposing the pedicle all the way to the profunda femoris.

Flap Elevation

- With the flap pedicle completely dissected out, elevation of the posterior half of the skin paddle can then be performed.
- The hip is flexed providing exposure of the posterior thigh, and incisions along the superior and inferior markings for the posterior half of the flap are made.
- A Bovie is then used to elevate the flap from the posterior toward the anterior aspect of the flap. All fat superficial to the semimembranosus and semitendinosus muscles is captured from the posterior thigh region, which is where most of the volume of the flap resides.
- Elevation over the adductor magnus to the posterior border of the gracilis ends the posterior flap elevation.
- Dissection underneath the gracilis muscle is then performed bluntly.
- Suprafascial dissection over the gracilis is performed distally toward the knee for the desired length of the gracilis to be harvested with the flap.
- On the more distal anterior border of the gracilis, the minor pedicle to the gracilis is identified, ligated with hemoclips, and divided.
- The gracilis is then divided distally underneath the medial thigh skin and proximally through the superior incision.
- At this point, the flap is fully elevated and only tethered to the thigh by its vascular pedicle (**TECH FIG 2**).
- The artery and veins (two venae comitantes) are ligated with clips just distal to the takeoff from the profunda femoris, and the vessels are divided with tenotomy scissors.

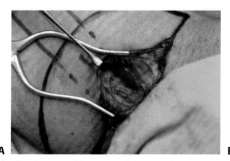

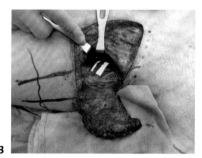

A   **B**

TECH FIG 1 • **A.** Early identification of the circumflex femoral vessels through a limited superior incision prior to proceeding with additional incisions and flap elevation. **B.** Isolation of the length of the circumflex femoral vessels as they run underneath the adductor longus muscle (retracted).

T E C H N I Q U E S

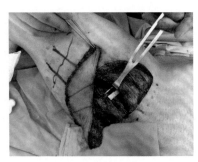

TECH FIG 2 • Fully elevated flap with division of the proximal and distal gracilis muscle.

Flap Preparation and Placement

- The flap is taken to a back table, where it is flushed with copious amounts of heparinized saline from the arterial end.
- Shaping of the flap is then performed on the back table, folding the superior border of the skin flap on itself and creating a circular-appearing flap (**TECH FIG 3A–C**).
- Flap skin edges are approximated with interrupted deep dermal sutures.
- The internal mammary vessels (the author's preferred recipients) are exposed with excision of the medial cartilaginous segment of the 3rd or 4th rib (see chapter on recipient vessel exposure).
- The flap is positioned on the chest wall such that the gracilis muscle will be inset in the superior pole of the breast. The flap is temporarily secured to the chest wall skin with Vicryl sutures (**TECH FIG 3D,E**).
- With the aid of an operating microscope, the veins are coupled and the arteries hand-sewn in an end-to-end fashion.
- Once reperfused, the flap is advanced into the mastectomy defect and secured to the pectoralis fascia with interrupted Vicryl sutures to avoid traction on the short pedicle.

Completion

- De-epithelialization of the flap skin is performed as needed, a drain is placed within the mastectomy defect, and skin edges are approximated in layers.
- A Doppler signal is identified and marked with a 5-0 Prolene suture.
- The donor site is then irrigated and a drain is placed in the upper thigh defect.
- Closure of the thigh donor site is performed in layers. Colles fascia (superiorly) is approximated to the deep fascia of the skin flap at the inferior border of the defect. The deep dermis and subcuticular layers are then approximated (**TECH FIG 4**).
- Skin glue is then applied to the donor-site incision to minimize dressings that have to be placed in this region of the thighs.

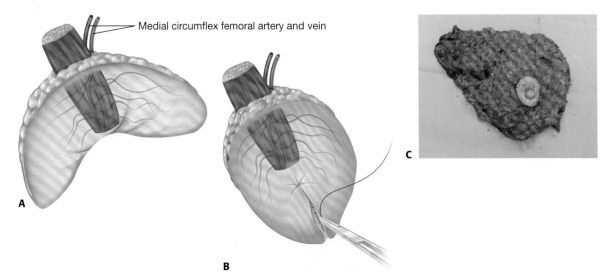

Medial circumflex femoral artery and vein

A

B

C

TECH FIG 3 • **A–C.** Shaping of the harvested flap to create a circular and conical mound that mimics the excised breast tissue.

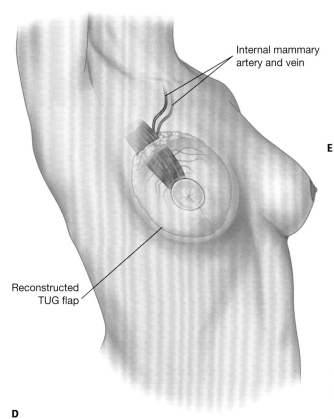

Internal mammary
artery and vein

Reconstructed
TUG flap

D

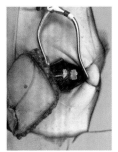

E

TECH FIG 3 (Continued) • **D,E.** An option for positioning of the shaped flap on the chest wall for the microvascular anastomosis. The flap is placed within the mastectomy defect in this orientation with the distal gracilis muscle placed in the upper pole of the breast.

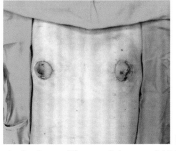

A

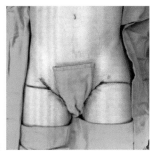

B

TECH FIG 4 • **A,B.** On table result after inset of flaps and closure of thigh donor sites.

PEARLS AND PITFALLS

Harvest technique	■ Early identification of the gracilis and the flap pedicle through the superior incision allows for rapid subsequent flap elevation.
Microsurgery	■ As the flap pedicle is relatively short, plan on providing exposure of at least the entire length of the internal mammary vessels between two adjacent ribs.
	■ To address the expected arterial size mismatch (medial circumflex femoral artery smaller than the IMA), consider exposure of the IMA at the 4th rib instead of the 3rd.
	■ Plan on spatulating the flap artery to account for the size mismatch.
Donor site	■ Efforts should be made to anchor the inferior thigh skin flaps to the Colles fascia to avoid inferior scar migration and widening.
Skin paddle	■ The TUG flap skin paddle is at times darker than breast skin and may grow hair in some patients.
	■ The darker color may obviate the need for tattooing in cases of immediate reconstruction where the skin paddle is used for nipple reconstruction.
	■ Laser therapy might be needed to limit hair growth.

POSTOPERATIVE CARE

- The head of the bed and consequently the patient's breasts are placed in slight elevation of 30 degrees or greater.
- Patients are transferred from the OR to the postanesthesia care unit and subsequently to a surgical floor where monitoring can be performed.
- Prior to leaving the operating room, flap monitoring is initiated with continuous near-infrared spectroscopy (NIRS) tissue oximetry. This is continued for 72 hours postoperatively.
- Serial Doppler assessments are also performed in addition to standard flap physical examinations (color, temperature, capillary refill) every hour for the first 24 hours. Flap evaluations are then spaced out to every 2 hours and 4 hours on postoperative days 2 and 3, respectively.
- Daily aspirin and DVT prophylaxis (subcutaneous injections) are the only forms of anticoagulation used routinely.
- Diet is advanced from clear liquids to a regular diet on postoperative day (POD) 1 with restrictions to caffeine intake.
- Patients are assisted out of bed to a chair on POD 1 and ambulate on POD 2; Foley catheters, intravenous fluids, and medications are discontinued on POD 2.
- Patients are discharged home on POD 3 to POD 5 with outpatient follow-up scheduled a week after discharge.

OUTCOMES

- Success rates ranging from 96% to 100% have been reported in larger series in the literature.[2–5]

- Soft and aesthetically pleasing breast reconstructions are achieved with the TUG flap (**FIG 4**).
- A good number of flaps, however, require some fat grafting to address contour abnormalities and volume deficiencies (**FIG 5**).
- Satisfaction with TUG flap reconstructed breasts from the patient's perspective is high; patient satisfaction with the donor site is similarly high, even when scars are visible[5] (**FIG 6**).

COMPLICATIONS

- Thigh donor-site wound dehiscence, delayed wound healing, and suture fistulae are common complications, particularly when the limits of skin paddle width are pushed.[5]
- Inferior displacement of donor-site scars results in scars that cannot be hidden (**FIG 7**); revisions might be necessary to reposition scars, anchoring the soft tissue to Colles fascia or the periosteum of the pubis.
- Pain along the scar, posterior thigh hypesthesia, and traction on the labia majora are also noted donor-site complications that have an impact on quality of life and sexuality.[5]
- Donor-site seromas are possible with disturbance of the upper thigh lymphatics but can be avoided by staying medial to the neurovascular bundle with the anterior flap elevation.

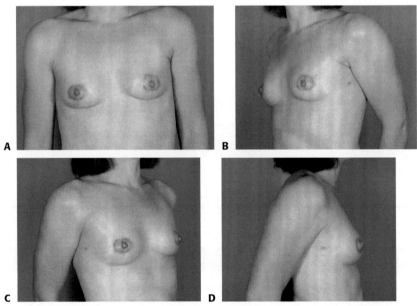

FIG 4 • **A–D.** Postoperative result after immediate TUG flap reconstruction with subsequent fat grafting and nipple reconstructions.

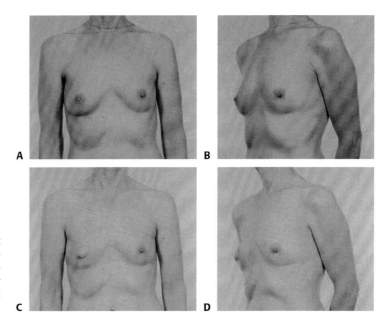

FIG 5 • **A–D.** Patient with right breast cancer who underwent a right mastectomy with immediate TUG flap reconstruction. Volume deficiencies at the superior and superolateral poles of the breast will require autologous fat grafting.

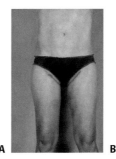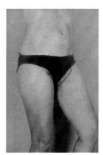

FIG 6 • **A,B.** Upper thigh donor-site scars that are visible in undergarments.

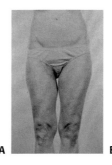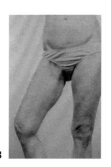

FIG 7 • **A,B.** Significant inferior displacement of an upper thigh donor-site scar.

REFERENCES

1. Wong CS, Mojallal A, Bailey SH, et al. The extended transverse musculocutaneous gracilis flap: vascular anatomy and clinical implications. *Ann Plast Surg.* 2011;67:170-177.
2. Schoeller T, Huemer GM, Wechselberger G. The transverse musculocutaneous gracilis flap for breast reconstruction: guidelines for flap and patient selection. *Plast Reconstr Surg.* 2008;122:29-38.
3. Fansa H, Schirmer S, Warnecke IC, et al. The transverse myocutaneous gracilis muscle flap: a fast and reliable method for breast reconstruction. *Plast Reconstr Surg.* 2008;122:1326-1333.
4. Vega SJ, Sandeen SN, Bossert RP, et al. Gracilis myocutaneous free flap in autologous breast reconstruction. *Plast Reconstr Surg.* 2009;124:1400-1409.
5. Graggs B, Vanmierlo B, Zeltzer A, et al. Donor-site morbidity following harvest of the transverse myocutaneous gracilis flap for breast reconstruction. *Plast Reconstr Surg.* 2014;134:682-691.

29 CHAPTER

Skate Flap for Nipple Reconstruction

Katie E. Weichman

DEFINITION

- Nipple-areolar reconstruction is the final stage of postmastectomy reconstruction. This procedure has been shown to positively influence overall satisfaction with breasts and outcomes in several series and transforms the mound to a breast.[1,2]
- The skate flap is a commonly performed technique in both implant and autologous reconstruction.
  - This local flap was first described by J. W. Little in 1994 for nipple reconstruction after mastectomy and breast reconstruction.
  - Further modifications of this flap have been described by Cordeiro for primary use in implant reconstruction and Hammond for use in autologous reconstruction.[3,4]
  - Although there are several additional iterations of the skate flap, the author prefers these two techniques.
- The Cordeiro modification to the skate flap has two main advantages.
  - It avoids elevating the body of the flap with a central wedge of subcutaneous fat as initially described by Little. The central wedge of subcutaneous fat creates a defect that requires primary closure, resultant fat undermining, and significant deformation of the remaining areola. The Cordeiro technique incises through only the epidermis, dermis, and subcutaneous fat without any undermining, resulting in a central subcutaneous stalk for volume without a secondary defect.
  - A tripoint stitch to the dermal platform is used when the two skate wings are sutured together at the 6 o'clock position.
- Hammond's modification to the skate flap provides the ideal nipple reconstruction for autologous reconstruction. This technique provides a nipple with adequate bulk and long-term projection but uniquely allows for primary closure of the donor site with minimal distortion of the breast.
  - This technique requires experience with the purse-string technique in breast reduction and mastopexy.

ANATOMY

- The skate flap is a local flap with a pedicle of epidermis, dermis, and subcutaneous fat centered at the site of the desired future nipple. The skate flap is named based on skin flaps that are shaped like wings of a skate fish (**FIG 1**).
  - Blood supply
    - Subdermal plexus
    - Subcutaneous plexus

PATIENT HISTORY AND PHYSICAL FINDINGS

- Patients undergoing skate flap nipple reconstruction have reached the end of the reconstructive process.
- Indications: A history of breast cancer requiring mastectomy, prophylactic mastectomy, congenital abnormalities, and transgender patients who have had mastectomy with complications associated with silicone injection
- History of radiation therapy or need for further radiation therapy should be considered when deciding timing of nipple reconstruction.
- Patients should not be actively smoking for at least 3 months prior to surgery.
- Patients should have a final breast mound without need for further revision.
- Nipple reconstruction should be performed when the breast has taken its final form and has adequately settled to prevent malposition.
  - This timing is least 3 months to 6 months after either the direct to implant reconstruction, tissue expander exchange for implant, or the autologous reconstruction. All revisions of the breast mounds should be performed prior to nipple reconstruction.
  - Revision of autologous reconstruction can often be performed synchronously with nipple reconstruction; however, assuring correct nipple position can be more challenging with an increased incidence of nipple malposition requiring further revision.

SURGICAL MANAGEMENT

- The authors perform skate flaps for nipple-areolar reconstruction when the nipple-areolar complex is absent.
- Patients who desire larger nipples and agree to harvest of full-thickness skin graft from a secondary donor site

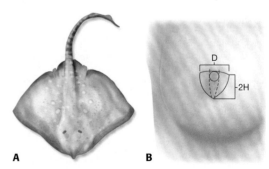

A   **B**

FIG 1 • **A.** Skate fish. **B.** Skate flap centered on breast mound. *D* represents the diameter of nipple and pedicle of nipple; *H* represents the desired height of the nipple. The length of the flap wings measures at least 3D, and the height of wings measures 2H.

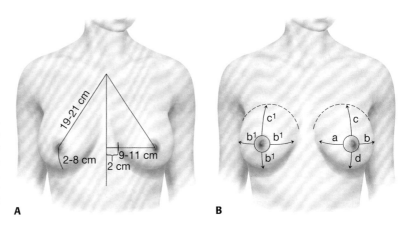

FIG 2 • A. Traditional landmarks for nipple position. Sternal notch to nipple distance of 19 to 21 cm. Distance from midline to nipple measuring 9 to 11 cm. Distance from nipple to inframammary fold measuring 7 to 8 cm. **B.** Ideal nipple position in asymmetric breasts. Maintain ratios of nipple in relation to the medial breast border, lateral breast border, inframammary fold, and superior breast extent.

(abdomen, inner thigh, or lateral chest wall roll) should be considered for the Cordeiro modification. Patients with autologous reconstruction should be considered for the Hammond modification.

- A 50% reduction of the nipple projection should be anticipated, and therefore, skate flap should be designed accordingly based on patient preference and contralateral nipple size in unilateral reconstructions.[5,6]

Preoperative Planning

- Patients are marked in the standing position with shoulders relaxed in the preoperative holding area.
- Nipple position should be centered on the breast at the point of maximal convexity and projection. Additionally, it should be symmetric to the contralateral nipple in unilateral reconstructions. In bilateral reconstructions, nipple position is often easier to match, and the location is less critical as long as it is symmetric and located on the center of the breast.
- Specific landmarks are often helpful in determining the correct position of the nipple-areolar complex on the breast. These include the level of the contralateral nipple-areolar complex, the position at the Pitanguy point (reflection of the inframammary fold), and triangle from the sternal notch to nipple/midsternal line (**FIG 2A**).
- When breasts are asymmetric, the surgeon should try to maintain the ratios of the nipple to the breast footprint. This includes midline, lateral breast, superior breast, and inframammary fold (**FIG 2B**).

Positioning

- The patient is positioned in supine position. Surgery should be performed in the operating room because a full-thickness skin graft is needed to cover the nipple site.

■ Cordeiro Modification of the Skate Flap

Flap Design

- Generally, the desired diameter of the nipple is designed to be 1 cm. The nipple is marked based on the above guidelines and is confirmed by both the surgeon and the patient as being in an acceptable position.
  - The use of an EKG lead, as a surrogate for the nipple-areolar reconstruction, is routinely used in the preoperative area (**TECH FIG 1A**).
- In unilateral reconstruction, the diameter of the areolar is matched to the contralateral breasts and is generally 38, 42, or 48 mm. A cookie cutter template is used to create a perfect circle (**TECH FIG 1B**).
- In bilateral reconstruction, choice between 38 and 42 mm is made by the surgeon and patient, and the cookie cutter template is used to create a perfect circle.
- The axis of the skate flap is designed so that the mastectomy scar does *not* cross either the wings or body of the flap.
- A horizontal line is then drawn cephalad or cranial to the desired nipple location depending on the mastectomy scar to form a hemicircle that will be de-epithelialized and the opposite hemicircle that will be used to construct the skate flap.
  - Based on this, the nipple reconstruction will be superiorly or inferiorly oriented based on the mastectomy scar (**TECH FIG 1C,D**).
- The body of the skate flap is the 1- x 1-cm square outlining the nipple centrally.
- The wings of the skate flap are the two triangles just outside the body peripherally.
- Full-thickness skin graft is designed using the same 38-, 42-, or 48-mm cookie cutter template used in skate flap design.
  - Donor sites include groin, abdomen, and lateral chest wall dog-ear. The groin has been shown to have the best areolar color match; however, donor site can be unacceptable to some patients.[4]

TECHNIQUES

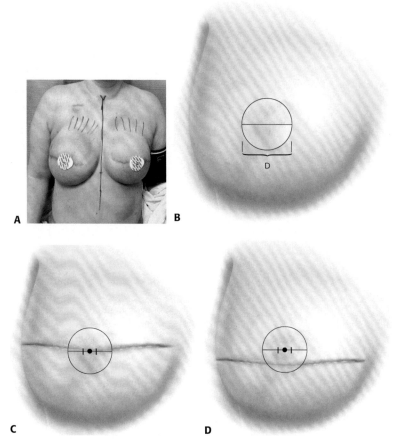

TECH FIG 1 • **A.** Preoperative use of ECG leads to confirm desired nipple-areolar position. **B.** Design of Cordeiro modification of the skate flap. Nipple position is marked with 1-cm diameter circle at the appropriate point. *D* represents the diameter of the areola, and the areolar is marked using a cookie cutter template of appropriate size (38, 42, or 48 mm) based on contralateral side. Base of the flap is the 1-cm representation on the line cranial to the nipple measuring the diameter of the circle. The superior hemicircle (*yellow*) is de-epithelialized, and the inferior hemicircle (*blue*) is elevated in the subcutaneous plane to become the skate flap. **C,D.** Position of nipple-areolar complex in relation to mastectomy scar. **(C)** Cranial scar position resulting in superiorly based skate flap. **(D)** Caudal scar position resulting in inferiorly based skate flap.

Elevating and Insetting the Flap

- The hemicircle that is opposite the base of the skate flap is incised and de-epithelialized (**TECH FIG 2A**).
- The wings of the skate flap are then incised and raised in the deep dermal plane until the peripheral margin of skate body is reached and then the plane is deepened into the subcutaneous plane (**TECH FIG 2B**).
- Subcutaneous fat is included to improve nipple projection.
- Once the skate body is fully elevated, the wings of the skate flap are wrapped around the skate body to form a cylinder 1 cm in height, with a diameter of 1 cm, using 4-0 chromic sutures (**TECH FIG 2C**).

- The cap of the nipple is then closed, and excess dog-ears are excised and closed using 4-0 chromic sutures (**TECH FIG 2D**).
- Full-thickness skin graft is marked in situ to proper positioning of 12, 3, 6, and 9 o'clock and the center of the graft.
- Adequate preparation and thinning of the full-thickness skin graft is necessary for complete skin graft take.
- The full-thickness skin graft is then sewn down onto the areolar bed using a running 5-0 Prolene suture (**TECH FIG 2E**).

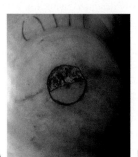
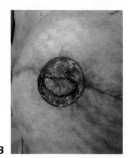
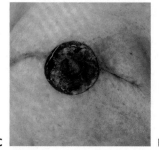
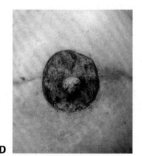

TECH FIG 2 • Intraoperative steps of skate flap elevation. **A.** De-epithelialization of superior hemicircle. **B.** Raising skate flap wings in subcutaneous plane. **C.** Wrapping of skate flap wings to create the nipple. **D.** Folding cap over nipple and trimming of lateral dog-ears.

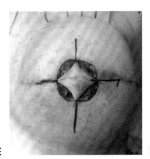
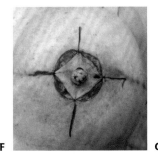
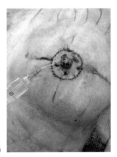

E   F   G

TECH FIG 2 (Continued) • **E.** Securing full-thickness skin graft into place over areolar bed. **F.** Delivery of nipple through areolar skin graft. **G.** Irrigation with angiocatheter under pie-crusted full-thickness skin graft.

- A circular hole is then made in the center of the skin graft to allow the delivery of the nipple through the areolar graft (**TECH FIG 2F**).
- The nipple is then sewn down to the graft with 4-0 chromic suture.

- Pie crusting of the graft is then performed with either small sharp scissors or a no. 11 blade scalpel.
- Irrigation with saline and a flexible 20-gauge angiocath is then performed to remove any debris (**TECH FIG 2G**).
- A bolster-type dressing is created and placed.

■ Hammond Modification of the Skate Flap

Flap Design

- The desired nipple diameter is generally 1 cm, and the flap is drawn with the measured vertical height designed to be 2 times the projection of the opposite nipple based on an approximate loss in projection in the long term of 50%[7] (**TECH FIG 3A**).
- The diameter of the skate flap (or horizontal width) is measured to provide the desired areolar diameter, usually between 40 and 50 mm.
- The vertical cap is drawn as a smooth oval and the height is generally equal to the vertical height of the skate flap wings (generally 1 cm) to allow this to come over the top of the flap without tension (**TECH FIG 3B**).
- The inferior areolar skin is marked from the midpoint of the skate flap wings at 90 degrees with the radius of the desired areolar diameter (eg, radius is 21 mm in a 42-mm desired areola)
  - A gentle arc connects the point to the medial and lateral limits of the width of the skate flap.
- The superior areolar skin is marked from the center of the cap extending superiorly with the same radius (eg, radius of 21mm in a 42-mm desired areola).

- Again, the gentle arc connects the superior extent to the medial and lateral limits of the width of the skate flap.

Elevating and Insetting the Flap

- All incisions are made full thickness through the dermis (**TECH FIG 4A**).
- The skate flap wings are elevated with an even layer of fat; usually only 1 to 2 mm of fat are included (**TECH FIG 4B**).
- The central cap of the skate is elevated just at the level of the dermis.
- The superior and inferior areolar skin islands are then further released and closed using 3-0 Monocryl sutures (**TECH FIG 4C**).
- The wings of the skate flaps are de-epithelialized or trimmed, depending on the desired amount of projection, and are then wrapped around the base and sutured together using 4-0 chromic sutures (**TECH FIG 4D**).
- The cap is then closed over the top and closed using 4-0 chromic sutures (**TECH FIG 4E**).
- Using a CV-3 Gore-Tex suture on a Keith needle, a purse-string suture is placed within the deep dermis of the surrounding peripheral edges of the periareolar pattern.
  - The knot requires at least 10 throws and must be buried.

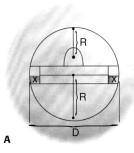
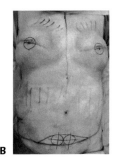

A   B

TECH FIG 3 • **A.** Design of Hammond flap modification. Routinely, the radius (*R*) is measured to be 21 mm and the diameter (*D*) is marked at 42 mm. The projection (*P*) is generally marked at 1 cm. In most instances, *C* (cap length) will equal the projection of the nipple to allow for a tension-free closure. Redundant flap is crossed out. The center of the nipple is indicated in *red*. **B.** Intraoperative markings of Cordeiro modifications of skate flap with abdominal harvest of full-thickness skin graft.

TECHNIQUES

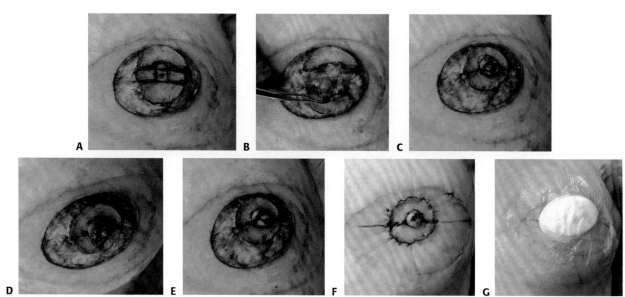

TECH FIG 4 • Intraoperative steps of Hammond purse-string skate flap elevation. **A.** Full-thickness incisions of construct, excluding base of skate flap. **B.** Skate flap wing elevation in the subcutaneous plane. **C.** Primary closure of superior and inferior areolar skin islands after elevation of skate flap wings. **D.** Wrap of skate flap wings to the midline and closure. **E.** Cap closure. **F.** Closure of periareolar purse string. **G.** Dressing with eye patch and adhesive dressing.

- After the purse-string sutures have been drawn closed, the skin is closed with a running, subcuticular 4-0 absorbable monofilament suture with a taper needle (**TECH FIG 4F**).

- Usual dressings are placed over the skin incisions, and the nipple reconstruction is covered with an eye patch and an adhesive dressing (**TECH FIG 4G**).

PEARLS AND PITFALLS

Physical findings	■ Nipple position on asymmetric breasts remains a great challenge. ■ Obtain breast symmetry PRIOR to nipple-areolar reconstruction. ■ Radiation proves challenging, and nipple reconstruction should be only undertaken if there was resolution of acute radiation changes, no evidence of late radiation changes, and appropriate thickness of mastectomy skin flaps.[8]
Technique	■ Preoperative marking in the standing position with shoulders relaxed is pivotal and the most important part of a successful operation. If markings are made with shoulders abducted, the nipple-areolar complex may be displaced superiorly and laterally, and if made with the shoulders hunched, the nipple will be too high postoperatively. ■ Preoperative markings must LOOK right. Proper appearance should supplant measurements. ■ It is far better for nipple position to be low and lateral rather than high or medial. ■ The axis of the skate flap must be designed so that the mastectomy scar does not cross the wings or the body of the flap. ■ Full-thickness skin grafts must be appropriately thinned for best take. ■ In the Hammond technique, using the Gore-Tex for the purse sutures requires at least 10 knots and buried knots. ■ Subcuticular running layer should be done with TAPER needle so as not to cut the Gore-Tex suture. ■ Tension-free closure of donor site is imperative and prevents both nipple flattening and distortion of breast mound.
Postoperative	■ The Cordeiro modification with full-thickness skin graft requires compressive bolster dressing to remain watertight and partial graft loss is possible. ■ Projection loss is estimated to be about 50%; therefore, nipples are often designed to be overprojecting. Occasionally, a minor revision in the office setting is necessary if the reconstructed nipple maintains too much projection.
Complications	■ Postoperative donor site problems remain the most common complication. ■ Early dressing changes and showers after 48 h are recommended.

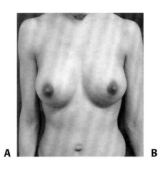 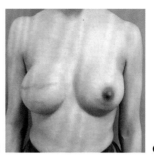 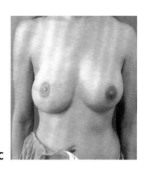

FIG 3 • This 47-year-old woman had cancer of the right breast and underwent right mastectomy with tissue expander reconstruction followed by breast reconstruction with the Cordeiro modification of the skate flap. **A.** Preoperatively. **B.** After mastectomy and implant exchange. **C.** Eight months after skate flap reconstruction of right breast.

POSTOPERATIVE CARE

- Patients routinely have occlusive dressings in place for 5 to 7 days.
- Avoid compression to the NAC, which can affect ultimate projection of the nipple.

OUTCOMES

- Skate flaps for nipple reconstruction provide good projection with minimal complications in patients undergoing nipple reconstruction after mastectomy.
  - Overall decrease in projection is noted to be between 50% to 75% over time.[4]
- Patients undergoing the Cordeiro modification have good long-term results and projection (**FIG 3**).
- Similarly, patients undergoing the Hammond purse-string modification have good long-term results and symmetry (**FIG 4**).
- Secondary revision in patients with too much projection is possible and requires a small in-office procedure to decrease the projection.

COMPLICATIONS

- Cordeiro modification complications
  - Major complications are possible but very rare and include
    - Complete necrosis of nipple or skin graft
    - Infection of the implant
    - Implant extrusion
  - In the Cordeiro modification, rates of minor complications are low and seen in around 7%.
    - These include donor site complications (dehiscence, infection, and cyst formation).
    - Recipient complications are very rare and include partial graft loss.
- Hammond modification complications
  - Donor site dehiscence and local wound problems can occur.
  - Additionally, the desired areola may become ovoid instead of round secondary to tension on the closure and tissue underneath. The tattoo can help with the problem.

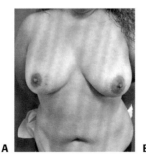 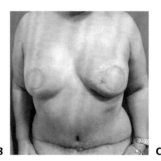 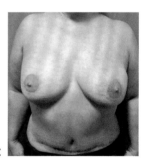

FIG 4 • This 43-year-old woman had cancer of the left breast and underwent bilateral mastectomy and DIEP flap reconstruction followed by Hammond flap reconstruction. **A.** Preoperatively. **B.** After mastectomy and DIEP flap. **C.** Eight months after skate flap breast reconstruction.

REFERENCES

1. Momoh AO, Colakoglu S, de Blacam C, et al. The impact of nipple reconstruction on patient satisfaction in breast reconstruction. *Ann Plast Surg.* 2012;69(4):389-393.
2. Wellisch DK, Schain WS, Noone RB, Little JW 3rd. The psychological contribution of nipple addition in breast reconstruction. *Plast Reconstr Surg.* 1987;80(5):699-704.
3. Hammond DC, Khuthaila D, Kim J. The skate flap purse-string technique for nipple-areola complex reconstruction. *Plast Reconstr Surg.* 2007;120(2):399-406.
4. Zhong T, Antony A, Cordeiro P. Surgical outcomes and nipple projection using the modified skate flap for nipple-areolar reconstruc-

tion in a series of 422 implant reconstructions. *Ann Plast Surg.* 2009;62(5):591-595.
5. Hallock GG, Altobelli JA. Cylindrical nipple reconstruction using an H flap. *Ann Plast Surg.* 1993;30(1):23-26.
6. Little JW 3rd, Munasifi T, McCulloch DT. One-stage reconstruction of a projecting nipple: the quadrapod flap. *Plast Reconstr Surg.* 1983;71(1):126-133.
7. Yang JD, Ryu JY, Ryu DW, et al. Our experiences in nipple reconstruction using the hammond flap. *Arch Plast Surg.* 2014;41(5):550-555.
8. Draper LB, Bui DT, Chiu ES, et al. Nipple-areola reconstruction following chest-wall irradiation for breast cancer: is it safe? *Ann Plast Surg.* 2005;55(1):12-15.

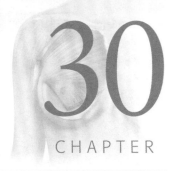

30

CHAPTER

C-V Flap for Nipple Reconstruction

Katie E. Weichman

DEFINITION

- Nipple-areolar reconstruction is the final stage in the process of postmastectomy reconstruction.
- This procedure has been shown to positively influence overall satisfaction with breasts and outcomes in several series and transforms the mound to a breast.[1,2] The C-V flap is the most commonly performed technique in both implant and autologous reconstruction.
- This local flap was first introduced in 1994 by Bostwick for use in nipple reconstruction after mastectomy and breast reconstruction.[3] Long-term results with this technique were further shown by Losken and Bostwick in 2001.[4]
- The C-V flap evolved from the skate flap but uniquely allows primary closure of the donor site.
- The main advantage of this technique is that the full-thickness skin graft is not required.
  - The main limitation is maintenance of projection of the C-V flap, as the thickness of the subcutaneous tissue and dermis is the main determinant of nipple projection. The loss of intraoperative volume has been shown to be up to 50%.[5]
- Further modifications of this flap to maintain and increase projection have been described and include using rolled triangular dermal fat flaps, a "Swiss roll" flap, V-V flap, CC-V flap, and C-V-M flap.[6–10]

ANATOMY

- The C-V flap is a local flap with a pedicle of epidermis, dermis, and subcutaneous fat centered at the site of the desired future nipple. The basic concept of the C-V flap is that the nipple consists of three flaps: 2 V flaps and 1 C flap.
  - Blood supply
    - Subdermal plexus
    - Subcutaneous plexus

PATIENT HISTORY AND PHYSICAL FINDINGS

- Patients undergoing C-V flap nipple reconstruction have reached the end of the reconstructive process.
- Patients having a history of breast cancer requiring mastectomy, prophylactic mastectomy, and congenital abnormalities and transgender patients who have had mastectomy with complications associated with silicone injection are indicated for the procedure.
- History of radiation therapy or need for further radiation therapy should be considered when deciding timing of nipple reconstruction.
- Patients should not be actively smoking at least 3 months prior to surgery.

- Patients should have a final breast mound without need for further revision.
- Nipple reconstruction should be performed when the breast has taken its final form and has adequately settled to prevent malposition.
  - This timing is least 3 to 6 months after either the direct to implant reconstruction, tissue expander exchange for implant, or the autologous reconstruction. All revisions of the breast mounds should be performed prior to nipple reconstruction.
  - Revision of autologous reconstruction can often be performed synchronously with nipple reconstruction; however, ensuring correct nipple position can be more challenging with an increased incidence of nipple malposition requiring further revision.

SURGICAL MANAGEMENT

- The authors perform C-V flaps for nipple-areolar reconstruction when the nipple-areolar complex is absent.
- A 50% reduction of the nipple projection should be anticipated, and therefore, C-V flap should be designed accordingly based on patient preference and contralateral nipple size in unilateral reconstructions.[4,5]

Preoperative Planning

- Patients are marked in the standing position with shoulders relaxed.
- Nipple position should be centered on the breast at the point of maximal convexity and projection. Additionally, it should be symmetric to the contralateral nipple in unilateral reconstructions. In bilateral reconstructions, nipple position is often easier to match and the location is less critical as long as it is symmetric and located on the center of the breast.
- Specific landmarks are often helpful in determining the correct position of the nipple-areolar complex on the breast. These include the level of the contralateral nipple-areolar complex, the position at the Pitanguy point (reflection of the inframammary fold), and triangle from the sternal notch to nipple/midsternal line (**FIG 1A**).
- When breasts are asymmetric, the surgeon should try to maintain the ratios of the nipple to the breast footprint. This includes midline, lateral breast, superior breast, and inframammary fold (**FIG 1B**).

Positioning

- The patient is positioned in the supine position and the procedure can be performed in the office under local anesthesia or in the operating room.

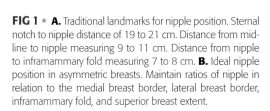
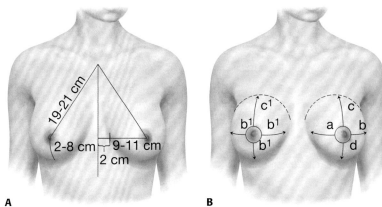

FIG 1 • **A.** Traditional landmarks for nipple position. Sternal notch to nipple distance of 19 to 21 cm. Distance from midline to nipple measuring 9 to 11 cm. Distance from nipple to inframammary fold measuring 7 to 8 cm. **B.** Ideal nipple position in asymmetric breasts. Maintain ratios of nipple in relation to the medial breast border, lateral breast border, inframammary fold, and superior breast extent.

■ C-V Flap

Flap Design

- Generally, the desired diameter of the nipple is designed to be 1 cm.
  - The nipple is marked based on the above guidelines (see **FIG 1**) and is confirmed by both the surgeon and the patient as being in an acceptable position (**TECH FIG 1**).
- The axis of the C-V flap is designed so that the mastectomy scar does NOT cross either the C or V flaps.
- The base of the nipple is marked to 1 cm in width and height.
- The V flaps are then marked measuring 2.0 to 2.5 cm in length
- The C flap is then marked 1 cm in width and 0.5 to 1 cm in height depending on the skin laxity.

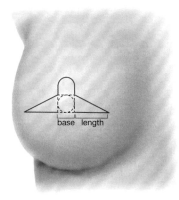

TECH FIG 1 • Design of C-V flap. A nipple with a base of 1 cm and height of 1 cm is designed. The lateral V flaps are marked measuring 2 to 2.5 cm in length, and the C flap is designed with a height of 0.5 to 1 cm depending on skin laxity.

Elevating and Insetting the Flap

- The incisions are made to define the C and V flaps with care taken not to transect the base of the flap or the attachment of the C flap to the vertical wall (**TECH FIG 2A**).
- The two V flaps are then elevated in a lateral to medial fashion with some subcutaneous tissue (**TECH FIG 2B**).
- Subcutaneous fat is included to improve nipple projection.
- The C flap is the elevated to the base of the desired nipple with care to maintain some fat at the base (**TECH FIG 2C**).

- The donor site is then closed primarily in two layers with 3-0 Monocryl deep dermal and running 5-0 Prolene suture (**TECH FIG 2D**).
- The V flaps are then wrapped around the base overlapping and secured using 4-0 chromic sutures.
- The C flap is then closed as the cap of the nipple (**TECH FIG 2E**).
- A bolster-type dressing is created and placed, using two eye patches and an adhesive dressing to avoid pressure on the nipple reconstruction.

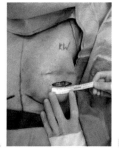
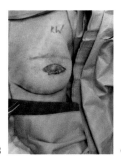
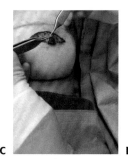
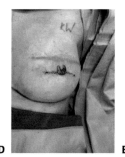
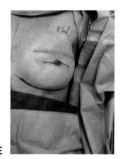

TECH FIG 2 • Intraoperative incisions of C and V flaps. **A.** Care made to not transect the base or the C flap attachment to the vertical wall. **B.** V flaps elevated in a lateral to medial fashion with subcutaneous tissue. **C.** C flap is elevated to the base with care to maintain fat along the base. **D.** Donor-site closure primarily. **E.** V flaps are advanced and wrapped around the base, and the C flap is closed over the top of the V flaps as a cap.

PEARLS AND PITFALLS

Physical findings	■ Nipple position on asymmetric breasts remains a great challenge. ■ Obtain breast symmetry PRIOR to nipple-areolar reconstruction. ■ Radiation proves challenging, and nipple reconstruction should be undertaken only if there was resolution of acute radiation changes, no evidence of late radiation changes, and appropriate thickness of mastectomy skin flaps.[11]
Technique	■ Preoperative marking in the standing position with shoulders relaxed is pivotal and the most important part of a successful operation. If markings are made with shoulders abducted, the nipple-areolar complex may be displaced superiorly and laterally, and if made with the shoulders hunched, the nipple will be too high postoperatively. ■ Preoperative markings must LOOK right. Proper appearance should supplant measurements. ■ It is far better for nipple position to be low and lateral rather than high or medial. ■ The axis of the C-V flap must be designed so that the mastectomy scar does not cross the flaps. ■ Tension-free closure of donor site is imperative and prevents both nipple flattening and distortion of breast mound.
Postoperative	■ Projection loss is estimated to be about 50%. ■ Dressing to avoid compression to the nipple reconstruction in the early postoperative period is imperative.
Complications	■ Postoperative minor partial flap loss and delayed wound healing problems are the most common. ■ Infection requiring implant removal is possible.

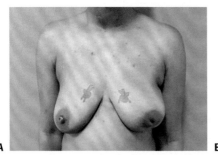 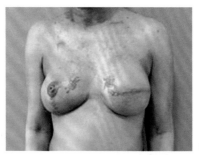 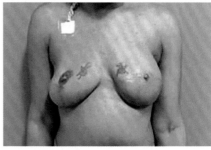

A   B   C

FIG 2 • A 55-year-old woman with a history of left breast cancer underwent left mastectomy and tissue expander reconstruction followed by implant exchange and right breast mastopexy. Three months after mastopexy and exchange, the patient had left nipple reconstruction with C-V flap. **A.** Preoperative appearance. **B.** Postoperative appearance after implant exchange and mastopexy. **C.** Appearance 12 months after C-V flap reconstruction.

POSTOPERATIVE CARE

■ Patients routinely have occlusive dressings in place for 5 to 7 days
■ Avoid compression to the NAC, which can affect ultimate projection of the nipple.

OUTCOMES

■ C-V flaps for nipple reconstruction provide good projection with minimal complications in patients undergoing nipple reconstruction after mastectomy.
  ■ Overall decrease in projection is noted to be between 50% over time.[4,5]
■ Patients undergoing C-V flaps have good long-term results and patient satisfaction (**FIG 2**).

COMPLICATIONS

■ C-V flap
  ■ Major complications are possible but very rare and include
    • Complete necrosis of nipple
    • Infection of the implant
    • Implant extrusion

REFERENCES

1. Momoh AO, Colakoglu S, de Blacam C, et al. The impact of nipple reconstruction on patient satisfaction in breast reconstruction. *Ann Plast Surg.* 2012;69(4):389-393.
2. Wellisch DK, Schain WS, Noone RB, Little JW III. The psychological contribution of nipple addition in breast reconstruction. *Plast Reconstr Surg.* 1987;80(5):699-704.
3. Jones G, Bostwick J III. Nipple-areolar reconstruction. *Operat Tech Plast Reconstr Surg.* 1994;1(1):35-38.
4. Losken A, Mackay GJ, Bostwick J III. Nipple reconstruction using the C-V flap technique: a long-term evaluation. *Plast Reconstr Surg.* 2001;108(2):361-369.
5. Valdatta L, Montemurro P, Tamborini F, et al. Our experience of nipple reconstruction using the C-V flap technique: 1 year evaluation. *J Plast Reconstr Aesthet Surg.* 2009;62(10):1293-1298.
6. Witt P, Dujon DG. The V-V flap—a simple modification of the C-V flap for nipple reconstruction. *J Plast Reconstr Aesthet Surg.* 2013;66(7):1009-1010.
7. O'Neill JK, Goodwin-Walters A. Modifications to the C-V flap for nipple reconstruction. *J Plast Reconstr Aesthet Surg.* 2010;63(4):e418-e419.
8. Macdonald CR, Nakhdjevani A, Shah A. The "Swiss-Roll" flap: a modified C-V flap for nipple reconstruction. *Breast.* 2011; 20(5): 475-477.
9. Temiz G, Yesiloglu N, Sirinoglu H, Sarici M. A new modification of C-V flap technique in nipple reconstruction: rolled triangular dermal-fat flaps. *Aesthetic Plast Surg.* 2015;39(1):173-175.
10. El-Ali K, Dalal M, Kat CC. Modified C-V flap for nipple reconstruction: our results in 50 patients. *J Plast Reconstr Aesthet Surg.* 2009;62(8):991-996.
11. Draper LB, Bui DT, Chiu ES, et al. Nipple-areola reconstruction following chest-wall irradiation for breast cancer: is it safe? *Ann Plast Surg.* 2005;55(1):12-15.

Nipple Reconstruction

Kasandra Dassoulas, Brendan Collins, and Bernard W. Chang

DEFINITION

- Nipple reconstruction is the final stage in breast reconstruction and allows the reconstructed breast to most closely resemble the natural breast.
- There are many different techniques used to reconstruct the projecting portion of the nipple-areolar complex; those reviewed in this chapter form the basis for many other techniques.

ANATOMY

- The nipple-areolar complex is an average of 4 cm in diameter, the nipple 1.3 cm in diameter, with the projecting portion 9 mm in length.[1]
- The aesthetic ideal for the location of the NAC is at the apex, or most projecting aspect of the breast mound.

PATIENT HISTORY AND PHYSICAL FINDINGS

- Nipple reconstruction should be offered to appropriate candidates, generally as the final step in the breast reconstruction process.
- Nipple reconstruction is typically performed at least 3 months after either autologous or final implant placement to allow incisions to completely heal and the shape of the reconstruction to stabilize.
- Presence and location of previous scars from breast reconstruction should be noted.
  - The presence of a scar across the breast mound and its location may influence the chosen reconstructive technique and decisions regarding placement.
- Thickness of the skin and subcutaneous tissue as well as a history of radiation should be noted.
  - In the case of implant-based reconstruction, if the soft tissue overlying an implant is excessively thin or damaged from prior irradiation, nipple reconstruction may carry a greater risk for skin necrosis, infection, and implant exposure.
  - Under these circumstances, surgical nipple reconstruction should not be offered or should be offered with caution. The patient may still be a candidate for tattooing alone.

NONOPERATIVE MANAGEMENT

- Tattooing without reconstruction of the projecting portion of the nipple is a nonsurgical option.

SURGICAL MANAGEMENT

- Once the decision has been made to pursue nipple reconstruction, the surgeon must decide whether this will be combined with other revisionary procedures. This may dictate the operative setting and anesthetic requirement, that is, office vs outpatient surgery.
- Nipple reconstruction alone can often be accomplished in the office with local anesthesia.

Preoperative Planning

- The location of the new nipple to be reconstructed is marked preoperatively with the patient standing, oftentimes in front of a mirror to allow for patient feedback.
- Silicone nipples or telemetry pads can help illustrate the reconstructed nipple location (**FIG 1A,B**).

Positioning

- For unilateral reconstruction, the nipple position will reflect the contralateral nipple position. If a contralateral symmetry procedure is needed, which will change the position of the native nipple, that is, reduction or mastopexy, the reconstructed nipple will reflect this new position.
- The operation is performed with the patient in a supine position with arms abducted 90 degrees or tucked at the patient's sides. The patient should be positioned with the option to elevate to a sitting position if desired.

Approach

- Chosen technique may be based on nature and location of existing scars, as well as surgeon preference. All techniques are associated with the tendency for soft tissue contraction and decrease in nipple projection.

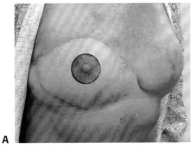
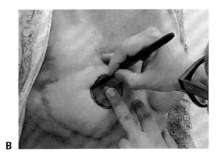

FIG 1 • A. Silicone nipples or telemetry pads can be used to mark the site of the new nipple. **B.** The silicone nipple can be traced to form the outside of the keyhole pattern.

A   B

■ Star Flap

- The star flap produces a moderately projecting nipple and minimal flattening of the breast mound but does not offer projection of an areola or circular border.
  - Three limbs are designed around a central portion (**TECH FIG 1A**). The central portion base width determines the width of the nipple. The length of the limbs of the star is based on the size of the contralateral nipple or a width of 4 cm if there is no nipple present. The scars can be included in a tattoo at a later point in time that will help to camouflage them.
  - The lateral wings of the flap are elevated sharply in a subdermal plane (**TECH FIG 1B**).

- The central wing of the flap is elevated distal to proximal including a gradient of subcutaneous fat with the most at the central base, serving as the bulk of the nipple (**TECH FIG 1C**).
- One lateral wing is the wrapped centrally, followed by the other lateral wing. Lastly, the central wing is closed over top. These are secured to each other with interrupted percutaneous, nonabsorbable monofilament suture (**TECH FIG 1D**).
- The donor sites of the three wings are closed primarily (**TECH FIG 1E**).

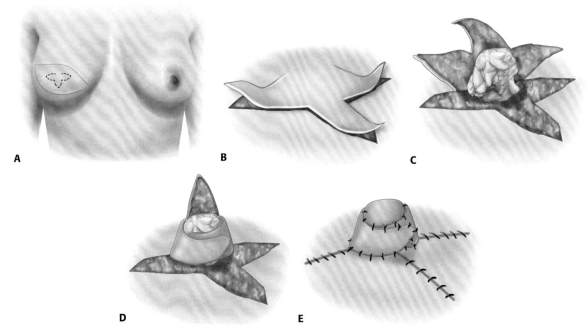

TECH FIG 1 • A. Basic design of the start flap. **B.** The lateral wings are elevated in a subdermal plane. **C.** The central wing is elevated subdermally, progressively recruiting subcutaneous tissue to add bulk. **D.** The lateral wings are wrapped around the central base. **E.** The central wing is closed over top. The donor sites are closed primarily.

■ C-V Flap

- Similar to the star flap, the C-V flap produces a moderately projecting nipple, no areolar projection, and no circular scar.
  - The C-V flap is composed of two lateral limbs (V shaped) and central component (C shaped). The lateral limbs are raised sharply in a subdermal plane (**TECH FIG 2A**).

- The central C-shaped portion is raised with subcutaneous tissue included to add bulk to the nipple (**TECH FIG 2B**).
- Each V-shaped lateral limb is then brought centrally and secured together, end to end or overlapping for greater nipple projection (**TECH FIG 2C**).
- The C-shaped central component is brought over the top of the reconstructed nipple and secured to form the nipple (**TECH FIG 2D**).
- The donor sites are closed primarily.

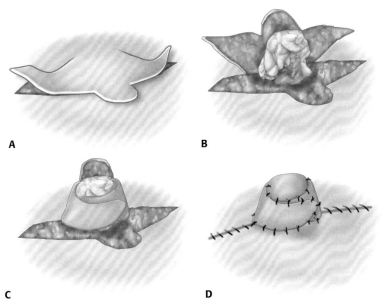

TECH FIG 2 • **A.** Lateral limbs are elevated subdermally. **B.** The central C-shaped portion is elevated, including a layer of subcutaneous tissue. **C.** Lateral limbs are wrapped centrally. **D.** The C limb is closed over top of the lateral limbs and donor sites closed primarily.

■ Keyhole Flap

- The keyhole flap produces a moderately projecting nipple and areola. It lends well to reconstruction on circular skin paddles of autologous reconstructions.
  - The nipple is based on a central wedge, which is shaped like a keyhole, surrounded by a semicircularly incised skin flap (**TECH FIG 3A**).
  - The keyhole and the border of the nipple are incised sharply. The keyhole is raised with some subcutaneous fat along the dermis (**TECH FIG 3B,C**).

- The keyhole is folded upon itself to create the projecting portion of the nipple (**TECH FIG 3D**).
- The remaining circular portion of the flap is advanced to fill the donor site, which is then closed primarily (**TECH FIG 3E–G**).
- The keyhole flap (or any of the techniques described in this chapter) can be combined with a tattoo after healing. Tattoo combined with keyhole flap is shown in **TECH FIG 3H**.

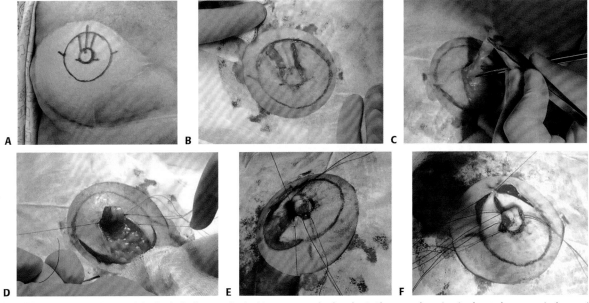

TECH FIG 3 • **A.** Basic design of the keyhole flap. **B.** The incisions are made sharply. **C.** The central portion is elevated, progressively recruiting subcutaneous tissue. **D.** The central portion is folded on itself and secured with 5-0 nylon. **E.** The apex of the remaining inner circular edge is secured as a tristitch with the central portion. **F.** The apex of the outer circular edge is secured with a tristitch.

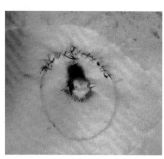
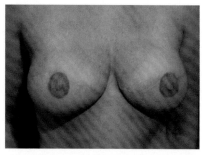

TECH FIG 3 (Continued) • **G.** The donor site is closed with interrupted deep dermal 5-0 Vicryl suture followed by running 5-0 nylon. **H.** Postoperative result of bilateral nipple reconstructions using the keyhole technique, followed by tattoo.

■ Nipple-Sharing Technique

- Patients with contralateral nipples greater than 5 to 6 mm may be candidates for this technique.
  - The location of the new nipple on the reconstructed breast is marked and de-epithelialized.
  - Then, a traction suture is placed through the distal end of the contralateral nipple, which is then placed on stretch. The distal 50% of it is removed sharply with a scalpel.

- The transected nipple is secured to the de-epithelialized recipient site with chromic sutures and dressed with a bolster, or a nipple protector is used to secure it.
- The donor site is closed with either a purse-string or interrupted sutures.
- Reconstruction of the areola may be accomplished with tattoo or skin graft from distant donor sites including excess skin from the abdomen or superomedial thigh.

■ Autologous, Allograft, and Alloplastic Materials

- A variety of autologous, allograft, and alloplastic materials have been described to augment and sustain projection of the nipple, including cartilage, acellular dermal matrix, silicone, hyaluronic acid, and prosthetic devices.
  - The chosen material must be manipulated into an acceptable size and shape to serve as a nipple.
  - Materials can be combined with a C-V flap, placing them under the C-shaped central portion of the flap. The lateral V-shaped limbs of the flap are wrapped around the material and secured with permanent suture.
  - Alternatively, a semicircular pocket can be dissected, the material placed within the pocket, and the skin

closed over top. This can then be combined with a tattoo for pigment after healing has been completed (**TECH FIG 4**).

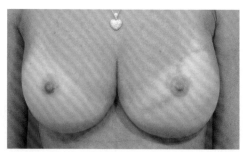

TECH FIG 4 • Postoperative results after left breast subdermal cartilage allograft placement, followed by tattoo.

PEARLS AND PITFALLS

Patient selection	■ Candidates with implants must have healthy skin of sufficient thickness to avoid major complications such as implant exposure.
Timing	■ Nipple reconstruction should be performed as the final procedure, ideally after results of other symmetry procedures and revisions have had time to stabilize, at least 3 months.
Technique selection	■ Star and C-V flaps work well for implant-based reconstructions. ■ The keyhole flap is ideal for autologous reconstruction with a round skin paddle and can also be used for implant-based reconstruction with a semicircular outer incision. ■ Consider nipple share for patients with excessive contralateral nipple length. ■ Use of foreign materials can be helpful with maintaining projection; however, patients should be counseled preoperatively that the projection is maintained continuously, unlike a native nipple with erectile function.
Outcomes	■ Patients should always be cautioned preoperatively that some degree of loss of projection is expected. ■ Always consider flap design relative to existing incisions, as this will impact blood supply.

POSTOPERATIVE CARE

- The reconstructed nipple is protected with a formal nipple shield or gauze with a central portion removed to accommodate the projecting nipple.
- In cases of nipple share and skin grafting to the areola, the bolster may be left for 5 to 7 days, similar to a full-thickness skin graft.

OUTCOMES

- The star flap is associated with a 43% loss in nipple projection at 12 months.[2]
- The C-V flap has been shown to have a 32% loss of projection at 12 months.[3]
- Nipple-sharing technique can be associated with some decrease in sensation of the donor site. This was a subjective finding in 47% of patients who underwent this technique.[4]

COMPLICATIONS

- Virtually all techniques are associated with loss of projection to some degree.

- Infection, asymmetry, malposition, graft loss, and wound separation are other potential complications.
- Nipple reconstruction performed over thin, compromised skin can lead to wound healing problems resulting in implant exposure.
- Using foreign devices for nipple augmentation may be complicated by exposure or extrusion, necessitating removal of the device.

REFERENCES

1. Sanuki J, Fukuma E, Uchida Y. Morphologic study of nipple-areola complex in 600 breasts. *Aesthetic Plast Surg.* 2009;33(3):295-297.
2. Shestak KC, Gabriel A, Landecker A, et al. Assessment of long-term nipple projection: a comparison of three techniques. *Plast Reconstr Surg.* 2002;110(3):780-786.
3. Valdatta L, Montemurro P, Tamborini F, et al. Our experience of nipple reconstruction using the C-V flap technique: 1 year evaluation. *J Plast Reconstr Aesthet Surg.* 2009;62(10):1293-1298.
4. Edsander-Nord A, Wickman M, Hansson P. Threshold of tactile perception after nipple-sharing: a prospective study. *Scand J Plast Reconstr Surg Hand Surg.* 2002;36(4):216-220.

32 CHAPTER

Low-Volume Fat Grafting for Contour Correction

Nolan Karp and Jordan D. Frey

DEFINITION

- The popularity of fat grafting to the breast has grown immensely since it was first described in the late 19th century with greater than 60% of plastic surgeons now utilizing fat grafting in reconstructive breast surgery.[1,2]
- Autologous fat grafting has proven to be extremely efficacious in correcting volume and contour deformities both after postmastectomy breast reconstruction and after breast-conserving therapy.[1,3–5]
- However, autologous fat grafting is most commonly employed in postmastectomy breast reconstruction as an adjunctive procedure after implant- or flap-based reconstruction.[1,4,5]

ANATOMY

- Contour deformities of the breast to be corrected with small-volume fat grafting may arise from a myriad of anatomical etiologies.
- In implant-based breast reconstruction, the gentle slope of the natural superior chest wall–breast junction is often difficult to reconstruct, resulting in a superior shelf contour deformity.
- Additional volume or contour abnormalities to be corrected may arise from size discrepancy between the implant and breast envelope or inadequate implant volume or due to complications of the initial reconstruction, such as mastectomy flap necrosis.[6]
- In autologous breast reconstruction, irregularities requiring fat grafting may develop due to inadequately sized flaps secondary to donor site paucity as well as from flap complications, such as fat necrosis.[6]
- Patients with small breasts or large tumors are particularly prone to contour irregularities that require fat grafting after breast-conserving therapy.[3]
- Possible anatomical donor sites for small-volume fat grafting of the breast include the abdomen, flanks, lateral and medial thighs, back, and buttocks.[5]
- Adipocyte viability does not appear to differ based on the donor site from which it is harvested.[1,7,8]

PATIENT HISTORY AND PHYSICAL FINDINGS

- The decision to proceed with fat grafting to the breast for contour correction after either breast reconstruction or breast-conserving therapy is based largely on physical examination and patient preference.

- Patients should be followed at regular intervals after their initial breast reconstruction to evaluate for evolving breast volume asymmetries or contour irregularities.
- In evaluating a subpectoral implant reconstruction, the breasts should be examined both statically and with pectoral contraction to observe for dynamic irregularities.
- Patient expectations should be assessed prior to proceeding with fat grafting; patients should be made aware of any prereconstruction breast asymmetries that will not be changed by fat grafting.
- Donor sites are chosen based on availability and patient preference to ensure that there is sufficient autologous fat to correct all breast deformities.[8]

IMAGING

- Patient photography should be obtained after breast reconstruction and compared with preoperative photographs to help plan for contour correction with fat grafting.
- Traditional radiographic imaging is typically not required prior to secondary breast reconstruction with small-volume fat grafting.
- MRI may at times be helpful in assessing the volume required for adequate contour correction; there is a substantial added cost with this technology, however.
- 3D imaging has recently been employed to assist with preoperative identification and quantification of breast volume deficiencies and asymmetries.[9,10]

SURGICAL MANAGEMENT

- Patients should wait a minimum of 3 to 4 months after their final implant placement, flap reconstruction, or breast-conserving procedure prior to proceeding with fat grafting for contour correction.
  - This will allow adequate time for tissues to heal and soften, both defining the final contour of the breast and increasing recipient bed vascularity.
- In general, small-volume fat grafting of the breast is best accomplished under general anesthesia given the multiple areas of surgery and need for position changes.

Preoperative Planning

- Physical examination, patient photography, and 3D imaging should be utilized preoperatively to precisely plan the location and amount of fat grafting required for adequate contour correction.[9,10]

- Given the fluctuating nature of adipose deposits, potential donor sites should be reassessed on the day of surgery to plan the volume of autologous fat to be harvested from each site.

Positioning

- Patient positioning in the operating room is dependent on the donor sites from which autologous fat will be obtained.
- Patients should be positioned on a bed permitting flexion at the hips so that the patient may be able to "sit up" during the procedure.
- A prone position with arms extended forward in a diver's pose is necessary if the back or buttocks are to be harvested.
- If required, the patient should begin in the prone position for autologous fat harvest prior to being placed in the supine position for additional fat harvest and recipient site grafting as indicated.

- A supine position is planned if the abdominal, flank, or lateral and medial thigh donor sites are to be harvested.
    - These sites are advantageous as both donor site harvesting and recipient site fat injection can proceed without position change.
- In the supine position, the arms should be abducted at approximately 90 degrees and secured to the arm boards in preparation for sitting the patient up during the procedure.

Approach

- The donor site areas from which the autologous fat will be harvested should be marked with concentric circles. Recipient site areas into which the fat will be grafted should be marked with cross-hatches on the patient.
- Markings for cannula access incisions should be placed in all donor and recipient sites within relaxed skin tension lines in areas typically hidden by clothing.

■ Tumescent Infiltration of Donor and Recipient Sites

- Tumescent solution is prepared using 20 cc of 2% lidocaine, 1 mg of 1:1000 epinephrine within one liter of lactated Ringer solution.[8]
- Lidocaine concentrations of 35 mg/kg have been proven safe using the tumescent technique.[11]
- Planned 2-mm stab incisions near donor and recipient sites are made with an 11-blade while pinching the skin to avoid damage to deeper structures.

- Tumescent solution is infiltrated using a tumescent cannula at rates ranging from 50 to 200 mL/min into all areas of autologous fat harvest as well as all planned recipient sites.[11]
- The end point of tumescent infiltration is judged on the basis of tissue turgor and skin blanching and is generally in the ratio of 2:1 infiltrate to aspirate.[11]
- Ideally, 15 to 20 minutes is allowed to elapse prior to liposuction fat harvesting to maximize the vasoconstrictive effect of the tumescent solution.[12]

■ Donor Site Autologous Fat Harvesting With Liposuction

- Given ease and efficacy of use, suction-assisted liposuction is the senior author's preferred method of donor site autologous fat harvesting.
    - Adipocyte viability with handheld and suction-assisted liposuction is equivalent when utilized with tumescent solution infiltration.[8]
- Generally, 3 to 4 mm cannulas are preferred as greater cannula size has been associated with improved adipocyte viability.[8]
    - Multiperforated or two-hole Coleman cannulas may be employed with similar outcomes.[8,13]
- Cannula length is chosen based on the reach required for each given donor site.
- Fat is harvested from the deep layer of subcutaneous fat, taking care to avoid the subdermal and superficial fat layers (**TECH FIG 1A**).
    - Liposuction of the subdermal or superficial fat layers can result in visible and unattractive skin dimpling.

- Within each donor site area, tissue is rolled between the thumb and index finger of the nondominant hand, while the liposuction cannula makes broad passes between the digits (**TECH FIG 1B**).
- After each 2 to 3 passes of the cannula in one area, the cannula is reoriented to an adjacent region to avoid overliposuction in any discrete area, which will result in donor site depressions and asymmetries (**TECH FIG 1C**).
- In the abdomen, posterior direction of the liposuction cannula risks perforation of the peritoneal cavity with concomitant intra-abdominal injury.
    - Caution must also be exercised in the epigastric and subcostal abdominal regions where inattentive technique can risk violation of the thoracic cavity.
- Fat harvesting proceeds until sufficient fat to correct all breast irregularities (estimated preoperatively) is obtained or all planned donor sites are depleted of useable autologous fat without the creation of donor site deformity.

TECHNIQUES

TECHNIQUES

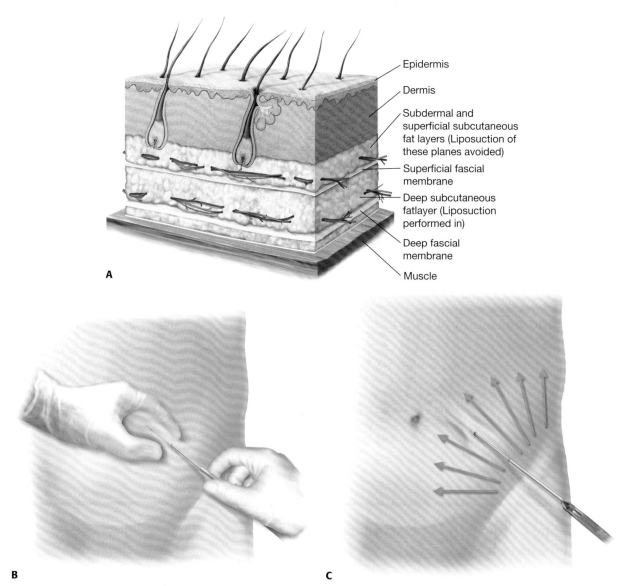

Epidermis

Dermis

Subdermal and superficial subcutaneous fat layers (Liposuction of these planes avoided)

Superficial fascial membrane

Deep subcutaneous fatlayer (Liposuction performed in)

Deep fascial membrane

Muscle

TECH FIG 1 • A. Cross-sectional anatomy of the skin and subcutaneous fat. Liposuction fat harvesting for small-volume fat grafting of the breast should be performed in the deep subcutaneous fat layer while the subdermal and superficial fat layers are avoided to prevent donor site contour abnormalities such as dimpling. **B.** Technique for donor site autologous fat harvesting. The donor site tissue (abdominal tissue in this figure) is rolled between the thumb and index finger of the nondominant hand while the liposuction cannula makes broad passes between the digits. This provides the surgeon with tactile manual feedback that will assist with maintaining the cannula in the appropriate fat plane. **C.** "Fanning" technique for donor site liposuction. After each 2 to 3 passes of the liposuction cannula in one area, adjacent tissue is taken up in a fanning pattern to avoid overliposuction in any one area.

■ Fat Aspirate Processing

- Autologous fat aspirate, once harvested, must be processed to separate the fat, stromal vascular fraction cells, and adipose-derived stem cells from tumescent solution and blood.[8]
- Fat aspirate may be processed by centrifugation, gravity separation, washing, and/or filtration.[8]
- Although animal studies suggest that centrifugation with filtration provides smaller fat grafts with impaired integrity, in vivo patient studies show no difference in fat graft retention based on different processing techniques.[8]

- Centrifugation forces greater than 50 g after suction-assisted liposuction have been shown to result in significant adipocyte damage; this effect is not observed after handheld liposuction.[8]
- After centrifugation, the lowest layer of the fat aspirate contains the most viable adipocytes for injection while higher layers progressively contain less viable cells.[8]
- The senior author currently prefers a combined hand washing-filtration system for autologous fat processing prior to small-volume fat grafting of the breast.

■ Recipient Site Fat Grafting (Video)

- Filtered fat is separated into 3- or 6-mL syringes and attached to the chosen cannula.
- Injection cannulas are generally smaller in diameter than harvesting cannulas and only have a single distal or lateral port for fat egress.[13]
- The cannula size utilized will depend on the body area to be grafted with 16- or 17-gauge cannulas most often employed for small-volume fat grafting of the breast.[13]
- The length, shape, and curve of the cannula chosen are based on the geometry of the recipient site and location of recipient site access incisions.[13]

- The cannula is inserted into the access incision and guided into the area to be grafted; fat is slowly injected as the cannula is withdrawn[8,13] (**TECH FIG 2A**).
- Approximately 1-2 mL is injected with each pass of the cannula.[13]
- Scar contracture release may be performed through multiple punctures with the beveled tip of an 18-gauge needle to prevent dimpling and undue tension at the site of fat injection[14] (**TECH FIG 2B**).
- After implant-based breast reconstruction, processed fat may be injected into both the subcutaneous fat and muscle planes as indicated to correct any contour deformities (**TECH FIG 2C**).

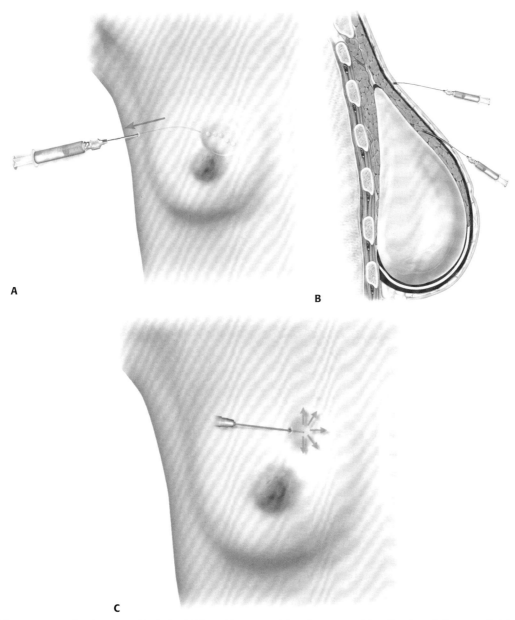

TECH FIG 2 • A. Harvested and processed fat is slowly injected into any recipient site contour deformities through the access incision as the cannula is withdrawn. In this figure, the recipient site access incision is hidden in the anterior axillary line. **B.** Scar contracture release is often performed prior to fat injection through multiple punctures with the beveled tip of an 18-gauge needle to prevent dimpling and undue tension at the site of injection. This is especially useful after breast-conserving therapy in order to create sufficient space for the fat to be grafted. **C.** After implant-based breast reconstruction, fat may be injected into both the subcutaneous fat and muscle layers as indicated to correct any contour deformities present. The decreased fat retention typically observed with injection into contractile muscle is obviated after breast reconstruction due to pectoralis disinsertion. Care must be taken to avoid trauma to the implant itself from the cannula that can result in rupture.

- In autologous breast reconstruction, fat may be injected into the subcutaneous fat plane or into the flap itself; care must be taken to protect the vascular pedicle if deeper fat injection is planned.
- After breast-conserving therapy, fat is typically injected into the glandular breast tissue and less often into the subcutaneous fat plane.

- Scar contracture release is usually required to create space for the fat in this circumstance.
- Slower injection speeds result in larger fat deposits; however, faster injection speeds increase the risk of adipocyte cellular injury.[8]
- Each planned recipient site is sequentially injected to the desired final effect and contour correction.

■ Wound Closure

- Donor site harvest and recipient site access incisions are closed with simple interrupted fast-absorbing sutures and dressed with adhesive bandage strips and semiocclusive dressings.

PEARLS AND PITFALLS

Preoperative planning	■ 3D imaging may be utilized preoperatively to analyze predicted volume requirements in the breast and aid in patient education.[9,10]
Donor and recipient site access incision placement	■ Recipient site access incisions for the breast can be hidden in the anterior axillary line, the medial and lateral breast folds, and the inframammary fold. ■ Avoid access incisions in the upper medial breast, abdomen or flanks above the bikini line, and lateral or medial thighs below the bikini line. ■ Particular care must be taken when donor site stab incisions are made in the groin; the femoral artery should be palpated with incisions made laterally to avoid both the femoral artery and more medial femoral vein.
Tissue planes of fat injection	■ Care should be taken to avoid overly superficial or subdermal injections that will result in unaesthetic visible and palpable deformities.
Initial fat injection	■ Care is taken to achieve optimal placement during initial fat transfer. ■ Alteration of any undesired fat accumulations is difficult to achieve with massage or manual manipulation and may require liposuction of the abnormal area.[13]
Intraoperative assessment of contour correction	■ The patient should be periodically sat up by flexing the operative bed during fat injection to assess breast volume and symmetry in both the supine and upright position. ■ Fat may even be injected with the patient in the upright, seated position.
Complications	■ Although not reported, intravascular fat injection resulting in devastating fat embolism with small-volume fat grafting to the breast is a theoretical risk of the procedure. ■ Utilizing blunt tip injection cannulas and injecting only during cannula withdrawal will minimize the risk of intravascular injection.

POSTOPERATIVE CARE

- Generally well tolerated, patients usually are discharged on the same day as their small-volume breast fat grafting procedure.
- Oral antibiotics with skin flora coverage should be provided for up to seven days; this is especially important in cases of secondary fat grafting after implant-based breast reconstruction to avoid prosthesis-related infections.
- Surgical bras may be provided to patients with instructions to avoid underwire bras or pressure on the areas in which fat was injected for at least 6 weeks.
- Compressive garments may also be worn over the abdominal, flank, back, or thigh donor sites according to patient and/or physician preference.

- Patients should be advised to expect some leakage of fluid from access incisions for 1 to 2 days and bruising of the donor site for the first 2 to 3 weeks postoperatively.[15]

OUTCOMES

- Secondary small-volume fat grafting as an adjunct to breast reconstruction and breast-conserving therapy has been shown to significantly improve aesthetic breast contour and volume.[3,15,16]
- Patient satisfaction after secondary small-volume fat grafting to the breast appears high.[4]
- The amount of fat retained long term after small-volume fat grafting to the breast ranges from near 40% to 50%.[1]

- Larger volumes of fat grafting appears to have increased retention, whereas the donor site likely has no significant influence on fat retention.[5]
- Abnormalities found on surveillance radiographic breast imaging after fat grafting are acceptably low and less than those seen after reduction mammoplasty.[17]
- Despite concern, the risk of locoregional breast cancer recurrence does not appear to be increased after secondary small-volume fat grafting to the breast.[18]

COMPLICATIONS

- Donor site issues, most frequently irregularities and depressions, represent the most common complications after this procedure.[15,19]
- Other donor site issues, such as hematoma and seroma formation, are less prevalent.[15,19]
- Donor or recipient site infection after small-volume fat grafting to the breast is rare, generally less than 1%.[4,15,19]
- Implant rupture, if fat grafting is performed after prosthetic breast reconstruction, is likewise rare but may occur due to cannula trauma.
- Fat necrosis and oil cysts may develop after small-volume fat grafting of the breast, more commonly if fat is injected in larger aliquots within the same tissue plane.
- Significant blood loss with this procedure is very rare, especially with the use of tumescent solution during which blood loss approximates 1% of the total fluid aspirated.[11]

REFERENCES

1. Choi M, Small K, Levovitz C, et al. The volumetric analysis of fat graft survival in breast reconstruction. *Plast Reconstr Surg.* 2013;131(2):185-191.
2. Kling RE, Mehrara BJ, Pusic AL, et al. Trends in autologous fat grafting to the breast: a national survey of the American society of plastic surgeons. *Plast Reconstr Surg.* 2013;132(1):35-46.
3. Biazus JV, Falcão CC, Parizotto AC, et al. Immediate reconstruction with autologous fat transfer following breast-conserving surgery. *Breast J.* 2015;21(3):268-275.
4. Kaoutzanis C, Xin M, Ballard TN, et al. Autologous fat grafting after breast reconstruction in postmastectomy patients: complications, biopsy rates, and locoregional cancer recurrence rates. *Ann Plast Surg.* 2016;76(3):270-275.
5. Small K, Choi M, Petruolo O, et al. Is there an ideal donor site of fat for secondary breast reconstruction? *Aesthet Surg J.* 2014;34(4):545-550.
6. Weichman KE, Broer PN, Tanna N, et al. The role of autologous fat grafting in secondary microsurgical breast reconstruction. *Ann Plast Surg.* 2013;71(1):24-30.
7. Rohrich RJ, Sorokin ES, Brown SA. In search of improved fat transfer viability: a quantitative analysis of the role of centrifugation and harvest site. *Plast Reconstr Surg.* 2004;113(1):391-395.
8. Strong AL, Cederna PS, Rubin JP, et al. The current state of fat grafting: a review of harvesting, processing, and injection techniques. *Plast Reconstr Surg.* 2015;136(4):897-912.
9. Patete P, Rigotti G, Marchi A, Baroni G. Computer assisted planning of autologous fat grafting in breast. *Comput Aided Surg.* 2013;18(1–2):10-18.
10. Tepper OM, Unger JG, Small KH, et al. Mammometrics: the standardization of aesthetic and reconstructive breast surgery. *Plast Reconstr Surg.* 2010;125(1):393-400.
11. Klein JA. Tumescent technique for local anesthesia improves safety in large-volume liposuction. *Plast Reconstr Surg.* 1993;92(6):1085-1098.
12. Mckee DE, Lalonde DH, Thoma A, Dickson L. Achieving the optimal epinephrine effect in wide awake hand surgery using local anesthesia without a tourniquet. *Hand (N Y).* 2015;10(4):613-615.
13. Coleman SR. Structural fat grafting: more than a permanent filler. *Plast Reconstr Surg.* 2006;118(3 suppl):108S-120S.
14. Khouri RK, Smit JM, Cardoso E, et al. Percutaneous aponeurotomy and lipofilling: a regenerative alternative to flap reconstruction? *Plast Reconstr Surg.* 2013;132(5):1280-1290.
15. Illouz YG, Sterodimas A. Autologous fat transplantation to the breast: a personal technique with 25 years of experience. *Aesthetic Plast Surg.* 2009;33(5):706-715.
16. de Blacam C, Momoh AO, Colakoglu S, et al. Evaluation of clinical outcomes and aesthetic results after autologous fat grafting for contour deformities of the reconstructed breast. *Plast Reconstr Surg.* 2011;128(5):411e-418e.
17. Rubin JP, Coon D, Zuley M, et al. Mammographic changes after fat transfer to the breast compared with changes after breast reduction: a blinded study. *Plast Reconstr Surg.* 2012;129(5):1029-1038.
18. Kronowitz SJ, Mandujano CC, Liu J, et al. Lipofilling of the breast does not increase the risk of recurrence of breast cancer: a matched controlled study. *Plast Reconstr Surg.* 2016;137(2):385-393.
19. Maione L, Vinci V, Klinger M, et al. Autologous fat graft by needle: analysis of complications after 1000 patients. *Ann Plast Surg.* 2015;74(3):277-280.

33 CHAPTER

Large-Volume Fat Grafting for the Breast

Wesley N. Sivak and J. Peter Rubin

DEFINITION

- Autologous fat grafting has become a common technique for addressing volume and contour deficiencies in plastic surgery.
  - A survey conducted in 2013 showed that approximately 80% of plastic surgeons have incorporated fat grafting into their clinical breast surgery practice.[1]
  - Fat grafting has been utilized for facial rejuvenation, breast augmentation, mitigating radiation damage, capsular contracture, post-traumatic deformities, congenital anomalies, and burn injuries.
- Autologous fat grafts have numerous beneficial characteristics including simple surgical procedure, low cost, and nearly universal accessibility.
- Although early use was largely as an aesthetic treatment, recent advancements have made fat grafting an attractive alternative for many reconstructive challenges.
- Contour abnormalities and volume defects of the breast routinely require large-volume fat grafting, often necessitating several sessions to achieve the desired result.

ANATOMY

- Female breasts are composed of glandular tissue that produces milk and adipose tissue; the amount and distribution of fat largely determine the size and shape.
- Milk production within the breast occurs within lobules that are organized into 15 to 20 lobes. Milk travels through a network of ducts that coalesce and exit the skin via the nipple.
- Adipose tissue, connective tissue, and ligaments provide support and shape to the breast. Nerves passing through these tissues provide sensation. The breast contains abundant blood vessels, lymph vessels, and lymph nodes.
- The breast due to its architecture and rich blood supply responds well to fat transfer; the architecture permits expansion of the tissues while ensuring close proximity to blood supply.
- Fat grafts are typically harvested from a donor region of abundance (eg, abdomen, flank, or thigh) and serially injected into the deficient recipient site.
- Harvested adipose tissue is composed of particles of tissue encompassing adipocytes and stromal vascular fraction cells, which include adipose stem cells (ASCs) or preadipocytes, fibroblasts, vascular endothelial cells, and a variety of immune cells.

- Clinical studies have demonstrated safety and favorable fat graft retention rates with strict adherence to basic principles and proper, rigorous technique (ie, Coleman technique).
- Stromal vascular fraction cells (and the ASCs within) improve fat graft survival, largely through their angiogenic properties.

PATIENT HISTORY AND PHYSICAL FINDINGS

- Patient selection must begin with a detailed history, noting pertinent medical comorbidities that may limit therapeutic potential.
  - Candidates must be able to withstand the anesthetic requirements of the procedure; it may not be prudent to offer fat grafting to those with significant systemic ailments.
  - Fat grafting to small areas can be performed under local anesthesia, but large-volume grafting will generally require sedation at a minimum.
- Physical examination entails a thorough assessment of the defect in question in addition to assessment of potential donor sites.
  - This allows the physician to formulate a plan for correction of the defect in question.
  - Patients must be informed that several rounds of fat grafting may be needed to achieve the desired results.
- For fat grafting to the breasts, significant fat volume is generally required; often, there is a limit as to the correction that can be made given the paucity of fat in some patients.
- Asking the patient to gain weight prior to the procedure is feasible only if the patient is willing and able to maintain that weight afterward. This strategy is generally not recommended as weight loss following fat grafting can lead to loss of volume and failure to maintain adequate correction.

IMAGING

- For breast fat grafting, screening mammography should be performed preoperatively consistent with current guidelines.
- Typically, no radiologic or other diagnostic studies are required; physical examination alone will suffice to formulate an effective grafting strategy.

SURGICAL MANAGEMENT

- It is not sufficient to merely graft fat diffusely in the breast. The grafted fat must be placed appropriately to accomplish the desired objectives of shaping the breast.
- The surgeon must be familiar with the potential levels of placement (eg, subdermal, subglandular, intramuscular, and supraperiosteal) and the amounts necessary at each level to accomplish a desirable change.
  - These amounts will vary across regions of the body as well as from patient to patient.
  - Determining the amounts of fat to place and the levels in which to place the fat in order to create subtle, lasting contour changes requires a sophisticated surgical plan.
- The Coleman method of fat grafting remains essentially unchanged since the original inception three decades ago.[2]
  - The process relies upon harvesting the fat gently to preserve its architecture, refining the fat with centrifugation to remove nonviable components and provide a predictable volume, and placement of the fat in small aliquots to increase the surface area and ensure a robust blood supply to the grafted tissue.
  - When these principles are adhered to, fat grafting can be a reproducible and safe procedure.
  - Histologic studies have shown that this method of harvesting and refinement with centrifugation yields fat with a high percentage of survival and near-normal adipose cellular enzyme activity.[3]
- However, this method of fat processing lacks efficiency for large-volume fat grafting. Therefore, the Coleman technique is used to refine results of large-volume fat grafting ("touch-up" procedures), and a simple method of harvesting large volumes of fat with machine-powered suction and decanting the aspirate is described below.

Preoperative Planning

- Patients should be marked in the standing position prior to surgery. When in the operating room, significant changes in breast shape can occur with changes in position.
- Areas of volume deficiency on the breast should be marked and the volume to be added estimated, keeping in mind that approximately 40% resorption of volume can be expected during healing. The plane of injection will depend on surgical goals. Superior pole fullness can be achieved predominantly with subcutaneous injection, whereas increasing central projection will require deep injection.
- A mastopexy can be performed concurrent with fat grafting, and we recommend a technique with minimal parenchymal dissection to preserve nipple/areolar blood supply after grafting.
- Concentric circles should be drawn around adipose depots that are going to be harvested to ensure areas are not overharvested.

Positioning

- With the patient in the supine position, both typical donor sites (eg, abdomen, flank, and thigh) and the breasts are easily accessible.
- Following fat harvest and processing, grafting can be done with the patient either supine or with the bed flexed into a sitting position with arms abducted.
  - Sitting position will allow for better assessment and correction of ptosis, clearly delineating the inframammary fold.
  - Supine position will make it more difficult to judge changes in shape during the fat injection.

Approach

- For large-volume fat injection, the principles of harvest and injection must be adapted to enable greater volumes of fat to be handled efficiently in the operating room.

■ Fat Harvest

- Access incisions should be hidden in skin creases, scars, stretch marks, or hair-bearing areas, if at all possible.
- For large-volume harvest, local anesthetic solution is then infiltrated using a blunt infiltration cannula.
  - Local anesthetic mixture consists of 0.025% lidocaine with 1:1 000 000 epinephrine and is a standard wetting solution used for liposuction.
  - The amount of solution infiltrated is equal to the amount of fat removed (1:1 ratio, superwet technique).
- After waiting approximately 10 minutes for the local anesthetic solution to take effect, fat is then harvested using a 3-mm harvesting cannula.
- The cannula may be utilized with any vacuum- or power-assisted liposuction equipment or simply attached to a syringe.

- For small-volume harvest, local anesthetic solution is then infiltrated using a blunt infiltration cannula.
  - Local anesthetic mixture consists of 0.1% lidocaine with 1:200 000 epinephrine and is a higher concentration of epinephrine than a standard wetting solution used for liposuction.
  - The amount of solution infiltrated is equal to approximately 25% of the amount of fat removed (injected sparingly).
  - After waiting approximately 10 minutes for the local anesthetic solution to take effect, fat is harvested using a Coleman bucket handled harvesting cannula attached to a 10-cc syringe barrel.
- Following harvest, incisions are closed with interrupted 5-0 fast-absorbing sutures.

TECHNIQUES

■ Fat Processing

- For small-volume Coleman technique, a Luer-Lok plug is used to cap the syringe.
- The plunger is removed, and the syringe is placed into a sterile centrifuge.
- Centrifugation at 3000 rpm (1200 g) for 3 minutes concentrates the fat so that the aqueous components (ie, local anesthetic and blood) can be removed and discarded by releasing the Luer-Lok plug.

- Any oil layer can be decanted off the top and/or wicked away with gauze pads.
- The processed fat is then ready for injection.
- For larger volumes, simple decantation from a large reservoir can be utilized in lieu of centrifugation (**TECH FIG 1**). Fat is collected into a sterile canister and allowed to decant for 5 to 10 minutes. Aqueous fluid is aspirated and the fat poured into 30-cc syringe barrels.

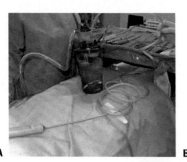 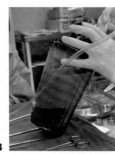 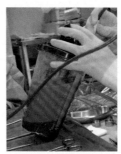 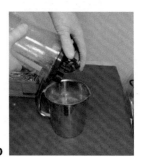

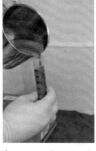 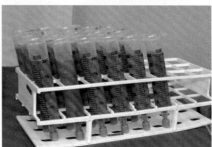

TECH FIG 1 • A. Large-volume fat harvest and processing represent a logistical challenge in the operating room. A simple apparatus consists of a sterile collection chamber set up in-line on the sterile field. Machine-generated suction from a standard liposuction aspirator is applied through the system, and a standard liposuction cannula of 3- or 4-mm diameter is used to harvest fat into the vessel. **B,C.** The aspirate is allowed to decant until the fat separates from the aqueous layer. The aqueous layer is then removed by aspiration with a suction cannula. Commercially available vessels for large-volume fat collection are also constructed with spigots at the base to drain the aqueous layer. (Reproduced from Sivak WN, Rubin JP. Repair and grafting fat and adipose tissue. In: Neligan PC, ed. *Plastic Surgery*. 4th ed. London: Elsevier, 2017, with permission.) **D.** The sterile graft material can be handled by placing it in a vessel with a pour spout **(E,F)** and then filling capped 30-cc syringe barrels from the back.(Reproduced from Sivak WN, Rubin JP. Repair and grafting fat and adipose tissue. In: Neligan PC, ed. *Plastic Surgery*. 4th ed. London: Elsevier, 2017, with permission.)

■ Fat Injection

- Planned incision sites are anesthetized with 0.5% lidocaine with 1:200 000 epinephrine, and small stab incisions are made for the placement of fat through 14- or 16-gauge injection cannulas.

- A blunt-tipped injection cannula is connected to the 30-cc syringe (**TECH FIG 2A,B**).
- Three to four injection sites are used, and these can be placed inferiorly and laterally so they are less visible.
- The success of the fat grafting procedure depends not only on the harvesting and refinement but also on the

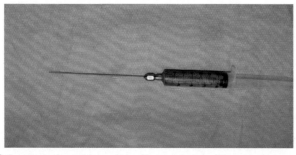 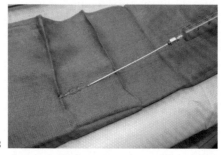

TECH FIG 2 • A. For large-volume fat grafting, a 16-gauge blunt-tipped cannula can be used with the 30-cc syringes, **(B)** and the fat should be easily flowable. (Reproduced from Sivak WN, Rubin JP. Repair and grafting fat and adipose tissue. In: Neligan PC, ed. *Plastic Surgery*. 4th ed. London: Elsevier, 2017, with permission.)

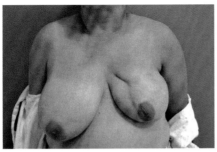
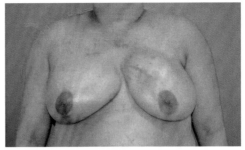

TECH FIG 3 • A. 54-year-old woman 3 years status post left breast quadrantectomy and radiation therapy for invasive breast carcinoma. **B.** Patient shown 5 months status post fat grafting with scar release of the left breast and concurrent reduction of left breast for symmetry. (Reproduced from Sivak WN, Rubin JP. Repair and grafting fat and adipose tissue. In: Neligan PC, ed. *Plastic Surgery*. 4th ed. London: Elsevier, 2017, with permission.)

placement of the fat in a manner that increases its chance for optimal survival.

- This means maximizing the contact surface area of the fatty parcel with the surrounding tissue, such that a blood supply can be conferred to the newly grafted fat.
- Transferring large globules of fat can result in central necrosis of the mass with subsequent resorption and loss of volume or possibly even cyst formation.

- The fat is gently placed during the withdrawal of a blunt infiltration cannula. Recall fat can be placed at different levels to accomplish different effects—determining where and at what level to place fat relies upon the skill and experience of the surgeon.

  - Grafting fat immediately beneath the dermis can improve the quality of the skin, decrease wrinkling, and decrease pore size and may even reduce scarring.

  - Deeper injection within the breast can be used to increase central projection.
  - Fat can be placed intramuscularly, as needed.

- Structure should be purposefully built up with tiny aliquots of fat rather than attempting to insert larger aliquots and then mold the tissue after it is placed.

- Manual molding of the shape should be considered if an irregularity is noted at the time of placement, as the surface must be smooth before leaving the operating room.

- The stab incisions used for placement of the fat can be closed with single interrupted 5-0 fast-absorbing sutures.

- Examples of large volume fat grafting are shown for lumpectomy defect (**TECH FIG 3**), replacement of implants (**TECH FIG 4**), and cosmetic mastopexy/augmentation (**TECH FIG 5**).

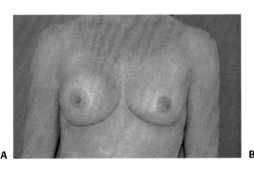
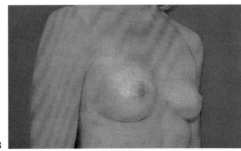
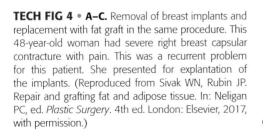
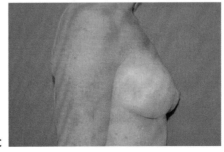

TECH FIG 4 • A–C. Removal of breast implants and replacement with fat graft in the same procedure. This 48-year-old woman had severe right breast capsular contracture with pain. This was a recurrent problem for this patient. She presented for explantation of the implants. (Reproduced from Sivak WN, Rubin JP. Repair and grafting fat and adipose tissue. In: Neligan PC, ed. *Plastic Surgery*. 4th ed. London: Elsevier, 2017, with permission.)

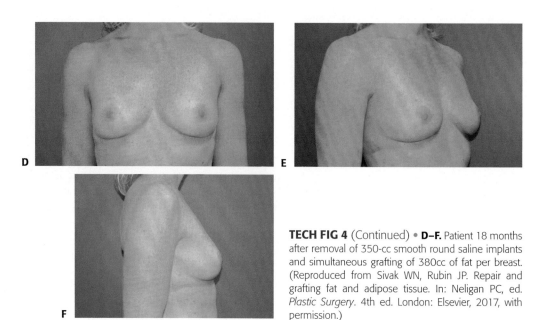

TECH FIG 4 (Continued) • **D–F.** Patient 18 months after removal of 350-cc smooth round saline implants and simultaneous grafting of 380cc of fat per breast. (Reproduced from Sivak WN, Rubin JP. Repair and grafting fat and adipose tissue. In: Neligan PC, ed. *Plastic Surgery*. 4th ed. London: Elsevier, 2017, with permission.)

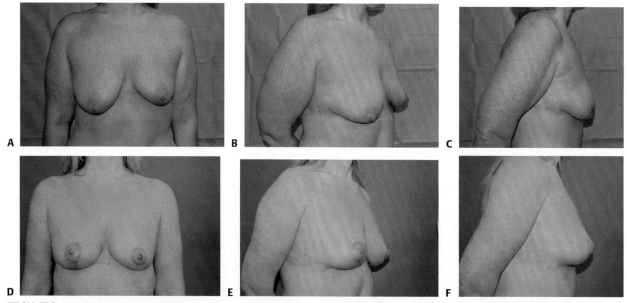

TECH FIG 5 • A–C. A 34-year-old woman with ptosis and asymmetry. Pre-existing flan scar is from a prior upper body lift. **D–F.** She underwent bilateral mastopexy with minimal parenchymal dissection and 350cc of fat grafting to the left breast to balance the asymmetry in volume. Postoperative views are shown at 4 months.

PEARLS AND PITFALLS

Fat harvest	▪ The fat harvest is, in itself, a procedure that must be done in a manner to avoid contour deformities and may also have aesthetic goals for that anatomic region.
Fat processing	▪ A sterile liposuction canister can be kept on the field for easy and efficient decanting. ▪ Large-volume canisters that include filters and outflow ports are commercially available. ▪ Workflow efficiency is key for large-volume fat grafting.
Fat injection	▪ Injection of local anesthetic solution with epinephrine at the injection site helps to reduce bruising. ▪ Special care must be taken when placing fat superficially, as surface irregularities are more apt to be apparent. ▪ Breast injection port sites can be kept inferior and lateral so they are less visible.

TECHNIQUES

POSTOPERATIVE CARE

- Care of the patient after fat grafting remains relatively simple.
- A loosely fitting surgical bra keeps the patient comfortable and avoids excessive pressure on the grafted sites.
- Direct pressure upon the grafted area should be avoided for 1 month (no sleeping on stomach).
- Donor sites may be dressed with compression garments or an abdominal binder if large volumes are harvested.
- Preoperative antibiotics are used, along with 5 days of antibiotics postoperatively.

OUTCOMES

- With fat grafting, secondary procedures, or touch-up procedures, are always possible because of unpredictable resorption.
  - Infiltration and swelling at the time of surgery, in addition to the unpredictable resorption of fat, make the precise estimation of final volume after healing difficult, especially when compared with silicone implants.
  - Patients should be instructed that multiple rounds of grafting might be required to achieve the desired end result.
- In reconstructive cases, the soft tissue envelope often limits the surgeon, and as tissue quality improves after initial fat grafting, the area may become more receptive to larger subsequent volumes.
  - It is far better to undercorrect a deficient area and return to the operating room for a second stage, if necessary, at a later date, than to overfill the tissues.

COMPLICATIONS

- Fat grafting procedures to the breast by and large are deemed to be low risk and are associated with low perioperative morbidity rates given proper patient selection. Soreness and swelling are common, but not every patient will experience them.

- The most significant risk remains the unpredictable nature of the graft, where the recipient site may simply reabsorb most of the transferred fat. The extent of resorption at this time cannot be predicted for a given individual, but some degree of resorption will happen in every patient.
- Rare but possible fat transfer risks and complications include allergic reaction to the local anesthetic, permanent discoloration caused by a ruptured blood vessel, fat necrosis, oil cyst formation, calcification, overcorrection, perioperative bleeding, hematoma at the treatment or donor site, a blood-borne infection (more likely if combined with another cosmetic procedure), scarring, and a fat embolism from direct fat injection into a blood vessel.
- The most problematic is the high potential for contour irregularities visible through the skin, which can occur in both the recipient and donor sites.
  - In the recipient sites, excess grafted fat will appear as lumps beneath the skin and is generally the result of placement of a volume that is too large just beneath thin skin.
  - Irregularities in the donor sites can be pronounced, particularly if too much fat is removed from a single area.
  - Significant changes in weight can also result in related changes in the size of the area grafted; therefore, patients are encouraged to have fat grafting procedures performed when they are at their ideal body weight and to maintain that weight indefinitely.

REFERENCES

1. Kling RE, et al. Trends in autologous fat grafting to the breast: a national survey of the American Society of Plastic Surgeons. *Plast Reconstr Surg.* 2013;132(1):35-46.
2. Coleman SR. The technique of periorbital lipoinfiltration. *Operat Tech Plast Reconstr Sur.* 1994;1(3):120-126.
3. Pu LL, et al. Autologous fat grafts harvested and refined by the Coleman technique: a comparative study. *Plast Reconstr Surg.* 2008; 122(3):932-937.

34
CHAPTER

Section IX: Lyphedema
Lymphedema Microsurgery for Breast Cancer–Related Upper Limb Lymphedema

Ming-Huei Cheng and Jung-Ju Huang

DEFINITION

- Lymphedema can be inherited or a complication after lymph node dissection. Breast cancer–related lymphedema (BCRL) is a potential complication after axillary lymph node dissection, particularly in patients who have or will receive adjuvant radiation.
- With the subcutaneous accumulation of lymphatic fluids, the typical early sign of lymphedema is swelling of the affected limb. Occasionally, patients may present with pain as the first symptom of lymphedema.
  - Definitive diagnosis can be confirmed by lymphoscintigraphy.

ANATOMY

- There are approximately 600 to 700 lymph nodes located in a human body, and the axilla is one of the most concentrated areas.
- Axillary lymph node dissection (ALND), as a procedure for breast cancer staging and treatment, often results in lymphedema of the upper extremity of the affected site, which is exacerbated by radiation therapy.[1,2]

PATHOGENESIS

- The lymphatic system maintains fluid homeostasis, absorbs dietary fat, and facilitates the host immune response. Once disturbed, fluid homeostasis is blocked and subsequent disease is initiated.
- Unbalanced fluid homeostasis can cause protein-rich fluid to leak into the interstitial tissue, resulting in swelling, local tissue inflammation, adipose deposition, and fibrosis.
- A compromised local immune defense makes a patient more susceptible to infection, and repeated cellulitis is one of the common features of lymphedema.
- Although breast surgeons have reduced the frequency of axillary dissection through the use of sentinel lymph node biopsy (SLNB), upper extremity lymphedema can still occur after SLNB or ALND.

NATURAL HISTORY

- BCRL is the major factor that compromises a breast cancer patient's quality of life after treatment.[1]
- The presentation time and symptoms of lymphedema are highly variable among patients.

- Risk factors that contribute to the severity of lymphedema other than radiotherapy include infection and obesity.
- The incidence of BCRL ranges from 12% to 49%.[1,2]
- As it differs from most traditional treatments that involve excision or other destructive procedures, microsurgical treatment for lymphedema aims to drain the accumulated fluid from the affected extremity.
- Lymphaticovenous anastomosis (LVA) is the first microsurgery procedure to treat lymphedema.
  - However, this approach has not been popular until recent years, as more accurate diagnostic tools to identify lymphatic vessels have become available, such as indocyanine green (ICG) lymphography. [3]
- Another microsurgical treatment is vascularized lymph node transfer, which was first developed in an animal study in the 1990s.
  - The idea of transferring healthy, unaffected lymph nodes from other donor sites to the affected extremities provides another approach for microsurgical lymphatic fluid drainage once the lymphatic vessels are destroyed and LVA is not possible.

PATIENT HISTORY AND PHYSICAL FINDINGS

- Patients with BCRL may experience discomfort, swelling, and recurrent cellulitis of the affected extremity.
  - The first sign of lymphedema is often swelling.
  - Occasionally, they present with intractable pain for an unknown reason or with repeated cellulitis.
  - The resultant problems may become both a physical and psychosocial problem.
- Physical examinations of a lymphedema-affected extremity often reveal nonpitting swelling and thickening of the skin (which can be peau d'orange skin or even woody in more advanced stage).
  - It is not uncommon to find skin erosion or ulceration or signs of infection on the skin.
  - Occasionally, brachial plexus dysfunction can occur.
- With long-term involvement, the skin of the affected extremity can present elephantiasis nostra verrucosa, which appears hyperkeratotic with cobblestonelike skin and some papillomatous plaques.
  - Clear or light yellow fluid can ooze from the skin.
  - The tissue may become malodorous in the setting of poor hygiene.

IMAGING

- Accurate diagnosis and grading of lymphedema help to identify suitable treatments.
    - Measurement of the limb circumference and calculation of the difference between the normal and diseased extremity often appears to be the first, easy diagnostic tool.
    - The level for measurement by the authors includes 10 cm above and below the elbow. The circumference difference can then be calculated accordingly (**FIG 1**).
- Lymphoscintigraphy remains the standard diagnosis for lymphedema.
    - With the injection of a tracer molecule with technetium-99m into the dermis of a distal hand, the traveling of Tc-99 can be traced. Information regarding the clearance of the injection tracer, obstruction status (such as total or partial obstruction), and possible obstruction level/presentation of dermal backflow can be provided.
    - With a similar injection technique, ICG (indocyanine) dye is intradermally injected into the distal hand (often the 2nd and 4th web spaces).
    - With an infrared light source and diagnostic devices, such as PDE (Hamamatsu Photonics, Hamamatsu City, Japan), SPY (Novadaq Mississauga, Canada), and infrared detector–incorporated microscopy, the traveling course of the ICG dye (mainly inside the lymphatic vessels) can be identified. ICG lymphography provides a dynamic and panoramic view of the lymphatic drainage with time. It is a powerful tool for both lymphedema diagnosis and intraoperative planning for lymphatic surgery.
    - The main drawback is that the detection of the ICG is limited to approximately 1 cm underneath the skin.

DIFFERENTIAL DIAGNOSIS

- Diseases other than lymphedema can present with swelling of extremities, such as mechanical obstruction and venous thromboembolism.
- Ultrasonography to assess the status of venous drainage is recommended.

NONOPERATIVE MANAGEMENT

- Nonoperative management strategies include manual massage, complex decongestive physiotherapy (CDP), and compression garments.

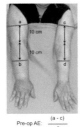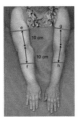

Pre-op AE: $\dfrac{(a-c)}{c}$ Post-op AE: $\dfrac{(e-g)}{g}$

A   Pre-op BE: $\dfrac{(b-d)}{d}$ **B**   Post-op BE: $\dfrac{(f-h)}{h}$

FIG 1 • Measurement of volume differentiation of circumference before (**A**) and after (**B**) lymphedema surgery. To do this, the circumferences of the upper arm and forearm are first measured at the level of 10 cm above and below the elbow.

SURGICAL MANAGEMENT

- Microsurgical treatment for BCRL includes LVA, vascularized lymph node transfer (VLNT), and the combination of microsurgical breast reconstruction and lymph node transfer using an abdominal flap with superficial groin lymph node transfer.
    - A "Barcelona cocktail" is a combination of microsurgical breast reconstruction with superficial groin lymph node transfer to the axilla and LVA in the forearm, which aims to complete surgical treatment at one stage.
- Early interventions provide better recovery because the pathological progress of adipose deposition and fibrosis can be better prevented. This is especially true when LVA is considered.
- Microsurgical treatments may not achieve the same degree of volume reduction as liposuction; instead, they gradually stop the disease progression by effectively draining lymphatic fluid into the venous system.
    - Patients with fibrosis may still benefit from surgery with adjuvant procedures, such as liposuction and/or partial soft tissue resection.
- The selection of treatment is based on the severity of lymphatic obstruction and clinical symptoms (**FIG 2**).

Lymphaticovenous Anastomosis

- Technological advancements in diagnosis and mapping have allowed LVA to become a popular procedure for lymphedema treatment in early-grade cases with promising results.
- Different surgeons have different preferences for performing LVA, including the method (end-to-end, end-to-side, and side-to-end), locations, and numbers of LVAs that have to be done.
- Supramicrosurgery, including anastomosis of vessels as small as 0.8 mm or less to small subdermal veins, has been recommended.[4] To prevent postoperative venous reflux, a suitable recipient vein should present with minimal backflow after it is cut. Strong backflow from the subdermal veins may result in venous blood backflowing into the lymphatics. This results in a limited chance for lymphedema recovery, ecchymosis, and discomfort.

Vascularized Lymph Node Transfer

- VLNT can be effective in patients with different stages of lymphedema, including advanced stage.[5,6]
- There are two different theories supporting its mechanism for lymphatic drainage.
    - One is based on lymphangiogenesis and spontaneous lymphatic connection.[7]
    - The other is based on the inherent lymphaticovenous connection inside the flap.[8]
- Cheng and colleagues demonstrated in animal studies and intraoperative images evidence to support their theory of this mechanism.[9] By injection of ICG dye into the subcutaneous tissue of lymph node containing flaps, ICG is eventually drained via the flap donor vein.
- Conversely, drainage is absent when the dye is injected into non–lymph node-containing flap.[9] They have demonstrated that the inherent lymphaticovenous connection is the main mechanism for lymphatic drainage. Combined with "catchment effect" and "gravity" effect, VLNT placed in the distal recipient site would offer the most benefit for lymphatic drainage.

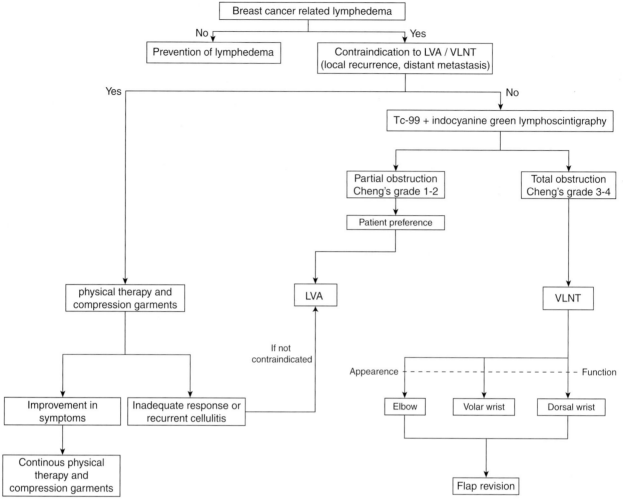

FIG 2 • Algorithm for surgical approaches of breast cancer–related lymphedema (BCRL).

Preoperative Planning

- Cheng and colleagues developed a disease grading system that includes both clinical symptoms and diagnostic results from lymphoscintigraphy[6] (Table 1). Based on the staging system, patients are graded from 0 to IV according to the lymphedema severity.
- By combing preoperative symptoms and diagnostic findings, mainly lymphoscintigraphy and ICG lymphography, an algorithm has been developed to more accurately assign the patients to appropriate treatment (see **FIG 2**).
  - If the lymphatic obstruction is partial and functional lymphatic vessels can still be identified in ICG lymphography, LVA can be considered a good surgical option.
  - However, if the lymphatic obstruction is complete and functional lymphatics are not identifiable, VLNT is the best surgical option.
- Patients who have stage III or IV lymphedema usually require additional procedures other than microsurgical treatment to optimize the results.
- Patients showing a linear pattern of lymphatic vessels with ICG lymphography can be selected for LVA with predictably good outcomes.
- The preoperative use of duplex ultrasonography aids in the selection of the optimal flap for VLNT.[8] Additionally, duplex ultrasonography can be useful in determining recipient vessels for VLNT.[8]
  - More detailed preoperative examinations, such as computer tomography (CT) scan or magnetic resonance imaging (MRI), can be helpful to further differentiate the disease pathology and identify the donor and recipient vessel quality.

Positioning

- Patients are in the supine position for both LVA and VLNT.
- Hyperextension of the neck is required if submental lymph node flaps or transverse cervical lymph nodes are selected as donor sites.

Approach

- For LVA, surgical approach includes one to several 3-cm incisions, depending on preoperative ICG lymphography.
- Surgical approach for VLNT includes flap harvest and recipient site preparation. There are many donor flaps for VLNT depending on preoperative evaluation and the surgeon's preference. Advance selection of appropriate recipient site is equally important (proximal vs distal on the extremity).
  - Some surgeons place the VLNT into the axilla where a previous axillary scar exists. The scar will need to be fully

released during VLNT. However, we prefer to place the lymph node flap in a more distal recipient site.

- A distally transferred lymph node flap may function better than proximally transferred lymph node flaps. One possible explanation could be that with disease progression, gravity draws the fluid to a more dependent site.
- In contrast to the need for a compression garment after surgery in patients receiving lymph node transfer to the axilla, the authors do not recommend a compression garment for patients with a distally transferred lymph node flap. We believe that omitting a compression garment is also an important part of enhancing the quality of life after lymphedema treatment.
- To balance the appearance and postoperative effectiveness of the surgery, the flap may be placed more proximal to the elbow, depending on the severity of lymphedema and area with the most fluid accumulation.
- Table 2 lists commonly used lymph node–carrying flaps and the pros and cons for each flap.
- The submental lymph node flap has a constant donor-site vascular anatomy and greater number of lymph nodes. As it was first introduced as a skin flap, Cheng and colleagues modified the submental flap harvest to include lymph nodes

at neck levels Ia and Ib and transferred it to a distal recipient site for treatment of lower extremity lymphedema.

- Compared to the groin lymph node flap, the submental flap has a longer vascular pedicle with a larger vessel size for microsurgical anastomosis and lymphatic drainage. The flap thickness is less than that of the groin flap, making it a better choice in terms of postoperative appearance of the recipient site when distal transfer is selected.
- The disadvantage of this flap is the potential injury to the marginal mandibular branch during flap dissection. To prevent this, meticulous dissection of the nerve off the facial vessels is required with the assistance of an operative microscope. Additionally, the platysma muscle may be completely or partially sacrificed, resulting in pseudoparalysis of the marginal mandibular nerve. For prevention, the authors recommend partial platysma preservation during flap harvesting.
- Unlike most of the available lymph node flaps with a cutaneous flap, the omentum flap is within the abdomen, and its harvest requires abdominal surgery.
  - An endoscopic approach has been well developed for omentum lymph node flap harvesting, with reduced donor-site morbidity and improved appearance.

Table 1 Cheng's Grading and Related Management for Lymphedema

Grade	Symptoms	Circumferential difference (%)	Lymphoscintigraphy	Management
0	Reversible	<9	Partial occlusion	CDP
I	Mild	10–19	Partial occlusion	LVA, liposuction, CDP
II	Moderate	20–29	Total occlusion	VLNT, LVA
III	Severe	30–39	Total occlusion	VLNT + additional procedure
IV	Very severe	>40	Total occlusion	Charles procedures and VLNT

Circumferential difference: circumference of the affected limb subtracted from the circumference of the healthy limb and divided by the circumference of the healthy limb, which is measured at 10 cm above and below the elbow. CDP, complex decongestive physiotherapy; LVA, lymphaticovenous anastomosis; VLNT, vascularized lymph node transfer.

From Patel KM, Lin CY, Cheng MH. A prospective evaluation of lymphedema-specific quality-of-life outcomes following vascularized lymph node transfer. *Ann Surg Oncol.* 2015;22(7):2424-2430.

Table 2 Comparisons of Various Donor Sites of Lymph Node–Carrying Flaps

	Cutaneous Lymph Node Flaps				
	Submental	**Groin**	**Supraclavicular**	**Lateral thoracic**	**Omentum flap**
Number of lymph node	+++	+++	+	++	+++
Artery/vein size	+++	++	+	+++	++
Pedicle length	+++	++	++	+++	+
Reliability of skin paddle	++++	+++	+	++	N/A
Ease of harvest	+++	++	++	+	+++
Donor-site scar	+++	+++	++	+++	+++
Advantages	Thin flap with concealed donor scar, reliable pedicle	Reliable pedicle Concealed donor scar	Thin flap	Lengthy pedicle	Rich in lymph nodes
Disadvantages	Risk of marginal mandibular nerve injury	Thick flap Short pedicle	Damage thoracic duct when the left side is selected, chest wall numbness	Injury of sentinel lymph node of upper extremity, sacrificing the thoracodorsal nerve	Risk of pancreatitis and internal bleeding, small size of vein

++++, great; +++, good; ++, fair; +, poor.

- The vascularized omentum flap contains numerous small lymph nodes and is currently our second-line lymph node flap. Its vascular pedicle is as small as 2 to 3 mm in diameter, but it is short and thin walled for microvascular anastomosis. Most of the lymph nodes can be found along the great curvature; therefore, the flap can be elevated with only the tissues around the pedicle, and most of them can be preserved in situ.

- Compared with the cutaneous lymph node flaps, the omentum flap lacks a skin paddle for replacing skin defects or flap monitoring after transfer.
- Care should be taken to avoid compressing the pedicle vein at wound closure.

Lymphaticovenous Anastomosis

- Before surgery, patients were treated with ICG lymphography to confirm the presence of functional lymphatic vessels.
- Functional lymphatic vessels presenting as a linear pattern in ICG lymphography are then selected and marked as the target for LVA. After ICG mapping, the linear lymphatic vessels are marked, and an incision can be transversely planned for 3 to 4 cm in length (**TECH FIG 1A**).

- After incision, another distal subdermal injection with blue dye is then performed, and lymphatic vessels can be identified accordingly under a microscope.
- A submental vein is then selected from the surrounding area. A good subdermal recipient vein for LVA should present with less venous backflow to prevent retrograde venous flow into the lymphatic vessels.
- Anastomosis can be performed with end-to-end, end-to-side, or side-to-end anastomosis, depending on the preference of

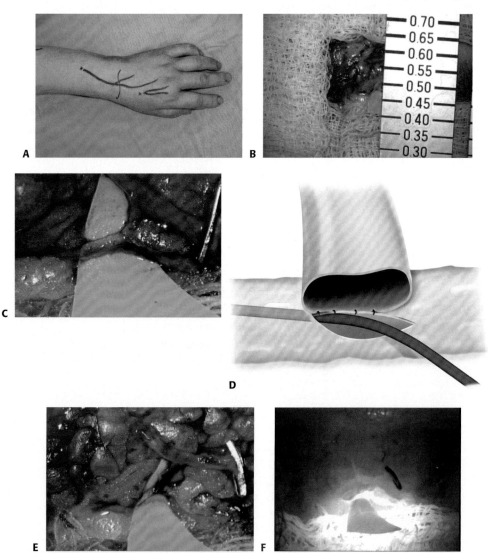

TECH FIG 1 • **A.** Before performing LVA, lymphatic vessels are detected by ICG lymphangiography, and the lymphatic vessels are marked. **B.** A lymphatic vessel sized 0.5 mm is identified. **C.** The lymphatic vessel is dissected. **D.** The technique of doing side-to-end LVA with a 6-0 nylon as stent inside the lymphatic vessel. **E.** Side-to-end LVA was performed. **F.** With the same view under ICG evaluation mode, ICG can be identified inside the lymphatic vessels, and the recipient vein confirmed the patency of the anastomosis.

the surgeon. The lymphatic vessels are usually small in caliber (0.5–0.8-mm diameter) (**TECH FIG 1B**).

- To see the lumen clearly and promote better visualization and anastomosis, an intravascular stent can be placed using 6-0 nylon suture under a microscope with 40× magnification (**TECH FIG 1C**).
- Multiple different techniques and methods of anastomosis have been used, such as T-shaped anastomosis, diamond-shaped anastomosis, octopus-shaped anastomosis, and ladder-shaped anastomosis. Many of these techniques were designed to simultaneously use a limited recipient vein for anastomosis with several lymphatic vessels.
- The authors recommended a side-to-end anastomosis to allow drainage of most of the lymphatic fluids from the same lymphatic vessel (**TECH FIG 1D–F**). Further large-scale series evaluating the outcomes of LVA are necessary.

Vascularized Lymph Node Transfer

Donor Site

- A lymph node flap can be selected among different donor sites. In general, the authors prefer subcutaneous lymph nodes over omentum lymph nodes.
- Subcutaneous lymph node flaps with a skin paddle are important for both flap monitoring and extra skin for tension-free wound closure. However, if the omentum lymph node flap is selected, a skin graft on the top of the flap should be considered instead of burying the flap

inside the subcutaneous pocket to avoid compression of the pedicle vein.

- In the example case, at the donor site, the midline of the neck and facial artery and vein are identified and marked (**TECH FIG 2A**).
- An incision is first made along the upper border of the flap and facial artery, and the facial vein and marginal mandibular branch of facial nerve are identified and carefully dissected out (**TECH FIG 2B,C**).
- The pedicle of the flap is then divided (**TECH FIG 2D**) and the donor site closed (**TECH FIG 2E**).

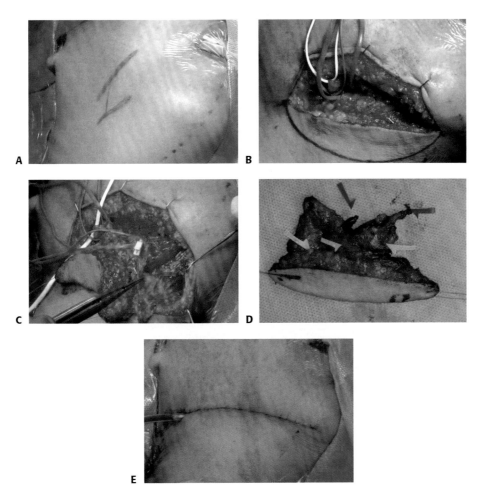

TECH FIG 2 • Example case of free submental lymph node flap transfer to treat upper limb lymphedema. **A.** Before surgery, the midline of the neck and facial artery and vein were identified and marked. **B.** Incision was first made along the upper border of the flap and facial artery; facial vein and marginal mandibular branch of facial nerve were identified and carefully dissected out. **C.** Flap dissection was completed. *Red arrow* showed the donor artery of the flap. **D.** The pedicle of the flap was divided. *Red arrow*, artery; *blue arrow*, vein; *yellow arrow*, lymph nodes. **E.** The donor site was closed primarily.

Recipient Site

- Recipient site selection is based on the severity of lymphedema.
  - The authors recommended transfer of the lymph node flap to the wrist in advanced lymphedema. ICG lymphography with the lymphatic drainage pattern can be a good reference for recipient site selection. The flap should be placed distally if severe dermal backflow is present.
- To use the wrist as the recipient site, the dorsal branch of radial artery in the snuffbox is often selected as a recipient artery, and the cephalic vein is often selected as a recipient vein.
- A lazy S incision is transversely made along the dorsal crease of the wrist (**TECH FIG 3A**).
- Subcutaneous dissection is then carried out. The fibrotic tissue should be removed to create a pocket with adequate space for a lymph node flap inset and adequate space to compensate for swelling of the lymph node flap after absorbing the lymphatic fluid inside the flap.

- The recipient vessels should be well prepared with removal of all the fibrotic adventitia to prevent restriction of blood flow from the fibrotic tissues.
- Microvascular anastomosis is performed first, following with tension-free flap inset and wound closure (**TECH FIG 3B,C**).
- The flap often becomes engorged after it is transferred to lymphedema recipient site because of transit of fluid into the lymph node in the first 7 days following the operation.
- Adequate pocket size for inset of the flap skin paddle will allow for tension-free wound closure, and avoidance of pedicle vein compression is critical for achieving an optimal result.

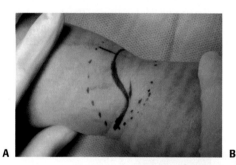 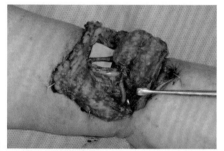

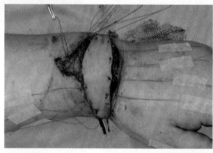

TECH FIG 3 • A. A lazy S incision was made along the wrist to identify the recipient vessels. **B.** The flap was transferred to the recipient site and anastomosis was accomplished. **C.** Flap inset.

PEARLS AND PITFALLS

Imaging	▪ Definitive diagnosis of lymphedema can be achieved using lymphoscintigraphy. ▪ ICG lymphography can be a good diagnostic and surgical guided tool. The results of ICG lymphography are used to separate the patients into LVA or VLNT groups. For LVA, it can provide good intraoperative lymphatic mapping.

LYMPHATICOVENOUS ANASTOMOSIS

Technique	▪ Do surgery only on patients presenting linear pattern of ICG lymphography. ▪ Selection of a small subdermal vein without venous reflux as a recipient vein ▪ Side-to-end anastomosis is recommended ▪ Intravascular stent of lymphatic vessel using 6-0 nylon to prevent back wall suture ▪ Tension-free wound closure to prevent compression
Postoperative care	▪ Restriction of ambulation for 3 days ▪ Compression garment is *not* recommended.

PEARLS AND PITFALLS (Continued)

VASCULARIZED LYMPH NODE TRANSFER

Technique	■ Recipient site selection should be based on the lymphatic obstruction; in general, distal transfer presents better results. ■ Subcutaneous lymph node flap is recommended to include its skin paddle for tension-free wound closure and flap monitoring. ■ Be sure to release all the fibrosis and create a subcutaneous pocket that is larger than enough for flap inset. ■ Release and adventitiectomy are important while preparing the recipient vessels. ■ Tension-free flap inset and wound closure are important. ■ Never hesitate to use therapeutic dose of anticoagulants.
Postoperative care	■ Intensive monitoring of the flap ■ Avoid ambulation for 7 days. ■ Prophylactic antibiotics for 7 days

POSTOPERATIVE CARE

Lymphaticovenous Anastomosis

■ After surgery, it is recommended that patients rest with limited ambulation for the first 3 days.

■ Parenteral prophylactic antibiotics are given for 3 days.

■ Movement is gradually increased after the first postoperative day.

■ Compression garments are not required after surgery.

Vascularized Lymph Node Transfer

■ After surgery, patients are admitted to microsurgical intensive care unit for postoperative monitoring of the flap.

■ Flaps are monitored using pencil Doppler detection of both artery and vein every 2 hours.

■ Postoperative prophylactic antibiotics are given for 1 week.

■ The use of anticoagulants depends on intraoperative findings. The authors found that there is a high tendency of thrombosis formation in lymphedema surgery. Therefore, the use of therapeutic dose of anticoagulation is not uncommon.

■ Patients are allowed to walk freely and move the upper extremity 1 week after surgery.

■ Compression garments are not required after surgery.

OUTCOMES

Lymphaticovenous Anastomosis (FIG 3)

■ The largest series of LVA for upper extremity lymphedema was reported by Chang and colleagues with significant improvement after LVA in 96% of patients.

■ Constant improvement of volume reduction was observed from 33% 3 months after surgery to 42% after 1 year.[10]

■ A better volume reduction after LVA was reported for earlier lymphedema stage for upper extremity lymphedema.

■ The most important consideration in performing LVA is that it is difficult to ensure a 100% patency rate after surgery.

■ Patency has been reported as low as 0% patency 3 weeks after surgery by Puckett[11] to 93% after 7 years of follow-up by Campisi et al.[12]

Vascularized Lymph Node Transfer (FIGS 4 to 6)

■ In patients with advanced stage lymphedema, it has been reported that VLNT has better results than does LVA.[5]

■ A reduction rate of 39% was with 18 months of follow-up using distal vascularized lymph node transfer.

■ With an average follow-up of 29 months, Brucker and colleague reported that 84% of the patients reported improvement of their lymphedema symptoms after vascularized lymph node transfer.[13]

■ Although distal transfer of the flap often results in an unsightly skin paddle in the beginning, revision surgery after the development of symptoms can significantly improve the appearance.

■ It is not uncommon for patients to require some other additional procedure to achieve better volume reduction and appearance after microsurgical approaches. These procedures often include liposuction, wedge resection of part of the proximal soft tissue, or debulking of the transferred skin flap.

Quality of Life After Lymphedema Microsurgery

■ VLNT helps to improve the patient-reported outcomes as soon as after the 1st week of surgery.

■ By using health-related quality of life (HRQoL) merits, Patel and colleagues prospectively evaluated patients undergoing vascularized lymph node transfer for upper or lower extremity

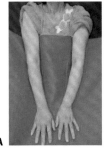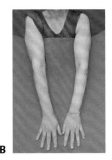

FIG 3 • **A.** This 60-year-old woman shown in **TECH FIG 1** underwent mastectomy and chemotherapy for left breast cancer and experienced BCRL. **B.** At 12-month follow-up after LVA, she had reduction rates of 5% and 20% at the above-elbow level and below-elbow level, respectively, in her left arm.

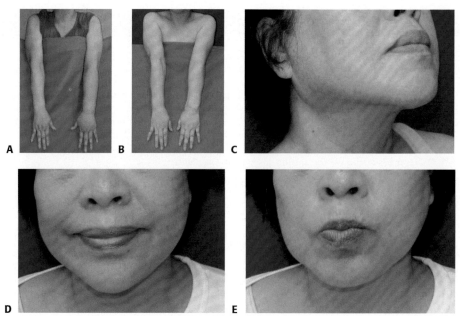

FIG 4 • This 56-year-old woman with left breast cancer is pictured in TECH FIGS 2 and 3. She received skin-sparing mastectomy and tissue expander reconstruction followed by chemotherapy for breast cancer. **A.** Left upper arm nonpitting edema presented 6 months after surgery. **B.** At 30 months of follow-up, she presented with reduction rates in her left arm lymphedema of 35% and 20% at the above-elbow level and the below-elbow level, respectively. **C–E.** Her donor-site scar was well concealed, and there were no donor-site morbidities.

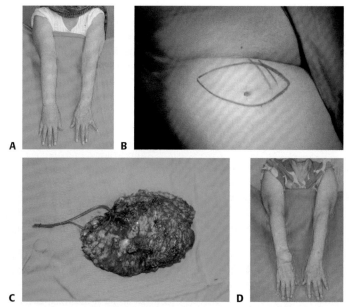

FIG 5 • This 79-year-old woman had a history of right breast cancer after modified radical mastectomy, radiotherapy, and chemotherapy. She started to experience right upper arm swelling 6 months after breast cancer treatment. She received vascularized groin lymph node flap transfer 14 months after the first presentation of lymphedema. **A.** Preoperative appearance of the upper extremities. **B.** Vascularized groin lymph node flap of 10 × 5 cm was designed on her left groin area. **C.** Vascularized groin lymph node flap was harvested based on the medial artery (*red arrow*) and vein (*blue arrow*). **D.** At 24-month follow-up, she had reduction rates of 30% and 35% in the upper arm and forearm, respectively.

lymphedema and reported improvement regarding the domains of function, body appearance, symptom, and mood in proportion to the improvement of limb circumference.[6]

■ The improvement in the HRQoL appeared as soon as the first month, and the improvement was continued and sustained during the 1 year of follow-up.

■ Gratzon evaluated the psychosocial outcome of vascularized lymph node transfer using the LYMQoL prospectively

and revealed early steady improvements with respect to the function, appearance, mood, and symptoms.[14]

■ Using Upper Limb Lymphedema Questionnaire 27, Brucker and colleagues evaluated the quality of life after simultaneous breast reconstruction and vascularized lymph node transfer with inspiring results.

■ With an average follow-up of 29 months, 84% of the patients reported improvement of their lymphedema symptoms.[13]

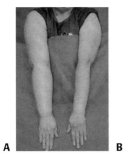
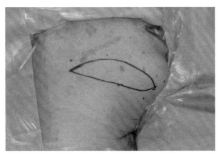
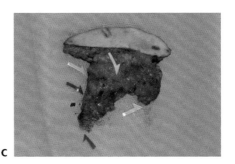

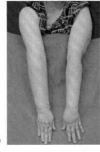

FIG 6 • This 52-year-old woman had a history of right breast cancer, stage II, after modified radical mastectomy, chemotherapy, and radiotherapy and lung metastasis after wedge resection of the tumor. She presented with right upper arm lymphedema 1 year after surgery and received vascularized submental lymph node flap transfer 4 years after her first presentation of lymphedema. **A.** Preoperative appearance of bilateral upper extremities. **B.** Vascularized submental lymph node flap of 8.5 × 2.5 cm was designed. **C.** Vascularized submental lymph node flap was harvested based on submental artery (*red arrow*) and facial vein (*blue arrow*). Lymph nodes were visualized during surgery (*yellow arrow*). **D.** At 18-month follow-up, she had reduction rates of 35% and 42% at the above-elbow level and below-elbow level, respectively.

- Although the different groups continue to have different preferences for recipient and donor-site selection, vascularized lymph node transfer seems to work by different designs and combinations of breast reconstruction with an abdominal flap.

COMPLICATIONS

- Complications of LVA include obstruction of the anastomosis and venous reflux into the lymphatics. To prevent this, the recipient vein should be a small subdermal vein with limited backflow.
- Common complications of vascularized lymph node transfer include early thrombosis of the vein, partial or total loss of the skin paddle, and infection.
- To ensure a safe flap transfer, inclusion of skin paddle for intensive monitoring is recommended.
- It seems that there is a higher incidence of thrombus formation in vascularized lymph node transfer. To minimize this risk, therapeutic dose anticoagulation is occasionally required.

REFERENCES

1. Lopez Penha TR, van Bodegraven J, Winkens B, et al. The quality of life in long-term breast cancer survivors with breast cancer related lymphedema. *Acta Chir Belg.* 2014;114(4):239-244.
2. McLaughlin SA, Wright MJ, Morris KT, et al. Prevalence of lymphedema in women with breast cancer 5 years after sentinel lymph node biopsy or axillary dissection: patient perceptions and precautionary behaviors. *J Clin Oncol.* 2008;26(32):5220-5226.
3. Mihara M, Hara H, Shibasaki J, et al. Indocyanine green lymphography and lymphaticovenous anastomosis for generalized lymphatic dysplasia with pleural effusion and ascites in neonates. *Ann Vasc Surg.* 2015;29(6):1111-1122.
4. Koshima I, Yamamoto T, Narushima M, et al. Perforator flaps and supermicrosurgery. *Clin Plast Surg.* 2010;37(4):683-689, vii-iii.
5. Akita S, Mitsukawa N, Kuriyama M, et al. Comparison of vascularized supraclavicular lymph node transfer and lymphaticovenular anastomosis for advanced stage lower extremity lymphedema. *Ann Plast Surg.* 2015;74(5):573-579.
6. Patel KM, Lin CY, Cheng MH. A prospective evaluation of lymphedema-specific quality-of-life outcomes following vascularized lymph node transfer. *Ann Surg Oncol.* 2015;22(7):2424-2430
7. Yan A, Avraham T, Zampell JC, et al. Mechanisms of lymphatic regeneration after tissue transfer. *PLoS One.* 2011;6(2):e17201.
8. Patel KM, Chu SY, Huang JJ, et al. Preplanning vascularized lymph node transfer with duplex ultrasonography: an evaluation of 3 donor sites. *Plast Reconstr Surg Glob Open.* 2014;2(8):e193.
9. Cheng MH, Huang JJ, Wu CW, et al. The mechanism of vascularized lymph node transfer for lymphedema: natural lymphaticovenous drainage. *Plast Reconstr Surg.* 2014;133(2):192e-198e.
10. Chang DW, Suami H, Skoracki R. A prospective analysis of 100 consecutive lymphovenous bypass cases for treatment of extremity lymphedema. *Plast Reconstr Surg.* 2013;132(5):1305-1314.
11. Puckett CL. Microlymphatic surgery for lymphedema. *Clin Plast Surg.* 1983;10(1):133-138.
12. Campisi C, Bellini C, Campisi C, et al. Microsurgery for lymphedema: clinical research and long-term results. *Microsurgery.* 2010;30(4):256-260.
13. De Brucker B, Zeltzer A, Seidenstuecker K, et al. Breast cancer-related lymphedema: quality of life after lymph node transfer. *Plast Reconstr Surg.* 2016;137(6):1673-1680.
14. Gratzon A, Schultz J, Secrest K, et al. Clinical and psychosocial outcomes of vascularized lymph node transfer for the treatment of upper extremity lymphedema after breast cancer therapy. *Ann Surg Oncol.* 2017;24(6):1475-1481.

PART 2
Trunk Reconstruction and Body Contouring

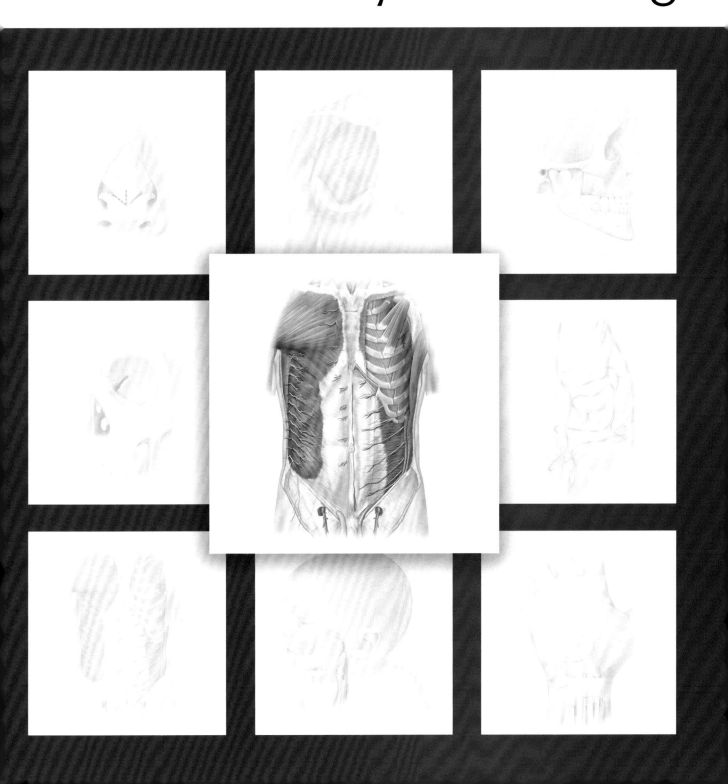

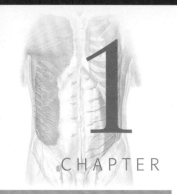

Section I: Reconstruction of the Chest Wall
Pectoralis Flap for Chest Wall Reconstruction

Jeff J. Kim and David H. Song

DEFINITION

- Chest wall defect: Most common etiologies include trauma, tumor resection, osteoradionecrosis, deep sternal wound infections, and chronic empyemas.
- Chest wall functions: Protection of visceral organs, support of respiratory mechanics, and base scaffold for shoulder/upper limb
- Basic defect management concepts: Adequate debridement of infection/nonviable tissue, reconstruct to re-establish form and function, replacing like with like whenever possible
- Reconstructive goals:
  - Stabilize thoracic skeletal defect to return proper respiratory mechanics.
  - Obliterate intrathoracic dead space that may predispose to infection.
  - Protect vital intrathoracic structures.
  - Provide soft tissue coverage for closure.
  - Recreate aesthetic contour.
- Defects requiring skeletal support to prevent paradoxical motion: 5 cm or more in diameter or two or more rib resection anteriorly, twice as much for lateral and posterior defect; radiated tissue can often tolerate larger defect due to rigidity from fibrosis.

ANATOMY

- Pectoralis major
  - Origin: Sternum, 1st to 6th costal cartilage, clavicle (**FIG 1A,B**)
  - Insertion: Lateral lip of bicipital groove of humerus
  - Innervation: Medial and lateral pectoral nerve from medial, lateral cord of brachial plexus
  - Function: Adduction, extension, and medial rotation of shoulder
  - Borders: Superficial to pectoralis minor, superior and superficial to serratus anterior, inferior to the subclavius; two heads converge laterally inferior to deltoids; lateral border forms the anterior axillary fold/wall
- Vascular anatomy (**FIG 1C**)
  - Mathes and Nahai classification: type V muscular flap—thoracoacromial artery (dominant) and internal mammary perforators (secondary segmental)

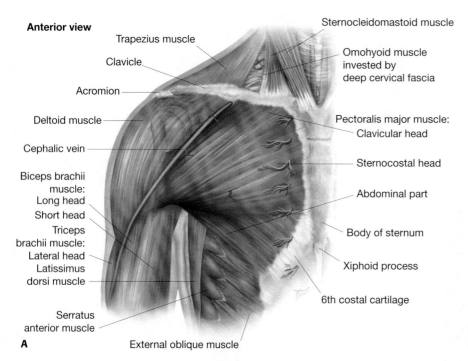

Anterior view

Trapezius muscle
Clavicle
Acromion
Deltoid muscle
Cephalic vein
Biceps brachii muscle:
Long head
Short head
Triceps brachii muscle:
Lateral head
Latissimus dorsi muscle
Serratus anterior muscle
External oblique muscle

Sternocleidomastoid muscle
Omohyoid muscle invested by deep cervical fascia
Pectoralis major muscle:
Clavicular head
Sternocostal head
Abdominal part
Body of sternum
Xiphoid process
6th costal cartilage

A

FIG 1 • A. Muscular anatomy of anterior chest and shoulder.

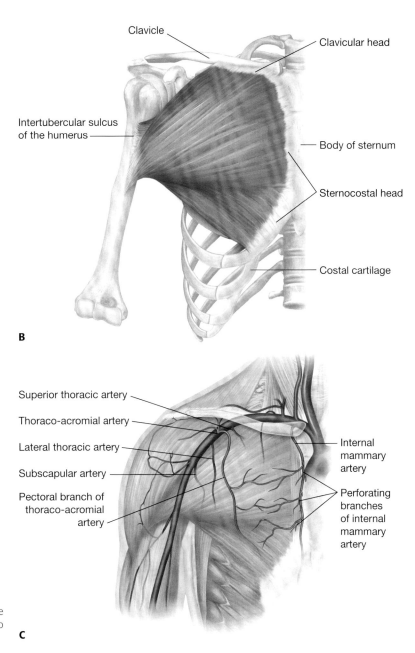

FIG 1 (Continued) • **B.** Origin and insertions of the pectoralis major. **C.** Vascular anatomy of blood supply to pectoralis major.

- Thoracoacromial artery arises from second portion of axillary artery deep to pectoralis minor, travels laterally and merges superomedially to pectoralis minor, and divides into four branches as it pierces the clavipectoral fascia. The dominant branch to the sternocostal portion is the pectoral branch, which courses deep to pectoralis major after piercing through the clavicopectoral fascia medial to pectoralis minor before dividing into muscular and cutaneous branches; clavicular branch arising lateral to pectoralis minor has much shorter pedicle (1 cm) before exclusively supplying the clavicular head, subclavius muscle, and soft tissue around the clavicle.
- Internal mammary artery (IMA) provides reliable secondary segmental pedicles through its perforating branches that pass through the intercostal spaces 1 to 2 cm lateral to the sternal edge; usually three perforators provide the muscle through the first to third intercostal space with branches coming through first or second space being the most dominant.

- Venous drainage: Muscle drains mainly via venae comitantes of the pedicles, through pectoralis branch into the axillary vein, while overlying skin drains through venules accompanying arterial perforators.

PATHOGENESIS

- Most common etiology and mechanism of chest wall defects requiring reconstructive interventions include injury from trauma, iatrogenic (radiation, cardiothoracic surgery), infection, congenital deformity, and neoplasm.

NATURAL HISTORY

- Tansini is often credited with first use of muscle flap in chest wall reconstruction using latissimus dorsi.[1]
- Jurkiewicz and others transposed the pectoralis major into the mediastinum either based on the thoracoacromial pedicle or as a turnover flap based on perforators of the IMA.[2]

- Nahai introduced a modification of the turnover pectoralis major flap by dividing the muscle medial to the thoracoacromial pedicle and using only the medial two-thirds of the pectoralis major for definitive coverage of the mediastinal wound.[3]
- Tobin suggested the splitting of the pectoralis major muscle into sternocostal, external, and clavicular segments and the preserving of the thoracoacromial pedicle.[4]
- Morain suggested the splitting of the pectoralis major muscle into segments but leaving some of the segments intact to preserve muscle function for smaller defects requiring only a small portion of muscle.[5]

PATIENT HISTORY AND PHYSICAL FINDINGS

- Preoperative evaluation for patients requiring pectoralis flap for chest wall reconstruction is mostly based on history and physical examination.
- History
- Etiology, chronicity
  - Important to note history of radiation and history of surgery, including history of coronary artery bypass grafting (CABG)/IMA harvest and other chest incisions. Also important to note pulmonary function and history of chronic obstructive pulmonary disease
  - Social: Smoking history
- Physical examination
  - Important to note size, location, and tissue composition of defect
  - Soft tissue: Size and location
  - Skeletal: Number of ribs and size of skeletal defect
  - Intrathoracic: Size and volume of dead space
  - Respiratory mechanics: Skeletal stability, presence of paradoxical motion, soft tissue compliance
  - Previous scars, radiation changes

IMAGING

- Preoperative computed tomography (CT) is not absolutely necessarily from a reconstructive standpoint, especially in wounds requiring further debridement where final size and composition of defect will invariably change.
- If a CT scan is available, however, it can provide some preoperative insight for operative planning in some cases.

DIFFERENTIAL DIAGNOSIS

- Trauma
- Empyema
- Poststernotomy mediastinitis
- Osteoradionecrosis
- Tumor resection of anterior chest wall

NONOPERATIVE MANAGEMENT

- For small and superficial wounds or defects with no exposed vital structure or functional defect, it may be possible and appropriate to manage using simple wound care methods with either traditional wet to dry gauze dressings or negative pressure wound therapy.
- In cases of heavily contaminated or actively infected wounds (except deep sternal infections), local wound care may be more appropriate initial method of management to prepare the wound bed prior to proceeding with definitive operative reconstruction.

SURGICAL MANAGEMENT

- Pectoralis major offers large muscular flap with robust blood supply, with arc of rotation based on thoracoacromial pedicle by allowing coverage of central, supraclavicular, and axillary or lateral chest wall defects, as well as being able to be transposed to an intrathoracic position for obliteration of dead space.
- The pectoralis major is most commonly used as an advancement flap to cover anterior chest wall defects in the upper part of the chest, classically for wounds resulting from an infected median sternotomy after open heart surgery.[6]
  - This technique allows for repeat subsequent procedures through the midline incision, including further debridement and costochondral resection, without sacrificing viability of reconstruction.[1]
- Turnover flap is based off its medial segmental blood supply from perforators of IMA allows coverage of wounds extending further inferiorly or to the contralateral side or to provide large bulk of healthy tissue to obliterate more significant area of dead space.
- Contraindications/disadvantages:
  - Low sternal and xiphoid defects may be out of reach for the pectoralis flap.
  - If IMA has been harvested for prior cardiac bypass procedure, secondary perfusion through segmental pedicles off IMA would not be available for a turnover flap.
- Other surgical options:
  - Local flaps: Latissimus dorsi, rectus abdominis, serratus anterior, omentum
  - Free tissue transfer

Preoperative Planning

- A good history and physical examination will usually suffice for preoperative purposes, as final size and extent of defect will often not be established until called on intraoperatively after resection/debridement.
  - Location, extent of defect, and availability of the pedicles (prior radiation, surgery) will primarily dictate whether reconstruction will be based off thoracoacromial vs internal mammaries, unilateral vs bilateral, or if at all.
- If size and extent of defect will not be fully established until intraoperatively, the surgeon should be prepared and comfortable to use alternative options, including other local flaps or even free tissue transfers.

Positioning

- The patient is positioned supine on the operating table.
- The arm should be adducted to the side and secured via tucking it on the side from which the flap is planned to be harvested (**FIG 2**).
  - This allows for ease of surgeon positioning and access, especially in case humeral attachments need to be divided.
  - It also allows for physiologic advancement where the pectoralis major muscle is not placed on passive stretch as in an abducted/arm out position.
- The opposite arm should be out.
- For ease of identifying landmarks, entire anterior chest surface should be prepped and draped into the field, with clavicle and acromial process of the scapula exposed superiorly and upper arm and midaxillary line laterally.

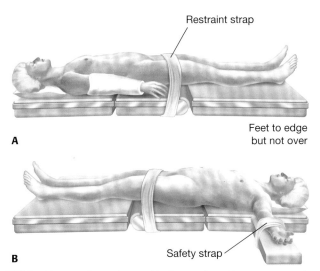

Restraint strap

Feet to edge
but not over

A

Safety strap

B

FIG 2 • Preoperative patient positioning: supine with arm on operative side adducted **(A)** and tucked and the other arm out **(B)**.

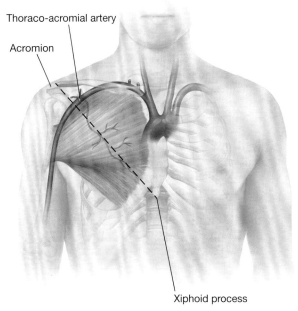

Thoraco-acromial artery

Acromion

Xiphoid process

FIG 3 • Markings for thoracoacromial pedicle.

Approach

- Pedicle landmarks
  - Thoracoacromial pedicle originates at the cross section of line drawn from the acromial process of the scapula to the xiphoid and perpendicular line originating at the junction between middle and lateral third portion of the clavicle (**FIG 3**).
  - Internal mammary perforators can be found piercing through within intercostal spaces, about two fingerbreadths lateral from the costosternal junction.
- Incisions
  - Depending on location of defect/wound, a separate incision may not be required to access around the muscle for necessary releases. Muscle can often be completely released through the wound.
  - For small median sternotomy wounds, lateral counterincision can often be helpful to more easily access insertion of the muscle at the anterior axillary fold.

- If not accessed through pre-existing wound, depending on the choice of vascular pedicle, location of defect, and plan for inclusion of cutaneous skin paddle, incisions may be varied.
  - Most useful incision is often placed along the lateral border of the muscle, with option to extend the incision curved inferomedially under the breast in subpectoral groove or inframammary fold (IMF) on females (this incision can be used for either pedicle and entire surface of the muscle can be accessed).
- Skin paddle
  - Design should be centered on a line drawn from tip of acromion to xiphoid process (approximate course of pectoral branch of thoracoacromial pedicle) on males or centered along the IMF for females.
  - Skin paddle width of up to 8 cm can be expected to be closed primarily.

■ Harvest for Rotation-Advancement Flap

- This flap is based off the primary thoracoacromial artery.
  - If accessed via medial sternal wound, skin incision can be extended vertically as needed. If a myocutaneous flap is planned, the muscle can be accessed superolaterally and inferomedially through the incision around the skin paddle.
  - Identify the plane between the subcutaneous tissue of the chest wall and the anterior surface of the pectoralis fascia.
  - Dissection should continue superolaterally toward the axilla until the entire anterior surface of the muscle is exposed.

Raising the Muscle

- Dissection of muscle off the chest along the medial insertion is generally more difficult so it may be helpful to raise the muscle off starting at the lateral edge, where the subpectoral plane is easier to identify.
  - It usually can be identified through blunt dissection just using the fingers (placement of counter skin incision over this area laterally on the chest surface may allow for easier access).
- Submuscular dissection can then proceed medially freeing the inferior attachment of the muscle along the rectus abdominis and external oblique aponeurosis and then subsequently proceed superolaterally toward the axilla/ pedicle.

T E C H N I Q U E S

- When dissecting the medial attachment of the muscle, care should be taken to ligate the intercostals and internal mammary perforators
  - It is important to leave some perforators from muscle to overlying skin to maximize healing potential of midline and to minimize postoperative seroma formation.
- As muscle is elevated toward superolaterally, care is to taken to find the right plane to avoid elevating the pectoralis minor and leaving it intact in situ.
  - Blunt finger dissection can be performed along the anterior surface of pectoralis minor, which will aid in identification of pectoralis minor branch from the thoracoacromial artery, which should be divided closely to the pectoralis minor muscle to avoid damaging the main pedicle (**TECH FIG 1**).
- Usually dividing the medial attachment and lifting the muscle off the chest wall thoracic cage is sufficient to mobilize the muscle to cover the sternotomy defect medially, but further mobilization can be achieved by releasing the clavicular attachments superiorly or dividing the sternocostal head from clavicular head of the muscle.
  - As the clavicular head of the muscle is dissected off the clavicle working in a medial to lateral direction, when approaching the lateral third of the clavicle, care is taken as subclavian vein can be found just deep to this landmark.

- Staying on the anterior surface of clavicle during release/dissection of muscle will minimize any risk of injuring critical structures.
- Humeral insertion can also be released laterally for further mobilization through separate incision near the humeral insertion at the lateral lip of bicipital groove; however, this usually accentuates aesthetic distortion of anterior axillary landmark.

Approaching the Pedicle

- An Allis or Babcock is used to grab the thick head of the muscle that has been freed of the clavicle, and careful dissection of the upper portion of the muscle can proceed.
  - The thoracoacromial artery should be identified as it exits the subclavicular space and enters the underside of the pectoralis major muscle.
- All muscle lateral to the pedicle is expendable and should be divided to maximize excursion and advancement of the flap medially.
- Careful inspection of the pedicle reveals initial lateral course of the pedicle prior to turning medially toward along fibers of the muscle. Careful dissection of the pedicle proximal to this "elbow" level can allow for straightening out of the vessel and maximize its length.

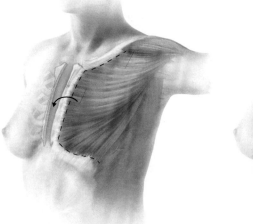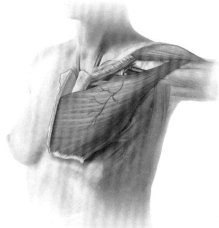

TECH FIG 1 • Rotation-advancement flap harvest. Release of medial, inferior, and lateral insertion of muscle while preserving thoracoacromial pedicle attachment.

■ Harvest for Turnover Flap

- This flap is based off perforating branches of internal mammary, often used when inferior pole of sternal wound requires coverage.
  - Disadvantages include relying on secondary blood supply.
- Entire anterior surface of the muscle should be dissected free off the overlying subcutaneous tissue.
- Raising of the muscle should begin laterally at the anterior axillary fold and proceed medially. A counter skin incision over this area can be very helpful for access.

- As the muscle is divided superolaterally, the humeral insertion of the pectoralis major muscle should be divided.
  - Modification can be made by dividing the muscle medial to the thoracoacromial pedicle and using only the medial two-thirds muscle.
  - Humeral insertion and anterior axillary fold can be preserved by dividing the muscle medial to it and anchoring the lateral portion of the muscle to the chest wall to preserve function and minimize donor-site morbidity.[7]

- Proceed to divide clavicular and inferior attachments, being mindful of the subclavian vessels deep to the clavicle.
- As medial attachment is approached, care should be taken to identify and protect the perforating vessels from

IMA, which will arise about 2 cm medial to the costosternal junction.
- No medial attachment beyond these vessels should be divided since the vessels themselves limit medial transposition of the flap (**TECH FIG 2**).

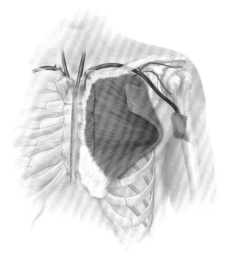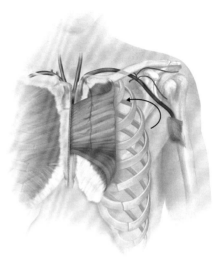

TECH FIG 2 • Turnover flap. Thoracoacromial pedicle is ligated to allow for turnover of the lateral portion of the muscle medially. Medial blood supply from internal mammary vessels is preserved.

■ Bilateral Advancement Flap

- This flap is often used for larger sternotomy wounds to obliterate deeper sternal dead space (**TECH FIG 3A,B**).
- Superiorly, dissection ends just below level of the clavicle.
- Laterally, elevation off the chest wall should be performed so just enough muscle can be mobilized from either side to approximate the two muscles together with minimum tension (usually between midclavicular to anterior axillary line; **TECH FIG 3C**).

- Humeral insertion, pedicle axis, innervation, and pectoralis minor should all be left intact.
- Inferiorly, dissection is continued deep to the muscle and deep to anterior rectus fascia, until level of xiphoid.
- The inferior insertion of the pectoralis major is elevated without detaching the muscle from the superior portion of anterior rectus sheath. The rectus muscle should be left intact (**TECH FIG 3D,E**).[8]
- The wound is closed (**TECH FIG 3F–H**).
- Three drains should be placed: one medial drain, two laterally (one under each flap; **TECH FIG 3I**).[6]

Sternal defect

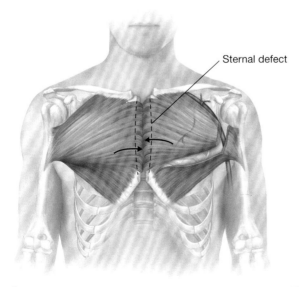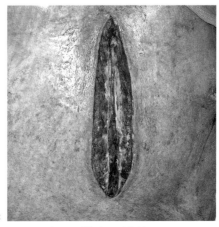

A   **B**

TECH FIG 3 • Bilateral advancement of pectoralis major. **A.** Design of flap. **B.** Large sternal wound before debridement.

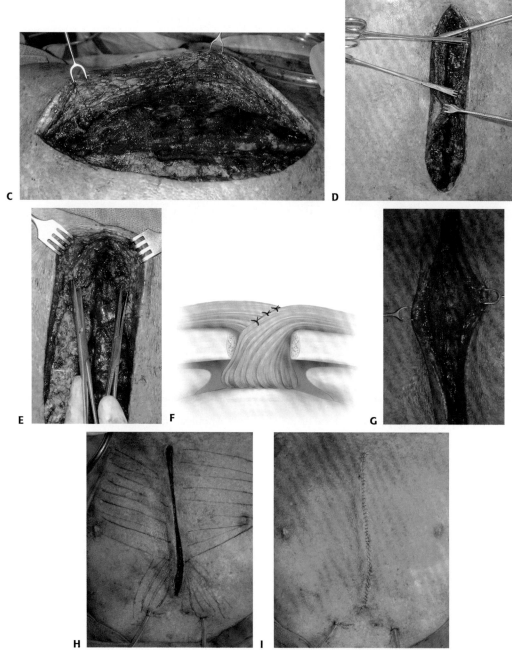

TECH FIG 3 (Continued) • **C.** Pectoralis major muscle dissected off the chest wall after complete debridement of sternum. **D.** Bilateral pectoralis major muscle advancement showing minimal tension. **E.** Raising the pectoralis major in conjunction with the superior portion of the rectus abdominis muscle as one single unit to close the xiphoid region. **F.** Pectoralis major advancement closure complete. **G.** Cross-sectional view of defect repair. **H.** Muscle layers closed. **I.** Closure completed with two drains in place.

PEARLS AND PITFALLS

Drains	▪ Placement of closed suction drains in spaces above and below the pectoralis muscle is critical to avoid seromas. Drains will typically stay in for up to 3 weeks. Care must be taken to avoid placing closed suction drains directly over the right ventricle. Closed suction drains that are well placed can also be set to continuous wall suction at –70 mm Hg or less to assist in obliterating the dead space.
Flap harvest	▪ Muscle harvest can be extended to the insertion of the pectoralis major into the humerus. For greater mobility, the humeral insertion can also be detached and the entire muscle can be transferred based on the thoracoacromial vessels with reliability.
Coverage	▪ The inferior portion of the sternal wound is the most difficult to cover. Developing the pectoralis major muscle in continuity with the superior origin of the rectus abdominis muscle can create greater vascularized coverage for the inferior most extent of the wound. This allows for an entire unit of both pectoralis major muscle and the superior origin of the rectus muscle to be advanced into the inferior sternal wound. Often, the superior epigastric artery must be ligated to gain greater mobility. This then allows for the entire unit to be based upon the thoracoacromial system above and the deep inferior epigastric system below.
Turnover flaps	▪ Turnover flaps are based on the secondary blood supply from the internal mammary system and thus are unreliable but can be used when the internal mammary vessels on the respective side have not been sacrificed. This maneuver mandates a close examination of the vasculature and blood supply with the use of either pencil Doppler probes or preoperative duplex.

POSTOPERATIVE CARE

- Keeping drains up to 3 weeks leads to decrease in seroma rate. Any drains in intrathoracic spaces should be put to low continuous wall suction to prevent possible pneumothorax.
- When wound dehiscence is encountered, wound irrigation and light gauze packing can be employed along with negative pressure dressings. Readvancement of the pectoralis myocutaneous unit can be considered once the wound is in bacteriologic control and all necrotic or infected tissues are removed.
- Other shoulder girdle muscles will compensate for weakened abduction, internal rotation, and flexion.
  - Starting 6 weeks, start consistent fair to moderate physical therapy for range of motion, flexibility, and strengthening only. Thereafter, full range of motion with resistance and weight training is allowed.

COMPLICATIONS

- Seroma/hematoma
- Skin/flap necrosis, wound dehiscence
- Infection
- Donor-site complications
  - Contour deformities
  - Impaired shoulder functions

REFERENCES

1. Bakri K, Mardini S, Evans KK, et al. Workhorse flaps in chest wall reconstruction: the pectoralis major, latissimus dorsi, and rectus abdominis flaps. *Semin Plast Surg.* 2011;25(1):43-54.
2. Jurkiewicz MJ, Bostwick J III, Hester TR, et al. Infected median sternotomy wound: successful treatment by muscle flaps. *Ann Surg.* 1980;191(6):738-744.
3. Naha, F, Morales L Jr, Bone DK, et al. Pectoralis major muscle turnover flaps for closure of the infected sternotomy wound with preservation of form and function. *Plast Reconstr Surg.* 1982;70:471.
4. Tobin GR. Pectoralis maor segmental anatomy and segmentally split pectoralis major flaps. *Plast Reconstr Surg.* 1985;75:814-824.
5. Morain WD, Colen LB, Hutchings JC. The segmental pectoralis major muscle flap: a function-preserving procedure. *Plast Reconstr Surg.* 1985;75(6):825-830.
6. Ascherman JA, Patel SM, Malhotra SM, Smith CR. Management of sternal wounds with bilateral pectoralis major myocutaneous advancement flaps in 114 consecutively treated patients: refinements in technique and outcomes analysis. *Plast Reconstr Surg.* 2004;114(3):676-683.
7. Arnold PG, Pairolero PC. Chest-wall reconstruction: an account of 500 consecutive patients. *Plast Reconstr Surg.* 1996;98:804-810.
8. Davidson SP, Clemens MW, Armstrong D, et al. Sternotomy wounds: rectus flap versus modified pectoral reconstruction. *Plast Reconstr Surg.* 2007;120(4):929-934.

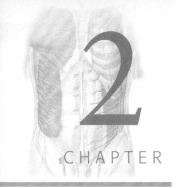

2 CHAPTER

Sternal Debridement and Application of Muscle Flaps

Sean M. Fisher, Jeff J. Kim, and David H. Song

DEFINITION

- Deep sternal wound infections (DSWIs) are a feared postoperative complication of open heart surgery, with a reported global incidence of 0.25% to 2.8%.[1]
  - Sternal infections may be classified based on the system popularized by Pairolero and Arnold[1-3]:
    - Type I: Demonstrate serosanguineous drainage without evidence of deep soft tissue, bone, or cartilage involvement.
    - Type II: Demonstrate purulent drainage, cellulitis, and mediastinal suppuration.
    - Type III: Osteomyelitis, costochondritis, and/or foreign bodies are commonly present.
  - Alternative classification systems are based on the extent of damage to underlying tissue or relative anatomic location of the wound.[2]
  - Sternal necrosis can result in critical-size defects in the thoracic wall with exposure of underlying thoracic structures, necessitating the involvement of reconstructive surgeons.
- Sternal nonunion is defined as pain or clicking with objective measures of instability lasting greater than 3 months, albeit in the absence of signs of infection.[4]

ANATOMY

- The thoracic cage has mechanical and protective properties, serving as an attachment point for a number of chest wall muscles and acting as a key protective barrier for thoracic organs.
- The sternum acts as a cornerstone of the thoracic cage and is composed of the manubrium, the body, and the xiphoid process.
  - Manubrium
    - Superior most aspect of the sternum, helping anchor the pectoral girdle via the sternoclavicular joints, and as the anterior aspect of the superior thoracic aperture (**FIG 1A**)
    - Sternal angle serves as a critical surface landmark, composed of the manubrium angled posteriorly to the body at the manubriosternal joint.
    - Contains articular surfaces at the superolateral aspect, allowing for articulation with the left and right clavicle
    - Facets inferior to the sternoclavicular joints represent the site of attachment for the first costal cartilage, whereas demifacets at the inferolateral aspect allow for articulation with the superior aspect of the second costal cartilage (**FIG 1B**).
    - Serves as the site of attachment for the sternocleidomastoid, pectoralis major, sternohyoid, and sternothyroid muscles

- Body
  - Narrow, flat bone that is oriented longitudinally with palpable transverse ridges
  - Contains facets along the lateral aspect, allowing for articulation with the 3rd to 6th costal cartilages
  - Demifacets at the superior and inferior aspect allow for shared articulation between the 2nd and 7th costal cartilages with the adjacent sternal components (see **FIG 1B**).
  - Serves as the major attachment for the pectoralis major
  - Xiphoid process
    - Inferior aspect of the sternum and demonstrates variable morphology
    - Along with the body of the sternum, the xiphoid process articulates with the 7th costal cartilage via superolateral demifacets.
    - Serves as an attachment point for the diaphragm and rectus abdominis

PATHOGENESIS

- The primary insult in DSWIs may begin as a site of focal sternal osteomyelitis without external evidence of infection when sternal fixation is inadequate or may be due to skin breakdown with subsequent penetration of bacteria to deeper layers.
- Presentation often demonstrates a highly variable time course, ranging from days to years following cardiac surgery.[2]
- In cases requiring surgical debridement, Gram-positive organisms, namely *Staphylococcus*, have been found to be overwhelmingly responsible for infection.[5]
- In addition to male sex, conditions associated with patients' habitual state have been shown to be risk factors in the development of DSWIs and associated morbidity and mortality.
  - Diabetes mellitus (DM), COPD, BMI over 30, chronic steroid use, and smoking are known predictors of DSWI.
  - Bilateral internal mammary artery (IMA) grafting for CABG also increases the risk of postoperative DSWI, as it may reduce sternal vascularity, and should be avoided in those patients with DM and other high-risk comorbidities.[1,2]
- Sternal nonunion represents a similar, yet separate, diagnosis that may necessitate sternal debridement as a treatment strategy.
- Both intrinsic and extrinsic factors may contribute to an increased propensity in developing sternal nonunion following median sternotomy or traumatic injury.
  - Factors that are dependent on patients' habitual state closely mimic those risk factors associated with DSWI.
    - These include DM, COPD, obesity, chronic steroid use, malnutrition, and osteoporosis.[4]
  - Intraoperative technical errors, as well as postsurgical factors, may also play a role in the development of sternal nonunion.[4]

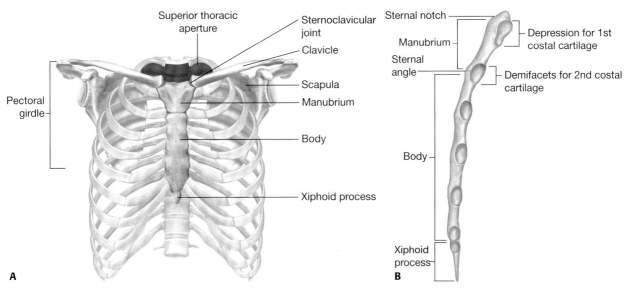

FIG 1 • A. The sternum represents an anterior anchor point for the pectoral girdle, attaching via the sternoclavicular joint bilaterally. The superior thoracic aperture, noted in *red*, houses the trachea, esophagus, and thoracic duct, as well as a variety of nerves and vessels. **B.** Lateral view of the sternum demonstrates the manubrium, the body, and the xiphoid process with corresponding facets and demifacets for articulation with corresponding costal cartilage.

NATURAL HISTORY

- Julian et al. first described the median sternotomy in 1957, which initially met resistance due to reported rates of infection exceeding 5%.[1]
- As the technique gained traction in open cardiac surgery, and advances were made allowing for surgical intervention in patients with more extensive comorbidities, DSWIs began being described with incidence ranging from 3% to 5%[1,6,7] and associated mortality as high as 50%.[1,2]
- Classification of the wound often typifies the time course to presentation[1,2]:
  - Type I: Often presents within the first few days following surgery
  - Type II: Typically occurs a few weeks following surgery
  - Type III: Can occur months to years following surgery
- A second classification system proposed by Jones et al. attempts to further qualify the severity of the wound by addressing the extent of involvement in underlying tissues[8]:
  - Type 1a: Superficial wound with skin and subcutaneous tissue dehiscence
  - Type 1b: Superficial wound with exposure of the sutured deep fascia
  - Type 2a: Deep wound with exposed bone and stable wired sternotomy
  - Type 2b: Deep wound with exposed bone and unstable wired sternotomy
  - Type 3a: Deep wound with exposed necrotic or fractured bone, unstable sternotomy, and exposed heart
  - Type 3b: Type 2a, 2b, or 3a wound with septicemia
- Marked improvement in outcomes has been demonstrated, due to the utilization of myocutaneous flaps for reconstruction, with more recent morbidity reported as low as 8% to 15%.[1,2]

PATIENT HISTORY AND PHYSICAL FINDINGS

- Surgical history, physical exam, and history of trauma are imperative in the initial assessment of patients suspected of

having a DSWI or sternal malunion, as well as complaints of ongoing pain, sternal clicking, or subjective instability.
- Signs of infection may vary based on the time of presentation in relation to patients' history of cardiac surgery, as laid out by Pairolero and Arnold.[3]
- Physical examination
  - Inspect the skin for median sternotomy scar.
  - Assess whether evidence of DSWI is present such as erythema, purulent discharge, fever, wound dehiscence, or frank necrotic tissue.
  - If an open wound is present, the extent of necrotic tissue should be assessed by evaluating the viability of different flap options based on the expected extent of excision.
  - Stability of the sternum can be assessed with direct palpation.
  - If sternal nonunion is suspected, clicking may be elicited with movement.

IMAGING

- Computed tomography (CT) is the mainstay of imaging support when suspicion of DSWI is high, allowing for the evaluation of the depth of dehiscence as well as sternal nonunion[5] (**FIG 2A**).
- ^{99m}Tc-leukocyte imaging also has value in the early detection of DSWIs (**FIG 2B**).

NONOPERATIVE MANAGEMENT

- Nonoperative management is based on the extent of the infection, evidence of instability, and clinic signs of systemic infection.
- Mainstay of nonoperative management includes long-term IV antibiotics and incision and drainage of limited/superficial abscess collection, followed by local wound care with frequent wet to dry gauzes, topical antibiotics, or negative pressure wound therapy (NPWT).[5]

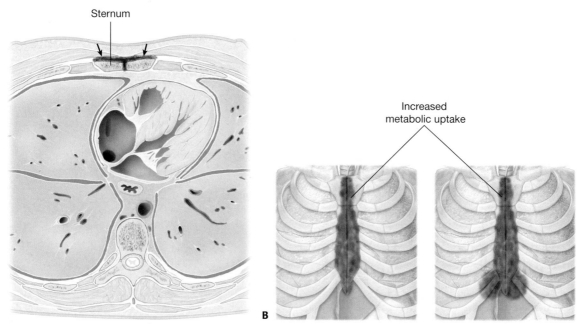

FIG 2 • **A.** Axial CT demonstrating fluid collection, as indicated by the *arrows*, resulting in the separation of the sternum into two distinct halves. **B.** 99mTc-leukocyte scan taken at 4 hours (*left*) and 20 hours (*right*) after leukocyte radiolabeling. Diffuse uptake of the distal sternum is noted at 4 hours, with lateral extension at 20 hours. Surgical intervention confirmed infection in areas noted to have enhanced signaling. 20 hours after leukocyte radiolabeling. Diffuse uptake of the distal sternum is noted at 4 hours, with lateral extension at 20 hours. Surgical intervention confirmed infection in areas noted to have enhanced signaling.

SURGICAL MANAGEMENT

- The need for surgical intervention is dependent on wound severity and may include complete debridement of devitalized tissue, removal of preexisting hardware, fixation of sternal fragments, partial or total sternectomy, and eventual reconstruction utilizing myocutaneous flaps.[2,8,9]
- Indications for sternal debridement include the presence of devitalized tissue, positive Gram stains of parasternal fluid, and notable sternal instability.[8,9]
- Timely surgical debridement has been shown to result in shorter hospital stays and fewer postoperative hospitalizations.[10]
  - Depending on the extent of devitalized tissue and time course since median sternotomy, either limited or complete debridement may be indicated.[8,11]
  - Single-stage intervention, with immediate flap coverage, has been shown to reduce the duration of hospital stays.[1,8,11]
  - Serial stage approaches utilizing bridging NPWT may avoid the need for a vascularized flap or reduce the total number of flaps needed.
- Consideration for flap selection is based largely on:
  - Anatomic location/extent of the defect
  - Prior surgical history, including prior CABG requiring IMA grafting, as this may prevent the use of pedicled flaps based on IMA perforators or the utilization of the IMA as recipient vessels in free flap transfer

Preoperative Planning

- Usually, a thorough history and physical examination are sufficient for preoperative planning. Evaluation of imaging studies can sometimes help elucidate less obvious infection and sternal nonunion.
- Given the extent of defect, adequacy of debridement may not be known until the time of the procedure. Surgeons should be prepared for all possibilities, including the need for sternal fixation, definitive closure/reconstruction after debridement, and various appropriate flap options given patients' surgical history (ie, previous IMA harvest for CABG) and location/size of defect.

Positioning

- In general, the patient is placed supine on the operating table with arms abducted and secured to an arm board.
  - If not already onboard, preoperative evaluation by cardiothoracic surgery should be performed, and need for groin prep or possible cardiopulmonary bypass should be discussed.
- If latissimus dorsi flap is planned, the patient will need to be positioned in lateral decubitus position and repositioned intraoperatively to supine once flap is raised.

Approach

- Sternal debridement should proceed from superficial to deep, carefully and continually reassessing the viability of tissues at the margins as further debridement is carried out.
- Depending on the location and extent of the final wound/defect following debridement, separate skin incisions/approaches frequently may be necessary for accessing local/regional muscles to be used for reconstruction.
  - Approaches for access/harvest of specific flaps will be discussed in subsequent respective chapters.

■ Sternal Debridement

- Generous debridement of all devitalized tissue is imperative to avoid complications and need for return to the OR for additional operations.
- Debridement should start superficially with soft tissue, continually assessing the viability of tissue at the margins and the need to continue further.

- Marginal/questionable tissue should be as aggressively debrided as safely possible down to clearly healthy, bleeding tissue.
- When in doubt, tissue/bone cultures should be sent to help tailor postoperative antibiotic regimen.
- In case of bony involvement or suspected osteomyelitis, any prior hardware should be removed before bone debridement is carried out using rongeurs and curettes.

■ Sternal Fixation

- Depending on the location/extent/etiology of sternal defect, a variety of techniques have been described for fixation of fragments and nonunions.
  - Obliquely oriented sternal wiring, figure-of-eight peristernal wiring, and parasternal wiring help by adding additional lateral support.
  - Steel banding, polymer tapes, and absorbable sutures can be used for repair of nonunions.

- Plate-based systems, such as the SternaLock System (Biomet Microfixation, Warsaw, IN), can be used when adequate bone stock is available for secure purchase from adjacent sides.
  - Requires close approximation of sternal halves using bone-reducing forceps
  - A variety of plate configurations can be used in conjunction with monocortical, self-tapping screws to allow for adequate union of sternal halves.
  - Provides rigid fixation and minimizes recurrence of nonunion/sternal wounds

■ Workhorse Muscle Flap Options for Reconstruction

- Detailed techniques of harvesting each flap will be discussed in their respective chapters.

■ Pectoralis Major

- Common choice of repair for ease of harvest and reliability of flap, especially for defects involving the superior aspect of the sternum
- Minimal functional donor-site morbidity especially compared to other options such as the rectus abdominis flap

- Can be used either as an advancement rotational flap based on the thoracoacromial pedicle for superior defects or a turnover flap based on IMA perforators for more distal and inferior defects, as well as for obliteration of significant dead space in the midline
- Secondary segmental blood supply may not be available in patients with history of IMA harvest.

■ Latissimus Dorsi

- Large, well-vascularized/reliable muscular flap is useful in the case of lateral defects—may not reach anterior midline defects especially superiorly

- Subscapular system can be used to harvest composite flap when concomitant bony reconstruction is also desired.
- Require intraoperative repositioning for harvest and inset

■ Rectus Abdominis

- Good for inferior midline defects
- Not available for patients with history of CABG and IMA harvest as pedicled flap would likely require a rotational flap based off the superior epigastric artery

- More significant functional donor-site morbidity (eg, hernias) when compared to pectoralis or latissimus flap

■ Omentum

- Can be useful in extensive defects with significant dead space/volume requirement for reconstruction as the omentum is able to conform to the recesses of deep wounds.
- Highly vascularized and has a high concentration of vascular endothelial growth factor, promoting extensive angiogenesis

- However, requires more invasive entry into the peritoneal cavity with risk of spreading infection and postoperative ventral hernia formation
- Use of omental flap for sternal defect reconstruction is largely of historical importance prior to rise in use/availability of various myocutaneous options.

PEARLS AND PITFALLS

Debridement	■ Early and aggressive debridement is imperative in decreasing the morbidity and mortality especially in DSWIs.
	■ In most cases, cardiothoracic surgery will already be involved, but if not, preoperative evaluation and intraoperative assistance/standby should be arranged prior to performing any excisional debridement.
Antibiotics	■ Empiric therapy should consist of broad coverage against Gram-positive cocci and Gram-negative bacilli with special consideration for methicillin-resistant *Staphylococcus aureus* based on its prevalence at individual institutions. Fluid and tissue cultures should be obtained when possible, to help tailor appropriate regimen.
Flap selection	■ For most sternal wound/defects requiring reconstruction, pectoralis major is a reasonable first choice given its ease of accessibility and reliability as a muscular flap; latissimus dorsi and rectus abdominis should be considered next if pectoralis is not available/contraindicated.
Negative pressure Wound therapy	■ In the absence of active infection or exposure of vital intrathoracic structures, NPWT can often be used to temporize urgent need for operative intervention.
	■ Well-documented efficacy in reducing wound size and promoting wound healing—can often reduce the complexity or all together need for surgical intervention.[7]

POSTOPERATIVE CARE

- After debridement without reconstruction
  - Frequent local wound care should be performed to keep wounds clean—wet to dry gauze or topical ointment dressings should be changed 2 or 3 times a day, whereas NPWT should be changed once every 2 to 3 days, especially if there is question of residual infection.
  - Wound cultures should be followed/repeated as necessary to tailor antibiotic regimen.
  - Depending on the presence of defect/exposure of critical structures that ultimately needs to be addressed with reconstruction, activity should be limited until repair is completed.
- General considerations after reconstruction with muscle flap (flap-specific postoperative care issues will be further discussed in respective chapters)
  - Drains: seroma is one of the most frequent complications following a large muscle flap harvest.
    - Conservative management regarding drain duration minimizes the chance of postoperative seroma.
    - Criterion of less than 25 mL per drain per day, for 2 successive days, is often used, though some reports note that 3-week duration regardless of output is associated with lower seroma rate.
  - Wound dehiscence:
    - Requires wound irrigation and light gauze packing
    - The presence of healthy, viable muscle tissue without evidence of vital structure exposure allows for secondary wound closure.
    - Consider supportive brassiere in those patients with large cup size breasts, as this population has been shown to have a greater risk of wound dehiscence following mediastinal operations.[12]
  - Activity:
    - Four to six weeks of rest following procedure
    - Consistent physical therapy for range of motion, flexibility, and strengthening should be started to rehabilitate and compensate for the loss of muscle function from donor site.

OUTCOMES

- Immediate consideration of sternal debridement with single-stage flap reconstruction has been shown to reduce morbidity and mortality when compared to those who underwent sternal preservation therapy with attempted rewiring.[13]
  - Reported mortality following immediate debridement has been reported as 0% to 1%, whereas mortality in those who underwent delayed debridement ranges from 14% to 47%.[12]
- No consensus as to whether single-stage intervention with immediate flap coverage or delayed debridement with bridging NPWT results in improved morbidity or mortality.
- Jones et al. retrospectively reviewed 186 patients who had undergone sternal wound reconstruction over a 20-year period.[8]
  - Flap closure complications (35), recurrent infection/wound dehiscence (24), and reexploration/wound necrosis (11) were among the most common complications noted.
  - Regression analysis showed that hypertension, smoking, previous sternotomy, IMA harvest, and previous sternal reconstruction were statistically significant risk factors in predicting outcomes.
  - Mortality was 9.1%, and those patients presenting with septicemia at the time of diagnosis had a risk of death 11 times greater than those who were not septic.
- Both early surgical debridement and single-stage repair have been shown to reduce the average hospital stay in patients with DSWI.[8,10]

COMPLICATIONS

- Hematoma/seroma
- Wound dehiscence
- Delayed union or nonunion following sternal fixation
- Partial or complete flap loss
- Donor-site complications (loss of muscle function, contour deformity, ventral hernia)
- Recurrent wound infection

REFERENCES

1. Juhl AA, Koudahl V, Damsgaard TE. Deep sternal wound infection after open heart surgery: reconstructive options. *Scand Cardiovasc J.* 2012;46:254-261.
2. Greig AVH, Geh JLC, Khanduja V, et al. Choice of flap for the management of deep sternal wound infection: an anatomical classification. *J Plast Reconstr Aesthet Surg.* 2007;60:372-378.
3. Pairolero PC, Arnold PG. Management of infected median sternotomy wounds. *Ann Thorac Surg.* 1986;42:1-2.

4. Chepla K, Salgado C, Tang C, et al. Late complications of chest wall reconstruction: management of painful sternal nonunion. *Semin Plast Surg.* 2011;25:98-108.

5. Singh K, Anderson E, Harper JG. Overview and management of sternal wound infection. *Semin Plast Surg.* 2011;25:25-33.

6. Zor MH, Acipayam M, Bayram H, et al. Single-stage repair of the anterior chest wall following sternal destruction complicated by mediastinitis. *Surg Today.* 2014;44:1476-1482.

7. Agarwal JP, Ogilvie M, Wu LC, et al. Vacuum-assisted closure for sternal wounds: a first-line therapeutic management approach. *Plast Reconstr Surg.* 2005;116:1035-1040.

8. Jones G, Jurkiewicz MJ, Bostwick J, et al. Management of the infected median sternotomy wound with muscle flaps: the Emory 20-year experience. *Ann Surg.* 1997;225:766.

9. Douville EC, Asaph JW, Dworkin RJ, et al. Sternal preservation: a better way to treat most sternal wound complications after cardiac surgery. *Ann Thorac Surg.* 2004;78:1659-1664.

10. Wu L, et al. A National study of the impact of initial débridement timing on outcomes for patients with deep sternal wound infection. *Plast Reconstr Surg.* 2016;137:414e-423e.

11. Preminger BA, Yaghoobzadeh Y, Ascherman JA. Management of sternal wounds by limited debridement and partial bilateral pectoralis major myocutaneous advancement flaps in 25 patients: a less invasive approach. *Ann Plast Surg.* 2014;72:446-450.

12. Copeland M, Senkowski C, Ulcickas M, et al. Breast size as a risk factor for sternal wound complications following cardiac surgery. *Arch Surg.* 1994;129:757-759.

13. Cabbabe EB, Cabbabe SW. Immediate versus delayed one-stage sternal débridement and pectoralis muscle flap reconstruction of deep sternal wound infections. *Plast Reconstr Surg.* 2009;123:1490-1494.

14. Moor EV, Neuman RA, Weinberg A, et al. Transposition of the great omentum for infected sternotomy wounds in cardiac surgery: report of 16 cases and review of published reports. *Scand J Plast Reconstr Surg Hand Surg.* 1999;33:25-29.

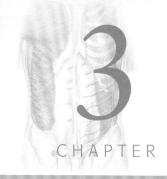

3 CHAPTER

Rectus Abdominis Flap for Thoracic Reconstruction

Maureen Beederman and David H. Song

DEFINITION

- Chest wall defects can involve the skin, subcutaneous tissue, muscle, rib, and underlying thoracic viscera.
- The rectus abdominis muscle flap (with or without overlying skin) can be used for chest wall defects and is especially useful for anterior, lower sternal, and parasternal defects.[1]
  - A vertical rectus abdominis myocutaneous (VRAM) flap contains both rectus abdominis muscle and overlying skin and subcutaneous tissue, supplied by a pedicle and its musculocutaneous perforators, with skin paddle oriented in a vertical direction.
  - A transverse rectus abdominis myocutaneous (TRAM) flap contains both rectus abdominis muscle and overlying skin and subcutaneous tissue, supplied by a pedicle and its musculocutaneous perforators, with skin paddle oriented in a horizontal direction.
- Rectus abdominis flaps can be used to fill a large amount of dead space or to cover prosthetic materials used for chest wall stabilization, such as methyl methacrylate, mesh, or titanium plates.

ANATOMY

- The rectus abdominis muscle is a Mathes-Nahai type III muscle with two dominant vascular pedicles: the superior epigastric artery and inferior epigastric artery.
  - The superior epigastric artery is a continuation of the distal portion of the internal mammary artery (IMA), which originally arises from the subclavian artery.
  - The inferior epigastric artery arises from the external iliac artery.
  - The rectus abdominis muscle has a predictable blood supply, making it a dependable option for reconstruction.
- Secondary blood supply also arises from intercostal arteries.
- Rectus abdominis muscle consists of two muscle bellies separated by the linea alba.
  - Each muscle is enclosed in fascia, which is formed from the aponeurosis of the external oblique, internal oblique, and transversus abdominis muscles.
  - Rectus abdominis muscle origin: xiphoid and 5th to 8th costal cartilages
  - Rectus abdominis muscle insertion: pubic symphysis
- The rectus abdominis muscle is thick, bulky, and durable and is good for filling dead space.
- One can raise the muscle in a vertical (VRAM) or transverse (TRAM) manner, depending on the size and orientation of the defect.

PATHOGENESIS

- Chest wall defects can occur as a result of trauma, tumor resection, infection, congenital disorders, or radiation-induced necrosis.
- Infectious sources include empyema, bronchopleural fistula, or mediastinitis after cardiothoracic surgery.
  - Sternal wound infection risk factors include obesity, diabetes, COPD, and bilateral harvest of IMAs during prior cardiothoracic surgery (compromising blood supply to the sternum and overlying tissues).[2]

PATIENT HISTORY AND PHYSICAL FINDINGS

- Patient history is important to consider when planning for chest wall reconstruction, as it will affect the reconstructive decision-making and options.
  - Consider previous attempts at chest wall closure and reconstruction, specifically if other local flaps have been used, including latissimus dorsi, pectoralis major, or omental flap.
  - Significant prior abdominal surgery, including autologous breast reconstruction or abdominoplasty, which could affect blood supply to the rectus abdominis muscle
  - One or both IMAs may have been harvested for prior cardiac surgery, which may adversely affect the superior epigastric artery blood supply to rectus abdominis musculature and need to be closely examined. However, owing to extensive intercostal collaterals, mostly a superiorly based flap is viable.
  - The presence of an ostomy or urostomy can potentially affect utility of rectus abdominis muscle.
  - A history of diabetes or history of smoking can affect small vessels and compromise blood supply to the skin of VRAM/TRAM flaps.
  - Other risk factors that can compromise reconstruction include obesity, malnutrition, older age, steroid use, and other comorbidities.
- Discussion of future treatment planning with thoracic surgeon
  - Determine whether the patient has had or will need to undergo future radiation therapy, as this will affect local tissue quality and flap options.
- Physical examination
  - Assess chest wall space requiring reconstruction, including the presence of mediastinitis or other localized infections, bronchopleural fistula, and exposure of vital organs.
  - Determine whether bony reconstruction is required.
    - Skeletal support is most often required for lateral and posterolateral wall defects.[1]
    - Number of ribs removed and history of chest wall radiation can affect the need for structural support.

IMAGING

- Imaging may not be required for all patients.
- CT of the chest and abdomen may be done to assess extent of tumor, invasion of surrounding structures, amount of dead space, and possible fluid collections or infection.
- Assess abdominal wall integrity, including the presence of any hernias.

NONOPERATIVE MANAGEMENT

- If no exposure of underlying vital structures, consider using negative pressure wound therapy (NPWT) to manage wound initially.
  - Should be used only in clean wounds; if infection is present, will require appropriate debridement of all infected tissues prior to use of NPWT.

SURGICAL MANAGEMENT

- Coverage of chest wall defects can either be immediate, commonly following tumor resection, or delayed, commonly following mediastinitis or other chest wall infections.

PREOPERATIVE PLANNING

- Must consider whether skeletal stabilization is required, especially if ribs are resected.
  - Skeletal chest wall reconstruction is outside the scope of this chapter but an important consideration when planning reconstruction and deciding the best reconstructive option.

- If more than four or five ribs are resected or if total sternotomy is performed, skeletal reconstruction is most often needed to prevent flail chest and maximize pulmonary function and to protect underlying vital organs.
- For pedicled rectus abdominis reconstruction, consider whether IMA (one or both) has been sacrificed during previous cardiac surgery and check for viability when raising flap. Typically, due to a rich network of collaterals from the 8th intercostal network, the flap should be suitable.
  - If IMA has been harvested, determine if enough time has passed for intercostal collaterals to form; consider basing flap superiorly off intercostal collaterals.[3]
- If rectus abdominis flap is being used for filling of dead space after infection, ensure that all devitalized and infected components of the wound have been thoroughly debrided prior to flap insetting.

POSITIONING

- For harvesting the rectus abdominis flap, supine positioning is optimal, with arms abducted on arm boards.
- Depending on the location of the defect, the patient may also be in lateral decubitus positioning, which still allows harvest of the rectus muscle.

APPROACH

- Based on the size and shape of the defect, consider whether muscle only or musculocutaneous flap is required.

■ Rectus Abdominis Musculocutaneous Flap

- Create a template to design your flap based on the proposed defect size.
- Design the flap either vertically (VRAM) or transversely (TRAM), depending on the location and size of defect (**TECH FIG 1A**).
  - The flap should be designed to capture periumbilical perforators (**TECH FIG 1B**).
  - Handheld Doppler can be used preoperatively to locate possible perforators prior to starting flap elevation.
- Make an incision just lateral to the midline on the side of the muscle to be harvested.
  - If a sternotomy incision is already present, simply extend this incision inferiorly.
- Make incision through skin and subcutaneous tissue and dissect to the medial and lateral perforators in order to spare as much anterior sheath fascia as possible.
- Incise fascia longitudinally, just lateral and medial to the perforators.
- Dissect laterally, superiorly, and inferiorly, until desired size is reached. Ensure that all suitable musculocutaneous perforators are identified and protected during flap elevation.
- Identify both the superior epigastric artery and the deep inferior epigastric artery.
- Once the deep inferior epigastric artery has been identified, ligate it close to its origin at the pubic symphysis.

- Divide the rectus abdominis muscle from its insertion on the pubic symphysis or more superior to the pubic symphysis if not using the entire muscle.
- Interpolate rectus abdominis myocutaneous flap into defect space (**TECH FIG 1C,D**).
  - Flap can either be tunneled below an existing skin bridge or interpolated into defect.
- Close anterior rectus sheath primarily in a figure-of-eight fashion.
  - If donor-site defect is too large, mesh may have to be used to prevent hernia formation.
- Inset the flap in a layered fashion, ensuring that there is no tension on the vascular supply.
- Place closed suction drains in both the donor and recipient sites.

Pedicled Rectus Abdominis Muscle-Only Flap

- Harvesting a muscle-only rectus abdominis flap is similar to the VRAM/TRAM harvest, with a few key distinctions.
- Consider using a rectus abdominis flap if there is enough local chest wall skin for coverage or if planning to harvest a split-thickness skin graft for coverage.
- Make a midline incision through the skin and subcutaneous tissue down to the anterior rectus fascia.
- Incise rectus fascia longitudinally, just lateral to the midline.
- Dissect laterally and inferiorly according to your template defect size until desired size is reached.
  - The entirety of the rectus abdominis muscle or just a portion may be used.

TECHNIQUES

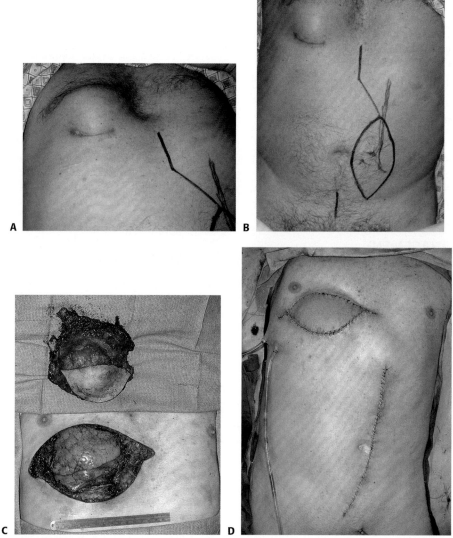

TECH FIG 1 • A. Large right chest wall chondrosarcoma to be resected, just inferior and medial to right nipple, measuring more than 5 cm. **B.** A contralateral vertical rectus abdominis musculocutaneous flap is designed based on the above defect. The flap is designed near the umbilicus to capture the periumbilical perforators, which are marked in *red*. **C.** Final defect was 13 × 8 cm with exposed lung and diaphragm. The resected mass involved two ribs and the parietal pleura. In this specific case, Gore-Tex mesh was used to prevent lung herniation prior to insetting of the rectus abdominis flap. **D.** Postoperative picture showing closure of the defect with the vertical rectus abdominis musculocutaneous flap and midline closure of the donor site. One Jackson-Pratt drain is seen in the recipient site, as well as a nearby chest tube.

- During dissection, identify the superior epigastric artery (which is the artery the flap will be based on) and the deep inferior epigastric artery.
- Ligate musculocutaneous perforators, if only harvesting muscle and not overlying skin and subcutaneous tissue.
- Once the deep inferior epigastric artery has been identified, ligate it close to its origin at the pubic symphysis.

- Interpolate rectus abdominis muscle into defect space, either tunneled below a skin and subcutaneous tissue bridge or directly into the defect.
- Close anterior rectus fascia primarily or using a piece of mesh if any significant tension is present or for added support.
- Inset rectus abdominis muscle flap into defect and close surrounding local skin in layers over the muscle.

PEARLS AND PITFALLS

Supercharging arterial supply or venous drainage	■ Consider performing microsurgical anastomosis to aid with venous drainage or arterial supply if recipient vessels are available by hooking up the divided deep inferior epigastric artery and/or vein.
Placement of Jackson-Pratt drains	■ It is important to place drains in the recipient site, and sometimes in the donor site, to prevent hematoma formation, which can lead to flap compromise.
Prior chest wall surgery or radiation therapy	■ Knowledge of prior reconstructive efforts and/or history of radiation is important prior to making a decision on flap design and elevation, as this could affect the blood supply and overall soft tissue coverage of the defect.
Intercostal artery–based rectus abdominis flap	■ If bilateral internal mammary arteries have previously been utilized or damaged (often the case with cardiothoracic surgery), consider harvesting rectus abdominis flap based on intercostal artery perforators.
Identify and protect key blood vessels	■ For superiorly based pedicled flaps, ensure that the superior epigastric artery is identified and protected. ■ It is also important to identify the deep inferior epigastric artery prior to dividing it.

POSTOPERATIVE CARE

- Jackson-Pratt drains are often placed in both the donor and recipient sites.
  - Abdominal drain (donor site) is typically placed oto wall suction.
  - Chest drain (recipient site) is typically placed oto bulb suction.
  - Discontinue drains once output is less than 30 cc for 2 consecutive 24-hour periods.
- Patient will often require a chest tube, if the pleural cavity is violated. This is managed by the thoracic surgery team.
- Flap monitoring, if possible
  - If skin paddle is present, monitor warmth, color, skin turgor, and capillary refill.
  - Tight inset may lead to arterial compromise or venous congestion, so clinical monitoring is important even though this is not a free flap.
- Avoid heavy lifting during immediate postoperative period to avoid hernias.

OUTCOMES

- Use of vascularized muscle flaps, including the rectus abdominis flap, has decreased morbidity and mortality associated with chest wall infections and tumor resection.
- Rectus abdominis flaps have been shown to be superior to other flap options (including pectoralis advancement flaps) for coverage of the inferior portion of the central chest wall.[4]

COMPLICATIONS

- Hematoma and seroma formation
- Compromise of vascular pedicle
- Partial or total flap lost
  - If flap is superiorly based, the prior harvest of IMA for cardiac surgery can lead to distal tip necrosis, most commonly located at the superior portion of the chest wall.
- Hernia formation
- Wound dehiscence of either the donor or recipient site

REFERENCES

1. Losken A, Thourani VH, Carlson GW, et al. A reconstructive algorithm for plastic surgery following extensive chest wall resection. *Br J Plast Surg*. 2004;57(4):295-302.
2. Clemens MW, Evans KK, Mardini S, Arnold PG. Introduction to chest wall reconstruction: anatomy and physiology of the chest and indications for chest wall reconstruction. *Semin Plast Surg*. 2011;25(1): 5-15.
3. Nguyen DT, Aoki M, Hyakusoku H, Ogawa R. Chest wall reconstruction of severe mediastinitis with intercostal artery-based pedicled vertical rectus abdominis muscle flap with oblique-designed skin paddle. *Ann Plast Surg*. 2011;67(3):269-271.
4. Davison SP, Clemes MW, Armstrong D, et al. Sternotomy wounds: rectus flap versus modified pectoral reconstruction. *Plast Reconstr Surg*. 2007;120(4):929-934.

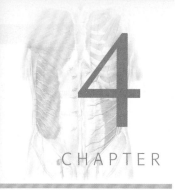

4

CHAPTER

Omental Flap for Thoracic Reconstruction

Amir Inbal and David H. Song

DEFINITION

- The omentum is rich in vasculature, lymphatics, and fat and serves an important immunologic function within the abdominal cavity.
  - The original anatomical term *epiploic* is derived from the Greek word *epipleein*, which means to float on. It was so named to reflect how the omentum "floated" anterior to the intestines.
- The omental flap can be harvested as a pedicled or free flap and is commonly used as a pedicled flap for thoracic reconstruction.
- These flaps are historically used to revascularize the myocardium and cover intra-aortic balloon pumps and ventricular assist devices.
- Thoracic and chest well defects are attributable to congenital malformations or acquired deformities and can cause significant physical and psychological morbidity.

ANATOMY

- The region of the thorax amenable to pedicled omental flap reconstruction includes the central and lateral thorax and its contents, most commonly the sternum, pericardium, pleural cavity, and at times the overlying skin. When needed, the flap can extend to reach beyond the chest.
- Thorax: Composed of the skin, muscles, bones, and internal organs/structures located between the neck and the abdomen
  - Muscles include pectoralis major, pectoralis minor, serratus anterior, serratus posterior, rectus abdominis, external oblique, intercostal muscles, latissimus dorsi, and trapezius.
  - Thoracic skeleton
    - Ribs—form the rib cage by attaching to vertebral bodies posteriorly and sternum anteriorly (variable)
    - Sternum—long, flat bone in the center of the chest composed of the manubrium, body, and xiphoid process
    - Thoracic vertebrae
  - Internal organs/structures that should be addressed when reconstructing the thorax include the lungs, heart, pericardium, pleura and pleural space, esophagus, trachea and bronchus, superior vena cava, thymus gland, diaphragm, liver, gallbladder, pancreas, duodenum, and pancreas.
  - Dominant blood supply provided by paired internal mammary arteries (branch of subclavian artery)
    - Run posterior to costal cartilage adjacent to sternum with one or two venae comitantes.
    - Interconnect with transverse cervical, thoracoacromial, lateral thoracic, and posterior intercostal arteries.
    - Cutaneous perforating vessels supply overlying tissues and skin

- Omentum
  - The omental flap is based on the greater omentum found in the abdominal cavity (**FIG 1A**).
  - It contains visceral peritoneum, fat, lymphatic tissue, a rich vascular arcade, and macrophage collections (milky spots).
  - It is a nonneurotized flap.
  - It originates from the peritoneum of the greater curvature of the stomach. From here, the two layers of the visceral peritoneum descend anterior to the small intestines, folding backward upon itself at a variable level within the abdominal or pelvic cavity to ascend and enclose the transverse colon before attaching to the posterior abdominal wall. With the two layers of visceral peritoneum folded upon itself, it effectively creates a four-layered structure.
  - The right border of the greater omentum may be attached to the second portion of the duodenum.
  - The left border of the greater omentum is continuous with the gastrosplenic ligament.
  - In a study of 200 cadavers and 100 patients who had abdominal surgery, the average omental length was 25 cm for men (range, 14–36 cm) and 24 cm for women (range, 14– 34 cm). The average omental width was 35 cm for men (range, 23–46 cm) and 33 cm for women (range, 20–46 cm). Size of the omental flap ranges from 300 to 1500 cm².[1]
- The greater omentum is supplied by the right and left gastroepiploic arteries, which communicate with a rich vascular network within the two layers of the greater omentum along the greater curve of the stomach (**FIG 1B**).
  - Vascular supply from the right: celiac trunk to common hepatic artery to gastroduodenal artery to right gastroepiploic artery
  - Vascular supply from the left: celiac trunk to splenic artery to left gastroepiploic artery
- The short gastric arteries originating from the splenic artery, superior to the left gastroepiploic artery, also serve as an additional source of blood supply to the omentum by multiple collateral vessels.
- The right gastroepiploic artery is usually the dominant vessel supplying the omentum. It is usually 2 to 3 mm in size, and the vein is typically larger.
- From the anastomoses of the right and left gastroepiploic arteries, the accessory, right, middle, and left omental arteries descend within the greater omentum. There is a rich connective arcade between these vessels within the omentum.
  - Five anatomic variations of the arcade have been described:[2,3]

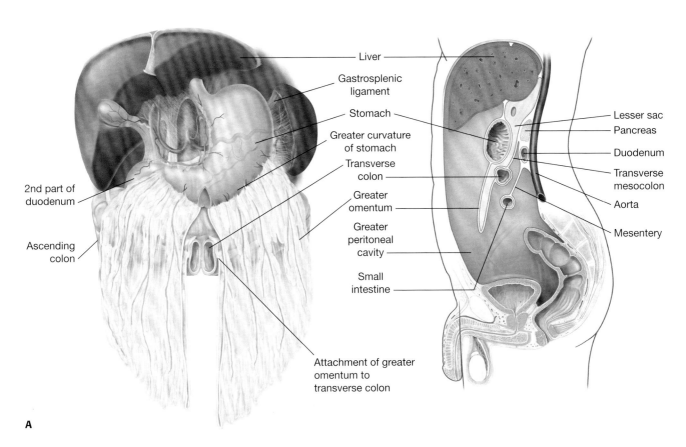

A

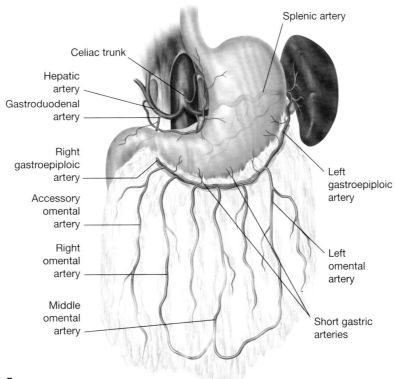

B

FIG 1 • **A.** Anatomy of the greater omentum within the abdominal cavity. **B.** Vascular anatomy of the omental flap.

- Type 1 (81.7%): middle omental artery bifurcation in the lower third, with anastomoses to the right and left omental arteries
- Type 2 (11.0%): middle omental artery bifurcation in the middle third, before anastomoses to the terminal branches of the right and left omental arteries
- Type 3 (4.5%): middle omental artery bifurcation in the upper third into two or three branches
- Type 4 (1.2%): middle omental artery absent and replaced by several short omental arteries
- Type 5 (1.6%): Left omental artery does not join the left gastroepiploic artery

- A robust venous system accompanies the arterial arcade and drains into the right and left gastroepiploic veins.

PATHOGENESIS

- Full-thickness defects of the anterior thoracic cavity can arise from a variety of causes:[4]
  - Infections
    - Necrotizing soft tissue infections
    - Mediastinitis
    - Sternal osteomyelitis
  - Fistulae
    - Bronchopleural
    - Esophagopleural
  - Trauma
  - Iatrogenic
    - Radiation injury
    - Postsurgical wound breakdown
    - Exposed hardware (eg, aortic grafts, breast implants, vertebral, sternal plates, or ventricular assist devices)
  - Neoplastic
    - Contour congenital defects of the chest wall
    - Poland syndrome
    - Other breast defects
- Flail chest: paradoxical chest movement during respiration of a portion of the rib cage after it loses continuity with the surrounding chest wall resulting in inefficient ventilation.
  - Most often the result of trauma or oncologic resection of a significant portion of the chest wall
  - May require reconstruction with soft and/or bony tissue
    - Defects 5 cm in diameter or larger generally require skeletal fixation.
- Risk factors for sternal dehiscence and infection include chronic obstructive pulmonary disease, obesity, diabetes, and bilateral harvest of the internal mammary vessels.
- Radiation-induced injury may cause significant scarring and nonfunctional tissue that will require debridement and reconstruction.

NATURAL HISTORY

- Without adequate treatment, defects of the anterior thorax can lead to devastating consequences including paradoxical breathing, osteomyelitis, mediastinitis, and death.
- The greater omentum can be harvested from the abdominal cavity without any major loss of function.
- Over time, the omental flap contracts slightly to "bed down" at the defect site.
- The omental flap provides soft tissue coverage only. In cases in which the chest wall is unstable due to loss of structural support, alternative methods such as wires, plates, mesh, or bony reconstruction are required.

PATIENT HISTORY AND PHYSICAL FINDINGS

- The preoperative evaluation for patients requiring thoracic reconstruction includes a detailed assessment of the etiology of the defect, the patient's underlying medical and functional status, the state of the pleural cavity, the extent of the soft tissue defect, and whether skeletal support is required and reconstructive options available.
- It is important to note whether the internal mammary vessels have been previously injured or sacrificed.
- The etiologic factors of the defect should be elicited in history taking, as well as its suitability for reconstruction.
  - Dirty or actively infected wounds or those with residual tumor are not amenable to reconstruction.
  - Bacterial cultures should be obtained and targeted antibiotic therapy started as necessary.
- A detailed medical history should be noted including cardiovascular problems, lung pathology, smoking, immunocompromise, and nutritional status.
  - As much as possible, any underlying medical condition should be corrected or optimized prior to undergoing definitive reconstruction.
- Special attention should be addressed with regard to history of previous abdominal surgery, trauma, and any other abdominal morbidity, as these may cause to preclude the omentum flap as a reconstructive option.
- Available reconstructive options or prior attempts at reconstruction should be noted.
- Physical examination
  - The skin is inspected for previous scarring, prior incisions, active infection, or radiation changes.
  - Hernias are noted. Laparoscopic surgical port site scars should be carefully searched. Any prior surgery in the abdominal cavity can lead to intra-abdominal adhesions, increasing the difficulty of omental flap harvest.
  - Missing tissues are noted.
    - Soft and/or hard tissue defects may be present.
  - Breathing mechanics are evaluated.
    - Pulmonary function tests are useful for evaluation of baseline pulmonary status.
- Routine preoperative laboratory testing should be performed.
- Obtain a baseline chest radiograph.
  - Computed tomography (CT) should be considered in cases of complex or extensive defects.
- The defect should be thoroughly examined again, if possible, under general anesthesia. The location, size, depth, and extent of the defect must be noted. Exposed vital structures such as the pericardium, major vessels, or hardware require more emergent coverage. Active infection or tumor should be excluded.
- Patients may present with postoperative sternal wounds after cardiac or mediastinal surgery.
  - Pairolero and Arnold classified wounds based on timing of presentation of infection:[4]
    - Type I—Occur soon after surgery, may contain incisional breakdown with serosanguineous discharge and/or sternal instability
    - Type II—Occur weeks after surgery, and cellulitis, mediastinal purulence, and positive cultures may be present
    - Type III—Occur months to years after surgery and contain draining sinus tracts and chronic osteomyelitis
  - Type II and III wounds often require operative reconstruction.

IMAGING

- Thoracic imaging
  - Chest radiographs in the anteroposterior and lateral dimensions can aid in assessment of the defect. Although lacking in sensitivity and specificity, they can be helpful in raising suspicions for other cardiac or lung pathology.
  - CT scans of the thorax are useful in preoperative evaluation of the thoracic structures, in delineating the extent of the defect, as well as in locating any underlying tumor or abscess.
  - Compared with CT scans, magnetic resonance imaging (MRI) scans are more sensitive at detecting osteomyelitis and evaluating the soft tissues. However, they are seldom required.
  - Vascular studies such as CT angiography may be warranted if tumor resection or trauma is thought to compromise the vascular anatomy or when extent of vascular involvement is unknown. In addition, if a free flap is planned, the vasculature anatomy can be assessed for recipient vessels.
- Abdominal imaging
  - In general, no investigations are needed to assess the omentum. In cases of previous abdominal surgery or trauma, where there may be significant adhesions or damage to the omentum, use of the omental flap would be avoided. An exception is previous laparoscopic surgery where no complications and minimal manipulation of abdominal contents have been confirmed.
  - CT of the abdominal wall may assist in evaluating patients with a history of surgery or trauma to the area.
  - Vascular studies such as CT angiography may be warranted if compromised vascular anatomy is suspected secondary to previous surgery or trauma.
  - Laparoscopic surgery enables a direct intraoperative "peak" at the omentum and its vascularity facilitating decision-making regarding its use.

DIFFERENTIAL DIAGNOSIS

- Other flaps that can be used to reconstruct defects of the anterior thoracic cavity include:
  - Pedicled flaps
    - Pectoralis major muscle flaps
      - Advancement based on the thoracoacromial blood supply
      - Turnover based on the internal mammary blood supply
    - Rectus abdominis flaps based on the superior epigastric artery
      - Muscle only
      - Myocutaneous
    - Latissimus dorsi flaps (usually for more lateral defects of the anterior thoracic cavity)
    - Internal mammary artery perforator flap
  - Free flaps

NONOPERATIVE MANAGEMENT

- When left long enough, any wound can heal without operative intervention. However, healing time, exposure of vital mediastinal structures or hardware, and the risk of intervening infection must be taken into consideration.

- There are a variety of wound dressings that can be used, ranging from simple wet-to-dry dressings to advanced silver-containing biomaterials, which are beyond the scope of this chapter.
- A useful bridge to reconstruction is the use of a negative pressure wound therapy (NPWT) system, which can aid in wound bed preparation and allow for patient and wound optimization prior to definitive wound coverage.

SURGICAL MANAGEMENT

Preoperative Planning

- The omental flap can be harvested as a pedicled or free flap. For defects of the thorax, it is commonly used as a pedicled flap.
- The size of the omental flap is variable and dependent on individual patient anatomy.[1] The reach of the pedicled omental flap depends on its size.
- Compared with muscle flaps, omental flaps allow better lining of the inferior third of the mediastinum, provide more bulk, and conform to the deep recesses of the mediastinum.[5]
- The general indications for the use of thoracic defects requiring omental flap reconstruction are[6]:
  - Full thickness in nature exposing the underlying bone, mesh (eg, ADM), hardware, or mediastinal contents
  - Where dead space obliteration in the thorax is required
  - Considered a good option for radionecrotic chest wounds, with its theoretical advantage of having immunogenic properties.
  - Foul-smelling, contaminated, or infected wounds
  - Provides a large surface area cover especially when extending the arc of rotation. If used for skin and subcutaneous tissue coverage, the omental flap can be skin grafted in the same sitting.
  - When covering a prosthetic material, musculocutaneous flaps are preferred to omentum and skin graft owing to a better seal by the former.
  - Good source of bulk providing volume for pleural defects or any dead space obliteration
  - Can plug and wrap around bronchopleural fistula.
  - Due to its donor-site morbidity risks by intra-abdominal incursion, the omentum is considered a second option when other fasciocutaneous or musculocutaneous options are unavailable and thus provides a secondary flap source when other flap options are exhausted.
- Risks of abdominal donor-site insult to the patient must be considered.
- Relative contraindications include previous abdominal trauma, surgery, or infection.

Preoperative Planning

- The thoracic defect requiring reconstruction needs to be assessed and optimized prior to definitive coverage. This may require multiple debridements and the use of NPWT and antibiotic therapy.
- We use the omental flap if there are no other pedicled flap options available to meet the reconstructive demands. Most commonly, no preoperative imaging is necessary for omental flap assessment.
- The omental flap can generally reach most of the central thorax up to the sternal notch and the lower parts of the pleural cavities (**FIG 2**). When detached only from the colon, it can reach the nipple in 75% of cases.[7]

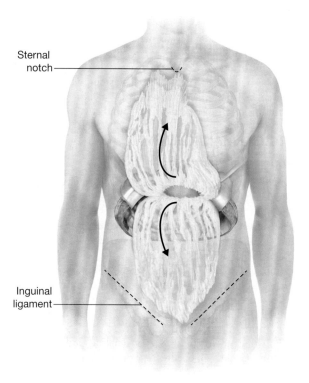

Sternal notch

Inguinal ligament

FIG 2 • Potential reach of the pedicled omental flap.

- If planned as a free flap, recipient vessel choice and preparation are required.
- Location and size of the defect are ideally identified prior to surgery to guide decisions regarding flap dimension, harvest technique, and required vascular pedicle length (ie, transposition or free flap).
- Ideally, microbiological and histological examinations should be established prior to flap harvest.
- Arc of rotation considerations when considering a pedicled omental flap:
  - Can extend to reach "knees to neck."
  - Arch includes the mediastinum and anterior, lateral, and posterior chest wall.[8]
  - A flap based on the left gastroepiploic pedicle has a greater arc of rotation compared to the right gastroepiploic vessel, which is the dominant of the two.
- Involved tissue types
  - Skin: identifying skin involvement is important for determining if a musculocutaneous flap or omentum with a skin graft is required. The decision to use omentum would be a very large surface area wound that requires skin graft use. Skin graft should be meshed to allow fluid transudation through.
  - Muscle:
    - Determine which muscles are involved and the level of functionality with remaining muscles.
    - If resection, radiation, or infection compromises a local musculocutaneous flap that would otherwise be available, this is critical to know prior to surgery as an omentum flap may be the best option for reconstruction.
  - Bony defects greater than 5 cm or involving more than 3 to 4 contiguous ribs are likely to benefit from structural support in addition to soft tissue coverage.

- Wound age
  - Acute vs chronic wounds often influences the quality of localized tissue vascularity, extent of fibrosis, and local wound healing capabilities as a result of inflammation-dependent changes.
  - This may indicate the use of the more distally located omentum with its known immunogenic properties.
  - Condition of the surrounding tissue. The presence of irradiated skin, previous scars/contractures, localized infection or inflammation, and acute trauma influences the regional tissue integrity and subsequently requires consideration while determining the reconstructive approach and complexity.
  - Patient lifestyle, general health, and functional status guide flap selection for those patients where preservation of muscular functionality is warranted.
- Prognosis
  - Life expectancy and patient-specific goals must be considered when determining complexity of reconstruction.
  - Abdominal morbidity must be considered in patients with poorer overall prognoses especially if their diseases or conditions involve abdominal morbidities.
- Preoperative patient preparation
  - Two days prior to surgery, mechanical bowel preparation is performed.
  - Patient is placed on clear liquid diet.
  - Preoperative prophylactic antibiotic regimen is given as indicated for laparotomy.
- Intraoperative considerations
  - Nasogastric tube is inserted and kept in place for 2 postoperative days.
  - Chest tube is considered for chest wall defects involving the pleura.
  - Deep venous thrombosis (DVT) prophylaxis is considered in accordance with major surgeries of the abdominal wall and thoracic surgery.
  - Two-team approach is possible and should be considered.

Positioning

- The patient is positioned supine for best exposure. This is done for both the open and laparoscopic harvest technique.
- Sterile preparation of the operative field should include the entire abdomen extending to the thorax where the defect is located.
  - Intraoperatively, the defect and donor site should be partitioned as much as possible to prevent cross-contamination.
- If skin grafting of the omental flap is required, the planned donor site should be prepared.
- The patient may be placed in partial or complete lateral decubitus position for posterior defects. For this approach, the laparoscopic approach can be considered.

Approach

- Laparotomy (open approach)
  - Partial upper midline (epigastric) incision is the most commonly used. It can be performed in a longitudinal or transverse fashion.
  - A complete midline incision is considered when a previous surgical scar can be used or in those cases demanding better exposure.

- We use the open technique when the thoracic defect is already communicating with the upper part of the abdominal cavity.
- Laparoscopic[9,10]
  - Considered in selected patients, especially if there is no communication between the thoracic wound and the abdominal cavity
  - Can assist in pedicle or free flap harvest with minimal size incisions
  - This technique has the advantages of reduced postoperative pain, shorter postoperative bed rest, lower rate of respiratory and wound complications, and earlier resumption of oral nutrition.[11]
  - After laparoscopic harvest, the pedicled omental flap can be delivered into the thoracic cavity in two ways:
    - Via a limited incision in the diaphragm
    - If harvested as a free flap, the omentum can be delivered via an extension of the infraumbilical laparoscopic access port.
  - There is a learning curve, and the surgeon must be competent at handling laparoscopic equipment within the abdominal cavity, as well as being equipped to handle any complications related to harvest, such as:
    - Intra-abdominal bleeding
    - Bowel perforation
    - Other visceral injuries
  - The laparoscopic approach requires carbon dioxide insufflation within the abdominal cavity. This can lead to increased cardiac afterload and decreased cardiac output, and can be detrimental to and precipitate arrhythmias in patients with significant cardiac disease, and should proceed with caution in this patient population.[12] Additional precautions can include:
    - Preoperative echocardiogram assessment and optimization
    - Intraoperative invasive hemodynamic monitoring
    - Slower carbon dioxide insufflation of the abdominal cavity
  - Partial or total harvest of the omentum can be done based on reconstructive requirement. Careful trimming of the omental flap can be done based on knowledge of its vascular anatomy.

■ Open Harvest of the Omental Flap

- After sterile preparation of the abdomen, incisions are made:
  - Upper epigastric incision is most commonly used and can be made in a transverse or vertical fashion.
  - For better exposure, a complete midline laparotomy incision is considered. This can be done via an extension of the existing thoracic defect or a separate incision.
  - Previous scars are considered for reuse.
- Dissection is continued, rectus fascia is divided, and once the parietal peritoneum is breached, the stomach and greater omentum come into view (**TECH FIG 1A**).
- At times, adhesions may be present and should be released if in the way of flap harvest.
- Commonly, the omentum will be visualized immediately under the peritoneum.
- The greater curvature of the stomach is identified and traced bilaterally along its gastric border.
- Right and left gastroepiploic vessels are identified, as well as their major descending branches to the omentum.
- The omentum is delivered out of the abdominal cavity and flipped upward to expose the posterior attachments of the transverse colon.
- The omentum is separated from transverse colon and great curvature of the stomach in the relatively avascular plane with the help of an assistant who keeps gentle traction on the omentum.
  - Care must be taken to secure the ligature of the short gastric vessels as coagulated vessels and insecure ligatures can dislodge postoperatively when they become distended and cause significant bleeding.
- Omental ligamentous attachments are freed, alongside meticulous collateral gastroepiploic perforating vessel ligation.
  - Any lateral attachments to the duodenum or gastrosplenic ligament are divided.
- Care is taken to avoid any injury to the appendices epiploicae when dissecting in the avascular plane adjacent to them.
  - Any possible colonic diverticula originating from the transverse colon must be avoided.
- Caution is taken to avoid injury to the middle colic vessels and the transverse mesocolon.

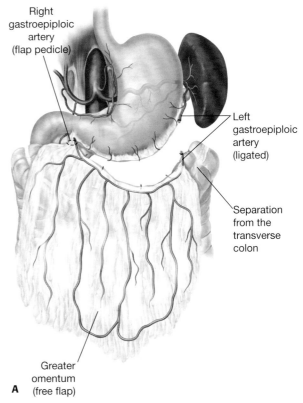

TECH FIG 1 • A. Open approach to omental flap harvest.

Right gastroepiploic artery (flap pedicle)

Left gastroepiploic artery (ligated)

Separation from the transverse colon

Greater omentum (free flap)

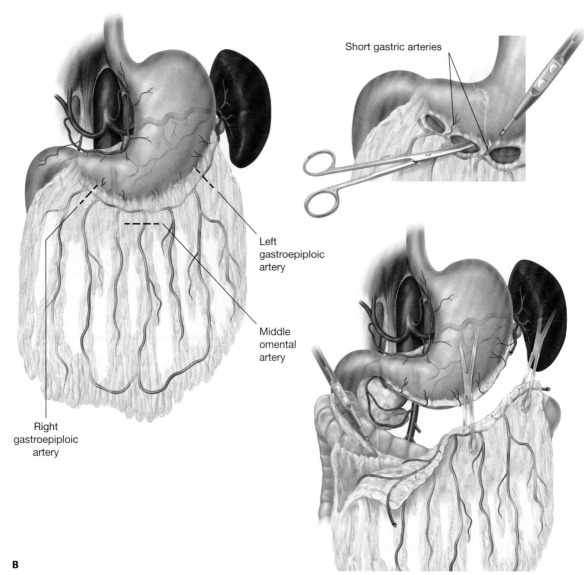

Short gastric arteries

Left gastroepiploic artery

Middle omental artery

Right gastroepiploic artery

B

TECH FIG 1 (Continued) • **B.** Harvest of omental flap and extension technique.

- Once the flap is isolated on its attachment to the stomach, a decision is made whether to harvest the flap based on the right or left gastroepiploic arteries.
  - This depends on the location of the defect as well as the size of the pedicle vessels, especially if it is being harvested as a free flap.
- Skeletonization of the pedicle is often not required or advisable and some perivascular tissue must be spared, to decrease the risk of vasospasm.
- Pedicle can be based on the commonly dominant right gastroepiploic artery originating from the gastroduodenal artery at the gastroduodenal junction.
  - Flap harvest based on the right gastroepiploic vessel is rapid because the leaves of the omentum usually are not fused to the body and tail of the pancreas and are easily dissected away.

- Alternatively, the pedicle can be based on the left gastroepiploic artery or short gastric arteries originating from the splenic artery.
  - The left gastroepiploic artery provides the greatest pedicle length and is more commonly used for extended arch of rotation and flap reach.[8]
- Elongation of the pedicle technique is performed by division of internal arcades and basing the flap on the right, middle, or left omental branch that arises from gastroepiploic system (**TECH FIG 1B**).
- Closure of the abdomen should be done in layers including robust rectus fascia closure.
  - A drain should be placed to detect any intra-abdominal hemorrhage.

■ Laparoscopic Harvest of the Omental Flap

- After sterile preparation of the abdomen, the laparoscopic ports are placed (**TECH FIG 2**).
- A 10-mm post is placed through an infraumbilical incision, and pneumoperitoneum is achieved.
- A 30-degree angled telescopic camera is then placed through this port, and three additional 2.5-mm ports are placed under direct vision.
  - One port is at the right hypochondrium, another at the right iliac fossa, and the third at the left flank.

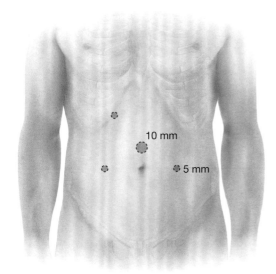

TECH FIG 2 • Laparoscopic approach to omental flap harvest.

- Although three ports are usually sufficient for instrumentation, additional ports can be added as required.
- The greater omentum is then identified. An instant look inside the abdominal cavity to check if the omentum has sufficient bulk and size, prior to flap harvest, is commenced.
  - Any pre-existing adhesions between the greater omentum and the parietal peritoneum are released with ultrasonic dissection.
- The omental flap is then dissected off the transverse colon.
  - A pair of atraumatic laparoscopic grasping forceps is placed through the right hypochondrium port to pull the greater curve of the stomach cranially toward the right, exposing the transverse colon.
  - The remaining ports facilitate the ultrasonic scalpel and additional atraumatic grasping forceps to pull the transverse colon caudally while dissecting the posterior attachments of the omentum off this structure.
- Once the flap has been isolated on its attachments to the greater curvature of the stomach, it is released from the left edge (for a flap harvested based on the right gastroepiploic artery), carefully ligating the short gastric arteries along the way.
- For delivery of the flap into the thoracic cavity, a communicating diaphragmatic incision measuring about 4 to 5 cm can be made either from the thoracic defect or laparoscopically.
- Care must be taken not to kink the pedicle when the flap is delivered into the defect.
- For external delivery as a free flap, the right gastroepiploic pedicle is divided, and the flap is delivered through an extension of the infraumbilical incision.
- Closure of the port sites can be done in a simple interrupted fashion. A drain should be placed to detect any postoperative intra-abdominal hemorrhage.

■ Transposition of the Omental Flap

Pedicle Transposition

- For extended arc of rotation, a left gastroepiploic artery–based flap is generally considered.[8]
- When transposing the flap, avoid overt pedicle compression against gastroduodenal area to prevent gastric outlet obstruction.
- Transposition to the thorax is done in one of three ways:
  - Extracutaneous tunneling over the costal margin, in which the exposed flap is skin grafted. This is associated with less risk of compression but with a higher infection rate that is contiguous with the abdominal cavity (**TECH FIG 3**).
  - Subcutaneous tunneling over the costal margin. This risks compression on the pedicle, especially when edematous.
  - Through the rectus sheath, facilitated by the laparoscopic approach. Lower hernia rates but risk of diaphragmatic hernia is increased. This is performed either through the diaphragm cruciate ligament on the right, where the liver buttresses the area, or to the left of the falciform ligament.[13]

- A small tacking suture may be placed where the omentum enters the chest wall to prevent pull or extrusion on the pedicle.

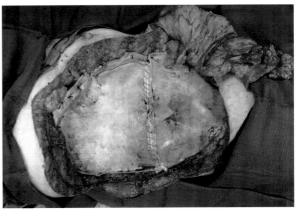

TECH FIG 3 • Pedicled omental flap harvest. Thoracic reconstruction for major resection involving all layers of the right thoracic cage. Resection included pleural cavity breach indicating ADM use for structural support. A pedicled omental flap was harvested based on the right gastroepiploic artery.

- Adequate pedicle length is ensured to avoid excessive tension on the pedicle during transposition and insetting.

Free Flap Transposition

- The omental flap has a relatively long ischemia time due to its low metabolic demand.
- The dominant right gastroepiploic artery is commonly used.

- Adequate preparation of the defect site and recipient vessels should be done prior to dividing the omental flap pedicle.
- Recipient vessels may include neck, thoracic, aortic, and vertebral arteries and their braches.
- Omentum is transferred and vascular anastomosis is commenced at the recipient site.

■ Flap Inset

- Attention is paid to pedicle positioning to avoid compression, kinking, or twisting, which may compromise blood flow to the flap immediately or early in the postoperative period (**TECH FIG 4A**).
- For the mediastinum and other external chest defects, the omentum can provide volume as well as a large surface area covered by a skin graft (**TECH FIG 4B**).

- Can be folded to fill dead space commonly present in the deep pleural cavity
- Can wrap around vessels or plug bronchopleural fistulas
- Multiple tucking or stay sutures are used to keep the flap in its place and prevent gliding or sliding.
- Drains are recommended for serous fluid accumulation, commonly associated with the omentum flap, and for early recognition of bleeding.

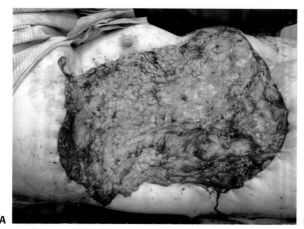 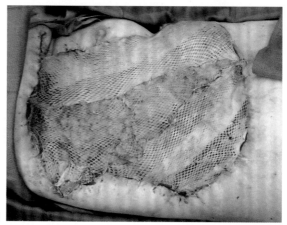

TECH FIG 4 • A. Pedicled omental flap inset. The omental flap covered the entire ADM. The flap was sutured all around for water seal closure. **B.** Skin grafting of the omental flap for complete cover.

PEARLS AND PITFALLS

Preoperative assessment	■ Past medical history of abdominal or pelvic surgery should prompt further investigation, and the omentum flap option should be reconsidered. ■ Adequate workup and precautions should be taken in patients with significant cardiac disease.
Port placement (for laparoscopic harvest)	■ First port to be placed should be the 10-mm camera port to allow pneumoperitoneum and placement of subsequent ports under direct vision.
Harvest technique	■ Special attention should be given to effective debridement of infected or necrotic nonviable bone and cartilage tissues (eg, sternum, ribs). ■ Laparoscopy allows a "peek" to assess the feasibility and dimension of the omentum flap. ■ Use of nontraumatic grasping forceps. ■ Keep the omentum flap wet at all times to prevent its desiccation. ■ Transillumination of the omentum allows visualization of its vascularity. ■ Minimal manipulation of bowel.

PEARLS AND PITFALLS (Continued)

Hemostasis	▪ Use of hemostatic ultrasonic scalpel for laparoscopic harvest. ▪ Avoid cautery use for vessels. Rather, ligate as you go to decrease the risk of bleeding, hematoma, and injury to vessels of the omental arcade. ▪ An intra-abdominal drain should be placed to detect postoperative hemorrhage. ▪ Sustained postoperative seroma should be anticipated and drains removed in time.
Delivery and inset of flap	▪ An incision in the diaphragm can be used for pedicle transposition but should be wide enough to avoid compression. ▪ Prior to ligating the main gastroepiploic vessel, the right and left arteries can be temporarily clamped alternatively to determine omental arch flow. ▪ Subcutaneous tunneling should be wide enough (4 fingers' wide or more) so that postoperative edema will not facilitate compression and venous congestion. ▪ Ensure that the pedicle is not kinked or compressed in the process of flap delivery and inset. ▪ If used for external coverage, the omental flap can be skin grafted. ▪ Sliding of flap postoperatively is a common difficulty and avoided by multiple tucking sutures. ▪ Gastric outlet obstruction should be thought of when the pedicle is transposed over the gastroduodenal area. ▪ Be alert for abdominal morbidities following surgery, especially infection and peritonitis.

POSTOPERATIVE CARE

- Immediate postoperative care should include flap care, monitoring, and postabdominal and thoracic surgery precautions.
  - A meshed skin graft is advised for externally placed flaps to avoid transudate under the skin graft. A dressing need not be applied to avoid flap compression.
  - Clinical monitoring of the omental flap is difficult. Changes within the flap are difficult to see until it is too late.
  - If used as a free flap, standard free flap protocols should be instituted including regular flap checks, nothing by mouth (NPO) for the first 24 hours, and bed rest.
  - As with any other flap, the 24- to 72-hour postoperative window requires particularly attentive flap monitoring in the form of clinical and/or US Doppler evaluations to identify any signs of pending flap failure.
- Monitoring options include the following:
  - An implantable Doppler for free flap monitoring.
  - Temperature probe placement.
  - A skin-grafted window directly over the omentum facilitates pedicled as well as free flap monitoring for direct flow signal monitoring with the use of a pencil Doppler.
- Postabdominal surgery precautions should include the following:
  - NPO followed by gradual clear fluids working up to normal diet over the first few postoperative days. Commonly,

a nasogastric tube is left in place until postoperative day 2 or 3.
  - Monitoring of drain output for early detection of intra-abdominal hemorrhage. The drain can be removed once output is less than 30 mL/d for 2 consecutive days.
  - Adequate pain control. The laparoscopic approach is associated with decreased postoperative pain.
  - Early mobilization of the patient on the first postoperative day is recommended, unless there are other factors preventing this.
  - Postoperative antibiotics are given in accordance with abdominal surgery and laparotomy.
  - Chest tube with an underwater seal may be indicated for deep thoracic defects involving the pleura. Chest tubes are removed following thoracic surgeon consultation.

OUTCOMES

- Remarkably very few complications are encountered in regard to donor-site morbidities and flap inset.
  - Most complications are minor and are addressed conservatively.
  - **FIG 3** shows an outcome in one patient after pedicled omental flap for thoracic reconstruction.
- In 135 patients undergoing use of the omental flap for extraperitoneal reconstruction (64 pedicled and 71 free flaps),

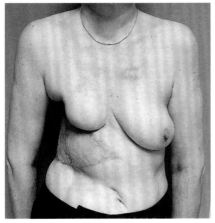 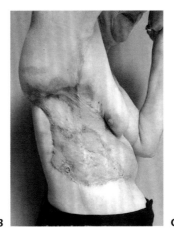 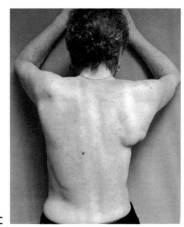

A   **B**   **C**

FIG 3 • A. Postoperative anterior view of the reconstructed thoracic defect. **B.** Postoperative lateral view of the reconstructed thoracic defect. **C.** Postoperative posterior view of the reconstructed thoracic defect.

there were 25 donor-site complications (18.5%).[1] All but one omental flap was harvested via an open technique.

- Twenty-six of 53 patients who had undergone previous abdominal surgery required extensive adhesiolysis, with 4 patients sustaining enterotomies.
- Eleven patients (8.1%) had partial flap loss and three patients (2.2%) had total flap loss.
- Factors associated with increased donor-site complications included:
  - Use of pedicled flaps
  - Mediastinitis
  - Advanced age
  - Pulmonary failure
- In a series of nine laparoscopically harvested pedicled omental flaps for chest wall and intrathoracic reconstruction, there were no major intra-abdominal complications postoperatively.[14]
  - One patient required conversion to a free omental flap due to the detachment of the pedicle, and another patient required conversion to an open harvest technique due to severe abdominal adhesions. One patient had a small transdiaphragmatic hernia treated laparoscopically.
- In a head-to-head comparison of omental flaps vs pectoralis major flaps in the treatment of 33 patients with sternal osteomyelitis, the sepsis-related mortality rate was higher in the pectoralis group (28%) than in the omentum group (0%). The authors concluded that the omental flap conferred greater immunologic advantage as compared with pectoralis major flap.[15]
- The open pedicled omental flap harvest technique was used successfully in 27 patients with deep sternal wound infections that had failed previous treatment including pectoralis major flap coverage. There was 1 abdominal wall hernia and 1 persistent fistula in this series.[16]

COMPLICATIONS

- In general, postoperative complications associated with chest wall reconstruction include hematoma, seroma formation (fluid transduction), infection, and pneumothorax.
- Skin graft nontake or separation could occur but is mostly only partial and self-resolving.
- If reconstructive plates are used for chest wall stabilization, foreign body reaction, extrusion, and infection can result. This occurs more commonly if the hardware is placed in a radiated field and insufficient soft tissue coverage is the case.
- Donor-site morbidity may include laparotomy-related complications. These include but are not limited to
  - Bowel obstruction
  - Gastric outlet obstruction
  - Peritonitis and other infections (eg, abscess)
  - Intra-abdominal hemorrhage
  - Viscera injury (eg, splenic, liver, bowel perforation)
  - Volvulus
  - Fascial dehiscence and hernia (eg, epigastric, diaphragmatic)
  - Late complications including adhesions and postoperative ileus
- In general, flap-related complications include flap loss secondary to vascular twisting, kinking, excessive tension, and vasospasm, as well as bleeding and infection.

- Specific complications related to the omentum flap include seroma formation (transudation), omental atrophy, flap sliding or migration, and avulsion.

ACKNOWLEDGMENTS

We thank Adrian S. H. Ooi, MBBS, MRCS, MMed, and Chad M. Teven, MD, for their contributions to the preparation of this chapter.

REFERENCES

1. Das SK. The size of the human omentum and methods of lengthening it for transplantation. *Br J Plast Surg*. 1976;29(2):170-44.
2. Alday ES, Goldsmith HS. Surgical technique for omental lengthening based on arterial anatomy. *Surg Gynecol Obstet*. 1972;135(1):103-107.
3. Upton J, Mulliken JB, Hicks PD, Murray JE. Restoration of facial contour using free vascularized omental transfer. *Plast Reconstr Surg*. 1980;66(4):560-569.
4. Pairolero PC, Arnold PG. Thoracic wall defects: surgical management of 205 consecutive patients. *Mayo Clin Proc*. 1986;61(7):557-563.
5. Puma F, Fedeli C, Ottavi P, et al. Laparoscopic omental flap for the treatment of major sternal wound infection after cardiac surgery. *J Thorac Cardiovasc Surg*. 2003;126(6):1998-2002.
6. Jurkiewicz MJ, Arnold PG. The omentum: an account of its use in the reconstruction of the chest wall. *Ann Surg*. 1977;185(5): 548-554.
7. Krabatsch T, Schmitt DV, Mohr FW, Hetzer R. Thoracic transposition of the greater omentum as an adjunct in the treatment of mediastinitis: pros and cons within the context of a randomised study. *Eur J Surg Suppl*. 1999;(584):45-48.
8. Alday ES, Goldsmith HS. Surgical qmy. *Surg Gynecol Obstet*. 1972;135:103.
9. Corral CJ, Prystowsky JB, Weidrich TA, Harris GD. Laparoscopic-assisted bipedicle omental flap mobilization for reconstruction of a chest wall defect. *J Laparoendosc Surg*. 1994;4(5):343-346.
10. Salameh JR, Chock DA, Gonzalez JJ, et al. Laparoscopic harvest of omental flaps for reconstruction of complex mediastinal wounds. *JSLS*. 2003;7:317-322.
11. Puma F, Vannucci J. Advantages of laparoscopic omental flap in the treatment of deep sternal wound infection. *Interact Cardiovasc Thorac Surg*. 2011;13(2):188.
12. El-Muttardi N, Jabir S, Win TS. Pearls and pitfalls of laparoscopic harvest of omental flap for sternal wound reconstruction in patients with significant cardiac dysfunction. *J Plast Reconstr Aesthet Surg*. 2013;66(12):e394-e395.
13. Vyas RM, Prsic A, Orgill DP. Transdiaphragmatic omental harvest: a simple, efficient method for sternal wound coverage. *Plast Reconstr Surg*. 2013;131:544-552.
14. Acarturk TO, Swartz WM, Luketich J, et al. Laparoscopically harvested omental flap for chest wall and intrathoracic reconstruction. *Ann Plast Surg*. 2004;53(3):210-216.
15. López-Monjardin H, de-la-Peña-Salcedo A, Mendoza-Muñoz M, et al. Omentum flap versus pectoralis major flap in the treatment of mediastinitis. *Plast Reconstr Surg*. 1998;101(6):1481-1485.
16. Eifert S, Kronschnabl S, Kaczmarek I, et al. Omental flap for recurrent deep sternal wound infection and mediastinitis after cardiac surgery. *Thorac Cardiovasc Surg*. 2007;55(6):371-374.

SUGGESTED READING

Hultman CS, Carlson GW, Losken A, et al. Utility of the omentum in the reconstruction of complex extraperitoneal wounds and defects: donor-site complications in 135 patients from 1975 to 2000. *Ann Surg*. 2002;235(6):782-795.

Latissimus Dorsi Flap for Chest Wall Defects

Essie Kueberuwa Yates and David H. Song

DEFINITION

- Composite defects of the chest wall can arise secondary to oncological extirpation, ablation due to infection, congenital defects, trauma, radiation, or iatrogenic causes such as surgical access and hardware extrusion.
- Methylmethacrylate (in a nonradiated wound bed), bioprosthetic mesh, vascularized bone, local myocutaneous flaps, and free tissue transfer are all routinely used in the reconstruction of chest wall defects.
  - The choice of technique is related to size, extent, and location of the defect and the availability of donor site.
- The latissimus dorsi flap (LDF) is a reliable flap with a robust and predictable vascularity. The proximity of the flap to the chest wall makes it an ideal choice for providing muscle, fat, and skin for use in reconstructing large chest wall defects.
- The thoracodorsal artery system nourishes the LDF and offers the possibility for incorporating multiple tissue types of its single vascular pedicle (chimeric flap).

ANATOMY

- The LD muscle has multiple origins (**FIG 1**):
  - Spinous processes of T7-T12
  - Thoracolumbar fascia
  - Posterior third of the iliac crest
  - Lowest six ribs
- The LD muscle inserts into the intertubercular groove of the humerus.
- It is a broad flat muscle, which is the most superficial back muscle overlying the paraspinous muscles medially and serratus anterior laterally. It lies deep to the trapezius superomedially.
- The LD is a type V muscle, with the dominant vascular pedicle being the thoracodorsal artery, a terminal branch of the subscapular artery, which arises from the third portion of the axillary artery.
- The thoracodorsal artery runs on the underside of the muscle, and the main pedicle divides into two main branches: an upper horizontal branch that travels medially along the superior border of the muscle and a descending oblique branch that runs inferiorly, parallel to the anterior border of the muscle about 2.5 cm from the edge.
  - The bifurcation is predictably found 4 cm distal to the inferior scapular border and 2.5 cm medial to the anterior border of the muscle.
- Thoracodorsal artery perforators exit the muscle and perfuse the subcutaneous tissue, one of these perforators is typically located 8 cm below the posterior axillary fold and 2 cm behind the anterior border of the LD muscle.[1]
- Secondary pedicles arise dorsally and mostly perfuse the distal part of the muscle. They are typically found about 5 to 10 cm lateral to the spinous processes and are arranged in a medial row (branches of the lumbar arteries) and a lateral row (branches of the intercostal arteries).
- The largest and most constant of these secondary blood supplies are the branches of the 8th to 11th intercostal arteries. They are typically not useful for large anterior chest wall reconstructions due to their location and short pedicle length.
  - These branches can be used, however, when the LD has been previously transected in a standard non–muscle-sparing thoracotomy incision, as the distal portion of the muscle can still be mobilized to provide coverage of limited posterior defects.

PATIENT HISTORY AND PHYSICAL FINDINGS

- When evaluating a chest wall defect, important considerations include the following:
  - Viability and quality of the wound bed (radiated, inadequately debrided; presence of contaminated hardware and large dead spaces result in poor wound healing)
  - Effect of the wound on respiratory mechanics
  - Exposure of vital structures
  - Aesthetics and contour of the chest

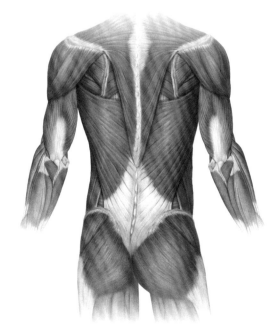

FIG 1 • Latissimus dorsi muscle.

- Typically, defects larger than 5 cm or involving more than three ribs require chest wall stabilization in addition to soft tissue coverage.
- In the postirradiated chest wall, larger defects can be tolerated without fixation due to the rigid scarring and fibrosis of tissue.

SURGICAL MANAGEMENT

- The LDF is ideal for chest wall reconstruction because the axis and length of the thoracodorsal pedicle afford this flap an excellent arc of rotation and virtually any part of the ipsilateral chest wall can be reached.
- The most common uses of the LD in chest reconstruction are as a muscle-only flap for intrathoracic obliteration of dead space or as a musculocutaneous flap for coverage of large chest wall defects.[2]

Preoperative Planning

- When planning chest wall reconstruction with an LD flap, the main considerations are as follows:
  - Ensuring vascularity and availability of donor site. (On occasions, the muscle is transected during thoracotomy.) Some syndromes (eg, Poland) are associated with congenital absence of the pectoralis and LD muscle.
  - Assessing defect size: The thoracodorsal artery provides branches to the serratus muscle, which can be taken in conjunction with the LDF if a larger flap is necessary.
  - Assessment of the need for rigid fixation in addition to soft tissue coverage for composite resections (involving more than three ribs). Vascularized bone can be harvested in conjunction with the LD flap.
  - Appropriate preoperative counseling: The LD is an external rotator of the shoulder, and patients should expect decreased strength and range of motion postoperatively.
- Preoperative markings: With the patient in the standing position, the borders of the latissimus dorsi muscle are delineated (**FIG 2**).
  - Inferior tip of the scapula
  - Anterior border (with the arm elevated, the anterior border extends from the posterior axillary line caudal to the iliac crest).
  - Upper border (with the arm elevated, the posterior border extends from the axilla over the tip of the scapula to the midline of the back).
  - Lower border (curves from the lower midline of the back lumbar region) to the anterior border of the muscle.

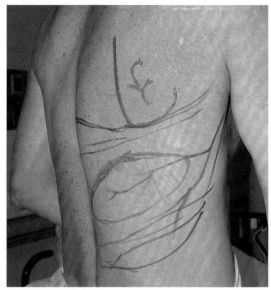

FIG 2 • Preoperative markings.

  - The inferior segment of the trapezius is also drawn out as it overlaps the upper medial border of the latissimus as a reminder of this important anatomic relationship.
- Once the limits of the muscle have been identified, the location and orientation of the skin island are planned.
  - The size of the skin island is a factor of the defect, and ability to close the donor site primarily.
  - The skin island is precisely centered on a dominant perforator that is identified using a handheld Doppler intraoperatively.

Positioning

- The LDF is typically harvested in the lateral decubitus position with an axillary support for respiration and with the arm prepped in and the shoulder flexed to 90 degrees.
- A beanbag with appropriate padding can be used, with a pillow placed between the knees and abducted and elevated arm placed on a Mayo stand.
- Lateral decubitus is the preferred positioning for a standard thoracotomy allowing posterolateral and intrathoracic reconstructions to be performed without position change.
- Anterior defects do require harvest, delivery, and closure of donor site, before inset performed when the patient position changes to supine.

■ Flap Elevation

- The skin paddle is incised down through the thoracic fascia to the loose fatty tissue overlying the LD muscle.
  - Caution is taken to bevel out circumferentially for a few centimeters to aid closure without dog-ears and to maximize flap bulk.
- Subcutaneous dissection is carried out inferiorly first, then superiorly keeping a thin layer of loose areolar fat on the muscle until the limits of the muscle are identified.
  - Care is taken to ensure the skin flaps are not too thin.

- The aponeurosis of the trapezius and latissimus muscles is identified, and the LD muscle is separated from underneath it.
- Submuscular dissection is carried down on the medial underside of the LD muscle from superior to inferior.
  - The fascial attachments to the paraspinous muscles are divided, and the lumbar perforators are ligated when encountered.
- Inferiorly, the muscle is divided through its attachments to the iliac crest.

- The anterior border is separated next, again identifying and ligating intercostal perforators and separating attachments from the serratus muscle.
- At this point, the muscle is totally freed and can be flipped upward on its pedicle. (The humeral insertion remains intact at this point.)
  - Any remaining attachments to teres minor or any other deep structures can be identified and divided.
  - The vascular pedicle is visible entering the muscle approximately 10 cm inferiorly from humeral attachment.

- In the case of a chimeric flap, other options involve harvesting the tip of the scapula (off angular branch), serratus muscle/fascia (off serratus branch), and rib based on perforator connections from the LD muscle (**TECH FIG 1**).
- Division of the humeral insertion above the entry of the pedicle greatly facilitates freedom of movement and ease of inset.
- The thoracodorsal bundle is readily identifiable at this stage of the procedure. Division of the nerve at this point minimizes dynamic movements in the flap postoperatively.

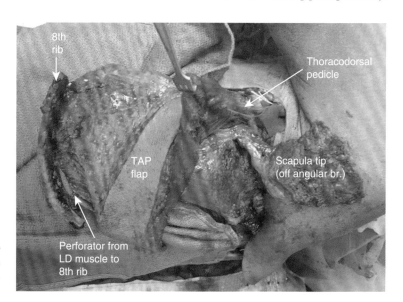

TECH FIG 1 • Chimeric thoracodorsal artery perforator (TAP) flap based on the thoracodorsal system. LD, latissimus dorsi muscle. (Courtesy of Lawrence J. Gottlieb, MD.)

■ Dissection of Axillary Tunnel

- The tunnel facilitates the passage of the myocutaneous flap into the chest for anterior defects.
- Care should be taken to ensure the tunnel has adequate width.
- The tunnel can be dissected from both the chest wall wound (recipient site) and from the donor site (flap side).

- Some surgeons like to predissect the tunnel prior to flap elevation.
- If the humeral origin was divided during elevation, care must be taken not to place tension on the pedicle as it passed through the tunnel.
- The donor site should be closed in layers over closed suction drainage.
- The flap is inset in layers over closed suction drainage

PEARLS AND PITFALLS

Minimizing seroma risk	■ Consider quilting sutures for donor site. ■ Use at least two large-caliber drains. ■ Minimize excessive arm elevation in early postoperative period.
Flap elevation pearl	■ If possible, leave the thoracodorsal branch to serratus intact. If you have an injury to the TDA high in the axilla, the serratus branch can nourish the flap via retrograde flow and intercostal communications.
Minimizing donor site morbidity	■ If only a small flap is required, consider a TAP flap or latissimus-sparing modification of the traditional procedure.
Stabilization of the chest wall	■ Posterior ribs can be elevated with this flap and used in the event when chest wall stabilization with autologous tissue is desired.
Optimizing success in chronic chest wall wounds	■ The LDF offers a good option for salvage in a chronic infected wound. Adequate aggressive debridement prior to flap coverage is essential to a successful outcome.

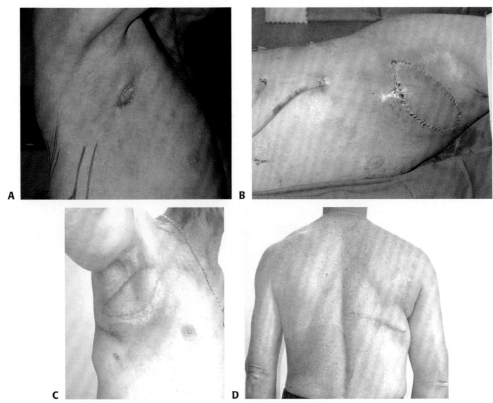

FIG 3 • A. This 53-year-old man had a history of fungating primary adenocarcinoma of anterolateral chest wall after radiation, with open draining wound and osteoradionecrosis of the underlying rib. **B.** After resection and reconstruction with LD flap. **C,D.** Recipient and donor sites, respectively, 6 months postoperatively.

POSTOPERATIVE CARE

- Most patients have an uneventful postoperative course specifically related to the LD flap.
- Early ROM is encouraged to minimize arm and shoulder stiffness.
  - Excess elevation and abduction of the arm are discouraged, however, because of significantly increased seroma formation risk.
- Drains should stay in situ until <30 cc/24-h period is recorded for 2 consecutive days. Drains are often required for many weeks.

OUTCOMES

- In the well-selected patient, the main outcomes for chest wall reconstruction are readily achieved using LDF (**FIG 3**).
- These flaps offer sufficient volume to fill the three-dimensional dead space, buttressing repair of hollow visceral leaks, maintenance of chest wall stability, restoration of aesthetic contour, covering of exposed prosthetic materials with vascularized flaps, and retaining the "right of domain" of abdominal and chest viscera while minimizing donor site functional deficits.[3]

COMPLICATIONS

- The most common complication from LD flap harvest is donor site seroma formation. Drains are often required for prolonged periods, on occasions up to 6 to 8 weeks.

- In the event of seroma accumulation, repeat in-office aspiration may be required. With time, fluid accumulation eventually stops, leaving behind an empty bursa of varying dimensions.
- Isolated arm strength can be diminished after flap transfer, although this is rarely a significant finding, as the other muscles of the back compensate for the absent muscle.
  - It takes 6 months to a year for the surrounding muscles to be fully compensatory, and patients often describe easy fatigability in activities requiring external rotation and elevation of the arm overhead (eg, swimming, climbing, painting).[3]
- The vascularity of the LD flap is robust, and vascular compromise or fat necrosis is rare after LD transfer.
  - However, donor site marginal skin necrosis can occur particularly in smokers, which might suggest avoiding excessive undermining.

REFERENCES

1. Bank J, Ledbetter K, Song D. Use of thoracodorsal artery perforator flaps to enhance outcomes in alloplastic breast reconstruction. *Plast Reconstr Surg Glob Open.* 2014;2(5):e140.
2. Bakri K, Mardini S, Evans K, et al. Workhorse flaps in chest wall reconstruction: the pectoralis major, latissimus dorsi, and rectus abdominis flaps. *Semin Plast Surg.* 2011;5(1):43-54.
3. Netscher D, Izaddoost S, Sandvall B. Complications, pitfalls, and outcomes after chest wall reconstruction. *Semin Plast Surg.* 2011;25(1): 86-97.

Serratus Anterior Flap for Chest Wall Reconstruction

Zachary J. Collier and David H. Song

DEFINITION

- Chest wall deformities arising from congenital malformations and acquired etiologies result in significant physical and psychological sequelae.
  - Regardless of the underlying etiology, failure to reconstruct chest wall deformities may result in debilitating respiratory abnormalities, risk of internal organ injury, and psychological ramifications.
- Serratus anterior flap (SAF)
  - SAF was first described in 1979 by Mathes and Nahai and later refined in 1982 by Takayanagi and Tsukie[1] for use as a muscle transposition flap based off of a type III (two major pedicles) vascular supply.
  - The SAF has been employed as a transposition and free flap for reconstructing defects of the upper and lower limbs, trunk, and head and neck.
  - It is a highly versatile small to medium-sized muscle flap that can be neurotized through the sensory branches of the intercostal nerves over the skin paddle as well as incorporated into a larger chimeric design for more complex reconstructions.

ANATOMY

- The chest wall is a complex musculoskeletal system that provides a rigid skeletal encasement for protecting vital organs while maintaining the flexibility to interact with multilayered and vectored musculature to facilitate respiration and upper extremity mobilization.
- The skeletal system is composed of 2 clavicles and 12 paired ribs, which in turn articulate posteriorly with the thoracic vertebrae's costal facets and transverse processes as well as anteriorly with the sternum via costochondral joints. The 8th to 10th ribs are referred to as "false" ribs as they lack direct sternal attachments, whereas ribs 11 and 12 are termed the "floating" ribs (**FIG 1**).
- The musculature is composed of two main groups—axial and appendicular muscles (**FIG 2**).
  - Most axial muscles can be divided into two subtypes based on their role in respiration—inspiratory (sternocleidomastoid and scalene) and expiratory (rectus abdominis, internal oblique, and external oblique)—although the trilayered intercostals participate in both respiratory processes.
  - The appendicular muscles are required for manipulation of the scapula (trapezius, serratus anterior) and humerus (pectoralis major/minor, latissimus dorsi).
- The serratus anterior originates from the superolateral borders of the first 8 or 9 ribs and inserts onto the costal surface of the medial scapular border to create 7 to 10 distinct digitations or slips (average dimension 10 × 20 cm).[2]
  - The distribution of serratus digitations is as follows: 7 (13%), 8 (48%), 9 (26%), and 10 (13%).[3]
- Arterial supply (Mathes and Nahai type III)
  - Superior 3 to 5 slips: The lateral thoracic artery (0.5 to 1.5 mm),[4] which originates from the axillary artery posterior to the pectoralis minor, follows the inferolateral border of the muscle to supply the first 3 to 5 slips.
  - Inferior 3 or 4 slips: The thoracodorsal artery (2 to 4 mm),[5] which originates from the subscapular artery, gives off one (40%), two (50%), or three (10%) serratus branches (1.5 to 2.5 mm)[6] to supply the inferior 3 to 4 slips. The average pedicle length is 11 cm but may be as long as 15 cm if taken to the subscapular artery.[3]
- Veins: Paired venae comitantes run parallel to their arterial counterparts (**FIG 3**).
- Nerves: Innervated by the long thoracic nerve, which arises from the C5 to C7 anterior rami and passes through the cervicoaxillary canal, it runs posterior to the brachial plexus and axillary artery/vein where it follows the inferior surface of the muscle and eventually diverges on the vascular pedicle as it travels inferiorly.[6]
  - Preserve the first 4 or 5 muscular slips to avoid damage to this nerve, which would produce a winged scapula deformity.
  - Innervation of the optional skin paddle is provided by the lateral cutaneous branches of the intercostal nerves (**FIG 4**).

PATHOGENESIS

- Congenital
  - Pectus excavatum (PE), pectus carinatum (PC), Poland syndrome, anterior thoracic hypoplasia, pentalogy of Cantrell, asphyxiating thoracic dystrophy, spondylothoracic dysplasia, and sternal clefts
- Acquired
  - Trauma, tumor resections, postoperative complications, wound infections involving musculoskeletal components, and chronic empyemas

PATIENT HISTORY AND PHYSICAL FINDINGS

- History
  - As with any other reconstructive procedure, a thorough evaluation of comorbidities, especially those that place the patient at risk for VTEs (ie, history of VTEs, obesity, diabetes, smoking, Caprini score greater than 8)[7] or vascular complications, is critical for preoperative medical and anesthesia optimization.

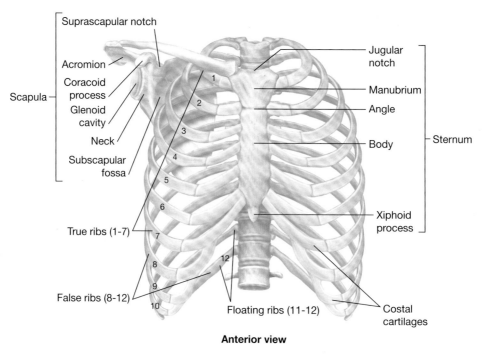

Anterior view

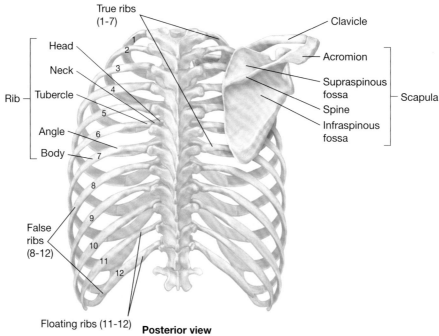

Posterior view

FIG 1 • Skeletal anatomy of the chest wall.

- Congenital: It is important to acquire any genetic workup or syndromic diagnoses in order to identify additional comorbidities and underlying structural abnormalities not readily apparent on physical exam that may complicate or alter the surgical approach.
- Acquired: History of insults to the chest wall soft tissue and skeletal integrity is critical for identifying the full extent of the defect as well as any factors that may influence the treatment plan.

- Trauma: Consider imaging (magnetic resonance imaging [MRI], computed tomography [CT], vascular imaging) studies if there is a potential for aberrant/obscured anatomy or foreign bodies.
- Infection: Consider tissue quantifications and cultures to identify any pathologic microbes and to guide preoperative planning regarding plating and/or other hardware utilization.

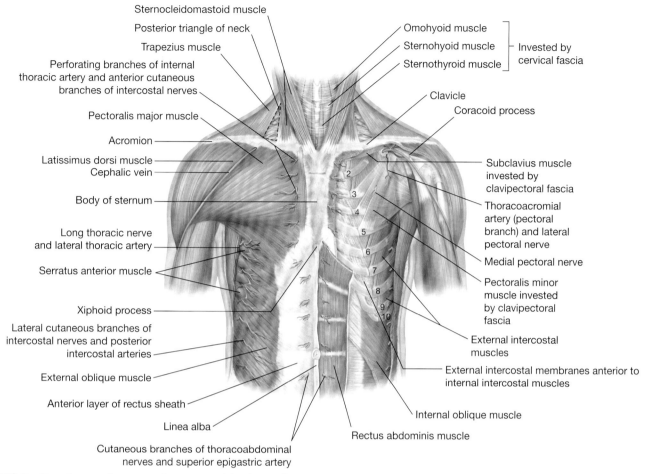

Sternocleidomastoid muscle
Posterior triangle of neck
Trapezius muscle
Perforating branches of internal
thoracic artery and anterior cutaneous
branches of intercostal nerves
Pectoralis major muscle
Acromion
Latissimus dorsi muscle
Cephalic vein
Body of sternum
Long thoracic nerve
and lateral thoracic artery
Serratus anterior muscle
Xiphoid process
Lateral cutaneous branches of
intercostal nerves and posterior
intercostal arteries
External oblique muscle
Anterior layer of rectus sheath
Linea alba
Cutaneous branches of thoracoabdominal
nerves and superior epigastric artery

Omohyoid muscle
Sternohyoid muscle   — Invested by
Sternothyroid muscle   cervical fascia
Clavicle
Coracoid process
Subclavius muscle
invested by
clavipectoral fascia
Thoracoacromial
artery (pectoral
branch) and lateral
pectoral nerve
Medial pectoral nerve
Pectoralis minor
muscle invested
by clavipectoral
fascia
External intercostal
muscles
External intercostal membranes anterior to
internal intercostal muscles
Internal oblique muscle
Rectus abdominis muscle

FIG 2 • Musculature and neurovascular anatomy of the chest wall.

- Oncologic: Ensure clear pathologic margins or identify additional resection requirements and treatment goals respective to tumor type.
- Radiation: Identify plans for postadjuvant radiation therapy to guide reconstructive decisions (ie, local/regional vs free flap design, timing).
■ Physical exam
  ■ In general, identification of defect dimensions and involved tissue types is critical for preoperative planning and flap design.
    • Skin: Note scars or contractures from prior procedures. Identify lacerations for potential utilization as or integration with incision design. Evaluate for skin integrity including turgor, elasticity, and signs of radiation damage or dermatologic disease.
    • Muscle: Assess muscle bulk and dimensions to identify tissue limitations and guide preoperative flap design.
    • Bone: Identify extent of skeletal defects to determine requirements for structural stabilization with plates, grafts, or bone-containing flaps.

IMAGING

■ CT or MRI studies may be beneficial in the preoperative evaluation of patients undergoing tumor resection as well as those with trauma to identify the extent of musculoskeletal defects and any complicating foreign bodies.

■ Vascular studies such as CT angiography may be warranted if tumor resection or trauma has compromised the natural vascular anatomy or extent of vascular involvement is unknown.
  ▫ Dynamic three- and four-dimensional CT imaging can facilitate individualized flap design by identifying angiosome filling patterns up to the subdermal plexus level, recruitment of neighboring angiosomes through communicating branches, and venous drainage.[8,9]
  ▫ As previously mentioned, three main serratus perforator branching patterns from the thoracodorsal artery have been identified in anatomical studies, so CT angiography can be utilized to identify patient-specific anatomical variants for facilitating intraoperative perforator identification and dissection.[3]

SURGICAL MANAGEMENT

Preoperative Planning

■ Location and size of the defect are ideally identified prior to incision to guide decisions regarding flap design (ie, transposition or free flap) and required vascular pedicle length.
  ▫ Direct closure of the donor site, stability of the thoracic wall, and protection of the thoracic viscera are all variables that need to be integrated into the decision to utilize a muscle transposition, myocutaneous, or chimeric flap.

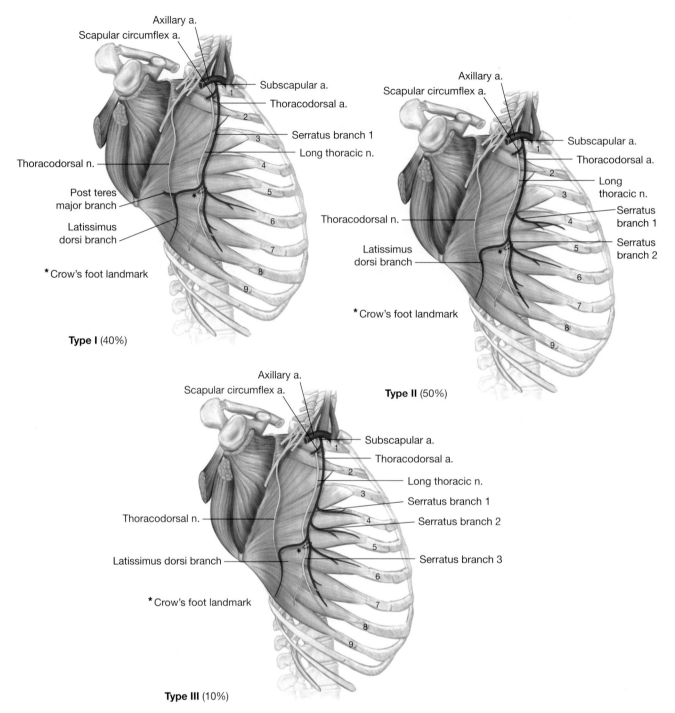

FIG 3 • Vascular branching patterns of serratus perforators from thoracodorsal artery.

- Involved tissue types
  - Skin: Identifying skin involvement is important for determining if a flap with a skin paddle or skin graft is required. The decision to include a skin paddle will alter the dissection to preserve the lateral cutaneous perforators of the posterior intercostals that would otherwise be transected during exposure of the serratus muscle.
  - Muscle: Determine which muscles are involved and the level of functionality that exists with the current muscular composition.
  - If resection, radiation, or infection compromises a muscle that would otherwise be available as flap, this is critical to know prior to taking the patient to the operating room so that a different flap or surgical approach may be chosen.
- Bony defects larger than 5 cm or involving more than 3 or 4 contiguous ribs are likely to benefit from structural support in addition to soft tissue coverage.[10]
- A defect's age (ie, acute vs chronic wound) often influences the quality of localized tissue vascularity, extent of fibrosis, and local wound healing capabilities as a result of inflammation-dependent changes in regional "physiosomes."

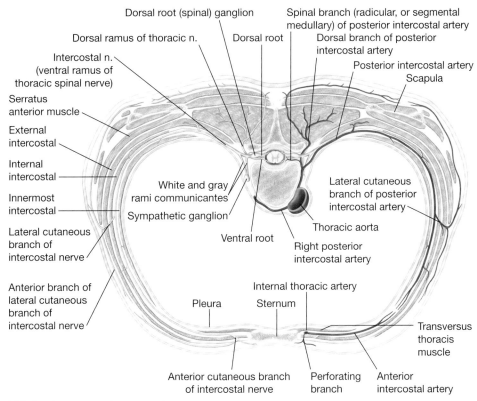

FIG 4 • Thorax anatomic cross section.

- The presence of irradiated skin, previous scars/contractures, localized infection or inflammation, and acute trauma all influence the regional tissue integrity and subsequently require consideration while determining the reconstructive approach and complexity.
- Patient lifestyle and functional status help to identify the measures to be implemented for preservation of postoperative muscular functionality and the overall type of reconstruction performed.
  - Certain activities (ie, boxing, golf, baseball, and swimming) and labor-intensive occupations (ie, construction) depend on the serratus anterior for full functionality, and this must be taken into consideration when choosing the donor muscle.
- Prognosis: Life expectancy and patient-specific goals vary significantly for each patient and, as a result, must be considered when determining the complexity of reconstruction.
  - Patient who have had the serratus anterior muscle harvested may have a "winged" scapula and discomfort.

- Those with poorer overall prognoses may be better treated with less complex reconstructive techniques that minimize intraoperative risks while facilitating faster recovery times.

Positioning

- The patient may be placed in partial or complete lateral decubitus position depending on the location of the defect relative to the donor site.
- Defects juxtaposed to the donor site allow for full lateral decubitus positioning with a beanbag setup.

Approaches

- Incisions overlying the anterior border of the latissimus muscle allow ready access to the serratus anterior muscle.
- Transverse or oblique incisions may lend to a more favorable donor site scar.
- Anterior access is necessary to adequately harvest the entire serratus muscle.

■ Landmarks and Markings

- It is important to identify the anterior border of the latissimus dorsi and the inferior border of the ninth rib to ensure the incision will appropriately expose the latissimus and inferior serratus slips.
- Create a template of the defect to identify the required dimensions for reconstruction.
- Trace the anterior border of the latissimus muscle as well as a straight line from the anterior axillary line to ASIS to delineate the ideal anteroposterior boundaries for the incision (**TECH FIG 1**).
  - If a skin paddle is going to be incorporated into the flap design, transpose the defect template into this defined region and identify perforators with US Doppler to optimize the flap position relative to underlying vasculature.

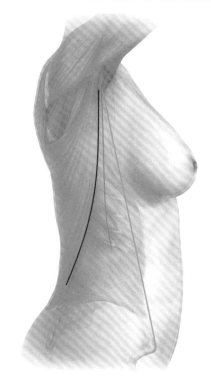

TECH FIG 1 • Preoperative markings.

■ Exposure

- Make a curvilinear incision from the axilla to rib 8 or 9 while avoiding anterior or posterior deviations beyond the previously identified A-P borders. The location and appearance are similar to those of a classic lateral thoracotomy incision.
- Dissect down to the deep fascia overlying the latissimus muscle.
- Following exposure of the anterior projection of the latissimus dorsi, reflect the latissimus posteriorly to expose the underlying serratus anterior muscle while preserving the thoracodorsal neurovascular pedicle (**TECH FIG 2**).
- Dissect out the thoracodorsal artery to identify and preserve the serratus artery branches.
- After isolating the serratus perforators, continue to expose the inferior 3 to 4 serratus slips.
  - The long thoracic nerve also travels superficial to the muscle and must be identified to avoid inadvertent damage.

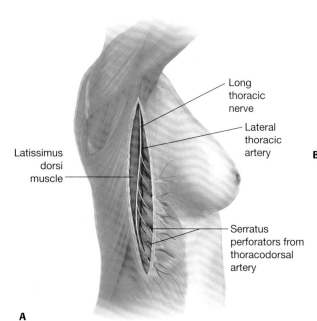

Long thoracic nerve

Lateral thoracic artery

Latissimus dorsi muscle

Serratus perforators from thoracodorsal artery

A

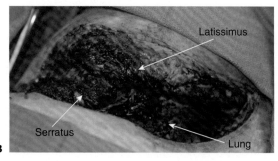

Latissimus

Serratus

Lung

B

TECH FIG 2 • **A.** Incision and initial dissection. **B.** Postdissection wound in a patient with a complicated empyema who underwent open window thoracomyoplasty.

T E C H N I Q U E S

■ Flap Harvest

- Dissect posteriorly and superiorly toward the axilla following the serratus slips to their scapular attachments.
- Identify and preserve the lateral thoracic artery and long thoracic nerve as the dissection travels posteriorly toward the axilla.
- Divide the muscular insertions on the scapula using electrocautery (**TECH FIG 3A**).
- Both the thoracodorsal perforators and lateral thoracic artery can be preserved for flap perfusion or selectively divided depending on the required pedicle length, arc of rotation, and vascular integrity.
- If skeletonizing the pedicle(s), it should be performed cautiously to preserve sufficient perivascular adipose tissue to reduce the risk for vasospasm and avoid damaging the paired venae comitantes that accompany the artery.
- Identify the origin for each slip on the corresponding rib.
  - For a muscle transposition or myocutaneous flap, this costal muscular insertion can be divided for elevation of the serratus muscle (**TECH FIG 3B**).

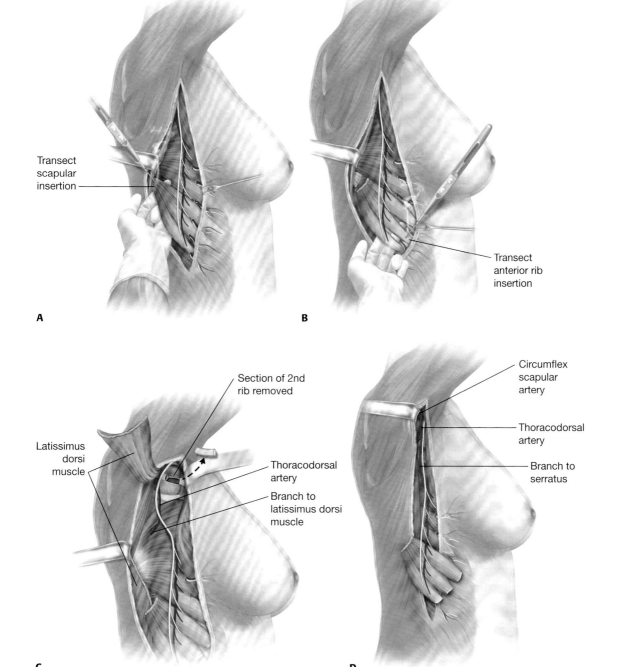

TECH FIG 3 • **A.** Retraction of latissimus and exposure of serratus. **B.** Serratus flap elevation. **C.** Optional rib harvesting step. **D.** Elevated serratus anterior flap on pedicle.

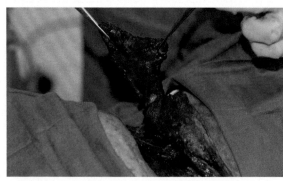

E

TECH FIG 3 (Continued) • **E.** Intraoperative photo of serratus anterior muscle flap elevated on lateral thoracic artery pedicle.

- If the rib is also desired for reconstruction, mark the anterior osteotomy site.
  - Sharply dissect onto the rib after identifying the superior and inferior rib boundaries.

- Dissect in the subperiosteal plane on the posterior costal border while ensuring the intercostal neurovascular bundle, posterior periosteum, and adjacent pleura remain intact.
- Perform the anterior and posterior osteotomies to elevate the flap (**TECH FIG 3C**).
- Following flap elevation, continue to proximally dissect the vascular pedicle to the desired length with or without skeletonization depending on inset goals.
  - Up to 15 cm pedicle length and 4 mm vessel diameter are possible if dissection is carried up to axillary insertion for the thoracodorsal-based pedicle (**TECH FIG 3D,E**).
- Ensure constant visualization and isolation of the long thoracic and thoracodorsal nerves to avoid injury.
  - The skin paddle is innervated by the lateral cutaneous branches of the intercostal nerves, which can be readily identified and preserved during flap elevation to preserve sensation to the skin flap.

Flap Inset

- Close attention must be paid during skeletonization to preserve some perivascular adipose in the pedicle, which will reduce the risk for vasospasm and pedicle kinking.
- Ensure sufficient pedicle length has been dissected to prevent excessive tension on the pedicle during flap transposition or insetting.
- Maintain awareness of the position in which the vascular pedicles lie to ensure that no kinking or twisting has occurred, which may compromise blood flow to the flap immediately or early in the postoperative period.
- **TECH FIG 4** depicts an intrathoracic transposition insetting.

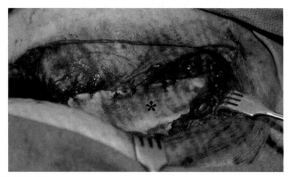

TECH FIG 4 • Intrathoracic flap insetting and subsequent coverage with acellular dermal matrix (*) for defect reconstruction.

PEARLS AND PITFALLS

Techniques	■ Limit harvest to inferior 3 or 4 slips to avoid damage to long thoracic nerve.
	■ The crow's foot landmark (around 7th to 8th slip) is the point at which the dominant serratus branch of the thoracodorsal artery enters the muscular fascia, crosses the long thoracic nerve, and arborizes anteriorly to supply the inferior slips that will be harvested for the flap.[3]
	■ The neurovascular bundle lies superficial to the muscle flap, which facilitates safe dissection from violating the posterior costal periosteum when harvesting a rib.
	■ The subscapular system can be further modified to create a chimeric flap involving the latissimus dorsi, scapular, parascapular muscle, and scapular spine.
	■ A skin paddle may also be taken by preserving myocutaneous perforators if needed for defect coverage.

POSTOPERATIVE CARE

- Occlusive-type dressings are preferred.
- Drains are necessary to avoid seroma.
- Local anesthetic block and muscle relaxant can be beneficial to mitigate postoperative pain.
- Thoracic epidural analgesia can also provide extended pain relief.

- Flap monitoring
  - As with any other flap, the 24- to 48-hour postoperative window requires particularly attentive flap monitoring in the form of clinical and/or US Doppler evaluations to identify any signs of pending flap failure.
  - Specific clinical findings point to the vascular etiology and can facilitate more efficient operative interventions.

- Arterial: Cold, pale, poor capillary refill, and minimal to absent bleeding with pinprick test
- Venous: Warm, edematous, dusky/purple, and dark blood with pinprick test
- Newer technology such as ViOptix tissue oximetry may be used to further enhance postoperative flap monitoring. These systems provide continuous flap monitoring with real-time feedback to support clinical decisions regarding flap compromise and the necessity for flap take backs.

OUTCOMES

- Depending on the number of serratus slips harvested, the donor site scar can be made relatively short and well hidden laterally parallel to the adducted arm.
- Limiting the harvest to the inferior 3 or 4 slips and preserving the long thoracic nerve result in good retention of muscular function and overall limited donor-site morbidity.

COMPLICATIONS

- Postoperative complications with chest wall reconstruction include donor and/or recipient site hematoma or seroma formation, infection, and pneumothorax.
- If reconstructive plates are used for chest wall stabilization, extrusion and infection can result if the hardware is placed in a radiated bed or has insufficient soft tissue coverage.
- Flap
  - Failure secondary to arterial or venous congestion is more likely to occur in cases where there was extensive skeletonization, excessive tension, and/or kinking of the pedicle during flap insetting.

- Donor-site morbidity may include chronic pain, loss of scapular/shoulder ROM or functionality, and winged scapula.

REFERENCES

1. Takayanagi S, Tsukie T. Free serratus anterior muscle and myocutaneous flaps. *Ann Plast Surg.* 1982;8(4):277-283.
2. Arnold PG, Pairolero PC, Waldorf JC. The serratus anterior muscle: intrathoracic and extrathoracic utilization. *Plast Reconstr Surg.* 1984;73(2):240-246.
3. Cuadros C, Driscoll C, Rothkopf D. The anatomy of the lower serratus anterior muscle: a fresh cadaver study. *Plast Reconstr Surg.* 1995;95(1):93-97.
4. Tashiro K, Harima M, Mito D, et al. Preoperative color Doppler ultrasound assessment of the lateral thoracic artery perforator flap and its branching pattern. *J Plast Reconstr Aesthet Surg.* 2015;68(6):e120-e125.
5. Jesus RC, Lopes MCH, Demarchi GTS, et al. The subscapular artery and the thoracodorsal branch: an anatomical study. *Folia Morphol.* 2008;67(1):58-62.
6. Godat DM, Sanger JR, Lifchez SD, et al. Detailed neurovascular anatomy of the serratus anterior muscle: implications for a functional muscle flap with multiple independent force vectors. *Plast Reconstr Surg.* 2004;114(1):21-29.
7. Caprini JA. Thrombosis risk assessment as a guide to quality patient care. *Dis Mon.* 2005;51(2):70-78.
8. Saint-Cyr M, Schaverien M, Arbique G, et al. Three- and four-dimensional computed tomographic angiography and venography for the investigation of the vascular anatomy and perfusion of perforator flaps. *Plast Reconstr Surg.* 2008;121(3):772-780.
9. Schaverien M, Saint-Cyr M, Arbique G, et al. Three- and four-dimensional arterial and venous anatomies of the thoracodorsal artery perforator flap. *Plast Reconstr Surg.* 2008;121(5):1578-1587.
10. Mahabir RC, Butler CE. Stabilization of the chest wall: autologous and alloplastic reconstructions. *Semin Plast Surg.* 2011;25(1):34-42.

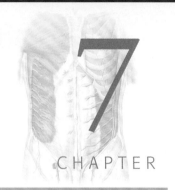

Section II: Reconstruction of the Abdominal Wall
Hernia Repair With Open Component Separation

Ibrahim Khansa and Jeffrey E. Janis

DEFINITION

- Traditional component separation, now termed "anterior component separation," involves separating the external oblique muscle from the remaining components of the abdominal wall.
- This requires two steps:
  - Incision of the external oblique aponeurosis
  - Delamination of the external oblique muscle from the underlying internal oblique muscle
- A third step (optional) is entry into and development of the retrorectus space.
- "Posterior component separation," also known as a transversus abdominis release (TAR), is another type of component separation. It requires two steps:
  - Entering and developing the retrorectus space
  - Transection of the posterior lamella of the internal oblique and transversus abdominis
  - Delamination of the transversus abdominis and transversalis fascia

ANATOMY

- The layers of the lateral abdominal wall, from superficial to deep, are the external oblique, internal oblique, and transversus abdominis muscles, transversalis fascia, and peritoneum.
- The segmental intercostal nerves to the abdominal wall musculature travel in the layer between the internal oblique and transversus abdominis muscles.
- Vascular perforators to the abdominal wall skin emerge from the deep epigastric vessels.
  - They are arranged into a medial and a lateral row.
  - The medial row is dominant, especially the periumbilical perforators.

PATIENT HISTORY AND PHYSICAL FINDINGS

- Assess if any indications for urgent surgery are present.
  - Bowel obstruction
  - Incarceration/strangulation
  - Infected mesh
- Assess effect of hernia on the patient.
  - Ability to carry out activities of daily living
  - Pain at hernia site
  - Difficulty with defecation
- On physical examination, look for:
  - Peritoneal signs
  - Reducibility of hernia

- Edges of fascial defect
- All scars on the abdomen (which will affect vascularity)
- Presence of skin graft
- Presence of a fistula
- Presence of an ostomy

IMAGING

- CT scan of the abdomen is useful to delineate:
  - The size, extent, and borders of the fascial defect
  - Whether component separation has been performed previously
  - The integrity of the musculofascial components (may have been previously resected)
  - An estimate of the loss of domain
  - Presence and position of prior mesh, if applicable
  - The thickness of soft tissue between the hernia (sac) and overlying skin

SURGICAL MANAGEMENT

Preoperative Planning

- Assess suitability of the patient for major surgery.
  - Smokers and tobacco users should completely abstain for at least 4 weeks preoperatively and 4 weeks postoperatively.[1,2]
  - Nutrition should be optimized before surgery (prealbumin greater than 15 mg/dL, albumin greater than 3.25 g/dL).[2,3]
  - Diabetes should be well controlled (HbA1c $\leq$ 7.4%).[2]
  - Body mass index should be 42 or less, and preferably less than 40.[2]
- After hernia dissection and lysis of adhesions, assess whether component separation is needed:
  - Apply Kocher clamps on the medial edge of the rectus complex on each side.
  - Attempt to simulate midline reapproximation of the rectus complexes by bringing the two sides toward each other.
    - If too much tension is present, which may result in fascial cheese wiring or inability to obtain primary musculofascial reapproximation, start with unilateral component separation and reassess.
    - If still there is too much tension after unilateral component separation, perform bilateral component separation.

Positioning

- Supine with arms abducted 90 degrees and all pressure points padded

Approaches

- Multiple approaches are possible for component separation.
  - Anterior component separation through the hernia defect itself:
    - Open
    - Minimally invasive
- Anterior component separation through separate lateral incisions: Endoscopic
- Posterior component separation: Transversus abdominis release (TAR)

■ Open Anterior Component Separation

- Identify the medial rectus reflection on each side.
- Using Bovie electrocautery, dissect from medial to lateral just above the anterior rectus sheath along the anterior rectus fascia. Multiple vascular perforators may be encountered depending on the extent of the dissection.
  - In the classic open anterior component separation, these perforators are sacrificed and wide skin flaps are developed.
  - In more modern perforator-sparing anterior component separation approaches, they are identified and preserved or remain undissected by limited undermining and preservation of composite tissue to decrease complication rates.

- Identify the semilunar line either by palpating the lateral rectus complex margin between your fingers (intraperitoneal) and thumb (extraperitoneal) or by displacing the rectus muscle laterally.
  - This latter maneuver, described by the senior author as the "tube of toothpaste maneuver" (**TECH FIG 1A**), accentuates the indentation of the semilunar line, making it more visible.[4]
- Once the semilunar line is fully exposed, make an incision in the external oblique aponeurosis 2 cm lateral to the semilunar line (**TECH FIG 1B**).
- Enter the plane between the external oblique and internal oblique muscles. This plane is identified by the presence of an avascular layer between the two muscles.

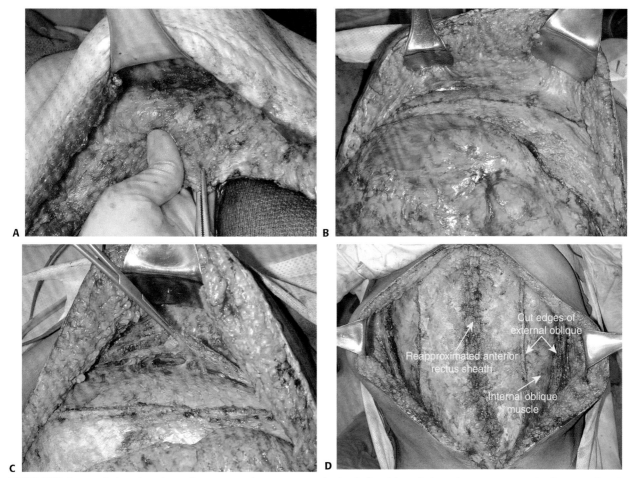

TECH FIG 1 • **A.** "Tube of toothpaste" maneuver: the rectus complex is displaced laterally in order to accentuate the linea semilunaris. **B.** Marking of the external oblique aponeurotomy in classic "Ramirez-style" open anterior component separation. **C.** Elevation of the external oblique muscle off the underlying internal oblique muscle in an areolar, avascular plane, up to the midaxillary line in classic "Ramirez-style" open anterior component separation. **D.** Closure of the anterior rectus sheath after bilateral classic "Ramirez-style" open anterior component separation. Note the degree of medial advancement obtained.

- Using a blunt dissection instrument (such as a plastic Yankauer suction), bluntly dissect the plane superiorly and inferiorly. Then use Bovie electrocautery to continue the external oblique aponeurotomy from the iliac crest inferiorly to 6 cm above the costal margin superiorly.
  - Superiorly, the aponeurosis is more muscular, and care must be taken to obtain adequate hemostasis as the muscle is incised.
- Apply two Allis clamps to the medial edge of the cut external oblique muscle, and lift it off the underlying internal oblique muscle.
- Place a wide malleable on the internal oblique to push it posteriorly, and use Bovie electrocautery or a spreader-dissector to dissect the plane between the external and internal oblique muscles from medial to lateral (**TECH FIG 1C**).
  - This plane should be dissected laterally until sufficient release is performed, varying between the anterior axillary line and posterior axillary line, if needed.
  - Near the posterior axillary line, the vascular pedicle to the external oblique muscle will be encountered along its undersurface and should be preserved.
- This technique allows advancement of 5, 10, and 3 cm in the epigastric, waistline, and suprapubic areas, respectively, on each side (**TECH FIG 1D**).[5]
- If needed, the retrorectus space can be entered by incising along the medial rectus reflection, identifying the rectus

muscle, and keeping the anterior rectus sheath and muscle together as a complex, as well as dissecting the space between the muscle and the posterior sheath.
  - Segmental neurovascular bundles (which enter laterally) should be visualized and preserved.
  - This maneuver theoretically adds 2 cm to the amount of possible advancement in addition to the numbers listed above.[5]
- After hernia repair is complete by primarily reapproximating the musculofascia, a closed suction drain should be placed into the space developed between the external and internal oblique muscles.
- Tension-free closure should be performed in layers with absorbable sutures:
  - Three-point sutures incorporating each side of Scarpa fascia and the underlying closed anterior rectus fascia
  - Deep dermal sutures
  - Running subcuticular suture
- Open anterior component separation requires widely undermined skin flaps, which can lead to seroma formation. The risk of seroma can be decreased by:
  - Closed suction drain placement in the midline, as well as at the external oblique aponeurotomy site
  - Progressive tension sutures between the underside of Scarpa fascia and the anterior rectus sheath
  - Spraying fibrin glue

■ Minimally Invasive Anterior Component Separation[6] (Video 1)

- Identify the rectus complex on each side.
- Using Bovie electrocautery, create a 5-cm-wide tunnel from medial to lateral just superficial to the anterior rectus sheath, located about 4 to 5 cm inferior to the costal margin.
  - This tunnel is meant to spare most vascular perforators to the abdominal wall, especially the periumbilical perforators, by preserving composite tissue.
- Continue medial to lateral dissection within the subcutaneous tunnel until 2 cm lateral to the semilunar line.
  - The semilunar line can be identified using the same "tube of toothpaste" techniques described above[4] (see **TECH FIG 1A**).
- Once the semilunar line is identified, make a limited incision in the external oblique aponeurosis 2 cm lateral to the semilunar line.
- Enter the plane between the external oblique and internal oblique muscles. This plane is identified by the presence of a fatty avascular layer.
- Using a blunt dissection instrument (such as a plastic Yankauer suction), bluntly dissect the plane superiorly and inferiorly.
- Now that the trajectory of the anticipated external oblique aponeurotomy is known by transposing the plastic Yankauer suction tip anteriorly, dissect a precise, narrow vertical subcutaneous tunnel overlying the planned location of the external oblique aponeurotomy (2 cm lateral to the semilunar line).
  - This is made with a combination of a narrow Deaver retractor, Bovie electrocautery, and spreader-dissector.

- Then use Bovie electrocautery to continue the external oblique aponeurotomy under direct visualization from the iliac crest inferiorly to 6 cm above the costal margin superiorly.
  - Superiorly, the aponeurosis is more muscular, and care must be taken to obtain adequate hemostasis as the muscle is cut.
- Apply two Allis clamps to the medial edge of the cut external oblique muscle, and lift it off the underlying internal oblique muscle.
- Place a wide malleable on the internal oblique to push it posterior, and use Bovie electrocautery or a spreader-dissector to dissect the plane between the external and internal oblique muscles from medial to lateral.
  - This plane should be dissected laterally, as needed, to anywhere between the anterior and posterior axillary lines.
  - Near the posterior axillary line, the vascular pedicle to the external oblique muscle will be encountered along its undersurface and should be preserved.
- If needed, the retrorectus space can be entered by incising along the medial rectus reflection, identifying the rectus muscle, and keeping the anterior rectus sheath and muscle together as a complex, dissecting the space between the muscle and the posterior sheath.
  - Segmental neurovascular bundles (which enter laterally) should be visualized and preserved.
  - This maneuver theoretically adds 2 cm to the amount of possible advancement in addition to the numbers listed above.
- After hernia repair is complete by primarily reapproximating the musculofascia, a closed suction drain should be placed into the space developed between the external and internal obliques.

■ Endoscopic Anterior Component Separation Through a Separate Incision[7]

- Make a 1-cm vertical incision 5 cm medial to the anterior superior iliac spine, and dissect down to the anterior rectus sheath (**TECH FIG 2A**).
- Create a vertical subcutaneous tunnel over the midaxillary line, using the Spacemaker balloon (Snowden Pencer, Franklin Lakes, NJ) (**TECH FIG 2B**).
- Use the port to insert a 10-mm, 30-degree, angled laparoscope (**TECH FIG 2C**).

- Under direct endoscopic vision, make a 0.5-cm incision 2 cm below the costal margin and another 0.5-cm incision 3 cm superomedial to the original incision.
- Use the additional ports to insert laparoscopic cautery and forceps.
  - Retract the external oblique muscle laterally while performing an external oblique aponeurotomy 1 to 2 cm lateral to the semilunar line.
  - Then dissect in the plane just deep to the external oblique muscle from medial to lateral (**TECH FIG 2D**).
- Modifications of this technique have also been described, with the use of laparoscopic instruments.[8]

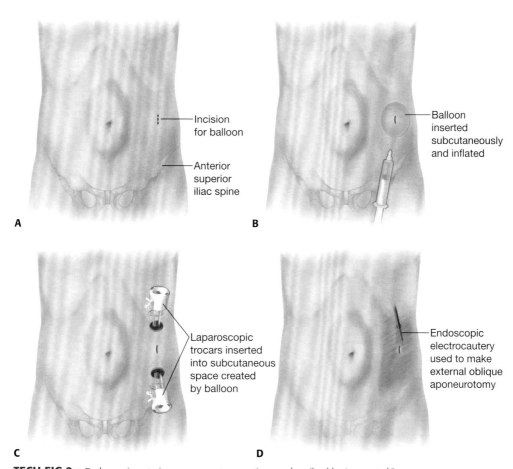

A   Incision for balloon / Anterior superior iliac spine

B   Balloon inserted subcutaneously and inflated

C   Laparoscopic trocars inserted into subcutaneous space created by balloon

D   Endoscopic electrocautery used to make external oblique aponeurotomy

TECH FIG 2 • Endoscopic anterior component separation, as described by Lowe et al.[7]

■ Transversus Abdominis Release[9,10]

- Identify the medial edge of the rectus complex on each side.
- Use Bovie electrocautery to incise the medial rectus reflection to enter the retrorectus space (**TECH FIG 3A**).
  - Note any small pre-existing rents in the medial aspect of the posterior rectus sheath through which the fibers of the rectus muscle are visible. If present, these constitute an ideal entry point into the retrorectus space.
- Apply a Kocher or Babcock clamp to the anterior rectus sheath/rectus muscle complex and retract it anteriorly and laterally while retracting the posterior rectus sheath posteriorly and medially.

- Using a combination of blunt dissection (Kittner) and Bovie electrocautery, or with a spreader-dissector, dissect on top of the posterior rectus sheath from medial to lateral, developing the space by elevating the rectus muscle and underlying fat.
  - The deep inferior epigastric vessels must be protected during this dissection.
  - The retrorectus fat must be elevated with the muscle, leaving behind the shiny white posterior rectus sheath. This facilitates protection of the deep inferior epigastric vessels.
- Continue this dissection laterally until the semilunar line is encountered. Segmental intercostal nerves to the rectus

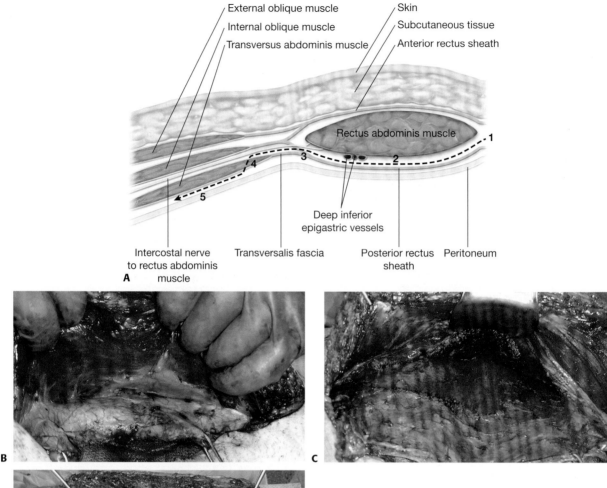

TECH FIG 3 • A. Transverse abdominis release steps. (*1*) Enter retrorectus space. (*2*) Elevate rectus abdominis muscle and fat off the posterior rectus sheath. (*3*) Incise posterior leaflet of internal oblique aponeurosis medial to the intercostal nerves. (*4*) Transect transversus abdominis muscle. (*5*) Dissect extraperitoneal plane deep to transversus abdominis muscle. **B.** Dissection plane in posterior component separation. **C.** Transection of transversus abdominis muscle fibers in transversus abdominis release (TAR) or "posterior component separation." **D.** Extended retromuscular plane after TAR. Note the degree of medial advancement obtained.

muscle will be visible and should be preserved. Blunt dissection can be performed around the nerves.
- Dissect this retrorectus plane superiorly up to the costal margin (or even posterior to it) and inferiorly to the pubic bone.
  - Care must be taken inferior to the arcuate line, as the posterior rectus sheath consists of only the transversalis fascia at this point and is very thin.
- Starting as superior as possible, and 0.5 cm medial to the intercostal nerves to the rectus muscle, incise the posterior lamella of the internal oblique aponeurosis. This will demonstrate the transverse muscular fibers of the transversus abdominis muscle (**TECH FIG 3B**).
- Using a right angle clamp, spread the fibers of the transversus abdominis muscle to separate them from the underlying fascia.

- Then, using Bovie electrocautery, incise the transversus abdominis muscle. Make sure the transversalis fascia and peritoneum are not injured. A saline-moistened bowel towel protector is also helpful.
- Continue this dissection from superior to inferior until the full length of the transversus abdominis muscle is incised.
- Apply two Allis clamps to the cut edge of the transversus abdominis muscle and enter the underlying avascular plane. This plane can be dissected from medial to lateral using a combination of blunt dissection (Kittner) and cautery (**TECH FIG 3C**).
  - The dissection can be taken superior to the dome of the diaphragm, inferiorly to the pubic bone and Cooper ligaments, and laterally to the psoas muscles.
- The posterior component separation allows advancement of 4 to 8 cm on each side (**TECH FIG 3D**).[9]

PEARLS AND PITFALLS

Techniques	■ Anterior component separation is only complete after the external oblique muscle has been completely elevated off the underlying internal oblique muscle laterally to the level of the anterior axillary, midaxillary, or posterior axillary line, depending on the patient. External oblique aponeurotomy alone does not constitute component separation. ■ Minimally invasive techniques for anterior component separation have been proven to have lower rates of wound healing problems compared to techniques with wide undermining. ■ When dissecting the retrorectus space, the fatty layer should be elevated with the rectus muscle, leaving behind the white posterior rectus sheath. This is very important to protect the deep inferior epigastric vessels from iatrogenic injury. ■ When performing a posterior component separation/TAR, start as superiorly as possible (where the transversus abdominis has the most muscle fibers and is easier to identify) and proceed inferiorly.
Visualization	■ When performing minimally invasive component separation, adequate visualization can only be obtained if the surgeons wear a headlight or use a lighted retractor.
Outcomes	■ Even in cases in which fascial reapproximation is not possible despite component separation, and where a bridged mesh repair is therefore necessary, the defect size should be reduced using component separation, as this has been shown to reduce recurrence rates.[11] ■ Mesh decreases recurrence rates in all cases and should be used in defects larger than 4 cm.

POSTOPERATIVE CARE

■ DVT prophylaxis: Patients should ambulate the evening of surgery and then at least 5 times daily thereafter.[2]

■ Pulmonary toilet: Patients should use incentive spirometry 10 times every hour while awake.[2]

■ Analgesia: The use of neuraxial blocks, intraoperative local anesthetic infiltration in the transversus abdominis plane, and postoperative use of nonopioid analgesics (gabapentin, celecoxib, ibuprofen, acetaminophen) reduce narcotic requirements, which improves mental status and pulmonary function and accelerates return of bowel function.

OUTCOMES

■ Minimally invasive techniques of component separation have lower rates of wound healing problems than techniques with wide undermining.

  ■ Ghali et al. compared minimally invasive technique to traditional component separation and found lower rates of skin dehiscence (11% vs 28%), seroma (2% vs 6%), abdominal bulge (4% vs 14%), and hernia recurrence (4% vs 8%).[12]

  ■ Saulis et al. compared minimally invasive technique to traditional component separation and found lower rates of wound necrosis/infection (2% vs 20%).[13]

  ■ Lowe et al. compared minimally invasive technique to traditional component separation and found lower rates of wound infection (0% vs 40%) and dehiscence (0% vs 43%).[7]

■ In cases in which fascia cannot be reapproximated and a bridged mesh repair is planned, component separation should still be performed to reduce the defect size.[11]

COMPLICATIONS

■ Surgical complications
  ■ Surgical site occurrences
    • Cellulitis
    • Abscess
    • Hematoma
    • Seroma
    • Dehiscence/necrosis
    • Fistula
  ■ Hernia recurrence
  ■ Bulge
  ■ Abdominal compartment syndrome
    • Suspect is intraoperative peak airway pressure increases by 12 mm Hg or more above baseline[6] or if intraoperative plateau pressure increases by 6 cm H_2O (4.4 mm Hg) or more.[14]
■ Medical complications
  ■ Pulmonary (atelectasis, pneumonia, reintubation)
  ■ Urologic (urinary tract infection)

REFERENCES

1. Sorensen LT. Wound healing and infection in surgery: the pathophysiological impact of smoking, smoking cessation, and nicotine replacement therapy: a systematic review. *Ann Surg.* 2012; 255: 1069-1079.
2. Harrison B, Khansa I, Janis JE. Evidence-based strategies to reduce postoperative complications in plastic surgery. *Plast Reconstr Surg.* 2016;137:351-360.
3. Kudsk KA, Tolley EA, DeWitt RC, et al. Preoperative albumin and surgical site identify surgical risk for major postoperative complications. *J Parenter Enteral Nutr.* 2003;27:1-9.
4. Janis JE, Khansa I. Evidence-based abdominal wall reconstruction: the maxi-mini technique. *Plast Reconstr Surg.* 2015;136:1312-1323.
5. Ramirez OM, Ruas E, Dellon AL. "Components separation" method for closure of abdominal-wall defects: an anatomic and clinical study. *Plast Reconstr Surg.* 1990;86:519-526.
6. Butler CE, Campbell KT. Minimally invasive component separation with inlay bioprosthetic mesh (MICSIB) for complex abdominal wall reconstruction. *Plast Reconstr Surg.* 2011;128:698-709.
7. Lowe JB, Garza JR, Bowman JL, et al. Endoscopically assisted "components separation" for closure of abdominal wall defects. *Plast Reconstr Surg.* 2000;105:720-729.
8. Rosen MJ, Jin J, McGee MF, et al. Laparoscopic component separation in the single-stage treatment of infected abdominal wall prosthetic removal. *Hernia.* 2007;11:435-440.
9. Gibreel W, Sarr MG, Rosen M, Novitsky Y. Technical considerations in performing posterior component separation with transverse abdominis muscle release. *Hernia.* 2016;20:449-459.

10. Novitsky YW, Elliott HL, Orenstein SB, Rosen MJ. Transversus abdominis muscle release: a novel approach to posterior component separation during complex abdominal wall reconstruction. *Am J Surg.* 2012;204:709-716.

11. Itani KMF, Rosen M, Vargo D, et al. Prospective study of single-stage repair of contaminated hernias using a biologic porcine tissue matrix: the RICH study. *Surgery.* 2012;152:498-505.

12. Ghali S, Turza KC, Baumann DP, Butler CE. Minimally invasive component separation results in fewer wound-healing complications than open component separation for large ventral hernia repairs. *J Am Coll Surg.* 2012;214:981-989.

13. Saulis AS, Dumanian GA. Periumbilical rectus abdominis perforator preservation significantly reduces superficial wound complications in "separation of parts" hernia repairs. *Plast Reconstr Surg.* 2002;109:2275-2280.

14. Blatnik JA, Krpata DM, Rosen MJ, et al. Predicting severe postoperative respiratory complications following abdominal wall reconstruction. *Plast Reconstr Surg.* 2012;130:836-841.

Ventral Hernia: Component Separation Technique

Mark W. Clemens and Charles E. Butler

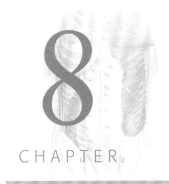

CHAPTER 81

DEFINITION

- The component separation technique is a type of rectus abdominis muscle advancement flap that reconstructs ventral hernia and large abdominal wall defects.
- Component separation is a fascial release of the external oblique fascia with creation of musculofascial advancement flaps.
- The general indications for performing a component separation of the abdominal wall include a deficiency of the abdominal wall fascia, which would require a bridged repair without fascial release.
- Ramirez and colleagues' description of the surgical technique of component separation moves the rectus musculofascia medially, to close midline defect by releasing the external oblique aponeuroses and posterior rectus sheath bilaterally.[1]
- Myofascial advancement techniques, or component separation, takes advantage of the laminar nature of the abdominal wall and the ability to release one muscular or fascial layer to enable medial advancement of another.

ANATOMY

- The lateral abdominal wall musculature is composed of three layers, with the fascicles of each muscle directed obliquely at different angles to create a strong envelope for the abdominal contents.
- Each of the muscles forms an aponeurosis that inserts into the linea alba, a midline structure joining the two sides of the abdominal wall.
- The external oblique muscle is the most superficial muscle of the lateral abdominal wall.
- The deepest muscular layer of the abdominal wall is the transversus abdominis muscle with its fibers coursing horizontally. These three lateral muscles give rise to aponeurotic layers lateral to the rectus abdominis muscle, which contribute to the anterior and posterior layers of the rectus sheath.
- The transversus abdominis muscle inserts into the transversus abdominis aponeurosis to form the posterior rectus sheath and continues as a muscular component laterally in the upper abdomen. This feature is important when considering the technical aspects of a posterior component separation.
- At the midline, the two anterior rectus sheaths form the tendinous linea alba. On either side of the linea alba is the rectus abdominis muscle, the fibers of which course vertically and run the length of the anterior abdominal wall.

- The arcuate line, located 3 to 6 cm below the umbilicus, delineates the point below which the posterior rectus sheath is absent and is composed of the transversalis fascia and peritoneum.
- The abdominal wall receives the majority of its innervation from the 7th to 12th intercostal nerves and the first and second lumbar nerves.
- The lateral abdominal muscles receive their blood supply from the lower three to four intercostal arteries, the deep circumflex iliac artery, and the lumbar arteries. The rectus abdominis muscles are perfused by the superior epigastric artery (a terminal branch of the internal mammary artery), the inferior epigastric artery (a branch of the external iliac artery), and the lower intercostal arteries.

PATHOGENESIS

- Indications for abdominal wall reconstruction include tumor ablation, congenital anomalies, and trauma.
- Abdominal defects and hernias may result from genetically impaired collagen formation, deposition, organization with sequelae from injury, failed laparotomy closures, or failed hernia repairs.
- Risk factors for the development of hernias included tobacco use and a strong family history of hernia, which suggests a genetic predisposition.

PATIENT HISTORY AND PHYSICAL FINDINGS

- The most common presentation to reconstructive surgeons is an incisional hernia as sequelae to a previous laparotomy.
- There are three general indications to repair an incisional hernia: the hernia is symptomatic, causing pain or alterations in the bowel habits; the hernia results in a significant protrusion that affects the patient's quality of life; and the hernia poses a significant risk of bowel obstruction (such as a large hernia with a narrow neck).
- Acquired hernias typically occur after surgical incisions and thus are commonly referred to as incisional hernias.
- Epigastric hernias occur from the xiphoid process to the umbilicus, umbilical hernias occur at the umbilicus, and hypogastric hernias occur below the umbilicus in the midline.
- Although not a true hernia, diastasis recti can present clinically as a bulge in the midline. In this condition, the linea alba is stretched, resulting in bulging at the medial margins of the rectus abdominis muscles. There is no fascial ring or true hernia sac. Unless significantly symptomatic, diastasis recti does not need to be corrected surgically.
- Previous rectus abdominis muscle flap harvest does not preclude the future use of component separation techniques.[2]

IMAGING

- Preoperative computed tomography to examine the defect characteristics and abdominal wall anatomy and vascularity is helpful for surgical planning.
- Computed tomography (CT) allows for visualization of intra-abdominal organs, and the abdominal wall, three-dimensional data sets, and multiplanar reformation capabilities.
- CT scans may assist in detecting fluid collections, bowel obstruction, incarceration, strangulation, and traumatic wall hernias.
- Magnetic resonance (MR) imaging also permits the detection of soft tissue defects and abdominal wall hernias though this modality does not usually offer further sensitivity and therefore may be cost-prohibitive.

SURGICAL MANAGEMENT

Preoperative Planning

- Physical examination should be performed to assess the patient's general condition, the abdominal wall integrity, and the extent and location of any abdominal wall abnormalities.
- The presence of scars that compromise blood supply could become an obstacle to raising reliable tissue flaps.
- Routine laboratory tests and a nutritional workup are advised.
- Patients should be marked in the preoperative holding area, and it is beneficial to evaluate patients in a recumbent and supine position for complete evaluation of abdominal wall defects.
- Markings may delineate anatomical boundaries such as the pelvis, midline, and costal margin as well as the fascial extent of any intra-abdominal defects.

- Bowel preps may be beneficial in patients with anticipated violation of the gastrointestinal tract.
- Intravenous antibiotics are initiated in the holding area.

Positioning

- Patients are placed supine on the operative table, sedated, and intubated.
- The abdomen is widely draped and prepped to expose the patient's flanks and from the pelvis to the midsternal area.
- Patients should receive sequential compression devices and or compression hoses for deep vein thrombosis prophylaxis.
- Patients requiring greater exposure should have room temperatures maintained above 75°F to minimize postoperative infections.

Approach

- All approaches to abdominal wall closure should be aimed at re-establishment of the abdominal domain integrity with complete fascial coaptation.
- All attempts should be made to avoid a bridged mesh repair because there is a clear trend toward higher recurrence rates compared with when the fascia can be reapproximated over a mesh repair.
- Component separation release can be done by open or minimally invasive component separation. A minimally invasive component separation can be performed in various ways, but all of the techniques (to a certain degree) maintain the blood supply to the skin from the underlying rectus abdominis muscles.

■ Open Component Separation

- An open component separation is performed by raising large subcutaneous flaps to expose the external oblique fascia[3] (**TECH FIG 1**).
- The cutaneous perforators emerging from the anterior rectus sheath are ligated and divided to facilitate exposure of the linea semilunaris in its entirety. These flaps are carried laterally past the linea semilunaris.
- An anatomically precise external oblique aponeurotomy is made 1 to 2 cm lateral to the linea semilunaris on the lateral aspect of the external oblique aponeurosis from several centimeters above the costal margin to the pubis. It is important to confirm that the incision is not carried through the linea semilunaris, as this would result in a full-thickness defect of the lateral abdominal wall, which is challenging to repair.
- The external oblique aponeurosis is then bluntly separated in the avascular plane away from the internal oblique aponeurosis to the midaxillary line, allowing the internal oblique and transversus abdominis muscles with the rectus abdominis muscle or fascia to advance medially as a unit.
- These techniques, when performed bilaterally, can yield up to 20 cm of mobilization in the midabdomen.
- Once the mesh inset and fascial closure are performed, the subcutaneous skin flaps are advanced and closed at the midline.

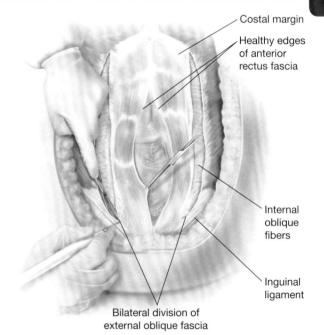

Costal margin

Healthy edges of anterior rectus fascia

Internal oblique fibers

Inguinal ligament

Bilateral division of external oblique fascia

TECH FIG 1 • Open component separation. Subcutaneous flaps are elevated off the anterior rectus sheath to expose the external oblique aponeurosis. The external oblique aponeurosis is released from the inguinal ligament inferiorly to above the costal margin superiorly. This allows exposure of the internal oblique muscle fibers once the external aponeurosis is incised.

T E C H N I Q U E S

- To reduce subcutaneous dead space, interrupted quilting sutures should be placed between the Scarpa fascia and musculofascial repair.
- This technique also decreases shear stress, which is thought to contribute to postoperative seroma formation, and decreases the total drain output, allowing the surgeon to place fewer drains and leave them in for a shorter period.
- After paramedian skin perfusion is critically assessed, a vertical panniculectomy may be performed so that the skin is reapproximated in the midline without redundancy.

■ Laparoscopic Component Separation

- Laparoscopically, component separation is performed through a 1-cm incision below the tip of the 11th rib overlying the external oblique muscle.[4,5]
- The external oblique muscle is split in the direction of its fibers, and a standard bilateral inguinal hernia balloon dissector is placed between the external and internal oblique muscles and directed toward the pubis (**TECH FIG 2**).[6]

- Three laparoscopic trocars are placed in the space created, and the dissection is carried from the pubis to several centimeters above the costal margin.
- The linea semilunaris is carefully identified, and the external oblique aponeurosis is incised from beneath the external oblique muscle at least 2 cm lateral to the linea semilunaris.
- The muscle is released from the pubis to several centimeters above the costal margin.
- This procedure may be performed bilaterally depending on the width of the defect and the amount of advancement required.

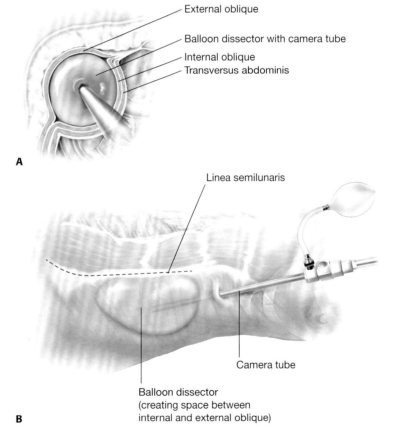

External oblique
Balloon dissector with camera tube
Internal oblique
Transversus abdominis

A

Linea semilunaris

Camera tube

Balloon dissector
(creating space between
internal and external oblique)

B

TECH FIG 2 • Laparoscopic component separation. **A.** Access to the external oblique aponeurosis is achieved through a small incision at the costal margin through which a balloon dissector is placed. The external oblique aponeurosis is then divided from the pubis to above the costal margin. **B.** This minimally invasive approach preserves the attachments of the subcutaneous tissue (including myocutaneous perforators) to the anterior rectus sheath throughout its course.

■ Periumbilical Perforator-Sparing Technique

- A periumbilical perforator-sparing technique of component separation may be performed to preserve the blood supply to the anterior abdominal wall skin near the midline and is based primarily on perforator vessels from the deep inferior epigastric vessels.

- Cadaver dissections and radiographic studies confirmed that the majority of these vessels are located within 3 cm of the umbilicus. With preservation of these vessels, ischemic complications involving the subcutaneous flaps are significantly reduced.
- To avoid injury to the periumbilical perforator vessels, a line is marked no less than 3 cm cephalad and 3 cm caudal to the umbilicus.

- The periumbilical perforator tunnels are begun at the epigastric and suprapubic regions. Subcutaneous tunnels are created using lighted retractors to identify the external oblique fascia.
- The superior and inferior tunnels are connected using cautery and retractors while maintaining the subcutaneous attachments of the periumbilical region.

- The linea semilunaris is identified by palpation, and the external oblique is incised 2 cm lateral to this junction.
- The aponeurotomy is extended several centimeters above the costal margin and to the pubic tubercle.
- The external oblique muscle is separated from the internal oblique muscle in an avascular plane toward the posterior axillary line for additional advancement to the midline.

■ Minimally Invasive Component Separation

- The MICS technique is designed to avoid division of the musculocutaneous perforators overlying the rectus sheath and thus maintain perfusion to the paramedian skin.[7-9]
- After lysis of adhesions and identification of the fascial edges, bilateral, 3-cm wide, subcutaneous access tunnels are created over the anterior rectus sheath from the

midline to the linea semilunaris at the level of the costal margin (**TECH FIG 3A**).
- Through these access tunnels, the external oblique aponeurosis is vertically incised 1.5 cm lateral to the linea semilunaris (**TECH FIG 3B**).
- The tip of a metal Yankauer suction handle (Cardinal Health, Dublin, OH), without suction, is inserted through the opening in the avascular plane between the internal and external oblique aponeuroses, separating them at their junction with the rectus sheath.

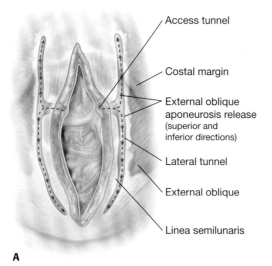

Access tunnel

Costal margin

External oblique aponeurosis release (superior and inferior directions)

Lateral tunnel

External oblique

Linea semilunaris

A

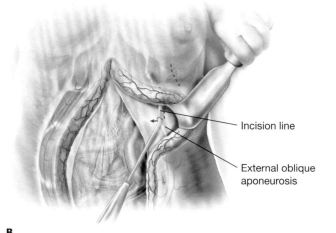

Incision line

External oblique aponeurosis

B

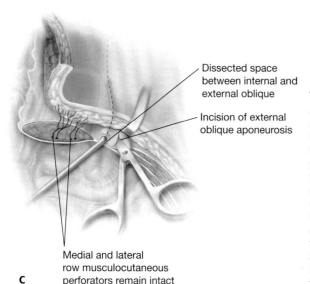

Dissected space between internal and external oblique

Incision of external oblique aponeurosis

Medial and lateral row musculocutaneous perforators remain intact

C

TECH FIG 3 • Minimally invasive component separation (MICS). **A.** Access to the external oblique aponeurosis is achieved through a small tunnel from the midline to the supraumbilical external oblique aponeurosis. Vertical tunnels are created dorsal and ventral to the planned release site of the external oblique aponeurosis. Periumbilical perforators and the subcutaneous tissue overlying the anterior rectus sheath are left undisturbed. **B.** The external oblique aponeurosis is then divided from the pubis to above the costal margin. The external oblique aponeurosis in the upper abdomen is released with electrocautery as the muscle is transected at, and superior to, the costal margin. **C.** Scissors are generally used to release the external oblique aponeurosis inferiorly. This MICS approach preserves the attachments of the subcutaneous tissue (including myocutaneous perforators) to the anterior rectus sheath throughout its course.

- The suction tip is advanced inferiorly to the pubis and superiorly to above the costal margin.
- Next, lateral dissection between the internal and external oblique muscles is performed to the midaxillary line (**TECH FIG 3C**).
- Minimal subcutaneous skin flaps are then elevated over the anterior rectus sheath circumferentially to the medial row of rectus abdominis perforator vessels, and a retrorectus or preperitoneal mesh inlay is generally used.
- If a preperitoneal inset is used, the preperitoneal fat is dissected from the posterior sheath circumferentially to allow the mesh to be inlaid directly against the posterior sheath or rectus abdominis muscle (below the arcuate line).
- Mesh is inserted to the semilunar line with no. 1 polypropylene sutures via the horizontal access tunnels and the cranial and caudal aspect of the defect.

- Next, the myofascial edges are advanced and reapproximated over the mesh with sutures placed through the myofascia and mesh.
- Interrupted resorbable 3-0 sutures are placed to affix the posterior sheath to the mesh, thereby obliterating dead space and reducing the potential for fluid collection.
- Closed suction drainage catheters are placed in each component separation donor-site area, in the space between the rectus complex closure and mesh, and in the subcutaneous space.
- The remaining undermined skin flaps are sutured to the myofascia with vertical rows of interrupted resorbable 3-0 quilting sutures to reduce dead space and potential shear between the subcutaneous tissue and myofascia.

■ Posterior Component Separation

- A posterior component separation is based on the retromuscular Rives-Stoppa approach to ventral hernia repair.
- The posterior component separation focuses on transversus abdominis aponeurosis release.
- By incising this myofascial aponeurosis, the surgeon exposes the preperitoneal space. This provides substantial advancement of both the posterior fascial flap and the anterior myofascial compartment.
- The initial release is completed by incising the posterior rectus sheath approximately 1 cm lateral to the linea alba, and the posterior rectus sheath is separated from the overlying rectus muscle (**TECH FIG 4A**).

- The transversus abdominis muscle is incised just medial to the intercostal nerves, and the underlying transversalis fascia and peritoneum are identified (**TECH FIG 4B**). This myofascial release is extended the entire length of the posterior rectus sheath.
- The potential space between the transversus abdominis muscle and the peritoneum is developed as far laterally as necessary, even to the psoas muscle if needed. This plane can be extended superiorly to the costal margin, retrosternally above the xiphoid, and inferiorly into the space of Retzius.
- The posterior sheath is then closed, to completely exclude any mesh from the viscera. An adequately sized piece of mesh is then secured, similar to a standard retromuscular repair but with greater overlap.

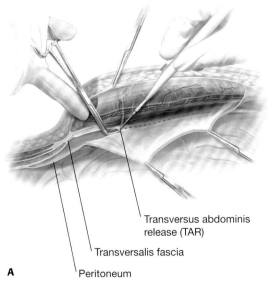

Transversus abdominis release (TAR)

Transversalis fascia

A Peritoneum

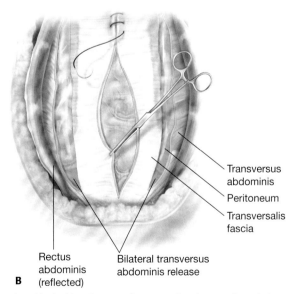

Transversus abdominis

Peritoneum

Transversalis fascia

Rectus abdominis (reflected)

Bilateral transversus abdominis release

B

TECH FIG 4 • Posterior component separation. **A.** The initial release is completed by incising the posterior rectus sheath approximately 1 cm lateral to the linea alba, and the posterior rectus sheath is separated from the overlying rectus abdominis muscle. Dissection is carried to the lateral border of the rectus muscle, and the perforating intercostal nerves are identified, marking the linea semilunaris. **B.** Next, the transversus abdominis muscle is incised just medial to the intercostal nerves, and the underlying transversalis fascia and peritoneum are identified. This myofascial release is extended the entire length of the posterior rectus sheath. The potential space between the transversus abdominis muscle and the peritoneum is developed as far laterally as necessary.

PEARLS AND PITFALLS

Abdominal compartment syndrome	■ Although every attempt to re-establish the midline is advisable, not all patients can tolerate the intraperitoneal compression required (which can result in intraperitoneal hypertension, pulmonary compromise, or abdominal compartment syndrome).
Seroma formation	■ Adequate drainage of the skin flaps should be performed with liberal use of drains and quilting sutures. Resection of a previous hernia sac is important to prevent seroma formation.
Hernia recurrence	■ All means necessary should be employed to avoid a bridged repair as primary fascial coaptation is essential to minimize hernia recurrence.
Mesh explantation	■ Tissue-based bioprosthetic mesh has gained popularity for its lower rates of mesh infection, fistula formation, and mesh explantation than the rates reported with synthetic mesh.
Skin coverage deficiency	■ Pedicled muscle flaps and free flaps are important to assist in soft tissue coverage for large abdominal wall defects.

POSTOPERATIVE CARE

- In general, abdominal wall reconstruction patients have prolonged postoperative healing periods due to the dynamic function and mobility of the abdominal musculature.
- Perioperative management of high-risk patients should include appropriate deep venous thrombosis (DVT) chemoprophylaxis according to the Caprini risk score.
- Sequential compression devices and early ambulation should be utilized with low molecular weight fractionated heparins administered postoperatively.
- Perioperative antibiotics are indicated, and cases with violation of the gastrointestinal tract should be offered broader coverage for anaerobic as well as Gram-negative bacteria.
- For ventral hernia, closed suction drains are used liberally and are kept in place on average 1 to 2 weeks until less than 30 cc/day.
- Abdominal wall reconstruction patients should refrain from strenuous activities and exercises that isolate the abdominal core for at least 6 to 12 weeks.
- Patients may gain comfort from the use of an abdominal binder for 3 months and then with any expected heavy physical activity thereafter.

- Routine follow-up includes a physical examination in an outpatient clinic, often performed weekly for 1 month after discharge, then every 3 months for 1 year, and then annually thereafter.

OUTCOMES

- Estimated incidences of hernia recurrence have a wide range from 2% to 54%, depending on the type of repair (mesh 2% to 36% vs suture repair alone 25% to 54%), patient comorbidities, and surgical technique[10] (**FIGS 1** to **3**).
- The number of prior attempts of hernia repair is predictive of the relative risk of recurrence. In a study of approximately 10 000 patients, 5-year reoperative rate was 23.8% after a primary repair, 35.3% following a secondary repair, and 38.7% after a tertiary repair.
- There are few comparative data to suggest the superiority of one myofascial advancement approach over another, and likely, each has a role in abdominal wall reconstruction. Open component separation often allows tension-free closure of large defects, and recurrence rates as low as 20% have been reported with the use of open component separation and mesh reinforcement in large hernias.

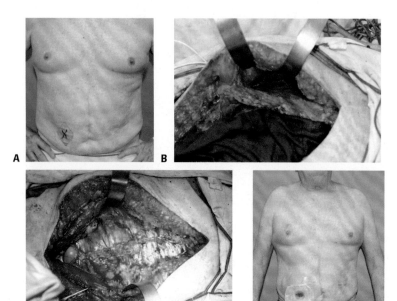

FIG 1 • Abdominal wall reconstruction. **A.** A 67-year-old diabetic man with a history of bladder cancer resection presented with recurrence invasive into his anterior abdominal wall. Following tumor ablation, he has an intraoperative defect of the abdominal wall 10 × 14 cm in size. **B.** Bilateral minimally invasive anterior component separation was performed (**C**) followed by creation of a retrorectus plane (Rives-Stoppa technique) and closure of the anterior abdominal wall fascia. **D.** Patient 18 months after abdominal wall reconstruction and ileal conduit construction with urostomy.

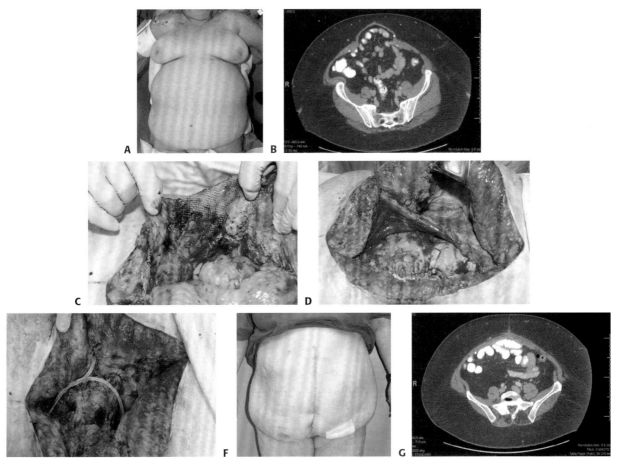

FIG 2 • Hernia repair. **A.** Patient was a 62-year-old woman with a history of colon cancer, morbid obesity with BMI 46, and previous midline hernia repair with mesh reinforcement. **B.** She had a recurrent hernia 12 cm in greatest diameter. **C.** Mesh failure. **D.** Bilateral minimally invasive component separation was performed, which allowed for complete fascial coaptation **(E)**. **F.** Patient at 1 month postoperatively and by CT scan at 1 year postoperatively **(G)**.

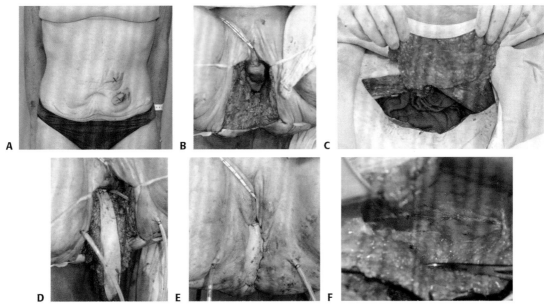

FIG 3 • Pelvic reconstruction and donor-site management. **A.** A 47-year-old woman with invasive cervical cancer required a total pelvic exenteration. **B.** Intraoperative defect. **C.** A pedicled vertical rectus abdominis muscle (VRAM) flap was elevated from the right hemiabdomen and passed through the pelvis **(D)** and inset for reconstruction of the perineum and posterior vaginal wall **(E)**. **F,G.** Patient was thin with minimal abdominal wall laxity, and therefore a unilateral component separation was performed to facilitate closure of the VRAM donor site.

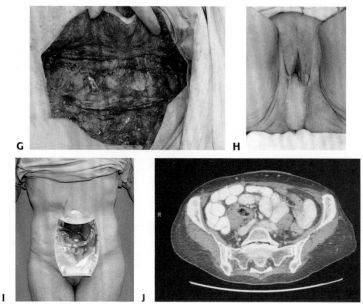

FIG 3 (Continued) • **H.** This allowed for complete fascial closure. **I.** One year postoperative photo and **J.** CT scan.

- Comparative data showed laparoscopic component separation to result in a lower rate of wound morbidity than open component separation. One series reported a significant reduction in wound morbidity with the periumbilical perforator-sparing technique compared with the standard open component separation technique (2% vs 20%; $P < 0.05$).
- A controlled study demonstrated that patients had significantly fewer wound healing complications (32% vs 14%, $P = 0.026$) and skin dehiscence (28% vs 11%, $P = 0.01$) with MICS than with traditional open component separation.

COMPLICATIONS

- Infection
  - In patients with clean-contaminated and contaminated wounds, a prospective multi-institutional study evaluating the role of a porcine ADM to repair abdominal wall defects reported a 34% rate of superficial surgical site infections. In contrast, studies of clean wounds have reported infection rates of 0% to 12%.
  - Mesh infections are reported to occur in 0% to 3.6% of laparoscopic ventral hernia repairs and 6% to 10% of open repairs employing mesh.
  - The most common organism infecting abdominal wall repair is *Staphylococcus aureus*, seen in up to 81% of cases; this suggests skin flora contamination.
  - Gram-negative organisms, such as *Klebsiella* and *Proteus* spp., have been implicated in up to 17% of mesh infections.
  - Management of abdominal wall infections is complex and requires patient individualization as well as a knowledge of bacterial susceptibility for a particular hospital.
- Seroma
  - Seroma formation can occur following abdominal wall reconstruction particularly in cases involving large undermined flaps, which create significant dead space.
  - If symptomatic, seromas can be aspirated percutaneously or under ultrasound guidance.
- In open ventral hernia repair, drains are often placed in an attempt to obliterate the dead space caused by the hernia and tissue dissection.
- Seroma formation is common after abdominal component separation and muscle flaps of the trunk owing to extensive tissue dissection, and drains may be necessary for up to 4 to 6 weeks.
- Intraoperative techniques, such as quilting sutures, fibrin sealant, and postoperative abdominal binders, may help to prevent or reduce seroma formation.
- Enterotomy and enterocutaneous fistulas
  - Appropriate management of an enterotomy during a hernia repair is controversial and depends on the segment of intestine injured (small vs large bowel) and amount of spillage.[11]
  - Options include aborting the hernia repair, continuing the hernia repair and repairing the enterotomy with local tissue or bioprosthetic mesh using a primary tissue or bioprosthetic mesh repair, or performing a delayed repair using mesh in 3 to 4 days.
  - When there is gross contamination, the use of synthetic mesh is generally contraindicated.
  - The treatment of patients with enterocutaneous fistulas (ECFs) is complex and approximately 1/3 of ECFs will close spontaneously with appropriate wound care, nutritional support, and medical therapy.
  - Depending on the location of the fistula along the gastrointestinal tract and the volume of output, significant electrolyte disturbances can occur. In particular, proximal high-output fistulas can result in substantial losses of bicarbonate, which must be adequately replaced.
  - Diligent protection of the surrounding skin is one of the most important and difficult aspects of ECF management. A dedicated enterostomal nurse is essential to the success of wound management as destruction of local skin can seriously affect eventual reconstructive options.

- In cases in which a fistula is already present, negative pressure wound therapy (NPWT) device can be helpful to isolate a fistula from the surrounding wound and to allow a skin graft to heal.
- In cases of uncontrolled intestinal leakage, a proximal diverting stoma can be lifesaving.
- Nutritional supplementation is one of the most important aspects of reducing deaths related to ECFs. During initial management of an ECF, parenteral nutritional support is preferred. However, once the sepsis is controlled and the patient is stabilized, enteral feedings are initiated.
- Hernia
  - The incidence of incisional hernia is approximately 11% following midline laparotomy.
  - Functional problems in hernia patients include poor respiratory effort, loss of abdominal domain, and weak abdominal musculature.

REFERENCES

1. Ramirez OM, Ruas E, Dellon AL. "Components separation" method for closure of abdominal-wall defects: an anatomic and clinical study. *Plast Reconstr Surg.* 1990;86(3):519-526.
2. Garvey PB, Bailey CM, Baumann DP, et al. Violation of the rectus complex is not a contraindication to component separation for abdominal wall reconstruction. *J Am Coll Surg.* 2012;214(2):131-139.
3. Shestak KC, Edington HJ, Johnson RR. The separation of anatomic components technique for the reconstruction of massive midline abdominal wall defects: anatomy, surgical technique, applications, and limitations revisited. *Plast Reconstr Surg.* 2000;105(2):731-738.
4. Itani KM, Hur K, Kim LT, et al. Comparison of laparoscopic and open repair with mesh for the treatment of ventral incisional hernia: a randomized trial. *Arch Surg.* 2010;145(4):322-328.
5. Rosen MJ, Jin J, McGee MF, et al. Laparoscopic component separation in the single-stage treatment of infected abdominal wall prosthetic removal. *Hernia.* 2007;11(5):435–440.
6. Mommers EH, Wegdam JA, Nienhuijs SW, de Vries Reilingh TS. How to perform the endoscopically assisted components separation technique (ECS) for large ventral hernia repair. *Hernia.* 2016;20(3): 441-447.
7. Butler CE, Baumann DP, Janis JE, Rosen MJ. Abdominal wall reconstruction. *Curr Probl Surg.* 2013;50:557–586.
8. Butler CE, Campbell KT. Minimally invasive component separation with inlay bioprosthetic mesh (MICSNIB) for complex abdominal wall reconstruction. *Plast Reconstr Surg.* 2011;128(3):698-709.
9. Ghali S, Turza KC, Baumann DP, Butler CE. Minimally invasive component separation results in fewer wound-healing complications than open component separation for large ventral hernia repairs. *J Am Coll Surg.* 2012;214(6):981-989.
10. Slater NJ, Knaapen L, Bökkerink WJ, et al. Large contaminated ventral hernia repair using component separation technique with synthetic mesh. *Plast Reconstr Surg.* 2015;136(6):796e-805e.
11. Visschers RG, Olde Damink SW, Winkens B, et al. Treatment strategies in 135 consecutive patients with enterocutaneous fistulas. *World J Surg.* 2008;32(3):445-453.

9
CHAPTER

Abdominal Hernia Reconstruction With Synthetic and Biologic Mesh

Sergey Y. Turin and Gregory A. Dumanian

DEFINITION

- A hernia is a defect in at least one of the layers of the abdominal wall, permitting intra-abdominal contents such as bowel and fat to protrude past their normal confinement layer of transversalis fascia. This is in contradistinction to a bulge, which is an imbalance between the outward force of the viscera and the containing force of the intact abdominal wall, as seen in denervation injuries or rectus diastasis.
- We will focus on the treatment of incisional hernias in this chapter—hernias due to a defect in the repaired abdominal wall after a prior laparotomy.

ANATOMY

- The key in a hernia defect is the disruption of the continuity of the abdominal wall—depending on the etiology of the hernia and the patient's surgical history, this may be one or many layers of the abdominal wall. In incisional hernias, this often means a midline defect at the site of the previous midline laparotomy incision (**FIG 1**).
- As shown in **FIG 2**, the abdominal wall lateral to the rectus muscle is intact, and we can clearly see all three layers—the external and internal oblique and the transversus abdominis muscles inserting onto the linea semilunaris. The defect is clearly between the rectus muscles (**FIG 2**).

PATHOGENESIS

- Coughing, the Valsalva maneuver, and contraction of the stomach muscles for postural stability all increase intra-abdominal pressure. This pressure is normally opposed by the abdominal wall, which is a muscular and elastic organ and can provide inward force to maintain the viscera in their domain.
- When one of the portions of the abdominal wall is unable to oppose the intra-abdominal pressure either due to denervation (as in a bulge) or due to discontinuity of the musculature (as in a hernia), the viscera are forced through that portion by the rest of the competent musculature. The abdominal wall functions uniformly as a pressurized cylinder, whereas sizeable hernias and bulges serve to lower intra-abdominal pressure.
- The abdominal wall is muscular but also elastic. This has great bearing on the choice of reconstructive technique, in that the reconstructed muscular and fascial components must be able to stretch, so they can absorb and dampen the sharp rises in intra-abdominal pressure that come with coughing, sudden exertion, and Valsalva.

- The most successful repairs occur in the most elastic abdomens, whereas a fibrotic, scarred abdominal wall that is unyielding will have more of a tendency for stitches tearing in the postoperative period. A bridging mesh (synthetic or biologic), besides its inherent inability to provide an inward force, is also inelastic and has a compliance mismatch with the intact abdominal wall, leading to a higher rate of dehiscence and suture pull-through, as shown in **FIG 3**.

PATIENT HISTORY AND PHYSICAL FINDINGS

- A full history and physical exam is performed, with a focus on prior abdominal surgeries and the means of closure. Patients are encouraged to obtain all previous abdominal operative reports. The medical history looking for bowel dysfunction and comorbid conditions such as diabetes, cardiac anomalies, and chronic obstructive pulmonary disease is obtained.
- Gestational history is important in order to ascertain if women have had their abdominal walls stretched previously.
- History of weight loss, prior abdominal wall sepsis, or peritoneal dialysis is a factor that will either increase or decrease the elasticity of the abdominal muscles.
- Examine the abdominal wall with the patient both standing and lying down. Attempt to reduce the hernia to assess the degree of bowel adhesions and the compliance of the abdomen.
- Document the scars of previous surgeries. Evaluate rectus diastasis by watching the patient on the descent phase of a sit-up—a maneuver that clearly shows muscle separation in all but the most obese patients.
- Evaluate the skin and subcutaneous tissues for scarring, excess, and wounds because this will need to be addressed for optimal closure.
- Social history is necessary, as return to work issues and help at home after surgery will need to be planned in advance.

IMAGING

- We routinely obtain a CT scan of the abdomen and pelvis using oral contrast to assess the layers of the abdominal wall, any implanted meshes, or biologic materials and measure the size of the defect for all major incisional hernias. If the patient has no kidney issues, we add IV contrast for an optimal study and to obviate the need to explore the abdomen at the time of hernia closure to save dissection time, limit tissue swelling, and avoid possible bowel injury.

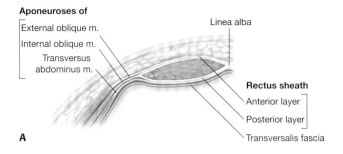

Aponeuroses of
External oblique m.
Internal oblique m.
Transversus abdominus m.

Linea alba

Rectus sheath
Anterior layer
Posterior layer
Transversalis fascia

A

Aponeuroses of
External oblique m.
Internal oblique m.
Transversus abdominus m.

Anterior layer of rectus sheath

Transversalis fascia

External oblique m.
Internal oblique m.
Transversus abdominus m.

Transversalis fascia

Latissimus dorsi m.

Psoas fascia
Psoas major m.

Lumbar fascia
Anterior layer
Middle layer
Posterior layer

Quadratus lumborum m.
Latissimus dorsi m.
Sacrospinalis m.

B

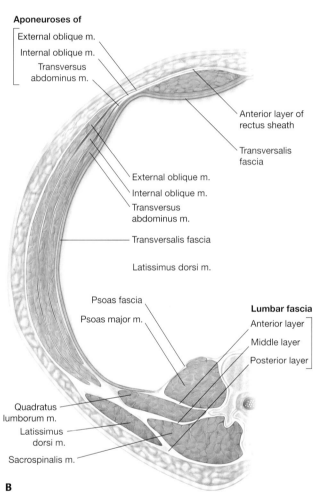

FIG 1 • **A,B.** Anatomy of the abdominal wall.

NONOPERATIVE MANAGEMENT

- The indications for repair of an incisional hernia are local hernia pain, a history of an obstruction, patient discomfort from an inability to raise core intra-abdominal pressure, unsightliness, and the need for intra-abdominal visceral surgery.
- Small asymptomatic defects can be observed (so long as the patient is not traveling to an area lacking modern medical care), as the risk of surgery approximates the risk of observation.
- For every patient, there should be a comparison of the expected benefits with the magnitude of the procedure required for repair.

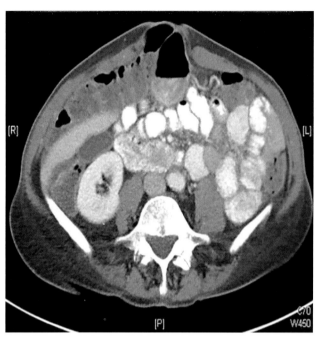

FIG 2 • CT Scan demonstrating an incisional hernia.

SURGICAL MANAGEMENT

Preoperative Planning

- These repairs are invasive procedures usually performed on an elective basis, so every patient should be optimized for surgery, including an appropriate perioperative evaluation, nutritional optimization and weight loss, and lifestyle changes such as smoking cessation.
- The Caprini risk stratification model is used to assess the individual patient's risk for DVT/PE and assign chemoprophylaxis if appropriate.
- Perioperative antibiotics are routinely given for 24 hours, and topical antibiotic irrigation is used during the procedure.
- The history and imaging must be reviewed and an operative plan put in place:
  - What incisions have been previously made? What layers of the abdominal wall are no longer continuous?
  - Is there mesh? If so, what kind, how large, and how was it affixed?

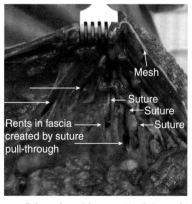

Mesh
Suture
Suture
Suture
Rents in fascia created by suture pull-through

FIG 3 • Suture pull-through or "cheese wiring" due to high focal stress placed by the suture on the tissues.

- Is there a concurrent procedure that needs to be performed (eg, stoma takedown or relocation or other bowel surgery)?
- Assume that some level of adhesiolysis will be required, and backup plans for an enterotomy repair or bowel resection should be in place.

Positioning

- The patient is in a supine position with the arms out to the sides. The field should extend from the xiphoid to pubis and down to the midaxillary line on the sides. Flank defects are repaired in the lateral decubitus position.

Approach

- We use the prior incision for access into the abdominal cavity. In general, the incision must be longer than the prior scar, and so extensions into an unscarred skin are the rule.
- At the end of the procedure, the prior incision, redundant skin and subcutaneous tissue, and hernia sac are excised so that healing will occur with unscarred tissue and so that the soft tissues will lie flat against the abdominal wall.
- For improved aesthetics and healing, the umbilicus is removed and a neoumbilicus created (see umbilicoplasty technique in associated chapter).

■ Laparotomy and Development of Tissue Planes

- Make a generous incision.
- Enter the abdominal cavity immediately rather than trying to preserve the hernia sac. In general, start where the hernia sac is most mobile and softest, as this is where adhesions will be least. After entry into the abdomen, extend the dissection in either direction until one reaches unscarred tissue, the xiphoid, and/or the symphysis pubis.
- Bowel adhesions to the hernia sac and the peritoneal surface of the abdominal wall should be widely taken down from the anterior abdominal wall, though a full abdominal exploration is not performed (**TECH FIG 1**).
- If there is a mesh, it must be removed completely at this point—it is a foreign body and will not contribute to the closure. We typically split the mesh for ease of dissection and take it off as two "halves." Alternatively, when there is infected mesh and an enterocutaneous fistula, the mesh is removed "en bloc."
- Using cautery, dissect through the hernia sac to identify the medial borders of the rectus muscle in their entirety. Clear 4 cm of anterior rectus fascia.
- To assess the need for a components release, the patient should be under general anesthesia and the patient fully muscle relaxed.

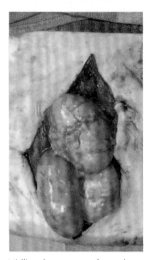

TECH FIG 1 • Midline laparotomy from the symphysis pubis to midepigastrium with division of hernia sac.

- Grasp the dissected rectus muscles in their midportion with two fingers on either side. If they cannot be brought together to the midline, the patient will require a components release.
- This occurs in a patient with normal compliance of the abdominal wall with a preoperative CT scan that shows a 6- to 10-cm separation.

■ External Abdominal Oblique Release (Anterior Components Release)

- In cases where a components release is required, palpate the inferior costal margin and make a 6-cm transverse subcostal incision in order to approach the linea semilunaris.
- Using a combination of cautery and spreading with curved Mayo scissors, the anterior-most external oblique fibers are identified as they blend into their insertion into the lateral aspect of the rectus sheath.
- Bluntly dissect a tunnel along the semilunar line going inferiorly and superiorly.
- Using electrocautery, make a small, finger-sized incision in the external oblique muscle just lateral to the rectus sheath. Then, bluntly dissect the plane between the internal and external obliques and use the cautery against your finger

to release the external oblique just lateral to the rectus sheath. A narrow Deaver retractor will help visualization.
- These incisions are continued in the tunnels going inferiorly and superiorly from the subcostal incision far above the rib cage down to the anterior superior iliac spine (ASIS). Especially superiorly, a deep fascia of the external oblique exists and should be divided for maximal movement—it is completely distinct from the internal oblique muscle.
- A suprapubic tunnel is brought into continuity with this lateral dissection, all with blunt dissection and remaining near the ASIS to avoid the periumbilical perforators.
- The external oblique release is completed inferiorly with "grabbing" the cut end of the muscle/fascia from the midline tunnel to allow it to be cut under direct vision. Once these releases are complete bilaterally, the rectus muscles should come together in the midline for the majority of hernias (**TECH FIG 2**) (Videos 1 and 2).

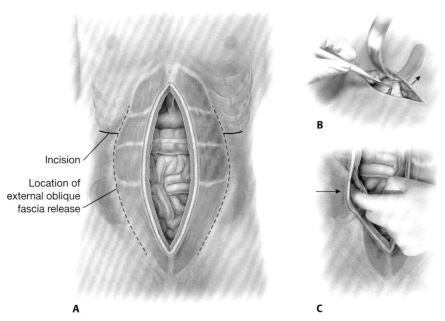

TECH FIG 2 • A. Transverse incisions for perforator sparing anterior components release located at the inferior aspect of the costal margins. **B.** Narrow Deaver retractor permitting release of external oblique muscle and fascia over the rib cage. **C.** From the suprapubic midline incision, a dissecting finger creates a tunnel and joins it with the dissections of the lateral incisions. The cut end of the external oblique muscle is captured by the index finger. The dissecting index finger pulls the external oblique fascia into the midline incision to be visualized and subsequently cut.

- This approach to releasing the external obliques preserves the periumbilical perforators that will be supplying the soft tissues overlying the midline closure and has been shown to decrease surgical site occurrences (SSO).
- Choice of mesh remains extremely controversial. General guidelines are that all hernias should be closed with a mesh to distribute forces and to limit suture pull-through.
  - Achievement of a "direct supported repair" with closure of biologic tissue over mesh has been shown to decrease hernia rates in comparison with a mesh that bridges a fascial defect.
  - For prosthetic meshes, coated meshes against adhesions are generally recommended when placed against bowel, whereas uncoated macroporous meshes with pore sizes greater than 1 mm to limit bridging scar and encapsulation are generally used in the retrorectus and onlay positions.

- Absorbable meshes distribute forces but for only a limited amount of time. Animal experimentation implies that the foreign body response recedes when the foreign body is absorbed. Whether absorbable meshes translate to improved long-term closure remains to be seen. Similarly, biologic meshes are known to incorporate into surrounding tissues.
  - Whether a net benefit exists or not of added long-term scar or even tissue regeneration of a fascia is completely unclear at the writing of this chapter.
- The retrorectus space is developed by incising the linea alba to mobilize the posterior rectus fascia (above the arcuate line) and the preperitoneal fat (below the arcuate line) off the rectus muscle for 4 cm. Care is taken to not injure the inferior epigastric vessels, blood vessels supplying this tissue layer, or intercostal nerves entering the muscles on their deep and lateral surface.
- The posterior sheath is then closed with a running 2-0 polydioxanone suture (**TECH FIG 3**).

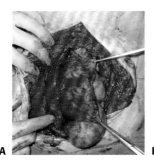
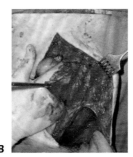
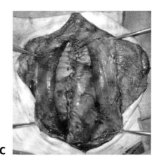

TECH FIG 3 • A,B. Development of retrorectus space. **C.** Closure of posterior rectus sheath.

■ Mesh Inset

- The key of the procedure is a well-fixed narrow mesh that is held flat and tight against the rectus muscles. Wrinkled mesh will not incorporate well into the tissues as a load-sharing component of the abdominal wall. Loose mesh is not load sharing and defeats the purpose of mesh placement.
- Cut a piece of uncoated midweight macroporous polypropylene mesh to a width of 7.5 cm and length equal to the length of the abdominal wall defect. Tension across the narrow width of mesh should maintain macroporosity, as opposed to allowing the holes of the mesh to close down. Macroporous meshes have improved tissue incorporation and biocompatibility in comparison with microporous meshes made of the same material.
- The mesh is then secured in place using #0 polypropylene sutures in an interrupted fashion. These stitches start at the lateral edge of the dissection superficial to the rectus muscle (approximately 4 cm away from medial edge), traverse the muscle and its anterior fascia, then take a small bite of the mesh near its edge before coming back out superficially and tying the knot.
  - Large bites of mesh will distort and wrinkle the mesh, hindering incorporation.
  - Bites should be spaced 2 cm apart or so.

- The undersurface of the rectus muscle should be well visualized to limit the injury of segmental nerves and blood vessels during placement of these transrectus sutures (**TECH FIG 4A–C**).
- Most techniques in the hernia literature that look to Rives-Stoppa repairs for inspiration use few or no sutures to fix the mesh in place. The mesh is held in place by its size and friction, with medial aspect of the rectus muscles approximated in the midline to cover the mesh.
- Placement of even larger meshes requires the release of the transversus abdominis muscles in what is called the TAR (transversus abdominis release or posterior components) procedure.
- Instead, we promote the use of a well-fixed narrow mesh and believe it has numerous advantages over wide meshes that require additional tissue dissection including less total foreign material, less opening of wide tissue planes, and speed of the procedure. SSO and surgical site infection (SSI) rates for a well-fixed narrow mesh are lower than that for large unfixed meshes in recently submitted data from our institution.
- As the mesh is 7.5-cm wide and the bites are taken 4 cm away from the medial rectus edge on both sides, once the lateral mesh sutures are in place, the medial borders of the rectus muscles should be able to be approximated with no tension with #0 polypropylene sutures (**TECH FIG 4D–F**).

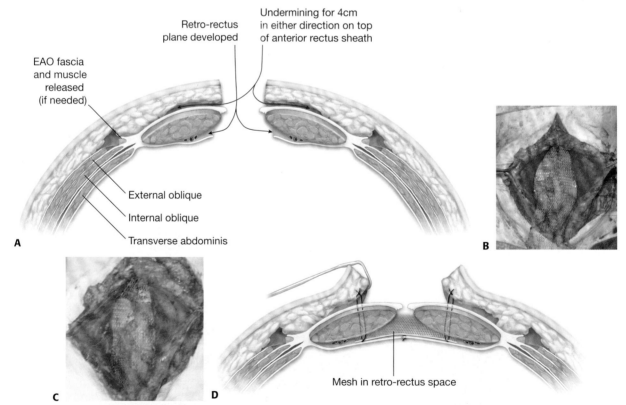

Retro-rectus plane developed

Undermining for 4cm in either direction on top of anterior rectus sheath

EAO fascia and muscle released (if needed)

External oblique

Internal oblique

Transverse abdominis

A

B

C

D

Mesh in retro-rectus space

TECH FIG 4 • A. Illustration of retrorectus mesh position. **B.** Mesh positioning in the retrorectus space with placement of upper transfascial sutures. **C.** Narrow mesh placed flat and tight in the retrorectus space. **D.** Diagram of placement of narrow mesh.

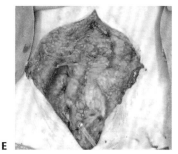
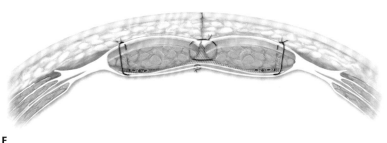

E F

TECH FIG 4 (Continued) • **E.** Rectus muscles and anterior rectus sheath closed over the mesh—one can see the lateral suture lines outlining the borders of the mesh and the midline closure of the rectus muscles over the mesh. **F.** Diagram of the abdominal wall reconstruction construct.

■ Closure

- We place at least 1 drain in the subcutaneous tissues, and for patients with BMI over 30, we place drains in each components release space.
- At this point, we turn our attention to the soft tissues of the abdomen. With the fascia closed, redundant skin and soft tissue are excised and yet still achieving a tension-free closure. This maneuver removes the poorest vascularized tissue and decreases the potential space where fluid can collect.

- We routinely excise the umbilical stalk and reconstruct the depression using "pumpkin-teeth" flaps as described in the umbilicoplasty chapter.
- Closure is performed with polyglactin dermal sutures and either staples or a running subcuticular stitch (**TECH FIG 5**).

Biologic Implant Placement

- In situations where wounds are contaminated and the clinical situation still requires abdominal wall closure, there are numerous options, though none of them are optimal.[1,2]

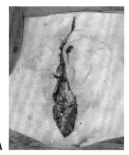
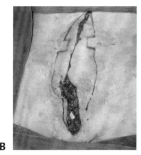
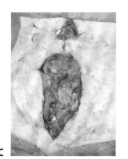

A B C

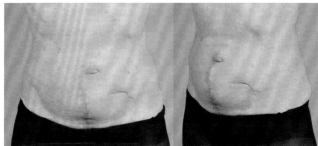

D

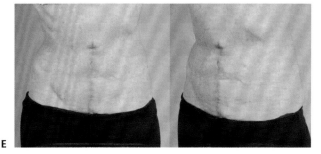

E

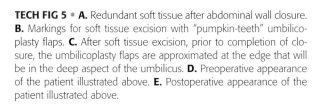

TECH FIG 5 • **A.** Redundant soft tissue after abdominal wall closure. **B.** Markings for soft tissue excision with "pumpkin-teeth" umbilicoplasty flaps. **C.** After soft tissue excision, prior to completion of closure, the umbilicoplasty flaps are approximated at the edge that will be in the deep aspect of the umbilicus. **D.** Preoperative appearance of the patient illustrated above. **E.** Postoperative appearance of the patient illustrated above.

■ A bridging piece of biologic mesh can be placed, with the idea of limiting further tissue dissection. These bridging biologics have extremely high failure rates and more likely than not will require a delayed hernia reconstruction.

■ Primary closure of the abdominal wall augmented by a components release, biologics, and retrorectus meshes has all been documented to have recurrence rates in the 20% range.

■ Our current management for contaminated closures is to perform a "mesh sutured repair."

• Strips of polypropylene 18 to 20 mm wide are introduced through the substance of the abdominal wall and tied as simple sutures.

• Conceptually somewhere between a suture repair and a planar mesh, these mesh sutured repairs in our hands have demonstrated SSI in the 6% range, SSO to be 18%, and a hernia recurrence rate of 4% with 7.6 months' follow-up.

■ In the interim, we would recommend that, when a biologic mesh is indicated, the surgeon use the technique as laid out above—the principles of flat and tight placement, scar excision, and lateral EAO release all apply in the same fashion. Secure attachment of the mesh is crucial to allow vascularization and integration of the material as quickly as possible. All manufacturer instructions must be followed regarding rehydration of the mesh and optimal tension of inset.

PEARLS AND PITFALLS

Scar is not your friend	■ Scar in the subcutaneous tissues, and even more so the scarred edges of the rectus muscles, may seem like strong tissue that can hold a stitch, but it is avascular, is inelastic, and has decreased potential to heal. With time, the suture will simply cheese wire through the noncompliant tissue leading to failure. We routinely excise all scar and make it a priority to close healthy tissue to healthy tissue.
Suture pull-through is the enemy	■ Not using enough suture fixation points to spread out the load of the closure along the suture lines will lead to disproportionately high force per unit area in the sutures that are placed, leading to a high risk of cheese wiring through the tissues.
Umbilicus management	■ Counsel the patient preoperatively that you may need to remove the umbilicus as part of the closure—if they do want an neoumbilicus, plan for the extra time needed for an umbilicoplasty.
Lysis of adhesions	■ As above, make sure that you or a colleague is prepared to deal with bowel adhesions and any intra-abdominal anatomy challenges, as well as the possible enterotomy and need for bowel excision.
Mesh sutured repairs	■ Are efficacious and efficient means to close abdominal wall, though long-term follow-up does not yet exist for this novel closure method. Strips of macroporous mesh 18 to 20 mm wide are passed through the abdominal wall and used as sutures. The strips of mesh use the same concepts of force distribution and reduction of pull-through as tenants of successful abdominal wall surgery. Despite the permanent material, they have been placed successfully in contaminated closures.

POSTOPERATIVE CARE

■ Diet management
  ■ Bowel preps do not decrease SSI or SSO, but a mechanical prep with Dulcolax that does not alter bowel flora may be helpful to reduce visceral volume and pressure during and immediately after surgery. An aggressive antiemetic regimen is necessary to prevent emesis and the associated high abdominal wall stresses. Patients are allowed to eat after passing flatus, typically on POD 3 or 4 for major hernias.
■ Activity
  ■ Patients are up to chair on POD no. 1 and instructed to ambulate on POD no. 2. Patients can ambulate as tolerated thereafter. They can begin nonimpact exercise (walking, swimming, elliptical training) at 6 weeks. They can do isometric abdominal exercise at 3 months and gentle impact exercise at 6 months. They have no restrictions at 9 to 12 months after surgery.
■ Foley and UOP monitoring
  ■ We routinely place and leave a Foley catheter for 24 hours to monitor urine output. A drop-off in urine output in a patient that otherwise appears adequately resuscitated raises concern for abdominal compartment syndrome—a

rare but possible complication. Rising intra-abdominal pressure by Foley catheter monitoring, low urine output, and difficulty with ventilation all point toward a compartment syndrome.
■ Tidal volume monitoring
  ■ Returning a large volume of viscera to the abdominal compartment can significantly impair ventilatory capacity by limiting diaphragm excursion. Pulmonary therapy is necessary during the immediate postoperative state to optimize the patient's respiratory status.
■ Valium
  ■ We routinely prescribe diazepam to patients postoperatively to reduce muscle spasms, improve pain control, and off-load the closure.
■ Pain management
  ■ We avoid the use of ketorolac given the fairly large dissection. Patients who we anticipate will have pain control difficulties undergo placement of an epidural catheter by the anesthesia pain team for the immediate postoperative period. Use of epidurals may help blunt the body's inflammatory response to surgical trauma but can lead to greater forces on abdominal sutures from greater patient activity.

- DVT prophylaxis
  - DVT prophylaxis must be administered as dictated by patient risk stratification on the Caprini score.

OUTCOMES

- In our series of 101 patients who have been treated with a narrow well-fixed mesh as described above, there was a 0% rate of hernia recurrence, SSO of 7.9%, and SSI of 3%. There were no enterocutaneous fistulae, and no meshes required removal. Minor complications included 3 infections, 2 hematomas, 2 seromas, 1 reoperation for a subcutaneous collection, and 5 readmissions within 30 days.[3]

COMPLICATIONS

- Hematoma/seroma
- Soft tissue infection and prosthetic mesh infection
- Bowel-related complications involving delayed return of bowel function and compartment syndrome
- Medical complications including DVT/PE, pneumonia, UTI, and coronary ischemia
- Abdominal wall pain

REFERENCES

1. Jason H. Ko, Edward CW, David MS, et al. Abdominal wall reconstruction lessons learned from 200 "Components separation" procedures. *Arch Surg.* 2009;144(11):1047-1055.
2. Chow I, Hanwright PJ, Kim John YS. A propensity matched analysis of 58,889 patients comparing ADM to synthetic mesh surgical site outcomes in ventral hernia repair. *Plast Reconstr Surg.* 2015;1364S:13-14.
3. Steven TL, Jennifer EF, Kyle RM, Gregory AD. Reliable complex abdominal wall hernia repairs with a narrow well-fixed retrorectus polypropylene mesh: a review of over 100 consecutive cases. *Plast Reconstr Surg Glob Open.* 2016;4(9 suppl):111-112.

10
CHAPTER

Rectus Femoris Flap for Abdominal Wall Reconstruction

Alexander F. Mericli and Charles E. Butler

DEFINITION

- The rectus femoris muscle can be used as pedicled or free flap for reconstruction of the abdominal wall.
  - The flap can be harvested as a myocutaneous or muscle-only flap, depending on the requirements of the defect.[1-4]
  - Several authors have had success employing the flap in an innervated fashion for abdominal defects.[5]
- Depending on the size of the defect, the rectus femoris muscle can be designed as an isolated flap or can be combined with other components of the lateral femoral circumflex vascular axis (vastus lateralis, anterolateral thigh skin and subcutaneous tissue, iliotibial band, and/or tensor fascia lata muscle) for the creation of a subtotal thigh flap.[1] For massive abdominal wall defects, bilateral flaps can be raised.
- As a rotational flap, the rectus femoris muscle will easily reach the lower abdomen, mons, lateral hip, perineum, and groin.
- Although the rectus femoris is recognized as a useful flap, debate continues regarding its associated donor-site morbidity.
  - There is disagreement in the literature as to whether the rectus femoris flap is associated with decreased range of motion or strength with knee extension.[6-8]

ANATOMY

- The rectus femoris is part of the quadriceps muscle complex. It is a bipennate muscle with two distinct muscle bellies (**FIG 1A**).
- It has two separate origins: the anteroinferior iliac spine and the anterior rim of the acetabulum. The muscle inserts onto the patella along with the other components of the quadriceps complex and both flexes the hip and extends the knee (**FIG 1B**).
- The motor innervation comes from the femoral nerve (L4 nerve root). The sensory innervation to the skin overlying the muscle is from the intermediate femoral cutaneous nerve.
- The vascular supply of the rectus femoris is consistent with that of a type 2 muscle flap, as defined by Mathes and Nahai.
  - The major pedicle is a medial branch from the lateral femoral circumflex artery (**FIG 1C**). The branch to the rectus femoris muscle emerges 1 to 2.5 cm distal to where the lateral femoral circumflex artery splits from the profunda femoris artery. The pedicle tends to enter the muscle on its deep and lateral surface. After sending a branch to the rectus femoris muscle, the lateral femoral circumflex

neurovascular bundle continues inferiorly, traveling in the septum between the vastus lateralis and rectus femoris muscle, to supply the tissue of the anterolateral thigh flap.
  - The minor pedicles are one to three small branches from the superficial femoral artery, distally. Generally, the minor pedicles are not independently sufficient to support flap viability.
- The muscle is bordered by the vastus medialis medially, the vastus lateralis laterally, and the vastus intermedius on its deep surface. The sartorius muscle crosses obliquely over the rectus femoris muscle proximally.

PATIENT HISTORY AND PHYSICAL FINDINGS

- Since the advent of the component separation technique, fascial approximation of defects up to 20 cm wide at the umbilicus can be achieved. Therefore, autologous reconstruction of the abdominal wall using thigh-based flaps is reserved for patients with total or massive subtotal defects of the full thickness of the abdominal wall.
- The etiology of these significant defects is variable and includes malignancy (tumor resection; **FIG 2A**), trauma (damage control of the abdomen or soft tissue loss due to ballistic or blunt injury), and infectious processes (necrotizing fasciitis, full-thickness abdominal wall resection due to extensive enterocutaneous fistula formation; **FIG 2B,C**).

IMAGING

- Imaging studies are not required before performing a rectus abdominis flap for abdominal wall reconstruction. However, imaging is often present for other reasons and can be utilized to the reconstructive surgeon's advantage.
- Computed tomographic scans of the abdomen and pelvis can be utilized for visualization of the abdominal defect size and associated anatomy.
- Computed tomographic angiography of the lower extremity—if present—can be used to confirm patency of the vascular pedicle (**FIG 3**).

SURGICAL MANAGEMENT
Preoperative Planning

- The patient should be seen preoperatively where a full history should be obtained and physical examination should be performed.
  - Special attention should be paid to a past history of any abdominal, groin, or thigh surgeries or injuries.

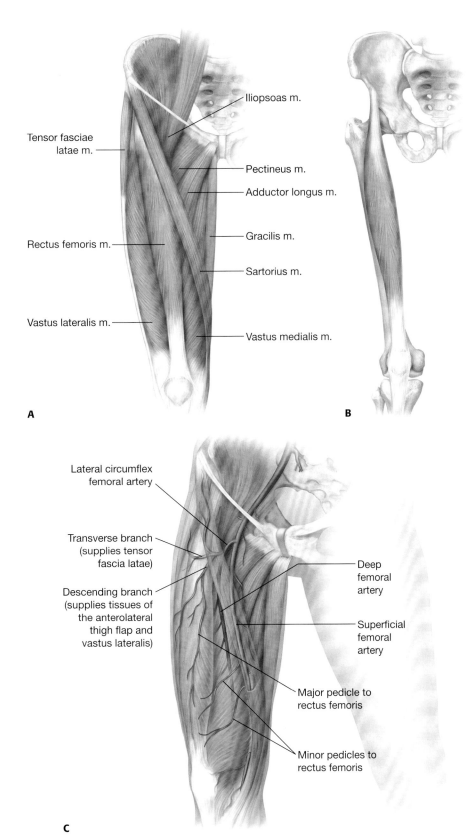

FIG 1 • A. Muscular anatomy of the thigh. **B.** The rectus femoris muscle originates from the anteroinferior iliac spine and the acetabulum. It spans both the hip and knee joints, thus serving as both a hip flexor and knee extensor. **C.** The rectus femoris muscle is supplied by the descending branch of the lateral femoral circumflex artery. The lateral femoral circumflex artery also supplies the tensor fascia lata, the vastus lateralis, and the overlying skin, allowing for a subtotal thigh flap to be designed, if necessary. Color code: rectus femoris muscle, *purple*; anterolateral thigh tissues, *blue*; tensor fascia lata, *green*.

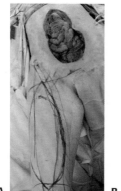 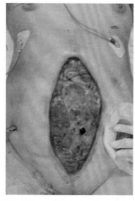 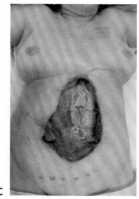

FIG 2 • Abdominal wall defects from various etiologies. Full-thickness defect after oncologic resection **(A)**, enterocutaneous fistula and associated soft tissue loss after evisceration **(B,C)**. (© Charles E. Butler, MD.)

- If vascular disease is suspected, a computed tomographic angiogram should be considered to verify perfusion of the rectus femoris muscle.
- Reconstruction of the abdominal wall is typically a multi-surgeon case involving both reconstructive and general surgeons. General surgeons should be available to assist with adhesiolysis or any enteral repairs, which might be needed during the exposure.

Positioning

- The patient is placed in the supine position with the bilateral legs internally rotated at the hip.
- The legs are secured in this position at the forefoot with a combination of tape and foam to relieve pressure.

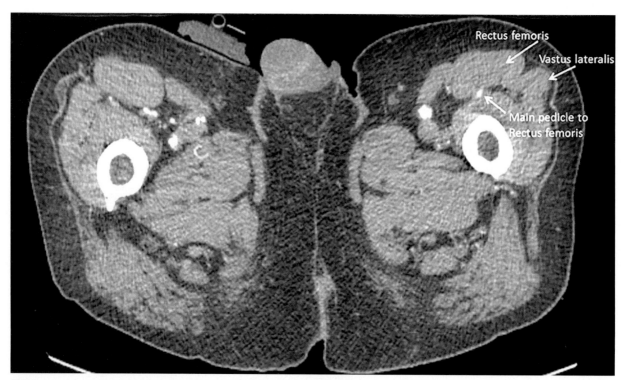

FIG 3 • Computed tomographic angiography demonstrating the cross-sectional anatomy of the thigh.

■ Markings

- With the legs internally rotated, markings are placed on the anterosuperior iliac spine and the superolateral border of the patella; a line connecting these two points approximates the lateral border of the rectus femoris muscle.
  - A line is extended superiorly from the midpoint of the patella to the anterosuperior iliac spine representing the central axis of the rectus femoris muscle (**TECH FIG 1**).
- For a muscle-only rectus flap, either one or two incisions are designed along the central axis of the muscle.
  - For a more minimally invasive approach, the two-incision technique is used: a short distal incision is planned for the distal thigh to allow disinsertion of the muscle from the patella. This incision is directly overlying the rectus femoris muscle and 6 to 8 cm in length. A separate incision is designed more proximally, over the region of the major pedicle. This incision will allow for more proximal dissection and will facilitate tunneling

of the muscle into the abdominal defect, if a pedicled flap is planned.

  - If a minimally invasive approach is not necessary, an incision is made over the central anterior axis of the thigh, directly overlying the rectus femoris muscle, from groin to distal thigh.

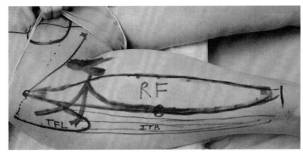

TECH FIG 1 • Surgical markings. RF, rectus femoris; TFL, tensor fascia lata; ITB, iliotibial band. (© Charles E. Butler, MD.)

■ Pedicled Rectus Femoris Flap

- If a skin paddle is desired, it is designed as an ellipse centered over the muscle on the anterior thigh.
  - An 8- to 9-cm skin paddle can generally be harvested without the need for skin grafting of the donor site.
- With a large skin paddle, it is useful to suture the edges of the skin to the muscle fascia once the flap is elevated to prevent any shearing of the skin during dissection.
- If no skin paddle is needed, an incision is made distally, along the midanterior line, directly over the rectus femoris muscle. This first incision should be made 4 to 6 cm proximal to the patella.
  - Dissection is carried down through the subcutaneous adipose tissue and through the deep fascia overlying the muscle belly. Blunt dissection is used to free the muscle along its medial and deep surfaces.
  - Laterally and distally, the transition between the rectus femoris muscle and vastus lateralis muscle is often indistinct. This part of the dissection must be performed

either sharply or with electrocautery to ensure accuracy; blunt dissection will likely not be possible.

- The distal muscle belly is disinserted from the patella, leaving 2 to 3 cm of tendon with the muscle flap to assist with insetting. The muscle is dissected proximally, freeing it from its medial, lateral, and deep attachments.
  - Several minor pedicles will be encountered entering the muscle's deep surface. These should be clipped and ligated as they are discovered.
- A lighted retractor may aid the surgeon in dissecting the muscle as proximally as possible.
- Either the incision is extended proximally up to the groin or, for a more minimally invasive approach, a separate incision is made overlying the groin, and the disinserted muscle is passed from the distal incision to the proximal incision.
  - The sartorius muscle will be found obliquely crossing over the muscle. The main pedicle enters the rectus femoris muscle on its deep and lateral surface at the level of the sartorius (**TECH FIG 2A**).
- Passing the flap deep to the sartorius will allow for approximately 5 cm of additional advancement (**TECH FIG 2B**).

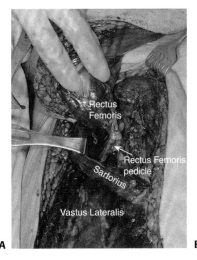
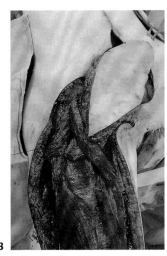

TECH FIG 2 • **A.** Main pedicle of the rectus femoris muscle (branch coming off the descending branch of the lateral femoral circumflex vessels). **B.** Passing the rectus femoris flap deep to the sartorius muscle in order to allow for greater advancement. (© Charles E. Butler, MD.)   **A**   **B**

- If the defect does not require skin, the rectus femoris flap can be buried as a muscle-only flap. If skin is required, the flap can either be designed with a skin paddle or a muscle-only flap can be skin grafted.
- Reconstructing the quadriceps tendon complex is an extremely important step of this operation and cannot be underestimated. Doing so will help to minimize the potential donor-site morbidity and loss of terminal knee extension.
  - Buried no. 1 polypropylene sutures are typically used to approximate the vastus lateralis tendon to the tendon of the vastus medialis, thus centralizing the moment arm of the remaining quadriceps tendon. It is not uncommon to extend this tenorrhaphy for 10 to 15 cm proximally.

Pedicled Subtotal Thigh Flap

- The rectus femoris muscle can be combined with other components of the lateral femoral circumflex vascular tree to create a subtotal thigh flap.
  - The skin paddle possible with this flap is larger than 400 cm² and can be used to reconstruct massive abdominal wall defects. Bilateral flaps can be used to reconstruct the entire anterior abdominal wall[1] (**TECH FIG 3A-C**).
  - The lateral femoral circumflex vessels supply the rectus femoris, vastus lateralis, and tensor fascia lata muscles and the overlying skin. All these structures can be incorporated into the flap, if needed.
- Just as for the rectus femoris flap, the ASIS and patella are marked. A template is made of the defect and its anatomic requirements (area of missing fascia; area of missing skin, dimensions, etc.). The template is then transposed onto the thigh.

- The iliotibial band can be included in the flap to reconstruct any abdominal fascial defect.
  - If an abdominal defect is significant enough to require a subtotal thigh flap for reconstruction, it is unlikely that the iliotibial band will be sufficient in and of itself to reconstruct the associated fascial defect.
  - Therefore, this flap is often combined with a mesh fascial repair for reinforcement of the abdominal wall.[1]
- The proximal extent of dissection is the branch point between the profunda femoris and the lateral circumflex femoral artery.
- Similar to the rectus femoris flap, the subtotal thigh flap should be passed deep to the sartorius muscle for an additional 5 cm of advancement. Because of the width of the flap, one or two segmental perforators to the sartorius will likely need to be divided to provide enough room for the flap to pass.
- A pedicled subtotal thigh flap will be able to reach to the level of the umbilicus.
  - If additional length is needed, the flap can be created into a free flap by way of a saphenous vein graft arteriovenous loop (see **TECH FIG 4C**).
- When a partial vastus lateralis muscle flap is included with the distal tendon intact, a vastus medialis to lateralis tenorrhaphy can be done. When the entire vastus lateralis is included in this flap, a vastus lateralis to vastus medialis tenorrhaphy is not possible as it is when only the rectus femoris muscle is used. Therefore, the patient should be counseled preoperatively that loss of terminal knee extension and strength is likely.
  - The patient should be maintained in a knee immobilizer for 6 weeks postoperatively and may complete

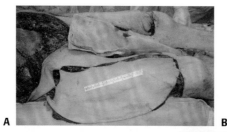
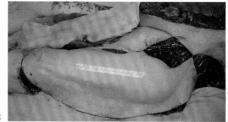
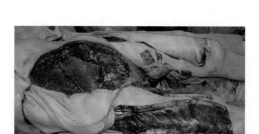
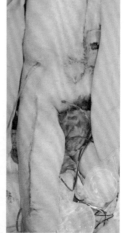
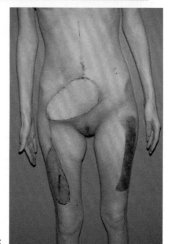

TECH FIG 3 • Bilateral pedicled subtotal thigh flaps can be used to reconstruct the entire surface area of the abdominal wall. **A.** Right subtotal thigh flap. **B.** Left subtotal thigh flap. **C.** Right subtotal thigh flap rotated to the abdomen with left subtotal thigh flap reflected to display abdominal defect. **D.** If the flap is less than 9 cm wide, primary closure is generally achieved. **E.** If the flap is wider than 9 cm, primary closure is typically not possible and a skin graft should be used. (© Charles E. Butler, MD.)

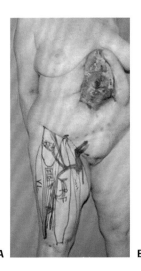
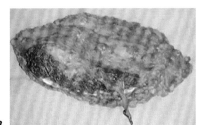
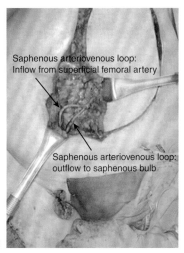

Saphenous arteriovenous loop:
Inflow from superficial femoral artery

Saphenous arteriovenous loop:
outflow to saphenous bulb

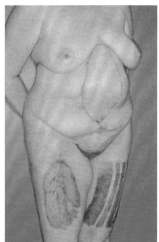

TECH FIG 4 • **A.** Full-thickness abdominal defect and preoperative marking. **B.** Free rectus femoris myocutaneous flap. **C.** Inset of flap to the abdomen via saphenous arteriovenous loop *(arrow)*. Distal saphenous anastomosed end-to-side to superficial femoral artery and venous outflow to saphenofemoral junction. **D.** Final result demonstrating healed flap and skin graft donor site. (© Charles E. Butler, MD.)

a formal postoperative physical therapy program for strength training and range of motion.
- The massive amount of skin taken with a subtotal thigh flap usually necessitates donor-site closure with split-thickness skin grafts (**TECH FIG 3D,E**).

Free Rectus Femoris/Subtotal Thigh Flap

- One significant shortcoming of the rectus femoris and subtotal thigh flaps is the associated short pedicle.
  - This disadvantage can be obviated by means of a free tissue transfer.
- If a free flap is required, but there is a short distance between the recipient vessels and the flap, the branch to the rectus femoris muscle can be transected as it emerges from the lateral femoral circumflex artery. This preserves the antero-lateral thigh flap and vastus lateralis muscle for future use.
  - Alternatively, for an additional 2 to 3 cm, the distal lateral femoral circumflex artery can be ligated just distal to the takeoff of the rectus femoris branch, and the pedicle can be transected where it emerges from the profunda femoris.
  - The disadvantage of this maneuver is it prevents future use of the anterolateral thigh and vastus lateralis muscle flap.

- If a subtotal thigh flap is being used, the pedicle is transected in the typical location for an anterolateral thigh flap, where the lateral femoral circumflex artery emerges from the profunda femoris.
- For abdominal wall reconstruction, potential recipient vessels include either of the deep inferior epigastric arteries and their associated venae comitantes.
- Of course, if a patient requires a large flap for reconstruction of their abdominal wall, it is likely that the deep inferior epigastric system is unavailable for use. In this situation, a femoral saphenous arteriovenous loop is a prudent choice (**TECH FIG 4**).
  - The loop is created by transecting the saphenous vein distally and leaving it intact proximally.
  - The distal end of the saphenous vein is then anastomosed in an end-to-side fashion to the superficial femoral artery. The loop is positioned on the abdominal wall adjacent to the flap's vascular pedicle. The loop is divided at its apex to provide both arterial and venous recipient vein grafts.
- Similar to the pedicled subtotal thigh flap and rectus femoris flaps, unilateral or bilateral flaps can be employed, depending on need.

PEARLS AND PITFALLS

Marking and positioning	■ The patient's legs should be internally rotated at the hip to ensure accurate markings. ■ The flap can be harvested easily in the supine, lithotomy, or lateral decubitus positions.
Flap design and reach	■ The rectus femoris flap can be employed as a muscle-only flap or myocutaneous flap. ■ A skin paddle wider than 8 to 9 cm will usually require skin grafting for donor-site closure. ■ The rectus femoris flap can also be utilized as a chimeric flap, including other elements of the lateral femoral circumflex vascular axis (vastus lateralis, tensor fascia lata, iliotibial band) for increased surface area coverage. ■ The flap should be passed deep to the sartorius muscle for an additional 5 cm of advancement. ■ The flap can reach the lower abdomen as a pedicled flap; if midabdomen or superior abdomen requires reconstruction, the flap should be elevated as a free flap.
Donor-site morbidity	■ Donor-site morbidity is limited to decreased eccentric quadriceps strength. Range of motion is unaffected. ■ Most donor-site morbidity can be obviated by performing a vastus medialis-lateralis tenorrhaphy, requiring a knee immobilizer during the postoperative period, and engaging in a physical therapy regimen.
Postoperative management	■ A knee immobilizer should be worn for 6 weeks postoperatively.
Therapy	■ Physical therapy for quadriceps strength training and lower extremity range of motion can be helpful.

POSTOPERATIVE CARE

■ The patient should be placed into a knee immobilizer postoperatively for 6 weeks, which should be worn at all times except when bathing.
■ Ambulation is encouraged as early as the first postoperative day with weight bearing as tolerated.
■ The affected lower extremity should be kept elevated at all times when not ambulating.

OUTCOMES

■ The rectus femoris muscle flap is an effective workhorse flap for abdominal wall reconstruction (**FIG 4**).
■ The donor-site morbidity is low.
  ■ Several authors have reported no loss of knee extension capacity or strength.[1,6–8]

■ The only quantitative assessment found knee range of motion to be unaffected after use of the rectus femoris flap; however, the extension power had decreased 10.3% (concentric contraction) and 19.3% (eccentric contraction). This decrease in strength can be obviated by participation in a postoperative physical therapy regimen.[2]

COMPLICATIONS

■ The rectus femoris muscle is a robust and reliable muscle flap with a low complication profile.
■ Published studies cite a 3% to 4% rate of donor-site wound separation and similar rate of donor-site hematoma.[1–8]
■ The flap loss rate is negligible as a muscle flap. If the flap is elevated as a subtotal thigh flap, there is a 2% rate of distal tip skin necrosis.[1]
■ The donor-site morbidity has been detailed in the outcomes section.

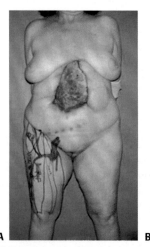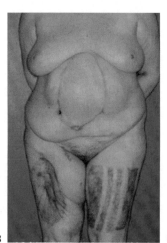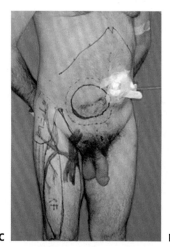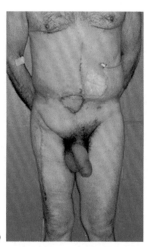

A   B   C   D

FIG 4 • Preoperative and postoperative photos of two patients who required rectus femoris flaps for reconstruction of the abdomen. **A,B.** This patient had a wide and superior defect, requiring a free flap with skin graft for donor-site management. **C,D.** This patient had a more inferior and narrower defect, allowing for a pedicle flap and primary donor-site closure. (© Charles E. Butler, MD.)

REFERENCES

1. Lin SJ, Butler CE. Subtotal thigh flap and bioprosthetic mesh reconstruction for large, composite abdominal wall defects. *Plast Reconstr Surg.* 2010;125:1146-1156.
2. Caulfield WH, Curtsinger L, Powell G, et al. Donor leg morbidity after pedicled rectus femoris muscle flap transfer for abdominal wall and pelvic reconstruction. *Ann Plast Surg.* 1994;32:377-382.
3. Koshima I, Nanba Y, Tutsui T, et al. Dynamic reconstruction of large abdominal defects using a free rectus femoris musculocutaneous flap with normal motor function. *Ann Plast Surg.* 2003;50:420-424.
4. Matthews MS. Abdominal wall reconstruction with an expanded rectus femoris flap. *Plast Reconstr Surg.* 1999;104:183-186.
5. Bostwick J III, Hill HL, Nahai F. Repairs in the lower abdomen, groin, or perineum with myocutaneous or omental flaps. *Plast Reconstr Surg.* 1979;63:186-194.
6. Sbitany H, Koltz PF, Girotto JA, et al. Assessment of donor-site morbidity following rectus femoris harvest for infrainguinal reconstruction. *Plast Reconstr Surg.* 2010;126:933-940.
7. Dibbell DG Jr, Mixter RC, Dibbell DG Sr. Abdominal wall reconstruction (the "mutton chop" flap). *Plast Reconstr Surg.* 1991;87:60-65.
8. Alkon JD, Smith A, Losee JE, et al. Management of complex groin wounds: preferred use of the rectus femoris muscle flap. *Plast Reconstr Surg.* 2005;115:776-783.

Lower Abdominal Wall Reconstruction With Lateral Thigh-Based Flaps

CHAPTER 11

Dhivya R. Srinivasa and Jeffrey H. Kozlow

DEFINITION

Abdominal wall reconstruction is required when partial- or full-thickness defects of the abdominal wall do not allow for primary fascial and/or skin closure. This situation can arise in a variety of clinical situations, sometimes presenting as an intraoperative consult requiring immediate closure. Defects should be evaluated for missing components of the abdominal wall including the skin, subcutaneous tissue, fascia, and musculature. Reconstruction should aim to close the intra-abdominal compartment while minimizing the risk of future hernia development. Techniques to reapproximate the midline fascia for a ventral hernia are reviewed in a separate chapter. Here, we will focus on restoring soft tissue where it is deficient in the lower abdomen.

ANATOMY

The anatomy of the abdominal wall is most readily described in layers. Most superficial is the skin and subcutaneous tissues. Within the subcutaneous tissues is the Scarpa fascia, a layer of variable thickness that provides some additional support to a repair. The critical component of the abdominal wall is the myofascial layer. This layer includes the paired, vertically oriented rectus abdominis muscles adjacent to the midline along with the internal oblique, external oblique, and transversalis muscles laterally. The investing fascia provides significant strength to the abdominal wall and includes both an anterior sheath and a posterior sheath. The central fascia around the rectus abdominis muscles extends from the oblique musculature. In the upper abdomen, the anterior and posterior sheaths are of similar strength; however below the arcuate line, the posterior sheath is much weaker as only the transversalis fascia contributes to the fascia deep to the rectus abdominis muscles. **FIG 1** depicts the layers of the abdominal wall.

Blood supply to the abdominal wall derives from multiple vessels with notable overlap in distribution. Centrally, the superior and inferior epigastric systems supply the abdominal wall. This is further enriched by branches from the internal mammary artery, specifically musculophrenic branches, as

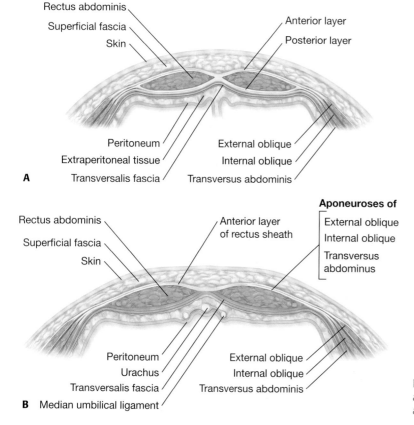

FIG 1 • Layers of the abdominal wall. **A.** Axial view of abdominal wall above the arcuate line. **B.** Axial view of abdominal wall below the arcuate line.

well as the superficial epigastric vessels. Laterally, the circumflex vessels from the iliac artery (deep and superficial) add to the redundancy in blood supply. Innervation is via subcostal nerves (from T12) and thoracoabdominal nerves from T7-T11. These ventral primary rami branches travel between the internal oblique and transverse abdominal muscles. This is the target for the TAP (transverse abdominis plane) block that is used to anesthetize the abdominal wall in select procedures.

A thorough understanding of the various meshes used in abdominal wall reconstruction (including the various synthetic and biologic materials) is critical for surgeons planning to use these materials. However, details on this topic are beyond the scope of this chapter.

PATHOGENESIS

Abdominal wall defects can arise from a variety of scenarios: trauma, cancer, and hernia reconstruction being the most common. Acquired hernias present as a fascial defect and often require abdominal wall myofascial advancement flaps and/or mesh-related techniques. This chapter will focus on closure of soft tissue defects that arise from traumatic injury and oncologic resections. However, some of the principles used for acquired hernia repair, such as component separation, can also play a role in traumatic and oncologic reconstructions. In trauma, all devitalized tissue should be debrided prior to closure. With respect to cancer, margins should be clear and the need for adjuvant radiation should be consider when choosing a reconstructive technique.

PATIENT HISTORY AND PHYSICAL FINDINGS

In addition to the usual key components of a patient's history, the following specifics should also be documented:

- Prior abdominal surgery
  - Include laparoscopic operations and cesarean sections
- Need for stoma postresection. If an ostomy is planned, the estimated location for the stoma should also be noted.
- History of radiation therapy or planned radiation therapy
- Medical comorbidities that will affect wound healing including diabetes mellitus, steroid use, tobacco use, or connective tissue disorders
- Prothrombotic disease states should be noted and a Caprini score should be calculated. Appropriate venous thromboembolism prophylaxis should be tailored accordingly.[1]
- Each patient should be examined thoroughly and all prior incisions should be noted.
- Evaluation of the thigh for adequate tissue to support transfer of the necessary tissue from this area to the abdomen.
  - Incisions within the estimated location of the donor flap should be noted. We also suggest an evaluation of body habitus in this region as thick or thin flaps may be harvested depending on the reconstructive needs.

IMAGING

No specific imaging is necessary for the reconstructive portion of the case. However, most patients will have an abdominal computed tomography (CT) scan, which can be used for planning purposes to understand the anticipated defect. In oncologic cases, specifically note involvement of the skin, anterior sheath, musculature, posterior sheath, and intraperitoneal or retroperitoneal contents. CT angiography of the thigh can be performed in select cases to evaluate perforator location or regional anatomy in complex situations.

SURGICAL MANAGEMENT

Preoperative Planning

- Preoperative planning is incumbent on anticipation of the size and depth of the defect. Whether full-thickness abdominal wall resection is necessary will dictate if fascial advancement and/or mesh will be necessary. The location of the defect is also important to note, as it will affect potential flap options. **FIG 2** illustrates various abdominal wall defects and how they can be covered with a thigh-based flap.
  - Inguinal defects can often be addressed with ipsilateral tensor fascia lata (TFL) based flaps. These flaps provide strong fascial tissue if needed for reconstruction of the inguinal ligament.
  - Lower abdominal (below the umbilicus) and flank defects can be addressed with flaps based off the descending branch of the lateral femoral circumflex system such as the anterolateral thigh (ALT) flap, vastus lateralis, or rectus femoris flaps.[2,3]
  - Midabdominal defects can be addressed with component separation techniques similar to ventral hernia repairs owing to the freedom of the abdominal wall tissue away from the fixed bony pelvis and rib cage.
  - Upper abdominal defects are the most difficult as thigh-based flaps will typically not transpose to the upper abdomen without vein grafts.

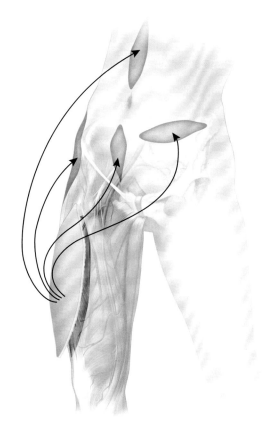

FIG 2 • Lateral thigh-based flaps are a versatile option for a variety of lower abdominal wall defects.

- Preoperative discussion with the patient should include possible donor sites, skin grafting, and potential use of mesh.
- Any planned stomas or existing stomas should be discussed so modifications can be made accordingly. Existing stomas likely pass through the rectus abdominis muscle. Future stomas should be marked preoperatively.
- In cases where primary myofascial repair may be possible, preoperative administration of Botox can be helpful if administered in advance. Typically, up to 100 units per side can be given at least 1 to 2 weeks prior to surgery to optimize the timing of neuromuscular blockade. The goal is to allow maximal relaxation of abdominal wall musculature in anticipation of myofascial advancement for closure.[4]

Positioning

- The patient will likely be positioned supine for the abdominal portion of the surgery. All of the lateral thigh-based flaps are most easily harvested in the supine position as well.
- A safety belt should be used for all cases, but this most often is placed around the chest area.
- A warming blanket should be placed to optimize normothermic core temperatures during the case.
- SCDs should be placed bilaterally as the critical areas of the thigh need to be prepped only to the knee and do not require intraoperative rotation of the leg.
- The thigh should be prepped circumferentially. The contralateral thigh should also be available in the event skin graft is needed for closure of the defect or donor site.

Approach

- Preoperative markings should be made in the preoperative area, prior to patient positioning in the OR.
- Anatomic Landmarks: The anterior superior iliac spine (ASIS) and the superolateral patella are identified. A line connecting these two points is drawn. For an ALT flap, the midpoint of this line will be near the central axis of the skin paddle. **FIG 3** depicts relevant anatomic landmarks and the axis of the skin paddle.
  - If a TFL flap is planned, the incision can be adjusted superiorly (cephalad).
  - If a rectus femoris muscle flap is planned, the incision can be adjusted medially.
- If an ALT flap is planned, there are two main approaches to identifying perforators and designing the skin paddle:
  - Some surgeons define the "A, B, and C" perforators. The perforators are most commonly found approximately 1.5 cm posterior to the line between the ASIS and superior lateral patella. The center point of this line should be marked as perforator "B." Perforators "A" and "C" are 5 cm proximal and distal to "B."[5]
  - Another approach is to draw a 3-cm-radius circle around the midpoint of the axis line, defining the most common location of skin perforators. A Doppler can be used to confirm and mark the location of these perforators. The

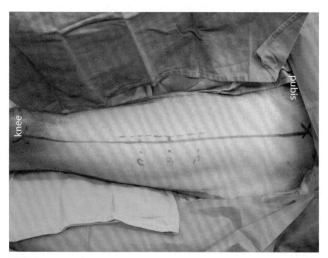

FIG 3 • External anatomic landmarks for an ALT flap from the left leg. The hip is on the right side of the photograph and the knee is on the left side.

skin paddle can be centered over these perforators. Most often the perforators are found in the inferolateral quadrant of the circle (**FIG 4**).
- The initial incision for perforator evaluation is drawn 2 cm anterior/medial to the line between the ASIS and superolateral patella. This is also 4 cm anterior to the expected location of the perforators for an 8- to 9-cm-wide flap. The incision is typically ~15 cm in length and centered near the region of the expected perforators (see **FIG 3**, dotted line). This initial incision is adjusted accordingly if a TFL or rectus femoris flap is planned.
- The final skin paddle is designed after the full nature of the defect is known and the planned perforators are identified. Delaying the design of the skin paddle after identification of the selected perforators can optimize flap perfusion and minimize donor-site morbidity.

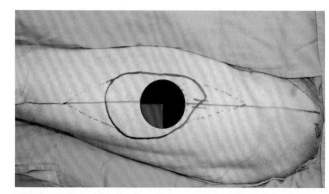

FIG 4 • Perforator location based on center of axis line. The red portion of the circle depicts the most likely location of perforators.

- The patient is marked while positioned supine as described earlier. Toes should be in neutral. Internal rotation of the foot can result in inadvertent rotation of the leg, which would affect markings.
- The marked incision anterior to the perforators is made and dissection is carried down to the fascia. After dissecting through the superficial fascia, care is taken to identify and preserve any medially directed branches of the lateral femoral cutaneous nerve to decrease the extent of postoperative thigh anesthesia.
  - In some situations, a suprafascial dissection can be performed with identification of the perforators above the fascia. We prefer including the fascia with the flap for abdominal reconstruction as it provides a robust layer for closure and anchoring of the flap in to the defect.
- The muscular fascia is then incised over the rectus femoris muscle. Three Allis clamps are placed on the fascia, roughly at the A, B, and C perforators, to gently retract the fascia and visualize the subfascial plane.[5]
  - It is advisable to place a few sutures to hold the skin edge of the flap down to the fascial edge to avoid pulling the subcutaneous tissue and skin off of the fascia inadvertently.
- Carry the dissection laterally in the subfascial plane until you encounter the septum between rectus femoris and vastus lateralis. A fat stripe is often visible here, denoting the correct plane of dissection and likely close proximity to the perforators. Proximal perforators are commonly septal perforators and more distal perforators travel intramuscular through the vastus lateralis (**TECH FIG 1**).
- Careful dissection is then performed posterolaterally over the vastus lateralis with preservation of any identified perforators.
- After identification of all potential perforators, continue the subfascial dissection behind the perforators as this will make the subsequent posterior flap dissection much easier.
- Next, retract the rectus femoris medially and separate the rectus femoris from the vastus lateralis. Care should be taken to dissect anterior to any septal perforators to avoid injury. Muscular branches to the rectus femoris can be divided (**TECH FIG 2**).

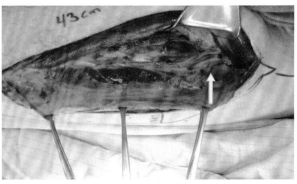

TECH FIG 2 • The rectus femoris muscle of this left leg has been retracted superiorly and an additional septocutaneous perforator (arrow) is seen on top of the vastus lateralis.

- Deep to the rectus femoris, the descending branch of the LCFA is identified. The investing fascial layer can be opened above the pedicle. This is continued proximally to the origin of the pedicle (**TECH FIG 3**).
  - The main branch to the rectus femoris is often near the origin and can often be preserved as well.
  - The main motor nerve to the vastus lateralis runs lateral to the main pedicle and can be dissected free to preserve muscle innervation.
- The flap perforators are then selected, and dissection is performed within either the septum or the vastus lateralis, back toward the descending branch of the LCFA. We recommend performing this dissection before clipping other branches of the main pedicle as the perforator course is not always direct to the main pedicle.
  - Distal perforators of adequate caliber are preferred due to the subsequent increase in functional pedicle length. However, flaps designed around the "B" or midthigh perforator will adequately reach the umbilicus in most patients.
  - The ALT can be harvested with vastus lateralis muscle if needed. The distal portion of the descending LCFA often runs within the muscle, and one can include the superficial portion of the muscle overlying the pedicle if a chimeric flap is needed.

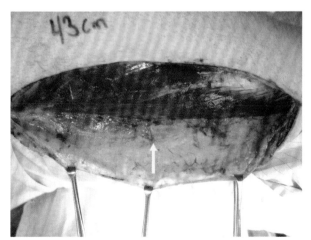

TECH FIG 1 • Allis clamps applied on fascia at the estimated perforator sites. Subfascial dissection has been performed over the rectus femoris back toward the vastus lateralis, and an initial perforator (arrow) has been identified.

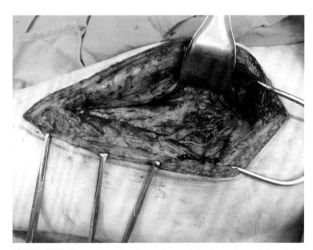

TECH FIG 3 • Dissection is performed back to the origin of the descending branch of the lateral femoral circumflex trunk.

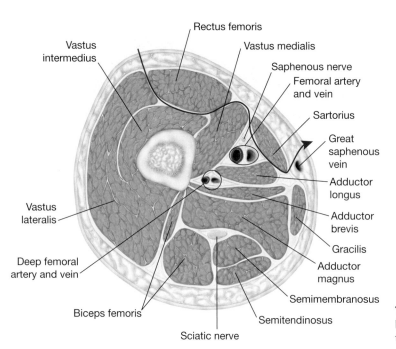

TECH FIG 4 • The tunnel for the flap should pass below the rectus femoris and sartorius and then through the soft tissue.

- The anterior incision is then tailor-tacked closed. A flap template is designed base on the abdominal defect. Positioning of the flap around the perforator is based on the defect and planned location for the tunnel between the thigh and the abdomen.
  - Flaps up to 9 cm wide and 22 cm long can typically be harvested while still allowing for primary closure of the donor site.
- The posterior incision is then made and dissection is performed through the subcutaneous tissue and muscular fascia with care taken to protect the perforators traveling into the flap. Prior dissection of the subfascial plan behind the perforators from the anterior incision allows for rapid flap elevation at this stage.
- With the distal pedicle now divided, the flap is isolated on only the main pedicle and can be evaluated for perfusion.
- Transposition of the flap from the thigh to the lower abdomen requires a wide tunnel. The typical tunnel is subrectus femoris, subsartorius, and then subcutaneous into the defect (**TECH FIG 4**).
  - The sartorius can also be transected to avoid potential compression in this area.
- The flap is transposed through this tunnel once wide enough to easily accommodate the flap. Note that chimeric flaps will require a much wider tunnel to accommodate the additional muscle bulk.
  - In cases requiring extended reach of the flap, the pedicle of the flap may kink around the vascular branch to the rectus femoris, which can be divided if needed.
- The flap is then inset into the defect using ideally a three-layer closure (the superficial fascia, deep dermis, and external skin) in addition to any abdominal fascia inset.

- We prefer to use dissolving sutures for the entire inset to avoid the removal of permanent sutures postoperatively.
- The donor site is closed in layers over a drain. A compressive dressing is not placed to avoid compression of the pedicle running across the medial upper thigh.

Resection of Soft Tissue Sarcoma

- Resection of a soft tissue sarcoma left the lower abdominal wall soft tissue defect is pictured in **TECH FIG 5A**. Preoperative markings for a left ALT flap are also shown. The subsequently harvested flap is seen in **TECH FIG 5B** with the vascular pedicle and two perforators seen in **TECH FIG 5C**. The flap is then transposed under rectus femoris and sartorius to the suprapubic defect as seen in **TECH FIG 5D** with final inset seen in **TECH FIG 5E**.
- A vastus lateralis flap in conjunction with a biologic mesh for reconstruction of a full-thickness lower abdominal wall defect following sarcoma resection is pictured in **TECH FIG 6**. There is an acquired defect of the lower abdominal wall with resection of all myofascial layers (**TECH FIG 6A**). After using the omentum to cover the bowel (**TECH FIG 6B**), a piece of acellular dermal matrix was used to close the peritoneum/residual posterior sheath (**TECH FIG 6C**). A vastus lateralis muscle-only flap was planned from the right thigh (**TECH FIG 6D**). After harvest of the vastus lateralis (**TECH FIG 6E**), it was transposed underneath the rectus femoris, under the sartorius, and then subcutaneously over the inguinal ligament to the lower abdomen (**TECH FIG 6F**). Inset was performed around the myofascial defect with the muscular fascia next to the acellular dermal matrix (**TECH FIG 6G**). The skin was closed primarily in this case.

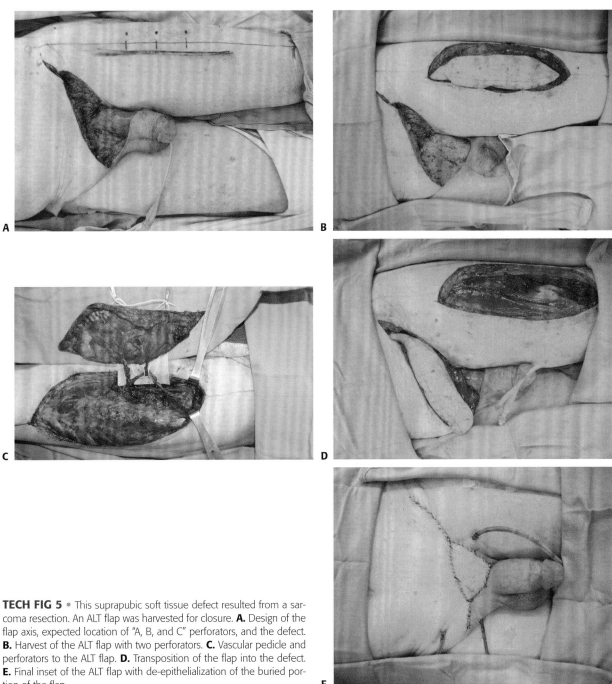

TECH FIG 5 • This suprapubic soft tissue defect resulted from a sarcoma resection. An ALT flap was harvested for closure. **A.** Design of the flap axis, expected location of "A, B, and C" perforators, and the defect. **B.** Harvest of the ALT flap with two perforators. **C.** Vascular pedicle and perforators to the ALT flap. **D.** Transposition of the flap into the defect. **E.** Final inset of the ALT flap with de-epithelialization of the buried portion of the flap.

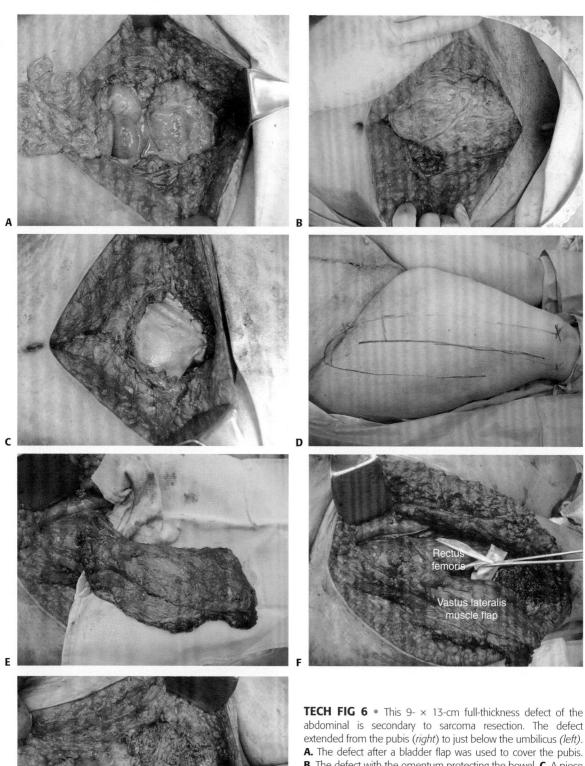

TECH FIG 6 • This 9- × 13-cm full-thickness defect of the abdominal is secondary to sarcoma resection. The defect extended from the pubis *(right)* to just below the umbilicus *(left)*. **A.** The defect after a bladder flap was used to cover the pubis. **B.** The defect with the omentum protecting the bowel. **C.** A piece of acellular matrix was used to close the peritoneum/transversalis layer of fascia. **D.** Markings for a right vastus lateralis flap. A vastus lateralis muscle flap was then harvested based on the descending branch of the lateral femoral circumflex system **(E)** and transposed under the rectus femoris muscle (with the Penrose drain around the muscle) **(F)**. **G.** The muscle was then inset into the abdominal wall defect with the fascial side down against the acellular dermal matrix. The overlying skin was closed primarily over the reconstruction.

PEARLS AND PITFALLS

Markings	■ Mark the patient *preoperatively*. ■ Toes should be maintained in neutral.
Positioning	■ Keep toes at neutral for flap harvest (slight internal rotation of the leg). ■ No bumps under thigh in the OR, as this can distort the soft tissue of the thigh
Skin paddle design	■ For an ALT, cutaneous perforators are most often located *1.5 to 2 cm posterior* to the axis line; keep this in mind when defining your skin paddle. The incision should be adjusted if other flaps are planned.
Surgical efficacy	■ Harvesting flaps from the right thigh is optimal for right-handed surgeons for dissection of this flap if the defect is midline; otherwise, the leg ipsilateral to the defect should be used if possible to minimize the distance for flap transposition.
Perforator selection	■ More distal perforators should be preserved and more proximal perforators can be sacrificed to optimize pedicle length.
Plan B	■ When using and ALT, expect pedicle variability. Follow the perforators in a systematic fashion. ■ Vastus lateralis and rectus femoris can be taken for additional bulk and/or muscle coverage. ■ If no adequate perforators are located, keep in mind that you can always convert to an anteromedial thigh flap (AMT) before committing to your lateral incision. The lateral incision should over the lateral border of the rectus femoris, as most of the AMT perforators are found there.
Avoid sensory deficits	■ Beware of the descending branch of lateral femoral cutaneous nerve. Preserve as many medial branches as possible to avoid undue numbness in medial thigh.
Tunnel for transfer to the lower abdomen	■ The shortest path for a lateral thigh flap to the lower abdomen is subrectus femoris, subsartorius, and then subcutaneous.

POSTOPERATIVE CARE

■ Drain management: Hematomas and seromas can place undue pressure on the flap and pedicle, therefore compromising flow. Pay careful attention to drain output, and any hematomas should be drained operatively.

■ Flap monitoring: Nursing staff should monitor the flap overnight, with checks for capillary refill, color, and warmth every 2 to 4 hours. A Doppler stitch can be used if needed. Evidence of congestion or ischemia should be noted immediately. Sometimes, release of sutures can help if undue tension is the source of the problem. Concerns for vascular compromise should prompt operative exploration to evaluate kinking or pressure on the pedicle

■ Review the pathology results to confirm margins are negative from the original resection for all oncologic procedures.

COMPLICATIONS

■ Flap loss: Complete flap loss is due to compromise of the vascular pedicle. Ideally, this would be discovered soon postoperatively with subsequent operative salvage. However, in the case of irreversible flap loss, the tissue should be removed and other reconstructive options should be explored.

■ Wounds: Recipient site wounds are relatively common and most often can be managed nonoperatively. This would include debridement as needed, local wound care, and close monitoring. The surgeon should avoid the urge to debride aggressively or perform additional procedures as most often, these wounds will heal secondarily.

■ Infection: Most infections can be managed with antibiotics. Interventional drain placement is helpful for formed abscesses seen on imaging.

■ Hematoma: Hematomas are possible at both the donor and recipient site. Drain output and physical exam are key. Hematomas should be drained surgically.

■ Seroma: Late seromas can develop at the donor site. Most can be managed with drains and compression.

REFERENCES

1. Charlton S, Cyna AM, Middleton P, et al. Perioperative transversus abdominis plane (TAP) blocks for analgesia after abdominal surgery. *Cochrane Database Syst Rev.* 2010;(12):CD007705.
2. Jang J, Jeong SH, Han SK, et al. Reconstruction of extensive abdominal wall defect using an eccentric perforator-based pedicled anterolateral thigh flap: a case report. *Microsurgery.* 2013;33(6):482-486.
3. Friji MT, Suri MP, Shankhdhar VK, et al. Pedicled anterolateral thigh flap: a versatile flap for difficult regional soft tissue reconstruction. *Ann Plast Surg.* 2010;64(4):458-461.
4. Ibarra-hurtado TR, Nuño-guzmán CM, Echeagaray-herrera JE, et al. Use of botulinum toxin type a before abdominal wall hernia reconstruction. *World J Surg.* 2009;33(12):2553-2556.
5. Yu P, Selber J. Perforator patterns of the anteromedial thigh flap. *Plast Reconstr Surg.* 2011;128(3):151e-157e.

Section III: Body Contouring

Abdominoplasty

Alan Matarasso and Darren M. Smith

DEFINITION

- Abdominal contour deformity results from relaxation of the abdominal wall and overlying soft tissues with childbearing, weight gain, aging, or a combination of the above.
- Rectus diastasis is the separation of the two rectus abdominis muscles in the midline; this separation, along with stretching of the abdominal fascia, constitutes the deepest anatomical layer responsible for the abdominal contour deformity.
- Lipodystrophy refers to excess adiposity, superficial to the abdominal wall, that contributes to the abdominal contour deformity.
- Skin excess (most frequently present after weight loss or pregnancy) is the most superficial anatomical component of the abdominal contour deformity.

ANATOMY

- The abdominal wall can be discussed in terms of three treatable tissue types, skin, fat, and muscle.
- Skin (from costal margin superiorly to mons pubis inferiorly, with lateral borders defined by the anterior axillary line)
- Fat in the abdominal region is either superficial or deep to the Scarpa fascia. Some surgeons aggressively excise subscarpal fat from the abdominoplasty flap, but this is not generally our practice.
- The rectus abdominis muscles are a paired midline structure that must be assessed in each abdominoplasty patient to determine the need for plication.
  - Plication is generally indicated except in men and in the massive weight loss population.

PATIENT HISTORY AND PHYSICAL FINDINGS

- Abdominoplasty patients should be low risk (eg, ASA I) healthy patients.
- Abdominoplasty patients should ideally have completed their childbearing, as future pregnancy will distort the result.
- Massive weight loss patients require heightened vigilance with regard to medical optimization given their unique risk profile.[1]
- In addition to ensuring general good health in the abdominoplasty patient, special attention should be paid to venous thromboembolism (VTE) avoidance given the risk of this potentially catastrophic event after this procedure.[2]
- In a survey of more than 1100 plastic surgeons on VTE occurrence and prevention in their practices, VTE was found to occur most frequently with abdominoplasty and abdominoplasty combined with another procedure (without a significant difference in frequency between the two).[3]

- Thorough history taking and patient-specific risk reduction strategies based on the literature are critical in VTE avoidance.[2,4]
- The physical exam should focus on identifying the degree to which the treatable tissues of the abdomen (skin, fat, and muscle) contribute to a given patient's abdominal contour deformity.
- Pre-existing scars should be evaluated with regard to their effect on blood supply to the abdominoplasty flap and to determine the best way to incorporate them into the incision design if they cannot be excised.

IMAGING

- No preoperative imaging is routinely performed prior to abdominoplasty.
- If hernias is suspected based on history or physical exam, an abdominal computed tomogram (CT) is indicated.

SURGICAL MANAGEMENT

- Choice of operation from the abdominolipoplasty system of classification and treatment[5] based on physical exam findings with respect to the treatable tissues of the abdomen (skin, fat, and muscle) (**FIG 1**):
  - Type I (liposuction alone): Minimal skin laxity, excess adiposity, minimal rectus diastasis
  - Type II (mini abdominoplasty): Mild skin laxity, excess adiposity, lower rectus diastasis
  - Type III (modified abdominoplasty): Moderate skin laxity, excess adiposity, lower with or without upper diastasis
  - Type IV (full standard abdominoplasty with or without liposuction): Severe skin laxity, excess adiposity, complete rectus diastasis
- Patients can be "downstaged" to less invasive options if they cannot accept a given scar or desire minimized recovery time, but it should be explained that a downstaged procedure cannot deliver the same result as the procedure that is indicated by the abdominolipoplasty system of classification and treatment.

Preoperative Planning

- Several red flag patient characteristics emerged from our experience that apply to combining abdominoplasty with any procedure.
  - Pulmonary conditions, history of or propensity for VTE, cardiac insufficiency, peripheral vascular disease, hypertension, obesity, bleeding diathesis, smoking, exposure to secondhand smoke, and diseases affecting microcirculation (diabetes, lupus, chronic fatigue syndrome) should be investigated and dealt with prior to abdominoplasty.

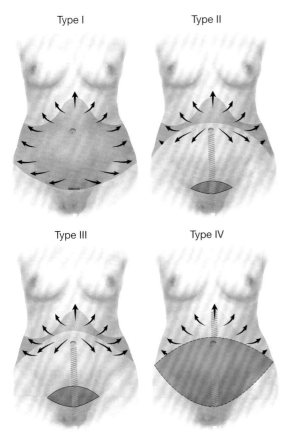

FIG 1 • The abdominolipoplasty system of classification and treatment. Type I, liposuction alone. Type II, mini abdominoplasty. Type III, modified abdominoplasty. Type IV, full standard abdominoplasty with or without liposuction. Types I and II are limited abdominoplasties. Pink, suction-assisted lipectomy; yellow, undermining; green, excision; blue cross-hatching, fascial plication; *arrows*, transitional area.

- A history of surgical site infections (especially involving methicillin-resistant *Staphylococcus aureus* [MRSA]) should also be addressed.
- With regard to VTE prevention, our patients discontinue the use of all female hormones (including drug-eluting patches and intrauterine contraceptive devices) and nicotine in the preoperative period. They are offered prothrombogenic blood test screening and postoperative venous Doppler testing.

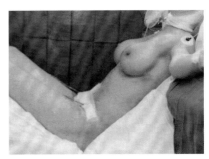

FIG 2 • The Miami beach chair position. The surgeon must verify that the operating table can reach full flexion prior to beginning the case.

- Those at high risk for VTE based on history (Rubin's group offers a good review of criteria with which to assess historical risk[6]) are referred for hematologic workup.
- All of our patients are liberally hydrated and placed in compressive stockings and sequential pneumatic compression devices prior to the induction of anesthesia.
- A history of surgical site infection (especially those involving MRSA) should also be addressed.
- We routinely utilize nostril mupirocin ointment (GlaxoSmithKline, Research Triangle Park, NC) in the perioperative period, along with oral and intravenous antibiotics and antimicrobial body scrubs. Alcohol-based prep solutions are utilized at the time of surgery.

Positioning

- Prior to surgery, it is confirmed that the operating room table can reach a full beach chair position (**FIG 2**).
- The operation begins with the patient in the supine position.
- The symmetry and angle of the arm boards is confirmed, and the arms are secured to the arm boards with a gauze wrap.

Approach

- The operation is performed under systemic anesthesia (spontaneous ventilation general anesthesia, or spinal/epidural) administered by a board certified anesthesiologist in a certified ambulatory surgery facility.
- A Foley catheter is inserted and thromboembolic precautions are taken as discussed above.
- If multiple procedures are to be performed, the abdominoplasty is usually performed last.

■ Abdominoplasty

Markings

- The abdominoplasty incision is marked with the patient wearing their preferred undergarment to ensure it covers the proposed incision.
- The abdominal excision, essentially an ellipse of tissue between the umbilicus and mons pubis, is determined by assessing the ease in which the lower abdominal skin (from umbilicus to hairline) can be excised after grasping the pannus with both hands in an attempt for the fingers to touch the thumbs.
- The pannus is held slightly upward and the lower incision is designed to traverse the natural lower skin

crease, slightly below its normal position extending in length to just beyond the lateral skinfolds (noted in a sitting position) and approximately 5 to 7 cm above the vulva cleft.
- The upper incision is demarcated passing over the umbilicus to encompass the old umbilical site and only higher if there is obviously sufficient loose skin, forming an ellipse when joining the upper and lower incisions; a flexible ruler bent to trace the lower incision and flipped along its horizontal axis can be helpful in designing this incision.
- Bisecting perpendicular lines are marked through it to line up the skin edges for closure.
- The incision for umbilical circumscription is drawn and its four quadrants marked.

TECHNIQUES

Liposuction

- The abdomen is infiltrated with approximately 1 L of superwet anesthesia (1 L Ringer lactate, 1 mL 1:1000 epinephrine, 20 mL 1% lidocaine).
- Liposuction is then performed as indicated.

Verifying Incisions

- The incisions are checked for symmetry by placing 0-silk sutures in the midline at the xiphoid and the mons below the lower incision.
- The sutures are crisscrossed and grasped with a clamp.
- The clamp is then moved to either side of the midline at various points on the upper and lower skin incision lines to confirm symmetry.

Incisions and Dissection

- The abdominoplasty commences by freeing the umbilicus from the rest of the ellipse to be excised during the abdominoplasty.
- The pannus is then prepared for pre-excision in a vest-over-pants fashion by sharply incising the upper limb of the ellipse to the level of the rectus fascia while beveling the cut inward at a 45-degree angle.
- The upper abdominal flap is then completely undermined with electrocautery in a narrow tunnel (inverted V) corresponding to red suction area 3 (the zone of complete undermining) (**TECH FIG 1**).

Selective Undermining and Suctioning

- An intact zone surrounding this tunnel (yellow area in **TECH FIG 1A,B,** which corresponds to suction area 2 or the zone of selective undermining in **TECH FIG 1C**) is undermined as necessary to decrease skin bunching after muscle closure.
- This pattern of dissection maintains intercostal blood supply sufficient to achieve rectus muscle plication.
- Dissecting in this manner maintains a broad intact subcostal perforator blood supply (green area in **TECH FIG 1A,B** or zone of discontinuous undermining in **TECH FIG 1C**, of axial blood supply corresponding to suction area 1) that has been discontinuously undermined by the liposuction.
- The entire flap can thereby be suctioned during full abdominoplasty, giving rise to the term *lipoabdominoplasty*.
- This operative sequence serves as a standard template and is adjusted according to individual patient needs unless they do not require liposuction, in which case it is not performed.

Confirming Height of Lower Incision

- The operating room table is then flexed and the upper skin flap is pulled over the pannus to verify that it reaches the proposed lower skin incision (**TECH FIG 2A**).
- If the flap does not reach, it can be stretched, further undermined as appropriate, Scarpa fascia scored, or adjustments in the height of the lower incision can be made, if necessary.
- The lower incision is made to the level of the fascia after it has been determined that the upper flap can reach it for closure.

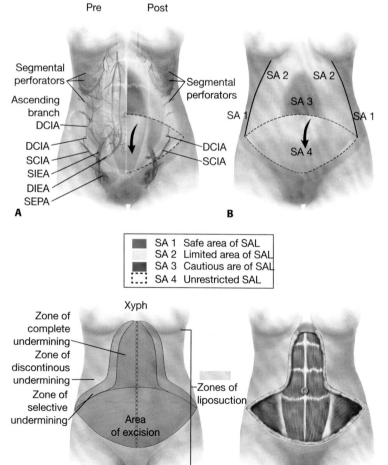

SA 1 Safe area of SAL
SA 2 Limited area of SAL
SA 3 Cautious are of SAL
SA 4 Unrestricted SAL

TECH FIG 1 • A. The abdominal blood supply before and after abdominoplasty. **B.** Suction areas (SA) 1 to 4 are determined by these patterns of blood supply. Suction area 4 is not suctioned; it is excised. **C.** The types of undermining in abdominoplasty can be divided into zones. Complete undermining is performed only as much as necessary to allow for abdominal plication. Note how these zones correspond to the abdominal blood supply detailed in **(A)** and **(B)**.

Excision of the Pannus

- Although some have suggested that leaving a thin layer of fibrofatty tissue on the fascia reduces seroma formation, this is not our practice.
- Special care must be exercised during the dissection in the massive weight loss population as a large pannus can distort the anatomy and bring the spermatochord into the field.
- The pannus is then grasped with Allis clamps and excised en bloc, from right to left.
- An ocular conformer is sutured to the umbilicus to facilitate later identification, and removed when the umbilicus is later exteriorized.
- The surgeon and assistants are actively achieving hemostasis at each step of the operation.

Rectus Plication

- Next, the rectus diastasis is marked in a long vertical ellipse from xyphoid to pubis such that it can be closed without excessive tension (**TECH FIG 2B**).
- The section above and then below the umbilicus is plicated in layers, first with running 0-loop nylon sutures and then a second layer of buried interrupted 2-0 Neurolon sutures.
- Puckering developing in the upper skin flap where it is still attached to the underlying muscle after fascial closure (**TECH FIG 2C**) is gently freed by selective blunt and sharp dissection (zone of discontinuous undermining).
- Small amounts of bunching (resolves in early postoperative period) are tolerated and indeed desirable as this is indicative of preserved lateral intercostal blood supply.

Preparing for Flap Inset

- At least 30 minutes after lidocaine administration and prior to wound closure, Exparel (1.3% bupivacaine liposome suspension, Pacira Pharmaceuticals, Parsippany, NJ) is injected linearly using a threading technique at strategic submuscular points and in the wound edges.
- The supplied 20-cc single-use vial of Exparel is diluted in 80 cc of preservative-free normal saline; 0.25% Marcaine can be added if desired and safe dosage levels allow.
- The cavity is irrigated, and final inspection and hemostasis are performed.

Closure

- The table is returned to the degree of beach chair position necessary for wound closure.
- Closure commences with placement of a 2-0 Vicryl suture in the midline.
- Staples are used to align the wound edges and minimize dog-ear formation.
- A 2-0 PDO bidirectional barbed suture (Quill SRS, Angiotech, Vancouver, Canada) is run in the deep layers from the Scarpa fascia to the dermis on either side of the midline.
- When most of the wound is closed, the ocular conformer on the umbilicus is palpated below the flap and marked on the skin in the midline slightly cephalad to its natural position.
- A second layer of 3-0 monoderm Quill is run in the subcuticular layer.
- Closed suction drains are placed in the incision (3 to 5 cm from the lateral extent of each side) and are secured with 3-0 nylon sutures.

Exteriorization of Umbilicus

- To exteriorize the umbilicus, the patient's midline is verified with the silk marking sutures and by observing the position of the vulva cleft.
- The new umbilical site is determined and marked as a 2.5-cm inverted V in the midline.
- The upper and (more so) lower skin edges of the umbilical opening are defatted.
- The umbilicus is exteriorized and the ocular conformer is removed.
- The umbilicus is sewn to the skin flap with deep absorbable sutures, and the umbilical skin is closed with 3-0 nylon sutures.

Application of Dressings and Binder

- A strip of Xeroform gauze is used to pack the umbilicus.
- The wound is covered with antibiotic ointment, and it is covered with a Telfa dressing.
- An abdominal binder can placed be used if desired.

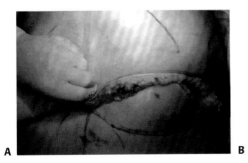
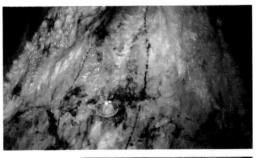
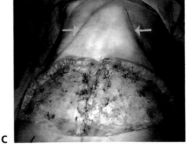

TECH FIG 2 • A. The upper flap is pulled down to the proposed lower incision before the lower incision is made so that the ability to close is ensured. **B.** The plication is marked as an ellipse above and below the umbilicus, shown here sutured to an ocular conformer. **C.** The *arrows* highlight skin puckering evident after abdominal wall plication. This is released selectively by blunt and sharp dissection (zone of discontinuous undermining).

TECHNIQUES

■ Achieving a Narrower Waistline

- Abdominoplasty patients frequently request a narrower waistline, but this result cannot be guaranteed.
- Appropriate rectus plication will achieve maximal waistline narrowing, although two maneuvers (selective waistline liposuction and, in patients with minimal visceral fat, horizontal waistline sutures) can contribute a modest improvement (**TECH FIG 3**).

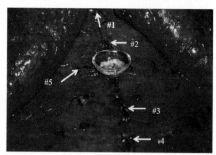

TECH FIG 3 • The rectus fascia has been plicated in two layers from xyphoid to pubis. Anatomic landmarks are highlighted: 1, toward the xyphoid; 2, supraumbilical region; 3, arcuate line of Douglas; 4, pubic bulge; 5, level of waistline suture (if indicated).

PEARLS AND PITFALLS

Multiple procedures	■ Abdominoplasty is frequently combined with other procedures.[2] ■ If multiple procedures are planned in a surgery, abdominoplasty is usually the last to be performed.
Venous thromboembolism	■ Abdominoplasty is the ambulatory plastic surgery procedure most frequently associated with venous thromboembolism; precautionary measures should be taken pre-, intra- and postoperatively.
Hemostasis	■ It is prudent to for the surgeon and assistants to ensure hemostasis at each stage of the procedure.
Communication	■ Review the areas so be addressed with the patient prior to surgery. ■ This conversation is critical in maximizing the chances of a positive outcome for the patient and success for the surgeon.

POSTOPERATIVE CARE

- The patient is transferred to a stretcher in the maximally flexed position used for closure.
- Patients should ambulate that day as if using a walker and over the next few days begin to walk fully upright.
- The first 24 to 48 hours after surgery are spent in a hotel-like facility under the care of an experienced registered nurse.
- Blood pressure management, pain control, fluid and foot intake, ambulation, hygiene, and pulmonary care are carefully protocolized.
- Drains are removed as early as permitted by character and volume of drainage.
- Patients are inspected frequently for seroma formation, as untreated seromas can result in a variety of sequelae and late contour irregularities such as pseudobursa formation.
- Any concern for thromboembolic events prompts an immediate workup.
- Appropriate pain management is essential not only in enhancing the patient's experience but also in avoiding a host of serious problems such is paralytic ileus and hematoma formation.[7]

OUTCOMES

- Abdominoplasty patients are generally very happy with the result of their operation.
- Perhaps the most common cause of dissatisfaction with abdominoplasty is poor communication between patient and surgeon prior to the operation.

- It is particularly important to discuss anatomic boundaries with patients so there is a clear mutual understanding of the areas to be treated (eg, soft tissue laxity in the flanks requires a flankplasty) (**FIG 3**).
- Clear communication is essential to ensure that:
  - The proper operation is selected and that if downstaging is to occur, its full repercussions are understood.

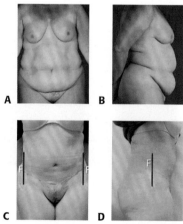

FIG 3 • Preoperative (**A,B**) and postoperative (**C,D**) images of a patient who underwent abdominoplasty with flankplasty. The flankplasty is a prime example of a procedure that underscores the importance of discussing anatomic boundaries with the abdominoplasty patient. To address the flanks (lateral to the vertical lines in **C** and to the left of the line in **D**), the abdominoplasty incision must be extended.

■ The anatomic limits of the abdomen and surrounding aesthetic units are defined, especially with regard to liposuction to avoid misplaced expectations in terms of areas to be treated.

COMPLICATIONS

■ Abdominoplasty carries the highest complication rate (4.7%) of all aesthetic surgery.[5]
■ Seroma is the most common complication after abdominoplasty[5] and is avoided by using closed suction drains and maintaining postoperative vigilance.
■ The most dreaded complication of abdominoplasty is pulmonary embolism, which occurs in 0.19% of abdominoplasties, underscoring the importance of the anti-VTE measures discussed earlier.[5]
■ Tissue ischemia can be minimized by exercising meticulous technique, an awareness of blood supply, and good judgment in reconciling the extent of liposuction with tension on wound closure.
■ Avoidance of tissue ischemia can be further ensured by paying close attention to the method and extent of undermining performed.
■ All wounds are examined for signs of ischemia the night of surgery and the next morning.

■ If ischemia is noted, any reversible causes such as fluid collection, cellulitis, infections, or wound tension (that can be relieved by suture removal) are addressed.
■ If signs of ischemia progress, dimethyl sulfoxide or nitroglycerine ointment may be employed.
■ Should frank necrosis evolve, standard wound management principles apply.

REFERENCES

1. Michaels J, Coon D, Rubin JP. Complications in postbariatric body contouring: strategies for assessment and prevention. *Plast Reconstr Surg.* 2011; 127(3): 1352-1357.
2. Matarasso A, Smith DM. Combined breast surgery and abdominoplasty: strategies for success. *Plast Reconstr Surg.* 2015; 135(5): 849e-860e.
3. Spring MA, Gutowski KA. Venous thromboembolism in plastic surgery patients: survey results of plastic surgeons. *Aesthet Surg J.* 2006; 26: 522-529.
4. Matarasso A, Smith DM. Strategies for aesthetic reshaping of the postpartum patient. *Plast Reconstr Surg.* 2015; 136(2): 245-257.
5. Matarasso A, Matarasso DM, Matarasso EJ. Abdominoplasty: classic principles and technique. *Clin Plast Surg.* 2014; 41: 655-672.
6. Friedman T, Coon DO, Michaels J, et al. Hereditary coagulopathies: practical diagnosis and management for the plastic surgeon. *Plast Reconstr Surg.* 2010; 125: 1544-1552.
7. Constantine FC, Matarasso A. Putting it all together: recommendations for improving pain management in body contouring. *Plast Reconstr Surg.* 2014; 134: 113S-119S.

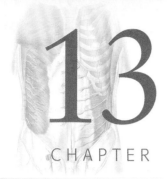

Abdominal Panniculectomy

Devra B. Becker

DEFINITION

- Abdominal panniculus derives from the Latin *pannus* (cloth, garment), the diminutive of which is *panniculus* (piece of cloth).
  - *Pannus* was used to describe "wrinkled or flabby skin" by the Roman Pliny, but is distinct from the Greek *panus*, meaning swelling (*panus inguinalis*). *Pannus* is defined in modern usage as an abnormal layer of granulation tissue covering the eye or synovial space.
- Panniculus morbidus was described in Petty and colleagues' 1992 article that reported on eight patients who had restored function after wedge resection.[1]
- A symptomatic panniculus can be graded by function[2]:
  - Grade I: chronic skin problems confined to the lower abdomen
  - Grade II: chronic skin problems around the naval or under a supraumbilical panniculus as well as an infraumbilical panniculus
  - Grade III: abdominal panniculus without chronic skin problem

ANATOMY

- An abdominal panniculus is so defined by redundant skin of the abdomen that can have both horizontal and vertical excess.
- There are three vascular zones of the abdomen as described by Huger.[3]
  - In Zone 1 (bounded craniocaudally from xiphoid to pubis and laterally by the lateral extent of the rectus sheath), the blood supply is the deep epigastric arcade.
  - In Zone 2 (bounded craniocaudally from a line drawn from the anterosuperior iliac spine [ASIS] to the pubis, and laterally by the inguinal creases), the blood supply is the superficial branches of the circumflex iliac and external pudendal vessels.
  - In Zone 3 (bounded craniocaudally by the costal margin to the ASIS and laterally extending from the lateral rectus sheath to the midaxillary line), the blood supply is intercostal, subcostal, and lumbar arteries.
- Nerve supply to the abdominal wall is segmental and dermatomal, from T7-L1.
- The lateral femoral cutaneous nerve from L2-L3 innervates the anterolateral thigh and travels medial to the ASIS.
  - The iliohypogastric and ilioinguinal nerves pierce the internal oblique muscle and travel along the external oblique muscle to provide sensation to the inner thigh and the groin and symphysis pubis.

PATHOGENESIS

- Risk factors for development of abdominal panniculus after bariatric surgery include a higher pregastric bypass body mass index (BMI) and advanced age.[4]

NATURAL HISTORY

- Symptomatic panniculitis is characterized by intertrigo that is refractory to conservative management with desiccants such as powder and topical antifungals.

PATIENT HISTORY AND PHYSICAL FINDINGS

- For patients who have had bariatric surgery, the surgeon should assess the type of bariatric surgery the patient had (restrictive, or restrictive and malabsorptive), time from surgery, total weight loss, and length of time that weight has been stable.
- Nutritional status should be addressed, including protein needs and any micronutrient deficiency.
- History should be assessed for patient reports of functional impairment, particularly with activities that require hip flexion such a cycling or walking up stairs, intertrigal rashes refractory to conservative management with desiccants and antifungals, and back pain.
- Physical exam should include inspection for scars and extent of panniculus, relationship of panniculus to the symphysis pubis, scars, abdominal striae, quality of skin, mons pubis edema and ptosis, intertrigal rashes or ulceration, intertrigal hyperchromia, vertical and horizontal excess, and asymmetry.
  - The abdomen should be palpated to assess for hernia, rectus diastasis, skin elasticity, and extent of subcutaneous fat (**FIG 1**).
- Factors important to surgeons are different from factors important to insurance companies.[5]
  - Surgeons value stability of weight for 6 months, and time from bariatric surgery of 18 months, whereas insurance companies value chronic maceration of skinfolds.
- There is no consensus on the most appropriate BMI at which to perform panniculectomy, but postoperative events increase with increasing BMI.
- Panniculectomy can be safely combined with other procedures.
  - In hysterectomy, panniculectomy can decrease wound dehiscence and increase ease of hygiene[6] without increasing complications,[16] as well as increase exposure of the pelvis.
  - In cases of uterine cancer, concurrent panniculectomy can result in greater total lymph node counts.[7]
  - When combined with hernia repair, it can decrease recurrence.[8]

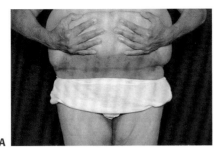 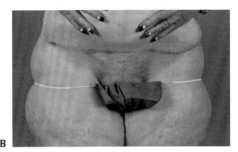

FIG 1 • Physical exam should include inspection as well as palpation. The relationship of the panniculus to the pubis should be assessed, as well as intertrigo. Photographs with the panniculus lifted help to identify hyperchromia and intertrigo.

IMAGING

- Routine imaging is not necessary in the presence of an adequate physical exam, but CT should be obtained in the case of hernia (**FIG 2**).

NONOPERATIVE MANAGEMENT

- Nonoperative management should be aimed at improving function.
- Weight loss, physical therapy for muscle rebalancing, and hygiene for intertrigo reduction are nonoperative strategies that should be trialed for several months.

SURGICAL MANAGEMENT

- If the umbilical stalk is greater than 5 cm or if it is involved in a hernia, it may need to be sacrificed. Discussion of the umbilicus should be frank (**FIG 3**).
- Blood transfusions are often not necessary, but some blood loss is expected. Transfusion rates have been reported from 9% to 12%.[9]
- Risks of the procedure include bleeding, hematoma formation, skin flap necrosis, fat necrosis, and asymmetry.[9]
- If a wedge excision is planned, whether the umbilicus will remain is determined based on its location cephalad to the panniculus.
- The main objective of the operation is to reduce the redundant skin and subcutaneous fat inferior to the umbilicus that creates the panniculus.

- The luminal diameter of vessels is increased in obese patients, and there is some evidence that the luminal diameter remains increased with massive weight loss.
  - Surgeons should be mindful of the larger caliber vessels encountered in panniculectomy, even in massive weight loss patients.
- The ability to close should be determined prior to resection.

Preoperative Planning

- Patients are assessed by Caprini score for deep vein thrombosis (DVT) risk assessment.[10]
- CT scans are obtained if there is clinical concern for hernia. If a hernia is present, a combined hernia repair and panniculectomy is planned.
- Patients often have some asymmetry of the panniculus; this is identified and discussed with the patient.
- Best practices in planning panniculectomy in the bariatric population are
  - Ensuring realistic expectations[11]
  - Allowing for at least 12 months after bariatric surgery to allow for nutritional and metabolic homeostasis
  - Allowing for a stable weight for at least 6 months
- Surgery should be performed by a board-eligible or board-certified surgeon.[11]
  - Postoperative events have been shown to be lower when the procedure is performed by plastic surgeons compared with general surgeons.[8]

Positioning and Anesthesia

- The operation is performed with the patient in the supine position.

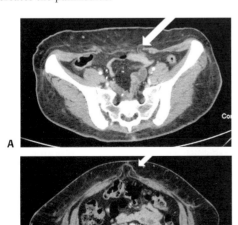

FIG 2 • CT scan can help delineate the extent of a hernia and can help with preoperative planning.

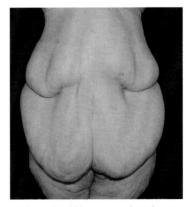

FIG 3 • The umbilicus should be assessed. In this case, the umbilicus is within the panniculus, and the stalk is likely greater than 5 cm. It may need to be sacrificed.

- If the lateral extent of the planned resection cannot be reached in the supine position, the patient is placed on a beanbag for intraoperative adjustment.
- SCDs are placed prior to induction of anesthesia.
  - The authors do not use a Foley urinary catheter unless the operation is going to be longer than 5 hours.

- General anesthesia is used.
- A transversus abdominis plane block can be used as an adjunct.
- Normothermia is important in the operating room. Operative hypothermia is associated with increased seroma formation and blood loss.

■ Abdominal Panniculectomy with Umbilical Transposition

Markings and Incision

- The patient is marked in the standing position, and the lateral extent of the panniculus is marked (**TECH FIG 1A,B**).
  - The authors use a measuring tape to confirm the distance of the lateral extent of the scars from the midline.
- To avoid a dog-ear, an inflection point is made, transitioning the scar from a horizontal vector to a vertical vector (**TECH FIG 1C–F**).
- Use staples to mark the midline cranial to the umbilicus and at the midline of the mons.
- The inferior incision is often placed in the lower abdominal crease.
  - The authors prefer to make the incision slightly cranial to that crease, which avoids a step-off between the abdominal skin and the mons pubis (**TECH FIG 1G**).

- Vessels are cauterized with electrocautery or tied with suture and divided. Vessels within the panniculus can often be large.

Dissection

- Scarpa fascia is identified and divided with electrocautery.
- The fat superficial to Scarpa fascia is often lobular, and deep to Scarpa fascia often has a stromal appearance. The deep fatty layer is often very thin (**TECH FIG 2A,B**).
- The rectus fascia is identified. Although the fascia itself can be skeletonized, we leave a thin layer of tissue over the rectus fascia.
  - Perforators are divided several millimeters superficial to the fascia, because once divided, they will retract, and bleeding can be better managed if they have not retracted within the muscle.
- Leave fat along the ASIS to protect the lateral femoral cutaneous nerve (**TECH FIG 2C**).

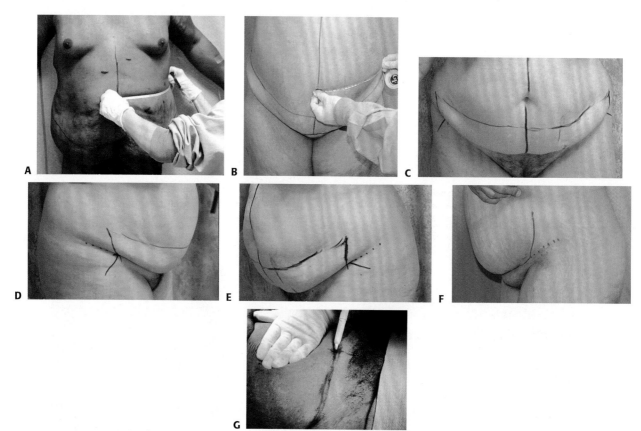

TECH FIG 1 • **A.** The lateral extent of the incision can be measured in both directions from the midline to increase symmetry. **B.** It can also be measured from the umbilicus, which provides a reference on both the mediolateral dimension as well as the craniocaudal dimension, although if the umbilical stalk is long, it may not be midline at the time of measurement. **C–F.** Creating an inflection point can help reduce dog-ears. Shown is the transition medial to the lateral extent or the panniculus. **G.** Marking the inferior incision slightly superior to the fold helps to avoid a step-off between the mons and the abdominal flap.

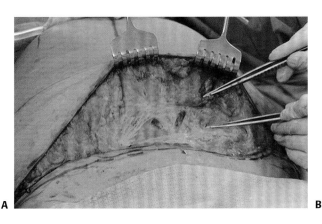

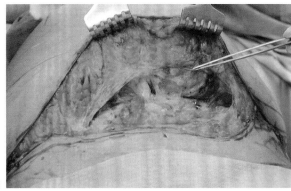

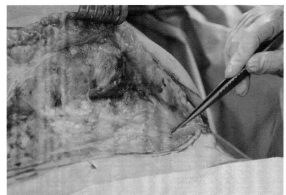

TECH FIG 2 • The fat superficial to Scarpa fascia is more lobular than the fat deep to it, and the deep fatty layer can be thin. **A.** Upper forceps demonstrate fat superficial to Scarpa fascia, and the lower forceps demonstrate fat deep to Scarpa fascia. **B.** The forceps indicate Scarpa fascia. **C.** A layer of fat can be left over the ASIS to protect the lateral femoral cutaneous nerve. It can also be identified visually. Forceps indicate level of ASIS.

Umbilical Transposition

- If umbilical transposition is planned, the dissection is continued cranially until there is approximately 2 cm of subcutaneous fat inferior to the umbilicus to prevent inadvertent disruption of umbilical blood supply.
- Use a surgical marker to mark out the umbilicus. The authors mark in the natural fold of the umbilicus (**TECH FIG 3A,B**).
- The stalk of the umbilicus is separated from the surrounding subcutaneous fat using either Metzenbaum scissors or electrocautery.

- ▫ The authors do not skeletonize the stalk, and if the stalk is long, they leave a generous amount of fat on the stalk to avoid separating perforators (**TECH FIG 3C**).
- Once the umbilicus has been isolated, the dissection continues superiorly to the xiphoid process.
  - ▫ The dissection plane becomes more difficult to identify as there is more adherence between the rectus abdominis fascia and the subcutaneous tissue.
- In the case of umbilical sacrifice, the umbilicus is taken as part of the resection specimen, and the stalk is cauterized or tied off.

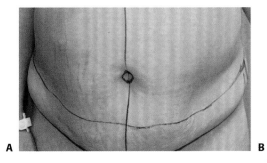

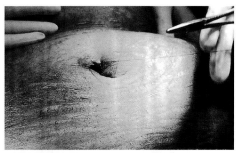

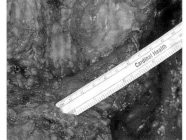

TECH FIG 3 • **A.** The umbilicus is marked in its natural fold. An umbilicus that is too small can be difficult to clean. **B.** A suture is placed at 12 o'clock to ensure proper orientation at inset and can aid in traction during incision. **C.** When the patient has a long umbilical stalk but the umbilicus is being preserved and transposed, a generous layer of fat can help preserve blood supply.

■ Flap Advancement and Skin Resection

- Once the flap is fully dissected (**TECH FIG 4A**), it is advanced inferiorly and the amount to be resected is determined. If needed, the patient can be placed in a slight reflex position.
- Indocyanine green can be used intraoperatively to assess viability of flaps and can predict wound healing complications.
- The excess panniculus is resected and passed off the table to be weighed.
- If there is a vertical component, the skin can be imbricated with staples to determine a safe amount of resection (**TECH FIG 4B-F**).
- Drains (19-French round hubless channel drains) may be placed underneath the flaps, although progressive tension closure using barbed suture has been demonstrated to be an alternative to drains.
- The receiving bed for the umbilicus is created by measuring the actual size of the umbilicus and drawing a template on the abdominal wall.

- The template is placed where the umbilicus is positioned when the stalk projects orthogonal to the abdominal wall, and the distance from the mons is measured to ensure that there is adequate skin (**TECH FIG 4G**).

Closure

- The Scarpa layer can be closed using either interrupted or running suture, but it is not always necessary.
- The skin is closed in layers using 3-0 poliglecaprone 25 or glycomer 631 for both the deep dermal and the subcuticular layers.
- The umbilicus is repaired using 3-0 poliglecaprone 25 or glycomer 631 for the deep layers and either 4-0 poliglecaprone 25 or glycomer 631 in a running subcuticular stitch of 5-0 fast as a running baseball stitch.
- All incisions are waterproofed with a cyanoacrylate tissue adhesive.
- An abdominal binder is placed.

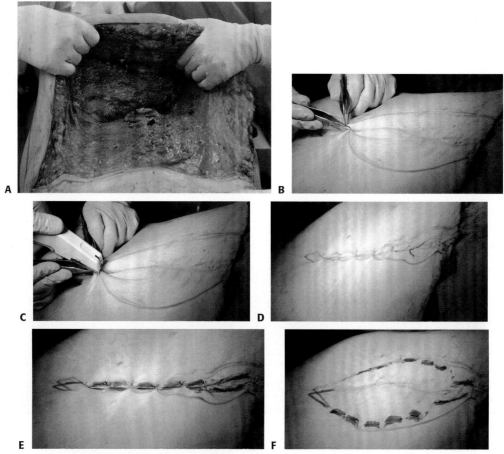

TECH FIG 4 • **A.** The fully dissected flap. **B–D.** If there is a fleur-de-lis component, the skin can be imbricated to determine a safe amount for resection. A marking pen is used to reinforce the boundaries **(E)**, and the staples are removed and the skin is resected **(F)**.

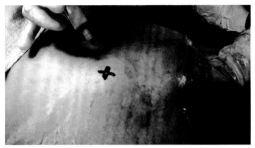

G

TECH FIG 4 (Continued) • **G.** The receiving bed for the umbilicus is placed at the position of the umbilicus as it projects from the abdominal wall. The surgeon places a hand under the flap to demonstrate the location of the umbilicus.

PEARLS AND PITFALLS

Physical findings	■ Intertrigo is common and should be assessed. Asymmetry of the panniculus is common and should be identified and discussed with the patient preoperatively.
Technique	■ Dog-ears can be reduced by transitioning the direction of the scar at its lateral extent.
	■ A layer of fat left on the ASIS can help prevent injury to the lateral femoral cutaneous nerve
	■ When performing an umbilical transposition, marking a receiving bed for the umbilicus based on the measured dimensions of the umbilicus will result in a natural-appearing umbilicus.
	■ Indocyanine green techniques can be employed to determine flap viability.
	■ The best position for the umbilicus is along a line drawn between the iliac crests. If the umbilicus is not transposed but remains in situ, a 10-cm flap of skin should remain between the umbilicus and the mons.
	■ Consider a fleur-de-lis approach if there is both vertical and horizontal skin laxity.[12]
Postoperative	■ DVT prophylaxis should be considered.
	■ Adequate fluid resuscitation is critical, particularly in bariatric surgery patients.

POSTOPERATIVE CARE

- Patient should wear an abdominal binder for 6 weeks.
- Drains should remain until output is less than 30 cc/d.
- Postbariatric patients should have fluid status monitored closely—because of decreased gastric volume, they cannot orally resuscitate at the same rate as nonbariatric surgery patients.
- Ambulate the day of surgery. Most procedures are performed as outpatient procedures or 23-hour observation.
- Postoperative analgesic medication as needed
- DVT prophylaxis should continue. American Society of Plastic Surgery consensus guidelines are 1 month of postoperative chemoprophylaxis.

OUTCOMES

- Functional outcomes of panniculectomy are often good (**FIG 4**).
- Patient satisfaction is high, regardless of technique used.[9]
- Body image and quality of life are improved after body contouring in bariatric surgery patients.[13,14]

COMPLICATIONS

- Some studies have shown that postoperative events are correlated with BMIs greater than 30.[9]
- Patients who have had weight loss surgery are at increased risk of postoperative events when compared to patients who have not; the most common events are wound healing problems, wound infection, hematoma, and seroma.[15]
  - It is unclear if the likelihood of bariatric surgery patients being more likely to have a history of diabetes mellitus, more likely to be smokers, or more likely to have a higher ASA class, is contributory.
- Undiagnosed vitamin deficiency can lead to postoperative events.
- Contour deformity can occur, and scar asymmetry can be seen. Scar asymmetry may be difficult to assess in initial marking, particularly with a large panniculus.
- The skin quality of the massive weight loss patient is not the same as in nonmassive weight loss patients.

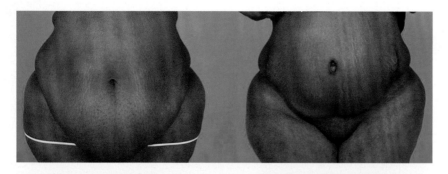
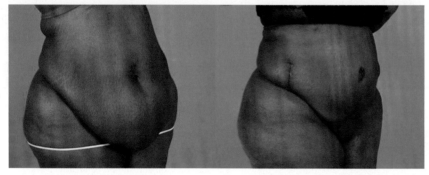
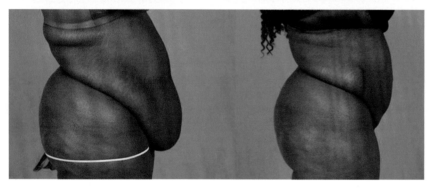

FIG 4 • Preoperative **(left)** and postoperative **(right)** views of a patient who had a combined panniculectomy and hernia repair. She noted improved mobility and decreased rashes after the procedure.

REFERENCES

1. Petty P, Manson PN, Black R, et al. Panniculus morbidus. *Ann Plast Surg.* 1992;28(5):442-452.
2. Gurunluoglu R, Williams SA, Johnson JL. A classification system in the massive weight loss patient based on skin lesions and activity of daily living. *Eplasty.* 2012;12:e12.
3. Huger WE Jr. The anatomic rationale for abdominal lipectomy. *Am J Surg.* 1979;45:612.
4. Chung CW, Kling RE, Sivak WN. Risk factors for pannus formation in the post-bariatric surgery population. *Plast Reconstr Surg.* 2014;133(5):623e-627e.
5. Stephanie E, Dreifuss SE, Rubin JP. Insurance coverage for massive weight loss panniculectomy: a national survey and implications for policy. *Surg Obes Relat Dis.* 2016;12(2):412-416.
6. Hardy JE, Salgado, CJ, Matthews MS, et al. The safety of pelvic surgery in the morbidly obese with and without combined panniculectomy: a comparison of results. *Ann Plast Surg.* 2008;60(1):10-13.
7. Eisenhauer EL, Wypych, KA, Mehrara BJ. Comparing surgical outcomes in obese women undergoing laparotomy, laparoscopy, or laparotomy with panniculectomy, for the staging of uterine malignancy. *Ann Surg Oncol.* 2007;14(8):2384-2391.
8. Koolen PG, Ibrahim AM, Kim K, et al. Patient selection optimization following combined abdominal procedures: analysis of 4925 patients undergoing panniculectomy/abdominoplasty with or without concurrent hernia repair. *Plast Reconstr Surg.* 2014;134(4):539e-550e.
9. Cooper JM, Paige KT, Beshlian KM Abdominal panniculectomies: high patient satisfaction despite significant complication rates. *Ann Plast Surg.* 2008;61(2):188-196.
10. Caprini JA. Thrombosis risk assessment as a guide to quality patient care. *Dis Mon.* 2005;51:70-78.
11. Apovian CM, Cummings S, Anderson W, et al. Best practice updates for multidisciplinary care in weight loss surgery. *Obesity.* 2009;17:871-879.
12. Friedman, T, Obrien Coon D, Michaels J, et al. Fleur-de-lis abdominoplasty: a safe alternative to traditional abdominoplasty for the massive weight loss patient. *Plast Reconstr Surg.* 2010;125(5):1525-1535.
13. Pecori L, Serra Cervetti GG, Marinari GM, et al. Attitudes of morbidly obese patients to weight loss and body image following bariatric surgery and body contouring. *Obes Surg.* 2007;17:68-73.
14. Song AY, Rubin JP, Thomas V, et al. Body image and quality of life in post massive weight loss body contouring patients. *Obesity (Silver Spring).* 2006;14:1626-1636.
15. Greco JA, Castaldo ET, Nanney LB, et al. The effect of weight loss surgery and body mass index on wound complications after abdominal contouring operations. *Ann Plast Surg.* 2008;61(3):235-242.
16. Forte AJ, Tuggle CT, Berlin NL, et al. Hysterectomy with concurrent panniculectomy: a propensity-matched analysis of 3-day outcomes. *Plast Reconstr Surg.* 2015;136(3):582-590.

Abdominal Panniculectomy in Super Obese Patients

David J. Rowe

DEFINITION

- Over 60% of the US population is overweight.
- Over 30% is obese by BMI stratification.
- Super obese is classified as BMI greater than 50, super-super obese is BMI above 60.

ANATOMY

- The anatomy of the abdominal panniculus is discussed in Chapter 13.

PATIENT HISTORY AND PHYSICAL FINDINGS

- The preoperative evaluation for a patient with super obese panniculus includes a detailed history as well as documentation of pertinent physical manifestations.
- Physical examination
  - Large abdominal panniculus
  - Intertriginous rashes
  - Chronic infection
  - Ulcerations
  - Fistulous tracts
  - Physical limitation
  - Presence of hernia: difficult given overlying tissue

IMAGING AND OTHER DIAGNOSTIC STUDIES

- If hernia is suspected, CT scan with contrast is warranted (**FIG 1**).

- Preoperative laboratory values: patients who have had previous gastric bypass will need a preoperative workup that will be discussed more in detail in other chapters. Given the likely comorbidities of the super obese, nutritional parameters may also be evaluated in the workup of all patients.
  - Nutritional parameters: albumin, prealbumin
  - Lab workup: CBC, basic chemistry

NONOPERATIVE MANAGEMENT

- The primary decision in the instance of panniculectomy in the super obese patient is the possibility of weight loss or gastric bypass prior to surgery.[1]
  - In the case of panniculus morbidus, the pannus may still be present following weight loss.[2]
  - In the case of combined surgery for cancer extirpation, etc., ideal weight loss may not be achieved.

SURGICAL MANAGEMENT

- Indications for surgery include overhanging panniculus interfering with ambulation and undergoing combined abdominal operations (eg, hysterectomy, tumor extirpation, hernia repair; **FIG 2**).
- Risks to the patient include an increase of overall complication rate given the extremely high BMI, increased risk of prolonged hospitalization, need for further surgical intervention, wound healing complications, and increased bleeding when compared to traditional panniculectomy.

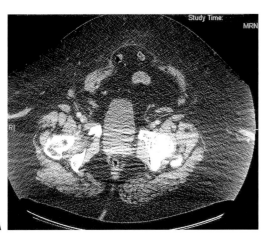
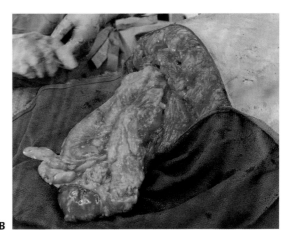

A **B**

FIG 1 • **A.** Presence of hernia on CT scan. **B.** Intraoperative view of hernia.

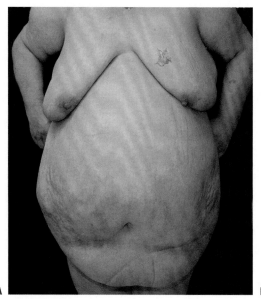 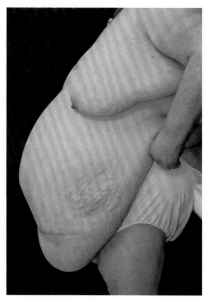

FIG 2 • **A,B.** Morbidly obese panniculectomy. Patient is a 53-year-old woman, BMI 52, with biopsy-proven cervical cancer and need for hysterectomy.

- Given the patient's preoperative risks, surgical intervention may include excision of the panniculus with closure or excision without total closure and use of negative pressure dressings.
- Brown et al. found that in instances of panniculectomy, patients who underwent excision and wound care via vacuum-assisted closure (VAC) therapy required significantly less readmissions and less reoperations.[3]
- The mons area is usually significantly redundant and must be assessed at this time as well.
- Given the risk of surgery in super obese patients, an anesthesia and medicine clearance is warranted prior to surgery.
- Deep vein thrombosis (DVT) risk assessment via the Caprini score is performed.

Preoperative Planning

- Markings
  - Midline
  - Inferior incision line to accommodate mons lift (if being performed) as well as general avoidance of attenuated skin at the actual crease. Given the actual size of the pannus, the surgeon may need additional assistance with this marking.
  - General area to be resected may also be marked with the understanding that this may change depending on intra-operative findings.
- Patients should be typed and cross-matched prior to the procedure.

■ Preparation and Transection of the Pannus

- Following induction and the administration of weight-based antibiotics, the pannus is prepped for elevation.
- At the most dependent portion of the pannus, several large Steinmann pins are placed through the pannus and attached to a mechanical lift (**TECH FIG 1**).
- A Foley catheter is now placed if it is warranted.
  - Access for the Foley placement is considerably easier following displacement of the large pannus.
- The caudal incision is then marked again approximately 2 to 3 cm above the pannicular crease.
- Sharp electrocautery dissection is performed through the skin; subcutaneous tissue to the abdominal fascia is performed in a caudal to cephalic direction.
- Given the large size of the superficial venous system, care is used in dissection in this plane.
  - The author uses medium and large clip appliers for ligation of these vessels; however, suture ligation may be used as well.

- Attention is then turned to the cephalic incision once visual inspection confirms enough skin to close the incision primarily.
  - In super obese panniculectomy, the umbilicus is usually transected, given the large and tortuous stalk.

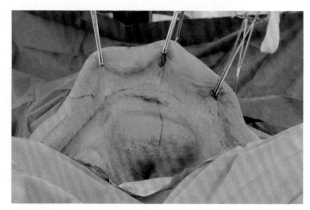

TECH FIG 1 • Hoyer lift is employed for retraction. Steinmann pins are placed under sterile conditions and attached to Kocher clamps.

■ Closure

- During closure, two 19-Fr Jackson Pratt drains are used.
- Meticulous hemostasis is performed with patient at the preoperative blood pressure.
- The Scarpa fascia is usually quite attenuated and may be approximated with 3-0 Vicryl suture if an adequate layer is available.

- Skin is closed with 4-0 Monocryl or staples depending on surgeon's choice (**TECH FIG 2A**).
- An incisional VAC may be used to aid healing (**TECH FIG 2B**).

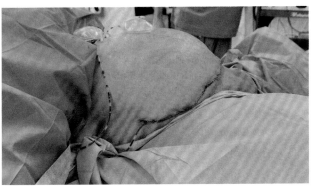 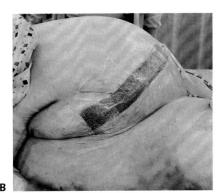

A   **B**

TECH FIG 2 • A. Closure of the skin. Note the continued protuberant abdomen consistent with an abundance of visceral adiposity. **B.** Incisional VAC placement.

PEARLS AND PITFALLS

Physical findings	■ Presence of hernia is difficult to clinically evaluate given patient's size. If there is concern, consider CT scan. ■ Intertriginous rashes are common and should be assessed prior to surgical intervention.
Hemostasis	■ Automatic clip appliers aid in effectively ligating the large vessels found in many of the large pannus specimens. ■ Careful evaluation of the dissected area with normalized blood pressure aids in decreasing reoperative rate due to hematoma.
Incisions	■ Caudal incision should be made above the pubic symphysis and above any areas of rash. This may decrease the possibility of incision-related infections as well as allow for closure in tissue that has not been overly attenuated. ■ Avoid "too low" an incision to decrease the seroma rate given the presence of lymphatic channels in the lateral abdomen/thigh.
Postoperative care	■ Consider DVT prophylaxis. ■ Encourage early ambulation.

POSTOPERATIVE CARE

- Use of chemoprophylaxis is warranted.
- Ambulation is encouraged early.
- Dehiscence of the skin and fat necrosis are common complications; patients are warned of the possibility of dehiscence, need for reoperation, as well as wound care.
- Depending on the preoperative functioning of the patient and the possible presence of wound healing complications by the time of discharge, some patients may benefit from a stay in a skilled nursing facility.

OUTCOMES

- The primary goal of the morbidly obese panniculectomy may vary depending on the patient population.
  - Restore ability to ambulate
  - Functional access for other surgical interventions

COMPLICATIONS

- Infection
- Fat necrosis
- Skin necrosis
- Hematoma
- Asymmetry of scar

REFERENCES

1. Natarajan B, Pallati PK, Bertellotti RP, Forse RA. Panniculectomy as a pre-bariatric surgery procedure. *Plast Reconstr Surg*. 2011;127:169e.
2. Manhan MA, Shermak MA. Massive panniculectomy after massive weight loss. *Plast Reconstr Surg*. 2006;117:2191.
3. Brown M, Adenuga P, Soltanian H. Massive panniculectomy in the super obese and super super obese: retrospective comparison of primary closure versus partial open wound management. *Plast Reconstr Surg*. 2014;133:132.

15
CHAPTER

Buttock Lift

Michele A. Shermak

DEFINITION

- Buttock lift describes excision of lax and/or redundant lower back tissue to improve lift and shape to the buttocks, as well as posterior waist contour. It is the basis for the posterior element to lower body lifting for individuals who have sustained massive weight loss. The procedure may be performed in combination with augmentation of the buttock using fat, autologous flaps, or implants or with lifts of adjacent body regions such as the abdomen or thigh to globally improve the lower body region.

ANATOMY

- The 10 gluteal aesthetic units, identified by Mendieta,[1] while not all in the buttock proper, impact the appearance of buttock (**FIG 1A**):
  - Sacrum
  - Flank
  - Upper buttock
  - Lower back
  - Outer leg
  - Gluteus
  - Diamond zone
  - Midlateral buttock
  - Inferior gluteal/posterior leg junction
  - Upper back
- Anatomic layers of the lower back/buttock (**FIG 1B**)
  - The skin can demonstrate varying degrees of redundancy, vertical excess, laxity, and collagen strength as manifested by striae. Thin skin may have greater recoil after surgery resulting in exacerbated loosening of the surgical result.
  - Subcutaneous fat varies in thickness. A thinner fat layer is more appropriate for buttock lift than a thick one, which might be more suitable for a liposuction contouring procedure or recommendation for weight loss. If subcutaneous fat is limited, an augmentation with autologous flaps, fat, or implant may be considered.
  - Scarpa fascia is the pseudofascial plane in the subcutaneous fat that varies in strength and is relied upon for closure and lift and may need more sutures to provide greater tension or better support for weak tissue.
  - Subscarpal fat is the layer in which dissection is performed for buttock lift.
  - Deep muscular fascia should not be cut during buttock lift. This layer protects the muscles and vital vessels and nerves.
  - Muscles of significance in this region include the paired gluteus maximus muscles, which should not be invaded during surgery so all structures deep to the gluteus

maximus are not dissected or visualized. Attenuated muscle may account for buttock deflation and may be improved with fat augmentation.
  - Circulation of greatest importance is provided by the superior gluteal arterial system and inferior gluteal artery system. Perforators from these arteries should be preserved, particularly when performing autologous gluteal augmentation[2] (**FIG 1C**).

PATHOGENESIS

- With skin laxity and/or weight loss of varying degrees, individuals can suffer from excess vertical dimension of skin in the lower back with deflation and flatness of the buttock area, an ill-defined infragluteal crease, cellulite, and lack of fullness.
- Ptosis may occur in the buttock and lateral thigh. This is associated with an aged look or with difficulty in wearing clothing.
- Lower backlift/buttock lifting surgery improves the posterior waist and shape and tautness of the buttock, in conjunction with improving adjacent areas, like the upper posterior thigh, outer thigh, and back.

PATIENT HISTORY AND PHYSICAL FINDINGS

- Patient history should be probed for significant weight loss, and if present in the history, the mode and degree of weight loss, as well as nutritional challenges that may exist.
  - Weight should be stable at the time of surgery at least 3 months.
  - Medical conditions that may impact outcome of backlift surgery should be queried, such as diabetes, peripheral vascular disease, heart disease, sleep apnea, autoimmune and endocrinological disorders, and coagulation disorders and venous thromboembolic history.
- Physical findings should note skin quality and degree of excess and redundancy, as well as adiposity.
  - Adjacent body regions such as the upper back, abdomen, and thigh anteriorly and posteriorly are examined to see if addressing these regions will improve overall lower body aesthetics.

SURGICAL MANAGEMENT
Preoperative Planning

- Preoperative planning depends on patient preference and deformities present.
- Limitations in patient state of health or finances may curtail extensive surgical procedure and mandate a staging plan.

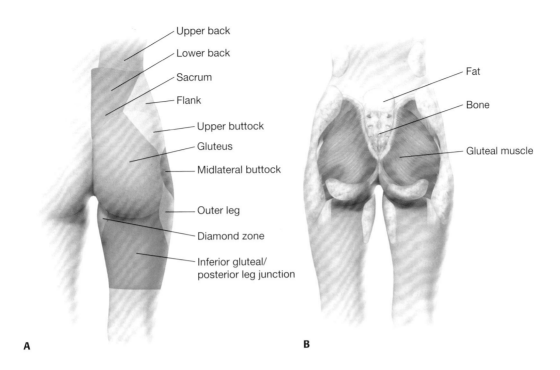

A

B

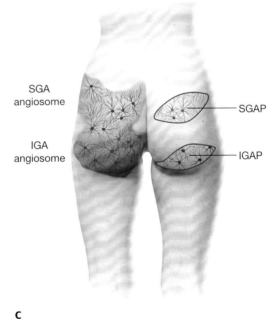

C

FIG 1 • **A.** The 10 gluteal aesthetic units are shown. The diamond zone includes the inner gluteal/leg injection. **B.** From superficial to deep, anatomy of the buttocks includes the skin, fat, pseudofascial plane in the fat, muscle fascia, and muscles. The subcutaneous fat layer may vary in thickness and deposition, and fascial layers may have varying degrees of strength. Thickness of each of these layers affects gluteal contour. **C.** Arterial supply of the gluteal region is primarily provided through the superior and inferior gluteal artery perforators. The autologous flap is primarily supplied by the superior gluteal artery perforator system as it is within the angiosome.

- Buttock lift is typically performed in continuity with abdominoplasty and may be performed either at the time of abdominoplasty or at a later stage.
- Planning and discussing possible augmentation in conjunction with buttock lifting should take place prior to surgery.[3]
  - Prediction needs to be made by the surgeon to determine whether excision of lower back tissue alone will provide adequate improvement to buttock position and contour or if additional tissue in the form of autologous flap tissue or fat graft should be harvested from the tissue that would otherwise be discarded to help amplify and shape a severely deflated buttock.

- Liposuction of the outer thigh also may be considered if it will improve contour and allow greater tissue resection.

Positioning

- Prone positioning is most optimal for buttock lift. It allows a symmetrical, safe, and stable approach.
- The patient is laid on two gel rolls laid horizontally across the OR table, one under the upper chest and axillae, and the other under the lumbar area (**FIG 2**).
  - Axillae and elbows are positioned at no greater than 90 degrees to limit traction on nerves and vessels.
  - The neck is in neutral position, and the face should be protected in a prone pillow, avoiding any pressure to the eyes.

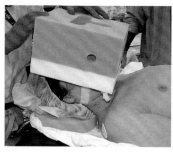 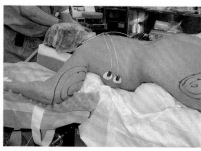 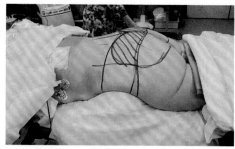

FIG 2 • Prone positioning helps provide the best access to the lower back, allowing symmetrical treatment. Safety measures must be followed to avoid blindness, stroke, neurapraxia, and pressure phenomena. **A.** Face in prone pillow with goggles protecting eyes from pressure and desiccation. **B.** Arms at 90 degrees and bumps under chest and lumbar region. **C.** Bump under lumbar region. Patient is warmed with forced warming blanket intraoperatively.

- These maneuvers in the head and neck limit the risk of kinking of arteries in the neck to prevent dissection and stroke, as well as blindness.
- The legs and arms should be padded with pillows or foam to avoid pressure to superficial nerves.[4]

Approach

- Landmarks including the posterior superior iliac crest and sacral depression guide markings for skin removal.

- The buttock down to the infragluteal fold should be marked and prepared in the field.
- Skin undermining and laxity is greatest laterally and extremely limited centrally.
- Markings made preoperatively with the patient standing allow for this and aim to create an incision that resembles a gull wing over the buttock to define and improve aesthetics of the buttock region.

TECHNIQUES

■ Buttock Lift

- The patient is marked while standing.
  - Excision is determined by movement and laxity of the skin, as well as goal of creating a symmetric, curvilinear incision that will border the upper gluteal region (**TECH FIG 1A**).
  - Skin is grasped, and pinching skin closed will guide the marks.
  - Midline should be marked.
  - Little will be excised centrally where there is strong tissue adherence, with increasing removal planned moving laterally.
  - Cross-hatches are made vertically across the proposed excision to aid in approximation.
- The patient is intubated on a stretcher and turned to the prone position with careful padding and protection of all potential pressure points.
- The patient is prepared with Betadine.
- If liposuction is planned in the outer thigh, tumescent solution is infused.
- Incision is made superiorly in skin, through subcutaneous fat to deep fascia.
- Dissection is then directed inferiorly toward the lower marked incision (**TECH FIG 1B,C**).
  - Minimal undermining is performed.
  - Careful hemostasis is performed, and the wound is irrigated.
  - Local anesthetic is injected above and below deep fascia; long-acting Marcaine is preferable.
- Prior to definitively determining the skin excision, if liposuction is going to be performed, it should be performed at this stage, as tissue may mobilize further and allow greater excision.

- Tailor tacking is performed to aid in precise skin removal, using the hatch marks as a guide.
  - The areas are stapled as skin is excised.
  - Tailoring often needs to take place at the sacral hollow in the middle of the incision, closing as a V in the cleft.
- A no. 10 flat Jackson-Pratt drain is placed within the wound and exited out laterally under the incision on each side. It is sutured to the skin.
- The wound is closed. No. 1 braided nylon is used to approximate Scarpa fascia, taking a bite of deep tissue with the fascial layer to close dead space.

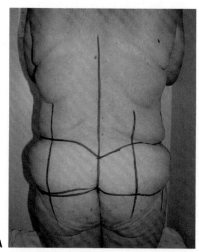

TECH FIG 1 • A. The patient is marked while standing. Markings are based on skin laxity as well as incision placement goal through a grasping technique and putting the skin on traction.

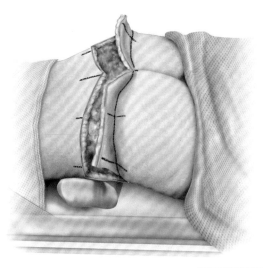

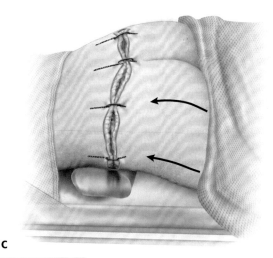

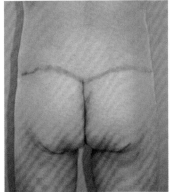

TECH FIG 1 (Continued) • **B.** Incision is made in the skin to the level of the deep fascia, leaving soft tissue intact, and dissection proceeds inferiorly. **C.** Skin removal is determined with tailor tacking. **D.** Closure of the lower back incision looks like a gull wing over the buttocks.

- The skin is closed with 3-0 monofilament absorbable suture to approximate deep dermis and running 4-0 monofilament absorbable suture as a running subcuticular suture.
- Skin is then better approximated with interrupted 4-0 nylon simple interrupted sutures (**TECH FIG 1D**).

- The wound is washed and dressed with cyanoacrylate glue.
- Attention can then be turned to another body region, such as the posterior thigh or abdomen.

Buttock Lift With Autologous Gluteal Augmentation

- The patient is marked standing.
  - A mirror image of the buttocks is drawn within the upper and lower markings of excision.
  - Err on the side of removing less over more to allow for closure over the flaps and avoiding undue tension on the closure or pressure on the flaps.
  - Also err on the side of elevating the lower incision to allow ease of closure over flaps.
  - Incision closure will be more transverse than gull wing at the end of the procedure.
- Cross-hatches are made vertically across the proposed excision, particularly in the midline and along the lateral buttock, to aid in approximation during closure (**TECH FIG 2A**).

- The patient is intubated on a stretcher and turned to the prone position with careful padding and protection of all potential pressure points.
- After preparing the area with Betadine, the areas marked for the buttock reconstruction flaps are de-epithelialized bilaterally and symmetrically.
- Superior incision marked on the back is made to deep fascia, whereas the lower incision is made to the subcutaneous fat.
- Tissue marked outside the flaps medially and laterally is then resected to deep fascia full thickness around the flaps.
- Deep fascia around the flap is incised, not to muscle, to allow release and movement of the flaps (**TECH FIG 2B,C**).
- Gluteal artery perforator blood supply is based on the superior gluteal artery, and this must be preserved when releasing the fascia around the flaps.

- Dissection of the skin flap over the buttock follows to create a pocket for the flap. Maintain subcutaneous fat on the skin flap and dissect inferiorly as marked to create a pocket for the flap (**TECH FIG 2D**).
  - Careful hemostasis is performed.
  - Local anesthetic is injected above and below deep fascia.

- The flap may then be moved without rotation under the skin.
  - The flap is tacked into position on deep fascia with 2-0 absorbable braided suture.
  - A 10-mm flat drain is then placed on each side in the dead space. It is sutured to the skin (**TECH FIG 2E**).

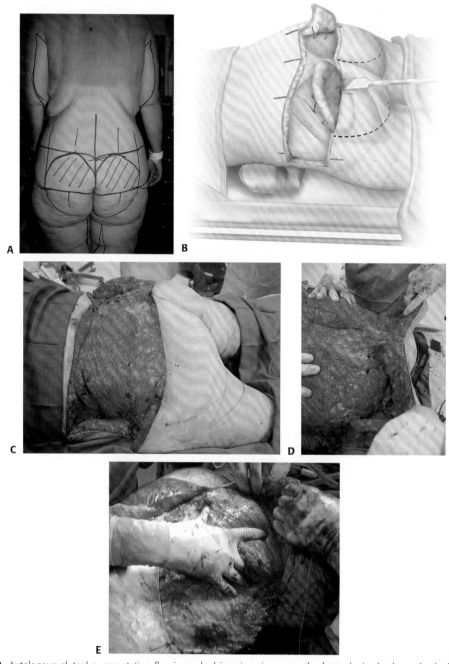

TECH FIG 2 • A. Autologous gluteal augmentation flap is marked in mirror image to the buttocks in the lower back skin excision marked. **B,C.** The tissue marked is de-epithelialized, and tissue between and lateral to the flaps is excised full thickness to deep muscular fascia. **D.** The pocket for the gluteal flap is dissected, maintaining subcutaneous fat under the skin to maintain circulation (see Video 1). The pocket must be dissected inferiorly toward the fold so the flap is not too highly placed. **E.** The flap freely descends under the skin designed for the flap pocket (see Video 2), and the flap is secured in place with 2-0 Vicryl sutures, prior to closing skin.

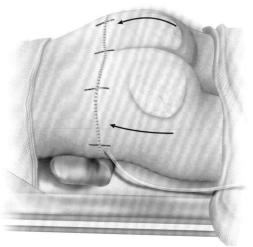

F

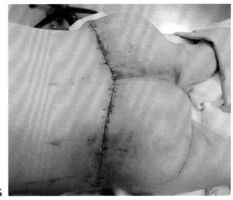

G

TECH FIG 2 (Continued) • **F,G.** Skin is closed in layers over the flap, with drains in place bilaterally.

- The wound is closed.
  - No. 1 braided nylon is used to approximate Scarpa fascia, with 3-0 monofilament absorbable suture to approximate deep dermis and running 4-0 monofilament absorbable suture as a running subcuticular suture.

- Skin is then better approximated with interrupted 4-0 nylon simple interrupted sutures (**TECH FIG 2F,G**).
- The wound is washed and dressed with cyanoacrylate glue.
- Attention can then be turned to another body region, such as the posterior thigh or abdomen.

PEARLS AND PITFALLS

Optimizing scar	■ The best scar results from reduction of tension on the wound, assured by limiting over-resection, and by scar location and symmetry. Without gluteal augmentation, the gull wing scar leads the eye to a focused, well-contoured gluteal region. Maintaining adequate subcutaneous fat on the skin flap for autologous augmentation is critical to avoid wounds.
Optimizing wound healing	■ Avoid high-tension closure and proactively address intraoperative issues such as hypothermia and anemia. Wounds are extremely common in the midportion of the incision at the lower sacrum and respond well to gentle cleansing and petrolatum application.
Seromas	■ These are not uncommon with this procedure, most often associated with large tissue removal. Maintaining a layer of tissue over deep fascia to assist in lymphatic and venous egress as well as limiting undermining and maintaining drains in place until output is low will best protect against seromas.
To augment or not to augment	■ This question needs to be addressed preoperatively as the most optimal tissue for augmentation will otherwise be discarded. This is a judgment call based upon the quantity of existing gluteal tissue: if there is very minimal tissue and significant flattening, then autoaugmentation should take place. This is a much bigger procedure from which to recover and requires hospital overnight stay and monitoring for anemia.

POSTOPERATIVE CARE

- Patients are followed on a weekly basis after surgery to assure optimal wound healing and drain care.
  - Drains can be removed when drainage is 30 to 40 cc or less per day.
  - Wounds that develop are typically superficial and respond well to gentle cleansing and topical petrolatum, with modification to topical antimicrobial medications for superficial wounds that may be infected, or debridement and packing for deeper wounds.

- Seromas are not uncommon and should be aspirated if there is concern about seroma presence to avoid chronic scar and possible abscess.
- Strenuous activity may be resumed about a month after surgery as long as healing is uncomplicated.
- Longer-term care is provided for scar management, including topical therapies to reduce scar visibility and massage to assist in dysesthesias and edema.
  - Compression with a pull-up girdle assists in reducing swelling through the day.

COMPLICATIONS

■ Seroma is one of the most common risks with this surgery and is best minimized by maintaining a layer of connective tissue over deep fascia to assure venous and lymphatic drainage, as well as maintaining drain tubes until output is less than 30 to 40 cc/d.
  ■ If a seroma develops, it is best to aspirate with a needle to assure no long-term pseudobursa and scar or abscess. More advanced techniques are helpful with chronic seromas.[5]
■ Wound healing problem: Addressing and planning how to compensate for preoperative risk factors like malnutrition, diabetes, peripheral vascular disease and smoking, and downstaging procedures for morbidly obese patients or patients with multiple medical problems.
  ■ Careful surgical technique and attention to maintaining circulation to the tissues and avoiding undue tension optimize wound healing.
■ Unsatisfactory scarring is best avoided by minimizing risk of wound healing problems, reducing tension, and closely monitoring postoperatively to innovate scar management depending on progress
■ Venous thromboembolism: It is necessary preoperatively to check on any history or elevated risk as per the modified Caprini scale.[6]

■ Infection is not common, and risk can be reduced by optimizing surgical conditions like addressing efficiency with reduced operative time and hypothermia, as well as initial dose of antibiotics prior to making incision.
  ■ Seromas can become sources of infection and should be treated.

REFERENCES

1. Mendieta CG. Classification system for gluteal evaluation. *Clin Plast Surg.* 2006;33(3):333-346.
2. Georgantopoulou A, Papadodima S, Vlachodimitropoulos D, et al. The microvascular anatomy of superior and inferior gluteal artery perforator (SGAP and IGAP) flaps: a fresh cadaveric study and clinical implications. *Aesthetic Plast Surg.* 2014;38(6):1156-1163.
3. Centeno RF. Autologous gluteal augmentation with circumferential body lift in the massive weight loss and aesthetic patient. *Clin Plast Surg.* 2006;33(3):479-496.
4. Shermak M, Shoo B, Deune EG. Prone positioning precautions in plastic surgery. *Plast Reconstr Surg.* 2006;117(5):1584-1588.
5. Shermak MA, Rotellini-Coltvet L, Chang D. Seroma development following body contouring surgery for massive weight loss: patient risk factors and treatment strategies. *Plast Reconstr Surg.* 2008;122(1):280-288.
6. Pannucci CJ, Barta RJ, Portschy PR, et al. Assessment of postoperative venous thromboembolism risk in plastic surgery patients using the 2005 and 2010 Caprini Risk score. *Plast Reconstr Surg.* 2012;130(2):343-353.

Circumferential Body Lift

Joseph Michaels and Jennifer Capla

DEFINITION

- A lower body lift is a combined procedure consisting of an abdominoplasty, lateral thigh lift, and buttock lift.
- Addresses the lower truncal skin redundancy in the massive weight loss patient in a circumferential fashion by removing skin excess from the abdomen, hips, lateral thighs, flanks, and buttocks.

ANATOMY

- Excess skin can distort a patient's anatomy.
- Knowledge of the superficial fascial system (SFS) as described by Ted Lockwood is important (**FIG 1**).[1]
- The SFS has zones of adherence. Posteriorly, this is to the spine; anteriorly, it is to the lower borders of the pelvis.
- The bony landmarks of the pelvis are commonly used as reference points, specifically the anterior superior iliac spine (ASIS) and the ischium.
- Preservation of the inguinal lymph node basin and knowledge of the course of the lateral femoral cutaneous nerve is important to minimize complications.
- Abdomen
  - The borders are the costal margins and xiphoid superiorly, the pubic symphysis inferiorly, and the ASIS laterally.
  - The blood supply to the abdomen is classically described as three zones (**FIG 2**):[2]
    - Zone 1: midabdomen supplied by the deep epigastric arcade
    - Zone 2: lower abdomen supplied by the external iliac artery
    - Zone 3: flanks and lateral abdomen supplied by the intercostal, subcostal, and lumbar arteries
- Buttocks
  - Landmarks include the posterior superior iliac spine, the ischial tuberosities inferiorly, and the greater trochanter laterally.
  - The gluteal fascia will serve as an anchor point for rotational flaps used to preserve and restore buttock volume.
- Thighs
  - This region overlies the greater trochanter and tensor fascia lata. Anteriorly, it extends to the ASIS.
  - The saddlebag deformity that is commonly seen is a combination of residual adiposity and loose skin.

PATIENT HISTORY AND PHYSICAL FINDINGS

- Patients generally present with massive weight loss (weight loss greater than 75 lb).
- This can lead to various degrees of skin laxity depending on the extent of weight loss, the rate of weight loss, and the patient's skin elasticity.
- Physical examination is focused on the abdomen, lateral thighs, flanks, and buttock.
- Patients often present with excess skin in the abdomen and may have an intertriginous rash (erythema intertrigo) in the skinfold. There is also commonly mons ptosis. Excess skin extends to the lateral thigh (saddle bag) region and continues onto the buttock. There is often a sense of deflation in the buttock region.
- Abdomen should be evaluated for degree of rectus diastasis, previous incisions, and any associated hernias.

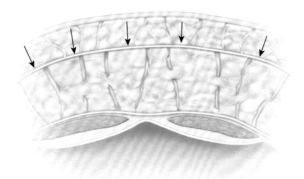

FIG 1 • The superficial fascial system between the superficial and deep fat compartments of the abdomen.

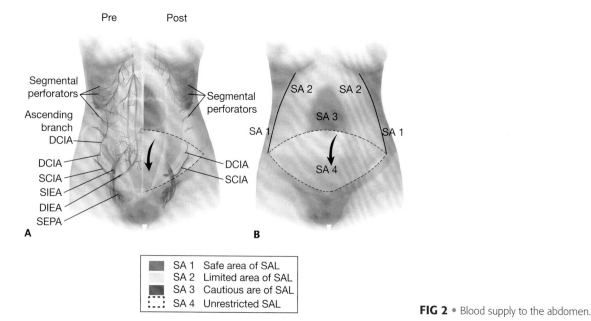

Pre Post

Segmental perforators
Ascending branch DCIA
DCIA
SCIA
SIEA
DIEA
SEPA

Segmental perforators
DCIA
SCIA

SA 2   SA 2
SA 3
SA 1   SA 1
SA 4

A   B

■	SA 1	Safe area of SAL
░	SA 2	Limited area of SAL
■	SA 3	Cautious are of SAL
⌐⌐⌐	SA 4	Unrestricted SAL

FIG 2 • Blood supply to the abdomen.

IMAGING

- An abdominal CT scan may be helpful if there are any concerns for an abdominal hernia—umbilical, ventral, or incisional. This will allow for better intraoperative planning and the possible need for a general surgeon.

SURGICAL MANAGEMENT

Preoperative Planning

- Patients should be at or close to their goal weight and weight stable for a minimum of 3 months.
- All massive weight loss patients should undergo a full preoperative evaluation in addition to a nutritional assessment.
  - Nutritional assessment is an important factor in wound healing and should include albumin, prealbumin, B12, folate, iron, and total iron binding capacity.
- Understanding and assessing the patient's goals is of primary importance.
- In front of a mirror, with the patient unclothed, the pinch technique can help provide the patient with a sense of how the tissues will translate and what will be achieved with this procedure. This can also be done with the patient lying down and showing them a picture of the projection (**FIG 3**).
- Determine whether the patient needs added volume in the buttock.
  - A lower body lift inevitably will flatten the buttock. Gluteal autoaugmentation is considered in patients who desire increased buttock volume and projection.
- The markings are the key to the procedure.
- Prewarm the operating and all IV fluids to minimize patient hypothermia.

Positioning

- The patient is intubated on a stretcher.

- The patient is transferred to the operating room table in the prone position with appropriate padding.
- Arm boards can be placed on the lower part of the table to widen the bed and to allow for additional abduction of the legs. This will help obtain the maximal lateral thigh lift.
- After the lower body lift is performed, the lateral dog-ears are tucked, stapled, and covered with a sterile dressing.
- The patient is then repositioned into the supine position for the abdominoplasty portion of the procedure.

Approach

- The determination of whether the patient requires additional buttock volume will ultimately determine the approach for the lower body lift.
  - If none is required, this procedure is simply a circumferential removal of skin, also known as a belt lipectomy.
  - If increased gluteal projection and volume is necessary, gluteal autoaugmentation or fat transfer will be required.

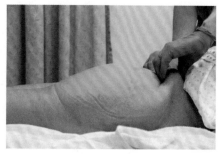

FIG 3 • Pinch test to evaluate buttock projection for whether autoaugmentation is needed during a lower body lift.

■ Lower Body Lift With Gluteal Autoaugmentation Flaps

Markings (TECH FIG 1)

- Patients are asked to bring an undergarment, and upper and lower borders are marked to try and keep the incisions hidden within these lines. Most people wear their undergarments at the level of the anterior superior iliac spine (ASIS).
  - The ASIS is also marked, and this height is also transposed to the back as a reference point.
- The next mark is made with the patient lying down. The lower abdominal incision is marked at 6 cm above the vulvar commissure in women or the pubic symphysis in men.
- The patient is then asked to stand up, and the posterior markings are done first. The posterior midline is marked, and the midaxillary line is marked. This represents the lateral extent of the posterior excision.
- In the midline, a mark is placed several centimeters above the gluteal cleft. This point will represent the top of the new gluteal cleft and should lie below the level of the ASIS.
- The superior marking is drawn as a gull wing from the midline mark to a point on the midaxillary line that lies below the ASIS on downward traction.
- A conservative pinch test is performed every 5 to 6 cm up to the superior line. These points are connected and represent the lower posterior marking.
- The area for autoaugmentation is marked. These flaps are designed within the area of resection and nearly encompass the entire area of resection except for the lateral few centimeters over the lateral thighs.
- The patient is then asked to turn around, and the anterior incision is marked with superior traction on the abdomen.
  - The previous marked lower abdominal incision is connected to the lower posterior marking at the midaxillary line.
  - This incision should also remain below the level of the ASIS on upward traction of the abdominal skin.

Gluteal Autoaugmentation

- The procedure starts in the prone position (**TECH FIG 2A,B**).
  - A towel clip is first used to approximate the upper and lower markings to confirm the area of resection. If too tight, adjust the lower marking superiorly.
- The area marked for autoaugmentation is de-epithelialized (**TECH FIG 2C**).
  - The flaps are further dissected with electrocautery to dissect down through the superficial fascial system (SFS) and down to the deep fascia at the superior and inferior margins.
  - Laterally, dissection continues through the SFS until the deep fat pockets are exposed; there is no deep fascia laterally.
- The tissue between the midaxillary line and the lateral extent of the flap is excised.
- Inferior to the flap, a pocket for the flap is dissected just above the gluteal fascia (**TECH FIG 2D**).
  - The gluteal tissue is elevated from the lateral aspect leaving a broad base to supply the flap.
  - The flap is raised just enough that it can be rotated inferiorly into the pocket to provide the desired projection.
- A Lockwood underminer is used to release the lateral thigh attachments to the greater trochanter allowing for additional upward movement of the lateral thigh and correction of the saddlebag deformity.
  - Liposuction can be used to remove any residual adiposity from this region at this time. Liposuction can also be performed in the lower back region as necessary.
- The SFS is reapproximated with 0-Vicryl sutures. The skin is closed in layers with 3-0 Monocryl (**TECH FIG 2E,F**).
- The lateral dog-ears are temporarily stapled and closed.

Abdominal Lift

- The patient is transferred to the supine position on the operating room table (**TECH FIG 3A**), dependent areas are again padded, and the patient is sterilely draped.
- The lower abdominal incision is made and connected to the posterior incision laterally.

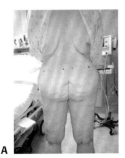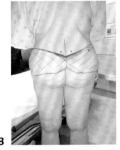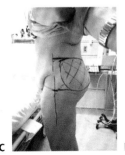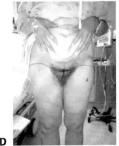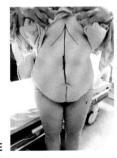

TECH FIG 1 • **A.** Transposition of ASIS to posterior aspect as a reference point. **B.** Superior and inferior markings of the resection with area of autoaugmentation marked. **C.** Lateral view of the markings showing the extent of the posterior excision, as well as the lateral aspect of the autoaugmentation flaps. **D.** Anterior markings of the lower abdominal incision connecting to the posterior markings. This line should remain below the ASIS. **E.** Anterior markings with the abdominal skin flap relaxed.

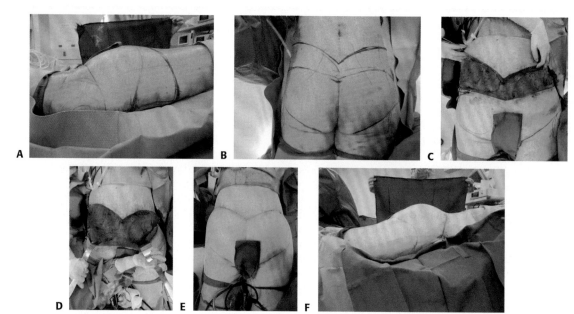

TECH FIG 2 • **A,B.** Patient in the prone position with superior and inferior body lift markings. **C.** De-epithelialized and dissected buttock flaps. **D.** Pockets made for the inferior rotation of the gluteal flaps. The left side shows the pocket dissected just superficial to the gluteal fascia. The right side shows the gluteal flaps inferiorly rotated and sutured to the gluteal fascia. **E.** Closure of the posterior incision line. **F.** Lateral view after gluteal autoaugmentation showing the change in gluteal projection. Compare with **A.**

- As this incision may lie below the level of the inguinal canal, care must be taken to avoid injury to the inguinal lymph node basin and the round ligament/spermatic cord during elevation of the abdominal flap.
- Care is taken to leave soft tissue on the deep fascia lateral to the rectus abdominis muscle. This helps preserve lymphatics and decreases the risk of seroma.
- Superior dissection continues to the level of the umbilicus.
  - The umbilicus is circumscribed, leaving adequate perforators, and dissection of the abdominal flap continues up to the level of the xiphoid process and costal margins.
- Any hernias are repaired along with repair of the diastasis recti with permanent sutures (0-Ethibond).
- The patient is sat up in the semi-Fowler position, and the skin excess is marked and excised. The new umbilical position is marked.

- Two no. 15 drains are placed and brought out laterally through the incision. These drains are placed in a crisscross fashion and extend to the opposite side to drain the back.
- The abdomen is closed in a similar manner as the back, and the umbilicus is sutured to the abdominal wall flap with 4-0 Monocryl sutures in layers (**TECH FIG 3B**).
- The markings are similar to the markings described above, except that there are no markings for the autoaugmentation flap (**TECH FIG 4**).
- This procedure is performed similarly to the above procedure except no dermoadipose flaps are dissected to provide added buttock volume.
- For this procedure, the tissue between the superior and inferior incision lines is removed at the level just deep to the SFS. There is no dissection performed outside the areas of resection.
- Posterior closure and the anterior steps are the same as described for the lower body lift with autoaugmentation.

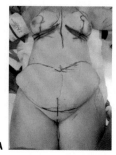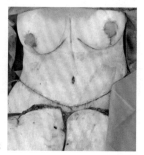

TECH FIG 3 • **A.** Patient now in supine position. Dog-ears from the back can be seen laterally on the abdomen. **B.** Closed abdomen following completion of the abdominoplasty and lateral dog-ear excision.

- Lower Body Lift Without Autoaugmentation (also Known as a Belt Lipectomy)

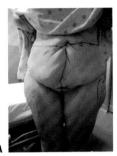 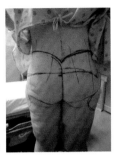 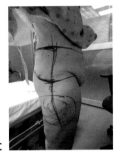

TECH FIG 4 • **A.** Anterior, posterior **(B)**, and lateral views **(C)** of preoperative markings for a lower body lift without autoaugmentation flaps.

PEARLS AND PITFALLS

Lower body lift	▪ Creating a dartoid point at the gluteal crease helps to avoid the appearance of the gluteal crease extension above the incision.
Lateral thigh lift	▪ Dividing the zones of adherence with the Lockwood underminer allows for a greater pull and redistribution of the tissues.
Mons pubis ptosis	▪ In marking the lower abdominal incision, be sure to lift the mons and resuspend at the time of closure.
Staging procedures	▪ Do not perform a vertical medial thigh lift or an upper body lift at the same time as a circumferential body lift because of the opposition of vectors on the pull of the tissues.
Lower body lift	▪ In the prone position, flex the table 5 to 10 degrees to take the tension off the posterior incision when the patient is in the semi-Fowler position.
Abdominoplasty	▪ Preserve tissue on the deep fascia to minimize the risk of seroma.
Lower body lift	▪ If patient has very heavy thighs, consider thigh debulking liposuction first to decrease pull on incisions.

POSTOPERATIVE CARE

- Patients should be maintained in the semi-Fowler position.
- Patients should ambulate the evening of surgery.
- Plan for hospital admission for 1 or 2 nights.
- Recommend postoperative venous thromboembolism chemoprophylaxis.
- No lifting over 10 lb for 6 weeks.

OUTCOMES

- Patients will see immediate improvement, but swelling will persist for up to 3 to 6 months.
- Long-term patient satisfaction is high (**FIG 4**).

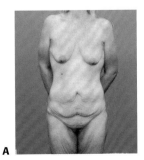 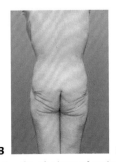 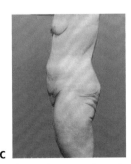

FIG 4 • Preoperative **(A–C)** and postoperative **(D–F)** views of patient who underwent a lower body lift with autoaugmentation.

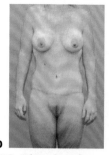 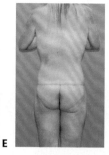 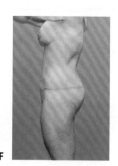

D   E   F

FIG 4 (Continued) •

COMPLICATIONS

- Seroma
- Wound dehiscence
- Infection
- Scarring
- Hemorrhage
- Residual laxity
- Skin loss
- Residual laxity

- Incomplete correction
- Need for revision
- Venous thromboembolism

REFERENCES

1. Lockwood TE. Superficial fascial system (SFS) of the trunk and extremities: a new concept. *Plast Reconstr Surg.* 1991;87:1009-1018.
2. Huger WE Jr. The anatomic rationale for abdominal lipectomy. *Am Surg.* 1979;45:612-617.

Lower Posterior Torso and Buttock Sculpting

Dennis J. Hurwitz

DEFINITION

- Harmonious sculpturing of a feminine lower back, waist, and buttocks is a new frontier in body contouring surgery. Because less attention has been focused on these regions than the breasts and abdomen, many plastic surgeons need training in advanced approaches to achieve femininity of the lower posterior torso.
- Although the public is increasingly requesting buttock enlargement, adjacent areas such as the flanks, hips, and lateral and posterior thighs should be also addressed when performing buttock augmentation. As there is minimal demand for augmentation of the male buttocks, the male situation will receive limited attention.
- A summary of this author's approach follows:
  - Back rolls with undersized buttocks are treated by third-generation ultrasound-assisted lipoplasty of the torso with lipotransfer to the buttocks in the young overweight female.
  - Posterior torso tissue laxity with flank rolls and buttock ptosis is the indication for lower body lift with de-epithelialized adipose fascial flap buttock augmentation. Liposuction harvest of fat from the flanks and abdomen followed by fat transfer to the inferior buttocks may be helpful to complete the lower torso buttock reshaping.
  - Maximum narrowing of the waist in the older female, especially when none ever existed and the most effective safe correction of oversized love handles in all males is achieved with direct oblique excision of the flanks, ie, a oblique flankplasty.
  - Silicone elastomer implants are reserved for buttock augmentation when harvestable fat stores are inadequate.
- The drawbacks of commonly accepted approaches have limited their use in favor of innovative solutions to be presented in this chapter.
  - Traditional liposuction is rather traumatic when applied to the fibrous posterior torso.
  - Hip-hugging circumferential lower body lifts with and without adipose fascial flaps for gluteal buttock augmentation often sag along the lateral gluteal region and fail to narrow bulging waists.

ANATOMY

- A sensuous woman's lower posterior torso, upper thigh, and buttocks and the procedures to create them are based anatomically (see **FIG 1** for an artistic rendering of role of underlying anatomy to feminine shape). The photographic results of the four case presentations of this chapter approximate aesthetic ideal.

- A subtle feminine S-shaped curvilinear midline is centered on the curving lumbar spine. Along with its paraspinous muscular ridges, this concavity bridges the convexities of the lower thoracic spine and sacrum.
- A tapering lower thoracic rib cage narrows to the pelvic brim. This gap is spanned by the latissimus dorsi and external oblique muscles with overlying adipose.

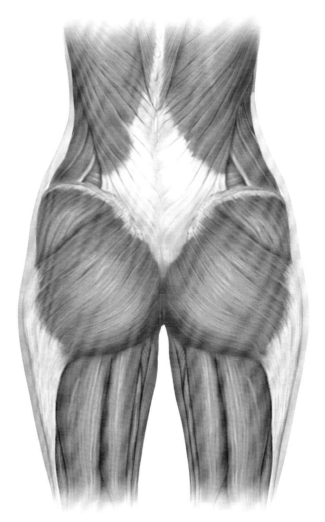

FIG 1 • Anatomy relationships in the aesthetic lower back and buttocks. The musculoskeletal structure and relationships are responsible for the underlying shape of the lower back, waist, and buttocks. Adipose fullness about the hips and buttocks accentuates femininity. The paramedian vascularity clearly nurtures advanced buttock flaps.

- At an ideal 0.7 transverse diameter, waist-to-buttocks ratio, the waist abruptly expands laterally over the posterior iliac spines to adipose rounded hips that are wider than her shoulders.[1]
- The maximal projection of the midbuttocks combines adiposity with the gluteus maximus muscle bulk and lies directly on a horizontal plane to the mons pubis.
- Buttock projection abruptly extends from back lordosis.
- From their widest diameter, lateral buttocks smoothly taper to slightly convex upper lateral thighs.
- Posterior medially, the curved buttocks abruptly end in horizontal folds about the ischial tuberosity to border the upper posterior thighs.
- Within those essential features, there are a variety of sensually pleasing sizes and shapes, but overall, the ideal 0.7 ratio of waist-to-buttock transverse diameter holds true.
- Preserved generous paramedian perforating blood supply allows for high-tension closures and limited mobilization of adipose fascial flaps for buttock augmentation.
- Android body build, massive weight gain and loss, aging, and lower body lifts may result in masculinization and/or undesirable contours.
  - Reducing of the curvilinear midline features
  - Dampening of lumbar lordosis
  - The lower back and waist undulating concavities are straightened and may even bulge.
  - Increased breadth of the back and waist dominates over the narrowing buttocks.
  - Lateral buttocks are flattened and even depressed.
  - Inferior buttock fold separations from the posterior thighs are obliterated.

NATURAL HISTORY

- The shape of the posterior torso and buttocks can be distorted by congenitally flared posterior costal margins, wide and high pelvic rims, localized flank adiposity, weight gain, weight loss, pregnancy, and menopause.
- Most commonly, aging with weight gain broadens the midtorso, deposits, and transverse rolls and narrows and flattens the buttocks. Buttock ptosis may obliterate the fold at the medial posterior thighs and leave sagging, wrinkled skin.
- Once acquired, increased girth of the flanks is hard to lose through exercise and weight loss, and narrow buttocks rarely expand.

PATIENT HISTORY AND PHYSICAL FINDINGS

- For the back and buttocks, women usually request elimination of sagging back rolls and filling flat buttocks. On occasion, they specifically mention a smaller back, a narrower waist with smooth contours bridging the lower chest and buttocks, and rounder buttocks. More commonly, they complain of sagging abdomen and/or breasts.
- They either ignore the back, waist, or buttocks or simply feel that little can be done to improve bulging or masculine features. Because of that, women considering breast reshaping or abdominoplasty should have their posterior torso, thighs, and buttocks examined. If those areas are sensually alluring, she should be complimented.

- As a rule, in all but morbidly obese patients or after extreme weight loss, the central back is feminine and need no correction. Her figure faults are presented, and if there is interest, the means for their correction are offered.
- In Western Pennsylvania and probably throughout most of America, candidates for body contouring of the back and waist rarely request improvement. Instead, they inquire about breast reshaping and are pleased to learn that the lateral breast roll and upper back can be reduced.
- They request a tummy tuck and are pleased to learn that their waist can be reduced by liposuction or direct excision. A deep and defined waist with rounded buttocks during youth suggests fertility, which is an aphrodisiac.
- With buttock augmentation requests, patients are pleased to learn that fat removed from around the buttocks not only can be processed to augment it but also the perimeter reduction can picture frame buttock prominence. Because their companions better see the posterior view, they tend to be enthusiastic about the anticipated improvement. For some, a lower body lift is the best approach to suspend the thighs and buttocks.
- The examination while standing exposes the entire aesthetic complex.
  - Overall and localized excess adiposity and skin laxity are noted.
  - Tightly bound skin expanded by underlying fat is noted as the contour can be improved by liposuction with the expectation of reasonable skin retraction.
  - Hanging tissues and rolls are described by location (lateral breast, scapular, midback, flanks, and hips) and magnitude.
  - Back rolls are characterized by transverse accumulations of adiposity within loose skin bordered inferiorly by transverse dense fibrous adherence from the dermis to the underlying muscular fascia through relatively thin subcutaneous fat.
  - Ptotic rolls, in most over 50 years of age, are best treated with direct or superior excisions.
  - Sagging and flat buttocks are congenital, age related, or the aftermath of severe weight loss.
  - Laxity with lateral flattening and even indentation are common with aging.
- While pointing out figure faults in front of a full-length mirror aids communication, reviewing standardized digital images is usually less awkward. In either case, lines can be drawn that indicate proposed excisions, liposuction or lipoaugmentation, and resulting scars.

IMAGING

- There are no supportive radiologic or other diagnostic studies.

NONOPERATIVE MANAGEMENT

- If the posterior torso and buttocks are obese, then a weight loss program is indicated.
- There are a variety of noninvasive treatments that apply energy to cause lysis of adipose for reduced volume. Topical treatments of proven but limited and somewhat variable reduced shaping are CoolSculpt, Thermage, VelaShape, Liposonix, and VASER Shape.

- They are intended to reduce small selected areas over repeated and rather painful treatments. Large contour adipose excess is difficult to reduce.
- The appeal is nonsurgery and minimal to no downtime.
- Smartlipo with YAG laser energy leads the list of recognized minimally invasive adipose lysis with some skin retraction, but this costly technology has not been widely embraced among plastic surgeons.
- Recently, minimally invasive treatments with subcutaneous thin probes delivering controlled radiofrequency energy, Thermi and InMode BodyTite, have shown consistent lipolysis with some shrinkage of the lower torso.

SURGICAL MANAGEMENT

Indications

- Patient recognizes correctable deformity of the lower posterior torso and buttocks.
- Patient is reasonable in goals and accepts the therapeutic recommendations and risks.
- Patient is in good health with control of chronic disease.

Preoperative Planning

- Medical, mental, and psychological conditions must be evaluated and acceptable for elective surgery.
- The roles of liposuction, fat grafting, tissue excision, adipose fascial flaps, and silicone implants toward reaching their aesthetic goals
- The functional working order of all equipment with special attention to high-technology instrumentation
- An awareness of the areas to be liposuctioned, lipoaugmented, and excised and the resulting scars
- The trade-off of scars for unwanted contour deformities
- Understanding of the unpredictable quality of scars and the likelihood of faded scars over many years

- The planned areas for liposuction and incisions for skin and fat excisions are drawn on the awake patient either the evening before or immediately prior to the operation.
- Patient understands the unpredictable magnitude of fat graft take.
- Patient understands the risks of implant malposition, exposure, and infection.
- Immediately prior to the procedure, the tissues are pushed together to simulate closures. Excessive width of resection is avoided. When closures are planned over buried adipose fascial flaps, the width of resection is appropriately reduced.
- Following neighboring liposuction and flap undermining, manual assurance of the proper width of resection is made during the operation for the final time with the plan to tangentially resect more tissue if needed to obtain mild tension at closure.

Positioning

- Surgery only on the posterior trunk is performed with the patient prone. The table is airplane towards lateral for deep liposuction of the flanks.
- When an abdominoplasty is part of the plan and fat harvest in the prone position is estimated inadequate for the buttock augmentation, then the operation starts supine with the lipoabdominoplasty followed by a turn prone with strategic placement of gel body rolls to obtain a jack-knife position.

Approach

- Some combination of the following advanced techniques are considered:
  - VASERlipo with optimal probe, mode, power, and cannula selections for extraction and harvesting of fat
  - Lower body lift with adipose fascial flap augmentation
  - Direct oblique excision of flank excess selectively replaces lower body lift.
  - Silicone soft elastomer gluteal implant augmentation

■ VASERlipo of the Posterior Torso With Lipoaugmentation of the Buttocks (Video 1)

- The demand for gluteal fat augmentation has increased in recent years, with 9993 reported procedures in 2013 and 11 505 in 2014 in the United States.
- VASERlipo is best indicated for flatten buttocks with mild to moderate torso adipose deposits in a previously well-shaped young woman (**TECH FIG 1A-D**).
  - The 1 year result of 3500-cc VASERlipo and 300 cc of lipofill of each lateral buttock reveals more pleasing feminine contours (**TECH FIG 1E-H**).

Markings

- Through visual and palpable cues, bulging and moderately ptotic back rolls are mapped with purple marker from one to three pluses for the extent of adiposity to be removed via liposuction.
- Excessive removal or etching is indicated in black. Depressed areas, such as adherences, should be avoided and are marked in red. Inadequate and depressed but-

tock projection is encircled with green marker with dashes indicating the extent of deficiency.

Power-Assisted Lipoplasty

- The densely fibrous adipose of the posterior torso makes traditional suction-assisted liposuction (SAL) arduous and traumatic. Popular power-assisted lipoplasty (PAL) reduces the surgeon's effort but not the damage to the retained tissue.
  - Excessive disruption of the connective tissue and neurovasculature intensifies the trauma and disrupts tissue elasticity.
  - With large volume removal, the patients are traumatized and intrinsic skin contraction damaged. Recovery can be prolonged for weeks.
  - Nevertheless, traditional liposuction and PAL are the most common means of fat shaping and the results can be dramatically excellent.

Fat Emulsification and Harvest

- VASER provides for the preliminary application of internal focused ultrasound. VASER is the acronym for Vibration Amplification of Sound Energy at Resonance.

TECHNIQUES

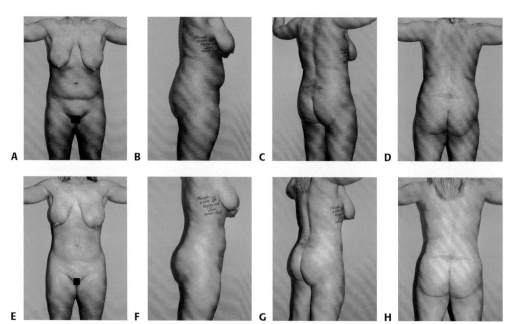

TECH FIG 1 • A–D. Preoperative frontal, right lateral, right posterior oblique, and posterior view presentation for 4400 cc VASERlipo of the torso, followed by 330-cc lipoaugmentation of each buttock. A 33-year-old woman desires a smaller, more sensual body with buttock roundness. **E–H.** One-year postoperative result of VASERlipo of the torso with lateral lipoaugmentation of the buttocks.

- Resonance is a natural phenomenon referring to the possibility to amplify up to nine times the input resonance versus the energy released. The use of ultrasound frequencies at resonance means that the energy release is most efficient, translating to less power needed to create the same effect, resulting in reduced adverse effects.
- VASERlipo emulsifies fat woven in dense connective tissue, with maximum preservation of supporting structures, neurovasculature, and adipose viability for immediate transplantation to the buttocks.
- Using a multiholed blunt cannula saline with Xylocaine and epinephrine is diffusely and meticulously infiltrated throughout the targeted fat until the tissues are turgid. Through a skin protector, a multiringed ultrasound probe is uniformly drawn back and forth to disrupt the fat through cavitation of microscopic bubbles introduced through the preliminary infusion of the wetting solution.
- The thrusts are lengthy and slower and more gentle than during typical liposuction. The concept is to achieve an even and thorough disruption of the fat.
- With the energy on, the push through the tissues is met with mild to moderate resistance. The cannula is then pulled back. Disruptive energy is being applied with both the push and pull of the cannula.
- The flattened helping hand stabilizes the skin and adipose, while the thrusting cannula traverses each level, usually from superficial to deep, as if the subcutaneous tissues were laminated.
- Solid titanium probes are available with 1, 2, 3, and 5 rings etched near the distal rounded tip. The greater the number of rings, the more the dispersion of energy. Initial ring selection is made based on the anticipated tissue resistance.
  - Firm or scarred tissue requires one ring, whereas soft fat is rapidly emulsified with 5 rings.

- When fat is being harvested for lipoaugmentation, the more gentle multiple rings are chosen if possible.
- Three- and five-ring cannulas tend to have just enough focused energy to traverse the tissue with minimal thrusting force. The power is set at 80%.
- When the adipose is soft, I prefer the speed of the 5-ringed probe set at 90%.
- The VASER mode, which rapidly alternates ultrasound energy, exudes negligible heat and is preferred when traversing the subdermis.
  - Superficial liposuction with retention of elasticity best leaves skin able to recontour to a smaller volume.
  - When the extracted fat is planned for lipofill, VASER mode is used throughout the procedure.
- Ultrasound is applied approximately 1 minute for every 100 cc of infiltration or until there is no longer resistance to the moving probe.
- Fat for discard is aspirated at one atmosphere (about 22 in. of mercury) through specially vented 3.0-, 3.7-, or 4.6-mm diameter VentX 4-holed cannulas. When the fat is being harvested for lipoaugmentation, the vacuum pressure is lowered to 18 inches of mercury, and a 24-holed grated cannula is chosen to aspirate fat into a 2200-cc capacity cylindrical glass harvester.
- The 24 two-millimeter openings reduce the vacuum pressure per opening and the size of the adipose particles able to enter each opening. Providing smaller fat packets that can be more easily injected through 1.5-mm diameter Coleman cannulas. When both intakes of the vacuum canister are used, the harvest is quickened and the pressure lowers to 18 in.
- Turning off the vacuum stops the agitation, allowing gravity to separate the denser fluids to the bottom of the canister (**TECH FIG 2**).

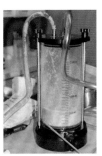

TECH FIG 2 • Harvester for aspirated adipose. In-line reusable glass collector with a heavy base traps sterile aspirate. After the suction is turned off, gravity settles the liquid, which is drained through a spout at the bottom. While the remaining fatty emulation can be syringe aspirated through the spout, we prefer and in this case removed the harvester lid and then poured the contents through a kitchen colander for drainage of excess liquid. The moist fat is then spoon-fed into 10- and 20-cc syringes. Through several stab wound incisions along the designated perimeter, fat is treadlike injected into the buttocks through 8-in.-long blunt Coleman cannulas. Initially, infiltration is fanned throughout the subdermis. Then the fat is evenly injected through the subcutaneous and superficial muscular layers, until a distinct firmness is palpated throughout the target.

Fat Processing and Injection

- Through a dependent spout, the infranate liquid is released. Then there are two reasonable ways to process fat for injection.

- Commonly, the canister lid is removed. The fat emulsion is awkwardly poured into a kitchen colander for drainage of the remaining fluid through multiple small holes. Within the open colander, long tissue strands are sliced and diced before the drained fat is spooned into 10- or 20-cc. syringes. The moist fat is pasty and may be difficult to pass through standard Coleman injection cannulas.
- Alternatively, the decanted adipose slurry is withdrawn through the dependent spout into 20- to 60-cc syringes, which are left standing in a tray. When ready to use, the dependent fluid is pushed out, and the syringe is attached to Coleman cannulas for fat injection. In the demonstration, 3200 cc of fatty emulsion was removed.
- Through stab wounds, fat is injected in a weavelike manner throughout the subcutaneous fat and superficial musculature of the buttocks. As deep, high-tension injections and sharp-pointed cannulas may be the source of fatal venous injections, they are avoided; 600 cc of fat was injected into each buttock.
- The diminution of the back and waist with shapely buttock augmentation is seen one year later (see **TECH FIG 1B,D,F-H**).
- The aesthetic male buttocks are narrow and centrally projecting, suitable for lipoaugmentation that includes infiltration into the gluteal musculature.

■ Gluteal Augmentation Through Lower Body Lift With Adipose Fascial Flaps and Lipotransfer From Flanks to Inferior Buttocks

- Following significant weight loss, sagging, flat buttocks are reshaped with de-epithelialized adipose fascial island flaps isolated within the lower body lift posterior tissue resection.[1] At the same time, reduction of flank adiposity by liposuction not only narrows the waist but also shortens apparent excess buttock height. Fat harvested from the flank is processed and then transferred to the lower buttocks by injection, where the de-epithelialized adipose fascia flap cannot reach.
- In this demonstrative case, a prior abdominoplasty has been done many years earlier, and so a circumferential lower body lift was not indicated. Due to a high rate of complications, there is a trend toward performing these two operations independently.[2]

Island Flap Harvesting and Placement

- A transverse anchor line is drawn along the posterior iliac crests over the lower lumbar midline. The width of resection, as determined by tissue gathering, leaves a transverse curvilinear line along the midbuttocks. Island flaps for augmentation are centered over the superior portion of each buttock (**TECH FIG 3A-C**).

- Reliable double set of paramedian perforator vessels vascularizes the tissues. The anticipated resection distance between the superior and inferior incisions is reduced about 20% to accommodate for the increased subgluteal volume created by the buried augmentation flap.
- The harvested island flaps are de-epithelialized and isolated for positioning under the gluteal skin flap (**TECH FIG 3D**). The perimeter of the flaps is undermined several centimeters. Restricting fascial bands are cut while trying to preserve perforating vessels.
- There are a variety of successful ways to advance the flaps. In this case, the adipose fascial flap was suture advanced to the gluteus muscle as distal under the gluteal skin flap as possible (**TECH FIG 3E**). The lateral fourth of the flaps are completely undermined so that tissue can be either rotated or flipped over the main body of the advanced flap to increase projection (**TECH FIG 3F**). Then the gluteal skin flap is sewn to the lower back and hip anchor incision line in two barbed suture layers (**TECH FIG 3G**).

Completion

- A Jackson-Pratt suction drain is inserted into each buttock pocket. Even a small seroma may allow re-epithelialization of the buried de-epithelialized flap, requiring an operation to decorticate the skin.

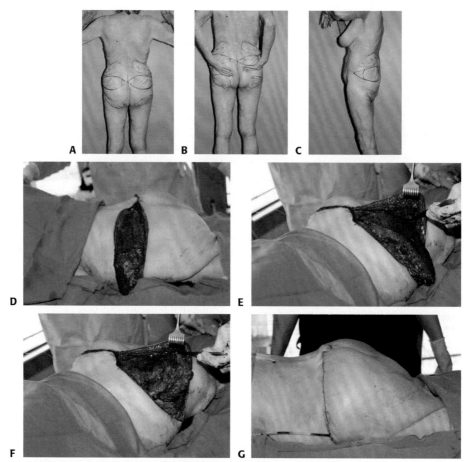

TECH FIG 3 • Operative planning for lower body lift with harvest of bilateral adipose fascial flaps, VASERlipo of the flanks, and lipoaugmentation of the lower buttocks. **A,B.** Posterior and left lateral standing views **(C)**. A beltlike excision, resembling the infinity symbol, starts at the posterior extent of her abdominoplasty scar. Spanning the posterior iliac crests, the low back side of the excision will anchor the advanced buttock skin flap. The width between incisions, indicated by obliquely oriented cross-hatched lines, is determined by the gap approximation of the excess upper buttock skin. Within these two incision lines lie the adipose fascial flaps for buttock augmentation. Plus marks within the encircled flanks indicate moderate depth VASERlipo. The inferior buttocks are narrow and deflated with loose skin, which will be lipoaugmented, as designated by the green rectangle, from fat harvested from the flanks. **B.** The same posterior projection of the flanks and buttocks leaves a flattened mega buttocks. **D.** The left side isolated de-epithelialized flap in prone position on operating room table. The flaps are initially deeply de-epithelialized manually or with the assistance of an electric dermatome set to cut thick at 32 000 of an inch thickness. The lower body lift (LBL) incisions form the perimeter of the planned buttock augmentation flaps. Her right LBL with a buried adipose fascial flap has been completed. The stuffed right buttock projects far beyond the unstuffed left. The LBL buttock skin flap needs to be closed over the buried flaps under mild tension. This left adipose fascial flap is isolated on an island pedicle with circumferential undermining. **E.** The flaps are suture advanced to the depths of the dissected space in prone position viewing from the head. After the left flap is fully mobilized, it is sutured advanced with large branded absorbable suture under the buttock undermined flap toward the inferior buttocks. Her right side LBL and buttock plasty have been completed. **F.** The lateral flap extension is flipped over and stacked. Most often, the lateral extensions are completely undermined in order to flip them over the more deeply positioned advancement flaps, providing more projection and lateral fill. **G.** The buttock flap is suture advanced to the lower back incision. The two-layer closure starts at the midline and progresses laterally with deep bites of double-armed no. 2 PDO Quill. Similarly, 2-0 Monoderm Quill closes the dermis. Compare the competed contour on prone left side with **TECH FIG 3F**.

- The final result in this 77-year-old woman shows a narrow waist with raised buttock and lateral thighs and modest augmentation of the buttocks (**TECH FIG 4**). The generalized skin laxity of the lower back and buttocks has been corrected. Lipoaugmentation of the lower buttocks has reduced the skin sag. Delayed healing of the left transverse suture line has left a depressed scar that may need revision.

- Adipose fascial flaps in men tend to unaesthetically broaden the buttocks and are prone to complications. The low-lying lower body lift tends to excessively depress the upper lateral buttocks. Male hirsutism tends to leave deep hair follicles in de-epithelialized flaps, which may lead to rapid re-epithelialization, which causes intractable seromas. Well-placed suction drains may obviate this complication.

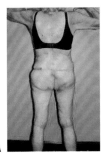 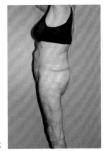 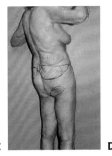 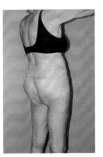

A   **B**   **C**   **D**

TECH FIG 4 • A. The 6-month result in this 77-year-old patient as seen in posterior and left lateral views **(B)**. After a limited dehiscence along the left buttock low back closure, she proceeded to heal with pleasing, hoped-for buttock shape, turgor, and projection, along with a deeper waist. The S-shaped curve from low back to prominent rounded buttocks is agreeable. **C.** Right posterior oblique, before and 6 months **(D)** following her LBL, adipose fascial flaps, VASERlipo of the flanks and lipoaugmentation of the inferior buttocks shows the improve contour best.

Oblique Flankplasty With Lipoaugmentation of the Buttocks (Video 2)

- Flank rolls widen the waist and lengthen the buttocks.
- When there is skin laxity, liposuction alone cannot adequately narrow the waist. Removing both excess fat and skin narrows the waist and reduces buttock height.
- A full-thickness obliquely oriented flank excision of broad adiposity covered by lax skin creates a narrow waist, especially welcomed when none ever existed. These posterior extensions of an abdominoplasty ascend from between the posterior iliac crests and posterior costal margins. The tapered femininity of the lower costal margin is best exposed through this deep and obliquely oriented resection.
- As the sagging skin along the lateral thigh and buttocks is pulled up with the helping hand, the inferior oblique incision line is drawn from the posterior iliac crests to just short of L1.
- The excess skin and fat are grasped between that line and the posterior costal margin for placement of the parallel superior incision. The two lines taper to meet near L1 **(TECH FIG 5A-E)**.
- The inferior perimeter incision is made vertically down along the iliac crests.
- The superior excision descends vertical to the lumbar fascia. The excision is deep, leaving some fat over the paraspinous muscles, and bares the fascia over the latissimus dorsi and external oblique muscles. The thickness of the specimen can be surprisingly large, like an oversized abdominal pannus.
- A no. 2 PDO Quill suture three-point closure encircling the most superficial subcutaneous fascia edges of the wound to the muscular fascia ensures a tapered deep waist. The quilting aspect of the closure inhibits seroma formation.
- Fat VASERlipo harvested from the excision site is processed to lipoaugment the buttocks.
- The one-year result shows a sensual posterior torso and buttocks in a 68-year-old woman, who is for the first time in her adult life pleased with the appearance of her waist **(TECH FIG 5F-J)**. The smooth transitions across her hip heightened the aesthetic appeal.

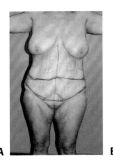 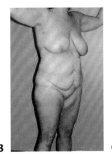 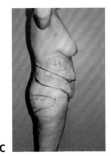 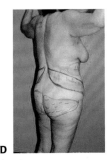 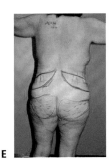

A   **B**   **C**   **D**   **E**

TECH FIG 5 • A–E. Surgical markings for Oblique flankplasty extension of an abdominoplasty.

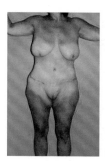 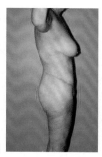 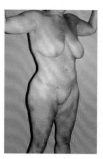 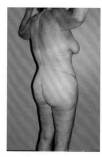 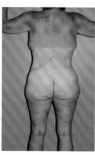

TECH FIG 5 (Continued) • **F–J.** The result of oblique flankplasty extension of an abdominoplasty. Multiple views show not only deep waists but also curvaceous transitions from the thorax and buttocks to the waist.

■ Silicone Soft Elastomer Intramuscular Augmentation of the Buttocks (Video 3)

- Buttock flattening with some skin laxity and normal BMI or less is the indication for implant augmentation of the buttocks. Often, coincidental liposuction of the flanks is performed.
- Based on the patient's desires and anatomy, an appropriate-sized and appropriate shape soft silicone elastomer gluteal implant is selected.
- In closed spaced vertical parallel intergluteal incisions, high intramuscular placement yields the best chance for complication-free aesthetic success.
- The case presentation is a 42-year-old, 5′7″, 135 lb self-employed home cleaner, who lost 100 pounds lb through

diet and exercise. She is disappointed with her sagging breasts and buttocks as well as generalized loose skin of her torso. She was tormented by her obesity since her adolescence.[4]
- Immediately prior to her buttock implant augmentation, she underwent a 330-cc textured round Sientra implant, Wise pattern implant augmentation mastopexy, and lipoabdominoplasty (**TECH FIG 6A-D**).
- After the gluteal outline is drawn, the perimeter of the chosen implant is outlined immediately inferior to the superior border of the buttocks (**TECH FIG 6E**).
- A large round implant, 14 cm in diameter and 350 cc in volume, is chosen to augment the central buttocks, take up skin laxity, and partially fill the depressed lateral buttocks.

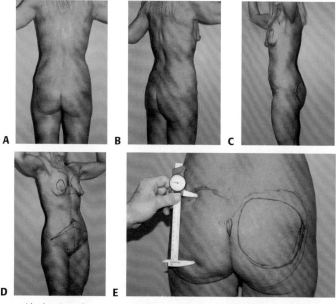

TECH FIG 6 • Preoperative views with drawings for mommy makeover in a 42-year-old include gluteal implant augmentation. Through diet and exercise, this 5′8″ woman has lost 150 pounds and is distressed by deflated breasts and buttocks and generalized sagging skin of the torso. **A.** Unmarked posterior view shows sagging torso and buttock skin. **B.** The left oblique posterior view best shows the flat and sagging buttocks, lower back, and lateral thighs. **C.** Left lateral view shows the markings in profile for correction of sagging breasts, abdomen, and buttocks. **D.** Right anterior oblique view has markings visible for periareolar mastopexy and 365-cc Sientra textured round implant augmentation and complete abdominoplasty, which will start with the lower of the two superior markings. **E.** In this posterior view, a caliper marks the 14-cm diameter of the implant within the boundary of the left buttocks. Implantech CCBS-NC-3 14 cm in diameter 330 cc. Contour flex gluteal "natural contour" implants were chosen to take up the skin laxity from pelvic rim to lateral gluteal regions without excessive projection. The gluteal implants are drawn extending from the pelvic rim. It is better to keep the placement slightly cephalad as the implants are likely to drop slightly.

Incision and Dissection

- Parallel 6-cm-long vertical incisions are drawn 1.5 cm on either side of the intergluteal cleft. A single midline incision is an alternative approach reserved for the most experienced operators, because without care the intragluteal cleft may be blunted.
- The incision and dissection are completed for one pocket and then the other prior to inserting the implants.
- After the 6-cm gluteal incision is made, dissection proceeds through the medial subcutaneous tissue, to enter the gluteal fascia. A partial-thickness electrocautery incision is made the medial gluteus maximus muscle.
- With the aid of electrosurgery and in-line suction, a tedious intramuscular dissection is continued for the entire pocket for the implant (**TECH FIG 7**).

Implant Insertion

- A plastic ruler cut to the diameter of the selected implant is inserted to assure adequate breadth of the dissected space. Alternatively, a sizer implant is inserted to assure fit. The Implantech buttock implant is pliable enough to roll up for insertion through the 6-cm opening.
- Immediately prior to inserting the implant into the pocket, Betadine-impregnated Ioban sheet is applied over the incision and operative area. The folded implant is shimmied into the dissected intramuscular space and then unfurled and spread out to precisely fill the intramuscular pocket.

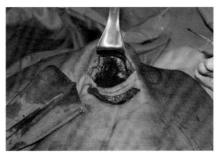

TECH FIG 7 • Intraoperative view of buttock surgery. With her head to the right, the right buttock dissection has been completed and a tail of a buried lap pad is seen. Through a left paramedian 6 cm long incision has been made through skin, and then tediously electrocautery intramuscular dissection is done as exposed by the Richardson retractor.

Completion

- The muscular incision is closed with interrupted absorbable braided suture (**TECH FIG 8A**), followed by two more layers in the subcutaneous tissues and dermis (**TECH FIG 8B,C**).
- Over 6 months, the slightly high positioned and large 14 cm in diameter round implants descend to the desired location.
- Immediately after her 350-cc intramuscular buttock implant augmentation, this 42-year-old woman also had 350-cc gel implant periareolar breast augmentation mastopexy and abdominoplasty. The transformation at 5 months is evident (**TECH FIG 8D-G**).

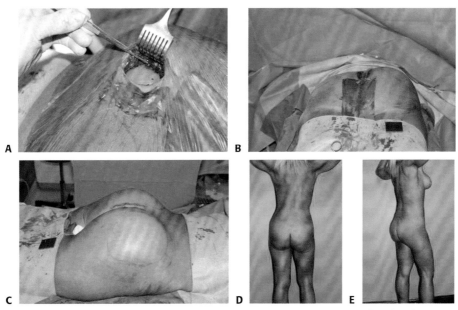

TECH FIG 8 • **A.** After placing an Ioban adhesive drape (3M Health Care, St. Paul Minnesota), the gluteal implant was folded, inserted into the dissected intramuscular space, and then unfurled. The carefully preserved muscular cuff is grasped by forceps for interrupted suture closure on the left side. **B.** Immediate intraoperative view of the augmented right buttocks. Compare the height and fullness of the just augmented right buttocks with the left. The 14-cm-wide implant gently fills the depressed lateral buttocks. **C.** Intraoperative view at the completion of the bilateral implant augmentation. **D.** The 6-month result of the periareolar mastopexy, 365-cc round textured breast implant subpectoral fascia augmentation, complete abdominoplasty, and 355-cc silicone elastomer buttock augmentation. Compare to **TECH FIG 6**. The entire buttocks are well shaped without any surrounding skin laxity. The parallel intergluteal vertical scar are hidden. **E.** Right posterior oblique view shows nicely projecting rounded buttocks that have taken in the slack of the lower back and upper posterior lateral thighs.

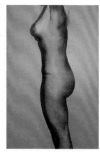 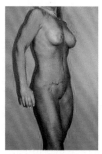

F G

TECH FIG 8 (Continued) • **F.** Lateral view shows proportionally youthful shape of the breasts, abdomen, and buttocks. **G.** Right anterior oblique view best shows the dramatic figure change with her implants, which along with the abdominoplasty adequately took up the slack. The well-shaped muscular abdomen with a low-lying and level scar complements her muscular upper torso.

PEARLS AND PITFALLS

Aesthetic evaluation	▪ The buttock evaluation is considered with lower torso and upper thighs. Liposuction about the perimeter of the buttocks enhances buttock appearance and provides donor grafts.
Buttock lipoaugmentation	▪ First choice when adipose donor sites are adequate. Take is generally very high, but unpredictable. Save potential donor sites.
Buttock adipose fascial flaps	▪ High rate of delayed wound healing. Avoid over-resecting with tight closure. Early overprojection is lost within months.
Silicone elastomer augmentation	▪ As implants in America are soft elastomer and not a firm gel, they are placed high and intramuscular to avoid uncomfortable inferior malposition. Minimize wound dehiscence and loss of intragluteal cleft with paramedian incisions.

POSTOPERATIVE CARE

▪ Immediate postoperative elastic garment that hugs the waist, supports the buttocks, and compresses the upper thighs is fitted according to size.
▪ Patient may not to lie directly on the incision closure. She may lie directly on the augmented buttocks for up to an hour at a time.
▪ Suction silicone drains are used after lower back liposuction and alongside adipose fascial flaps but not worth the risk of infection near silicone implants. Meticulous drain care maintains function and exit site cleanliness.
▪ Extreme hip flexion is avoided.

OUTCOMES

▪ When properly informed, patients tend to like the outcomes, even when falling somewhat short of expectations.
▪ Repeat lipoaugmention for inadequate buttock fullness is anticipated and accepted if performed at reasonable costs.
▪ Buttock implant failure needs a complete reoperation, which is hard to accept, even when forewarned.
▪ Adipose fascial flap augmentation, in most instances, settles considerably, causing considerable loss of projection.
▪ Prolonged secondary healing after adipose fascial flaps may be followed by painful depressed scarring and considerable disappointment.

COMPLICATIONS

▪ Infection following lipoaugmention is a difficult and fortunately rare problem to clear, due to the large reservoir of necrotic fat. Numerous small drainage procedures and intravenous administered antibiotics are indicated.
▪ Forceful injection of fat into the deep gluteal tissues is to be avoided, as sudden death through large vein fat deposits followed by pulmonary embolism has been reported in Latin America.[3]
▪ Adipose fascial flaps placed added tension to the lower body lift closure, which may lead to skin and fat necrosis along the closure.
▪ If limited, debridement is a minor office procedure. When extensive, debridement has been in hospital under general anesthesia procedure, usually followed by application of VAC.

REFERENCES

1. Robert FC, Leroy VY. Clinical anatomy in aesthetic gluteal body contouring surgery. *Clin Plast Surg.* 2006;33:347-358.
2. Small KH, Constantine R, Eaves FF III, Kenkel JM. Lessons learned after 15 years of circumferential body contouring surgery. *Aesthet Surg J.* 2016;36(6):681-692.
3. Condi-Green A, Kotamari V, Nini KT, et al. Fat grafting for gluteal augmentation: a systematic review of the literature and meta-analysis. *Plast Reconstr Surg.* 2016;138(3):437-446.
4. De la Peña JA, Rubio OV, Cano JP, et al. History of gluteal augmentation. *Clin Plast Surg.* 2006;33(3):307-319.

Gynecomastia Procedures After Massive Weight Loss

Michele A. Shermak

DEFINITION

- Gynecomastia technically is defined as enlargement of breast tissue in men. Often with massive weight loss patients, there is pseudogynecomastia, with skin redundancy and ptotic nipple-areolar complex (NAC) position, which might be associated with true breast tissue.

ANATOMY

- In male massive weight loss patients, there may be underlying musculoskeletal deformity with barrel chest. Glandular breast tissue may be present. Skin is excessive vertically and horizontally, with a visible inframammary fold (IMF), and skin excess may extend posteriorly to the upper back. Standard position of the NAC is just lateral to the pectoralis muscle, 20 cm from the sternal notch and 10 cm from midline. With gynecomastia, nipple-areolar position is lower, oftentimes beneath the inframammary fold.

PATHOGENESIS

- Most male neonates have some amount of palpable breast tissue. The next chronological peak for gynecomastia occurs during puberty, with the last peak occurring in men between 50 and 69 years of age.
- Physiological gynecomastia in pubertal male teens is benign and self-limited; on the other hand, several conditions and drugs may induce proliferation of male breast tissue. Most cases result from estrogen excess and/or androgen deficiency as a consequence of different endocrine disorders.
- Thyroid and testicular disease may cause gynecomastia.
- Biochemical evaluation should be performed once physiological or iatrogenic gynecomastia has been ruled out. Nonendocrine illnesses, including liver failure and chronic kidney disease, are other cause of gynecomastia that should be considered.
- Medications associated with the onset of gynecomastia are spironolactone, cimetidine, ketoconazole, hGH, estrogens, hCG, antiandrogens, GnRH analogs, and 5-α reductase inhibitors.
  - Medications probably associated with gynecomastia include risperidone, verapamil, nifedipine, omeprazole, alkylating agents, HIV medications (efavirenz), anabolic steroids, alcohol, and opioids. Cessation of these medications may result in resolution of gynecomastia.[1-3]

PATIENT HISTORY AND PHYSICAL FINDINGS

- History should be queried regarding potential causes of gynecomastia that may be reversible, such as use of medications or marijuana. Medical history including hyperthyroidism or testicular disease should be checked, in addition to family history of breast cancer. Symptoms such as pain and nipple discharge should be checked.
- Physical examination should emphasize on the chest as well as other body regions elicited on medical history. Examination of the chest wall should focus on symmetry, presence of breast tissue, skin quality, underlying thoracic/skeletal deformities, and any masses on palpation. Testicular physical examination is warranted.
- Examination of the massive weight loss patient may also assess other body regions that may be directly or secondarily addressed at the time of gynecomastia correction.

IMAGING

- Mammogram should be considered in a male with breast asymmetry, palpable mass, or family history of breast cancer.[4] If there are any suspicious findings on mammogram, ultrasound and MRI studies may follow, with PET/CT if concerns are present for metastatic breast cancer.

SURGICAL MANAGEMENT

Preoperative Planning

- After physical examination and any necessary assessments rule out cancer concern, planning for gynecomastia follows. Lack of skin redundancy and good skin quality lend themselves to limited incision approaches.[5] Massive weight loss patients with skin excess, stretch marks, and NAC ptosis require skin reduction techniques and possibly NAC grafting.[6] Scars associated with skin reduction must be discussed with the patient who should weigh in on the technique chosen.

Positioning

- Positioning for surgery is standard supine with arms lateral to the body at 90 degrees. Sequential compression devices and lower body warming are optimal.

Approach

- Approaches range from liposuction to limited scar with glandular resection and liposuction to skin reduction, glandular resection, and nipple-areolar grafting.

▪ Liposuction

- Patient is marked preoperatively.
- Small stab incisions are created medially and laterally on the inframammary fold (IMF).
- Superwet tumescent liposuction technique is followed, aiming for 1:1 match with tumescent fluid volume instilled and lipoaspirate volume removed.
- After adequate time is allowed for hemostatic effect, liposuction with traditional approach (suction-assisted liposuction [SAL]), power-assisted liposuction (PAL), or ultrasound/VASER-assisted liposuction (UAL) is performed, reducing adipose and glandular elements, with particular attention to treating the IMF and axillary regions (**TECH FIG 1**).

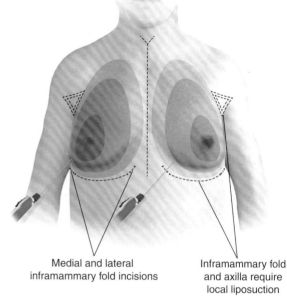

Medial and lateral inframammary fold incisions

Inframammary fold and axilla require local liposuction

TECH FIG 1 • Liposuction of the chest includes small incisions at the inframammary fold medially and laterally on each side, utilizing preferably PAL or UAL to remove the full tissue and gland.

▪ Limited Scar Glandular Resection With Liposuction

- Technique for liposuction of the chest is followed.
- Semicircular incision around the lower NAC is made and the NAC is dissected off of the glandular tissue, maintaining glandular tissue within the NAC to avoid NAC deformity.

- The glandular tissue is completely removed, maintaining appropriate subcutaneous tissue on the chest wall skin.[5] (**TECH FIG 2**).
- The lateral IMF stab incision may be utilized to place a drain tube.
- The incision is closed in layered fashion with dermal and subcuticular layers.
- The patient is dressed with foam compression and a vest to aid in contour and reduce swelling and bruising.

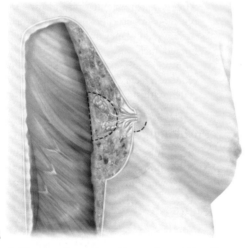

A

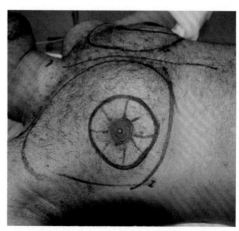

B

TECH FIG 2 • A. Diagram of resection of breast tissue. This will occur after fat surrounding the *red* area is liposuctioned out. **B.** Markings for liposuction with glandular excision (*outer circle*) include an added incision (marked with a *semicircle*) at the lower edge of the areola from 3:00 to 9:00. The *inner circle* marks palpable breast tissue. Liposuction is performed first, followed by incision of the NAC and glandular excision. It is important to maintain some tissue behind the NAC to create the most optimal contour.

■ Mastectomy With Skin Reduction After Massive Weight Loss

- Wise pattern is marked on the patient standing, aiming for nipple-sternal notch distance of 21 cm and distance of 20 cm between nipples.
  - The new NAC goal is for small ovoid NAC just along the border of the pectoralis major muscle (**TECH FIG 3A**).
- NAC is harvested to superficial dermis and stored on the side table in saline-moistened gauze.

- Wise pattern breast reduction follows, removing glandular and pseudoglandular tissue while maintaining appropriate-thickness skin flaps (**TECH FIG 3B**).
- A drain is placed and the skin is approximated in layered fashion, including the Scarpa fascia, deep dermis, and subcuticular suture layers.
- The new NAC recipient site is de-epithelialized and the NAC harvested is sutured to the site with interrupted and running no. 4-0 chromic sutures (**TECH FIG 3C**).
- Compression dressing is created over the NAC with nonstick gauze and foam stapled into place.

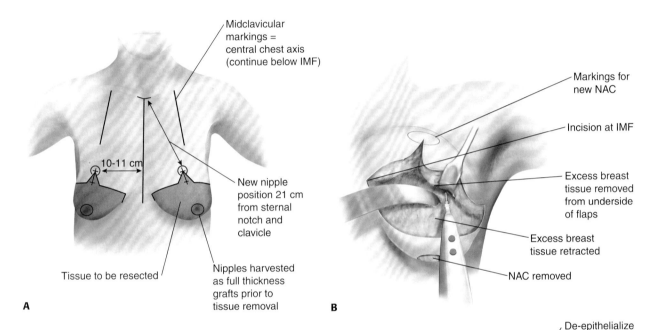

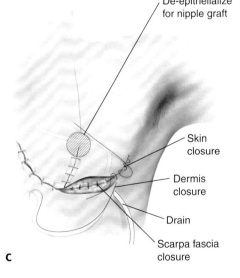

TECH FIG 3 • **A.** Markings for Wise pattern mastectomy with nipple grafting for gynecomastia. The NAC is 21 cm from the sternal notch and 10 cm lateral to the midline, and 7 cm is allowed for the distance between the nipple and IMF. **B.** The breast tissue is dissected under the skin flap, which includes the full thickness of the subcutaneous fat layer. The breast tissue is then elevated off the pectoralis fascia after the NAC is harvested and stored, and the breast tissue is removed at the IMF. **C.** The Scarpa fascia is closed with 2-0 or 3-0 interrupted braided absorbable suture, the dermis is closed with 3-0 interrupted absorbable monofilament suture, and the skin is closed with 4-0 continuous intracuticular monofilament suture. A no. 10 flat Jackson-Pratt drain is placed. After approximating the medial and lateral skin flaps to the IMF, the new NAC position is de-epithelialized and grafted with the NAC harvested earlier in the procedure.

PEARLS AND PITFALLS

Unsatisfactory contour	■ Avoid overthinning the NAC and chest skin to create best aesthetic result. Assure if liposuction is performed that the surgeon avoids over- or under-resection and aims for symmetry.
Completely resolve chest fullness	■ Aim to add glandular tissue resection to liposuction. Men generally do not like to palpate, let alone see, any chest fullness after surgery. In massive weight loss, the surgeon should consider grafting the NAC rather than maintaining the NAC on a pedicle to avoid residual chest fullness.
Contour takes precedence over scar	■ In massive weight loss patients, skin removal is critical to contour. Scars fade over time. Scars range from inframammary scars to anchor incisions to transverse or oblique incisions in the midchest. Scar outcomes may be optimized with patient engagement and counseling.
Individualize care	■ Presentation of gynecomastia runs a wide spectrum. Each patient should be evaluated and treated specifically for his or her presentation and scar tolerance.
Other procedures pair well with gynecomastia treatment	■ Massive weight loss patients may choose to also undergo abdominoplasty, liposuction, and/or brachioplasty, which may be safely performed together and will complement aesthetic results of the gynecomastia surgery.

POSTOPERATIVE CARE

■ Surgery is most often performed as an outpatient.
■ Patients are seen within days of surgery at which time any drain tubes are removed.
■ After this, patients are seen the following week for suture removal and counseling for optimal scar, which may include compression, topical therapies, and activity limits for 4 to 6 weeks.

OUTCOMES

■ Scar therapy is managed and cosmetic outcome should be excellent. There should be no functional deficit (**FIGS 1–3**).

COMPLICATIONS

■ Contour irregularity—This may result in need for revisions, which are typically performed under local anesthetic. Focal minimal liposuction or fat transfer may be necessary, as well as excess skin removal. If a liposuction-only technique is

performed, patients may be able to palpate or see residual breast tissue after surgery, resulting in patient dissatisfaction and desire to undergo definitive glandular excision in a subsequent surgical procedure.
■ Visible scarring—After conservative topical management of scars for 4 months, scar management may require injectable steroid, with consideration for later scar revision under local anesthesia as needed.
■ Seroma—If seroma results, this is initially treated with needle aspiration, which may be performed several times. If this does not fully resolve the seroma, a drain may be replaced to more optimally treat residual fluid.
■ Infection—This is not common and may be treated with antibiotics, beginning with oral antibiotics that cover gram-positive organisms. Local wound care with topical antibiotics may provide adequate treatment of cellulitis.
■ Wound healing problems—Local wound care tends to be adequate, with local debridement as needed and moisture with coverage. Antibacterial topical medications such as mupirocin are helpful if there is cellulitis.

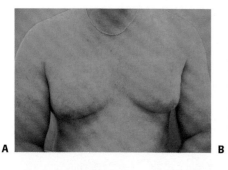
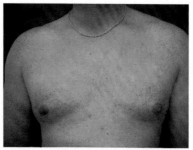

FIG 1 • A,B. Pre- and postoperative photos of a male who underwent treatment of gynecomastia with liposuction.

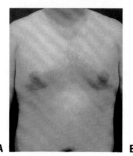
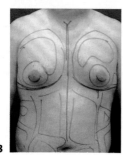
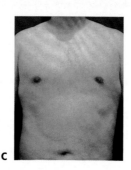

FIG 2 • A-C. Pre- and postoperative photos of a male who underwent liposuction and glandular resection of liposuction. He also underwent liposuction of his torso while being treated for his chest.

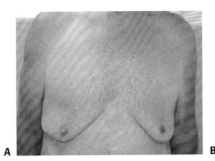 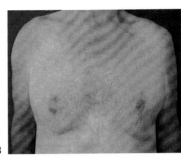

FIG 3 • A,B. Pre- and postoperative photos of a male who underwent Wise pattern mastectomy with nipple grafting after massive weight loss. He also underwent abdominoplasty while being treated for his chest.

- Nipple-areolar pigmentation irregularity—This may occur with nipple grafting and is first allowed a year to improve with moisturizers. If there is residual hypopigmentation, then local excision for small areas or tattoo for larger areas resolves pigment issues.

REFERENCES

1. Sansone A, Romanelli F, Sansone M, et al. Gynecomastia and hormones. *Endocrine.* 2017;55(1):37-44.
2. Deepinder F, Braunstein GD. Drug-induced gynecomastia: an evidence-based review. *Expert Opin Drug Saf.* 2012;11(5):779-795.
3. Narula HS, Carlson HE. Gynaecomastia—pathophysiology, diagnosis and treatment. *Nat Rev Endocrinol.* 2014;10(11):684-698.
4. Yen PP, Sinha N, Barnes PJ, et al. Benign and malignant male breast diseases: radiologic and pathologic correlation. *Can Assoc Radiol J.* 2015;66(3):198-207.
5. Kim DH, Byun IH, Lee WJ, et al. Surgical management of gynecomastia: subcutaneous mastectomy and liposuction. *Aesthetic Plast Surg.* 2016;40(6):877-884.
6. Gusenoff JA, Coon D, Rubin JP. Pseudogynecomastia after massive weight loss: detectability of technique, patient satisfaction, and classification. *Plast Reconstr Surg.* 2008;122(5):1301-1311.

Mons Pubis Reduction

Michele A. Shermak

DEFINITION

- The mons region is defined as a part of the vulvar anatomy, which also includes the labia majora and labia minora.
- Monsplasty is performed as an isolated procedure or in conjunction with abdominoplasty and/or medial thighplasty. The goal of monsplasty is to create a smooth mons with attractive dimensions vertically and horizontally and appropriate fat composition, with harmonious continuity with the abdomen.
- The mons is often affected by massive weight loss (MWL) and pregnancy, with descent of the pubic area, lengthening of the distance between umbilicus and the vulvar cleft, and residual adiposity.
- Although shortening of vertical dimensions and thinning and resuspension of the mons may be performed with abdominal contouring procedures, narrowing horizontal dimension can occur in conjunction with medial thigh lift.
- Monsplasty has been shown to improve hygiene, urinary continence, and confidence in sexuality.

ANATOMY

- The vulva includes the mons pubis, labia majora, labia minora, vaginal vestibule, and bulb of the vestibule (**FIG 1**).
- The mons pubis is superficial to the pubic bone.
- The labia majora are paired cutaneous folds that extend posteriorly from the mons pubis and contain variable fatty tissue. The labia majora converge with the labia minora at the posterior commissure or fourchette.

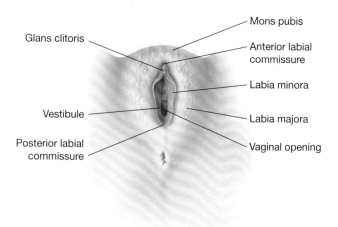

Glans clitoris

Vestibule

Posterior labial commissure

Mons pubis

Anterior labial commissure

Labia minora

Labia majora

Vaginal opening

FIG 1 • The female genitalia, with anatomic areas indicated: 1, labia majora; 2, labia minora; 3, mons pubis; 4, clitoral hood; 5, glans clitoris; 6, urethra; 7, vaginal opening.

- The labia minora are cutaneous folds located medial to the base of the labia majora. The visible rounded portion of the clitoris is located near the anterior junction of the labia minora, above the openings of the urethra and the vagina.
- The vasculature of the female external genitalia includes the anterior labial arteries, branches of the external pudendal arteries, the posterior labial arteries, and branches of the internal pudendal artery. The labial veins drain to the pudendal and femoral veins.
- The vulva is innervated anteriorly by the anterior labial nerves and branches of the ilioinguinal nerve and by the genital nerve, which extends from the genitofemoral nerve. The vulva is innervated posteriorly by posterior pudendal branches.

PATHOGENESIS

- Mons pubis and labia majora morphology are impacted by aging, pregnancy, and weight changes that in turn impact fat composition, dimensions, and ptosis.
- The youthful mons pubis is narrow, with good skin tone, and has a moderate amount of fat in the subcutaneous plane to provide padding against the bony symphysis.
- With age, pregnancy, or weight fluctuations, the mons pubis can appear wide and protuberant with poor skin tone (**FIG 2**). The labia majora may be deflated, and there is ptosis of the external genitalia with increasing distance from the abdomen inferiorly.
- With obesity, the mons becomes increasingly protuberant with a relatively high composition of fat, which often lends itself to surgical correction with liposuction alone. Difficulty with sexual intercourse and maintenance of hygiene as well as discomfort when wearing pants and swimsuits may result. This situation can also impact self-esteem.
- Techniques to correct the protuberant mons and pubic descent with excess skin address these issues with pubic lifting, fat excision and liposuction, and/or elevation and suspension of the fatty layers to the rectus abdominis fascia.

PATIENT HISTORY AND PHYSICAL FINDINGS

- The surgical consultation should begin with discussion of patient concerns and desired outcomes. Discomfort or dissatisfaction with sexual intercourse, bladder control, problems with exercise or wearing certain clothing, and hygienic concerns could result in a patient initiating a surgical consultation.
- Medical history should be explored for any medical conditions and history of weight gain or loss and pregnancies, as well as surgical history.

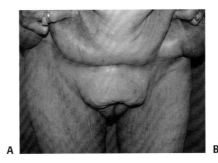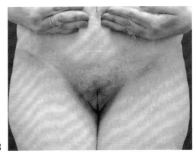

FIG 2 • **A.** Mons pubis in MWL demonstrates significant ptosis and excess fat. **B.** Abdominoplasty with removal of the upper part of the mons pubis will allow a rejuvenated appearance.

- Physical examination is comprehensive and involves the abdomen as well as the external genitalia.
- A surgical plan is then developed to address patient desires and goals, as well as physical findings, adjusting treatment to health and safety concerns.

IMAGING

- This is not applicable to monsplasty management.

SURGICAL MANAGEMENT

Preoperative Planning

- After history and physical examination, planning for monsplasty takes place. Considerations for the pubic region include fat composition and skin quality and excess, as well as height and width dimensions. In most abdominal contouring procedures, the mons pubis is treated with the abdomen with liposuction.
- With varying degrees of mons distortion beyond excess fatty tissue, excisional procedures including horizontal and vertical wedge excision with or without abdominal or thigh contouring are necessary.
  - Horizontal excision shortens vertical distance and may be performed in continuity with abdominoplasty, allowing 6 to 7 cm of distance between the vulvar cleft and the lower abdominal skin incision.
  - Vertical excisions of the mons and labia majora as a central ellipse or as lateral wedges may be included in medial thighplasty to narrow the mons pubis, by restoring a more youthful triangular configuration.
- Lipoplasty through liposuction or excision in conjunction with central wedge excision techniques allows for thinning a protuberant mons pubis and aids in final contouring to provide better harmony with the abdomen. When contouring of the mons pubis and/or labia majora is complete, the pubic tissues may be suspended up to the fascia of the rectus abdominis to prevent them from recurrent descent.

Positioning

- Positioning for surgery is standard supine with arms lateral to the body at 90 degrees, with appropriate padding and heating for the body to optimize safe surgery without complicated outcomes. Sequential compression devices are mandated as well. Some surgeons like to perform monsplasty in stirrups, which may increase VTE risk.

Approach

- Allowing for a distance of 6 to 7 cm from the vulvar cleft to the top of the mons pubis is necessary to avoid distortion and overelevation of the mons pubis. The mons pubis when performed in conjunction with abdominoplasty should strive for the same depth of skin to deep fascia as is present in the abdomen to create harmony between the abdomen and mons pubis.

▪ Liposuction

- Patient is marked preoperatively. Small stab incisions are created. Superwet tumescent liposuction technique is followed, aiming for 1:1 match with tumescent fluid volume instilled and lipoaspirate volume removed. After adequate time passes for hemostatic effect, liposuction with traditional approach (SAL), power-assisted (PAL), or ultrasound/VASER-assisted (UAL) liposuction is performed, reducing adipose content (**TECH FIG 1**).

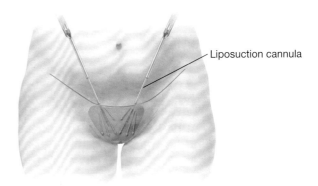

Liposuction cannula

TECH FIG 1 • Liposuction of the mons pubis may be performed with augmented technologies such as ultrasound and power to provide skin tightening.

T E C H N I Q U E S

Central Wedge Excision of the Mons Pubis

- Elliptical width is determined for appropriate narrowing of the pubis. Surgical resection includes skin and fat, working the dog-ear inferiorly into the vulvar cleft and avoiding injury to the region of the clitoris (**TECH FIG 2**).

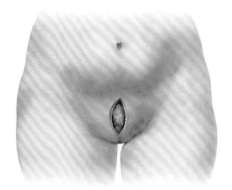

TECH FIG 2 • Central wedge excision is marked, centered around the central vertical axis of the mons pubis and short of the convergence of the labia majora.

Horizontal Excision With Lipoplasty and Suspension to the Rectus Fascia in Conjunction With Abdominoplasty

- Markings for abdominoplasty establish 6 to 7 cm of distance between the lower abdominal incision and the vulvar cleft.
- Abdominoplasty proceeds with elevation of the lower skin flap for upper mons excision in continuity with the abdominal skin flap.
- After completion of the abdominoplasty, subcutaneous fat of the mons is excised, leaving a layer of fibrofatty tissue on the abdominal wall and allowing for skin thickness congruent with the abdomen.
- The deep fat on the mons skin flap is then suspended to the rectus fascia with 3 to 4 braided absorbable sutures (**TECH FIG 3**).
- The abdominal incision is closed over drains in layered fashion with superficial fascia, deep dermal and subcuticular layers.

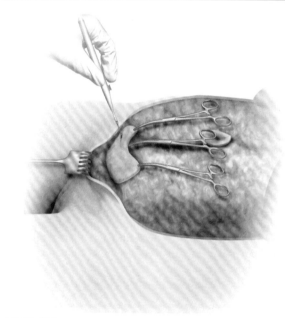

TECH FIG 3 • Horizontal wedge excision of the superior mons pubis in conjunction with abdominoplasty includes defatting of the mons pubis with suspension to the rectus abdominis fascia.

Lateral Wedge Excision of the Labia Majora and Mons Pubis in Conjunction With Medial Thighplasty (See Thigh Lift chapter)

- In marking the anterior aspect of the APEX thigh lift or vertical extended thigh lift into the inguinal region, a central axis is marked on the mons pubis.
- The width of the pubis is determined and should be consistent with dimensions of the underlying bony pubic

symphysis, with symmetry of the mons result around the central axis measured and marked.
- In performing the anterior excision of the thigh lift along the inguinal crease, markings along the lateral pubis are commitment excisions, with excision of the redundant lateral pubis and anterior medial thigh dependent on avoiding tense closure and performed in stepwise fashion (**TECH FIG 4**).

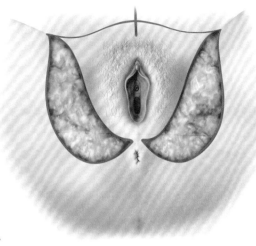

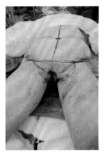

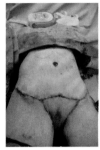

A   **B**   **C**

TECH FIG 4 • A. Lateral excision of the mons pubis and labia majora is carefully marked preoperatively, in order to create a symmetrical pubis centered around the central axis. **B.** Intraoperative photo of the anterior aspect of medial thigh lift, with pubis markings and extent of thigh lift excision to occur superiorly. **C.** Intraoperative photo of completed medial thigh lift with contoured, thinned mons dimensions.

PEARLS AND PITFALLS

Contour irregularities and skin laxity secondary to liposuction	▪ Avoid overthinning and assure uniform treatment, recording "ins and outs" of tumescent fluid infiltrated and lipoaspirate removed to create best aesthetic result. Augmented technologies such as PAL and UAL assist in avoiding tunneling deformities and may tighten the skin beyond what is achievable with SAL.
Horizontal skin resections rejuvenate the mons pubis, but they may descend with time	▪ Suspend the upper mons deep fatty tissue to the rectus fascia with several absorbable sutures to promote prolonged suspension of the mons pubis.
Avoid asymmetrical or shortened mons pubis dimension	▪ Asymmetry in skin dimension horizontally or vertically is best avoided through careful preoperative markings, working around a central axis, and allowing for symmetry around the axis and the vulvar commissure. Patient presentation may be asymmetrical, so asymmetrical treatment may be mandated. Using the vulvar cleft as a fixed point, the mons should be no shorter than 6–7 cm to avoid overly high labia majora placement.
Lateral pubic wedge excision during medial thighplasty with vertical reduction through abdominoplasty can lead to a puffy mons pubis due to pincushion effect of circumferential scar	▪ Markings should not create overly full or overly shortened pubis at the outset. Lymphatic injury should be avoided and superficial excision leaving tissue above deep fascia and vascular and lymphatic structures helps optimize edema prevention. Pincushion effect is often unavoidable. Compression with foam and a support girdle and massage help. Secondary liposuction may be necessary.
Individualize care	▪ Presentation of mons pubis and labia majora deformity cover a wide spectrum. Each patient should be evaluated and treated specifically for her presentation, surgery on adjacent areas such as the abdomen and medial thigh, and scar tolerance.
Avoid damage to the clitoris	▪ Knowledge of external genital anatomy and limiting excision inferior to the superior convergence of the labia majora will help avoid clitoral injury, which is very difficult to fix.

POSTOPERATIVE CARE

▪ Surgery is most often performed as an outpatient. Patients are seen within days of surgery. After this, patients are seen the following week for suture removal and counseling for optimal scar, which may include compression, topical therapies, and activity limits for 4 weeks. Follow-up may then take place months later for scar management reinforcement.

OUTCOMES

▪ Scar therapy and compression are managed expectantly, and cosmetic outcome should be excellent. There should be no functional deficit, and in fact there may be improvement in sexual satisfaction and urinary continence.

COMPLICATIONS

- Asymmetry and contour irregularities—Markings are most important to proper symmetry and mons dimensions, and suspension of the mons pubis will protect against recurrent ptosis. Focal liposuction or fat transfer may be necessary, as well as excess skin removal.
- Visible scarring—After conservative topical management of scars for 4 months, scar management may require injectable steroid, with consideration for later scar revision under local anesthesia as needed. The hair-bearing pubis is a setup for hypertrophic and keloid scarring.
- Injury to external genitalia—Surgery should not be performed below the level of the upper pubic symphysis internally, and tissue should be maintained on deep fascia. More superficially, the anterior labia majora converge over the clitoral hood, and the clitoris should be protected from surgical injury.

REFERENCES

1. Alter GJ. Pubic contouring after massive weight loss in men and women: correction of hidden penis, mons ptosis, and labia majora enlargement. *Plast Reconstr Surg.* 2012;130:936-947.
2. Alter GJ. Management of the mons pubis and labia majora in the massive weight loss patient. *Aesthet Surg J.* 2009;29(5):432-442.
3. Bloom JMP, Van Kouwenberg E, Davenport M, et al. Aesthetic and functional satisfaction after monsplasty in the massive weight loss population. *Aesthet Surg J.* 2012;32(7):877-885.
4. Davison SP, LaBove G. Going in the wrong direction with monsplasty. *Aesthet Surg J.* 2013;33(8):1208-1209.
5. Matarasso A, Wallach SG. Abdominal contour surgery: treating all aesthetic units, including the mons pubis. *Aesthet Surg J.* 2001;21(2):111-119.
6. Shermak MA, Mallalieu J, Chang D. Does thighplasty for upper thigh laxity after massive weight loss require a vertical incision? *Aesthet Surg J.* 2009;29(6):513-522.
7. Triana L, Robledo AM. Aesthetic surgery of female external genitalia. *Aesthet Surg J.* 2015;35(2):165-177.

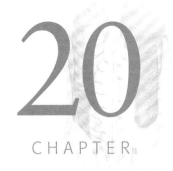

Upper Arm Lift (Brachioplasty)

Jennifer Capla and Joseph Michaels

DEFINITION

- A brachioplasty or upper arm lift is a procedure that targets the skin excess from the axilla to the elbow.
- The "hammock"-like effect of loose skin is sometimes known as "bat wings."

ANATOMY

- With the arm abducted and flexed at 90 degrees, the important landmarks for assessment are from the apex of the axillary crease to the olecranon (**FIG 1**).
- The bicipital groove is the area between the biceps brachii above and the long head of the triceps below.
- In the bicipital groove, below the brachial fascia, lie several important neurovasculature structures including the median and ulnar nerves and the axillary artery and vein.
- In the midportion of the upper arm over the bicipital groove, superficial to the brachial fascia, lies the medial brachial cutaneous nerve.

- In the distal portion of the upper arm over the bicipital groove, superficial to the brachial fascia, lies the medial antebrachial cutaneous nerve and the basilic vein.

PATHOGENESIS

- Factors that can produce laxity of the upper arm soft tissue:
  - Significant weight changes
  - Aging
  - Previous liposuction
  - Sun damage
- Despite a good exercise regimen, skin may not retract. This is likely due to weakness of the connections of the superficial fascial system to the axillary fascia.

PATIENT HISTORY AND PHYSICAL FINDINGS

- A history of significant weight loss, aging, or previous liposuction can lead to skin excess of the upper arms.
- Patients complain of loose hanging skin of the upper arms that interferes with daily activities, difficulty with finding shirts that fit, and the need to wear long sleeves even in the summer to cover up due to embarrassment of the tissue excess.
- Physical examination:
  - Examine the patient with arms abducted at 90 degrees and the forearm flexed at 90 degrees.
  - Visible skin excess from the axilla to the elbow that drapes like a hammock.
  - Determine residual adiposity vs skin laxity.
  - Assess for any arm swelling or lymphedema.
- Contraindications: chronic swelling from lymphedema or venous incompetence

IMAGING

- No radiologic imaging or diagnostic testing is necessary.

SURGICAL MANAGEMENT

Preoperative Planning

- Assess the patient's goals—in front of the mirror with the arm abducted and flexed at 90 degrees, use the pinch technique to demonstrate what the arm lift will achieve.
- If the patient has significant residual adiposity, an arm lift alone may leave the patient with a heavy arm. Consider liposuction prior to debulk the arm, and then return for an arm lift at a second stage. If the majority of fat is in the posterior compartment of the arm, then liposuction can be combined with the procedure.

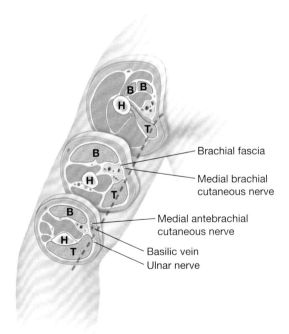

Brachial fascia

Medial brachial cutaneous nerve

Medial antebrachial cutaneous nerve

Basilic vein
Ulnar nerve

FIG 1 • Arm serial sections over bicipital groove. The blue dotted line approximates scar position in the bicipital groove. B, biceps tendon; T, triceps muscle; H, humerus.

- Weight loss patients should be weight stable for a minimum of 3 months. Nutritional assessment is an important factor in wound healing. Labs should include albumin, prealbumin, TIBC, and folate.
- Managing expectations: Preoperative discussion with the patient about the scar ensures that the patient understands the trade-off. Brachioplasty scars can be red, raised, thickened, and cordlike. Take a black sharpie and mark the approximate position of the scar on the patient. This allows them time to go home and look in the mirror to make sure that they are willing to trade for the scar.
- Scar position: The brachioplasty scar can be positioned in either the bicipital groove or the posterior arm. A patient should be given the opportunity to choose. We prefer the bicipital groove for scar location. There are patients in certain professions, like teachers, who raise their arms a great deal and have opted for the posterior scar.
  - Bicipital groove scar—visible from the front view when the arm is abducted and flexed, but when the arm is down at the patient's side, it is not seen.
  - Posterior scar—not visible from the front or back when the arm is abducted and flexed, but when the arm is down at the patient's side, it can be seen from behind.
- Marking the patient preoperatively is of utmost importance.

- Using the pinch technique, a guide to the excision pattern can be determined. Pay careful attention to the pull in the axilla and the lateral chest wall to ensure that there is no distortion on the chest/breast area.
- If any arm bands are present, then resection may lead to worsening of the bands ("Popeye deformity") that you must make the patient aware of before surgery.
- Speak with your anesthesiologist:
  - IV placement in the hand, not the antecubital fossa
  - Blood pressure cuff on the leg or forearm
  - If performing more than one procedure, it is best to start with the arms. If not, discuss with the anesthesiologist about the possibility of limiting IV fluid to decrease overall swelling until the arm resections are performed.

Positioning

- Patient should be in the supine position with arms abducted laterally at 90 degrees on arm boards.
- Prep arms circumferentially to maintain full mobility and include chest and lateral chest wall.
- Sterile self adhesing wrap (Coband) is helpful to cover any tubing or wiring to maintain a sterile field.

Approach

- Bicipital Groove Scar Brachioplasty.

TECHNIQUES

■ Full Scar Brachioplasty-Bicipital Groove Scar

Marking

- Mark the patient in the standing position with the arm abducted and elbow flexed at 90 degrees.
- Ask the patient to flex the biceps and palpate the bicipital groove.
- Draw a horizontal line from the apex of the axillary crease to a point about 2 cm proximal to the olecranon, marking the final scar position.
- With a marker positioned over your line in place, distract the arm tissue downward to obtain the superior marks.
- The next point is essential to the marking.
  - First mark the apex of the axilla (x).
  - Find a point on the low hanging skin that can be distracted inward and upward to the apex point marked in the axilla. It may take several attempts until it appears right.
  - Once this point is chosen, mark it with a distinguishable circle point and call it (x') (**TECH FIG 1A**).
- While holding the x' point to the axillary apex point (x), do a pinch test at several places in the arm distal to the axilla to mark the estimated lower border.
- The mark in the apex point in the deltopectoral groove (x) is carried inferiorly on the lateral chest, posterior to the lateral pectoralis border to carry out the dog-ear or to excise excess lateral chest wall tissue.[2]
  - With the arm extended, carry the marking from x' and connect it to the inferior aspect of the above marked axillary marking.

- The length of this line should be estimated using a pinch technique to determine where the skin excess tapers. Careful attention to the pull on the chest/breast area should be noted.
- Last, place hash marks perpendicular to the previous marks as a guide to line up the closure. Assess both arms from a distance to ensure symmetry (**TECH FIG 1B,C**).

Liposuction

- If combining this technique with liposuction, perform the liposuction of the posterior arm and then begin the excision. Important, do one arm at a time.
- Do not liposuction of both arms first, because the swelling will alter the ability to excise on the other side.

Incision and Flap Elevation

- Infiltrate with local anesthetic.
- Incise the superior portion of the marked incision.
- Elevate a subcutaneous flap above the brachial fascia. Recognize that the arm is a cylinder, so check the thickness of your flap for consistency. It is easy to get too deep.
- Raise the flap just past the inferior border marking.
- In the axilla, stay superficial to avoid injury to underlying lymphatics and neurovasculature structures.
- When approaching the elbow, stay superficial to avoid injury to the medial antebrachial cutaneous nerve. If you see the basilic vein, the nerve will be close.

Resection, Stapling, and Closure

- Once the entire flap is elevated, place two towel clips on the flap and have an assistant distract the flap superiorly and medially.

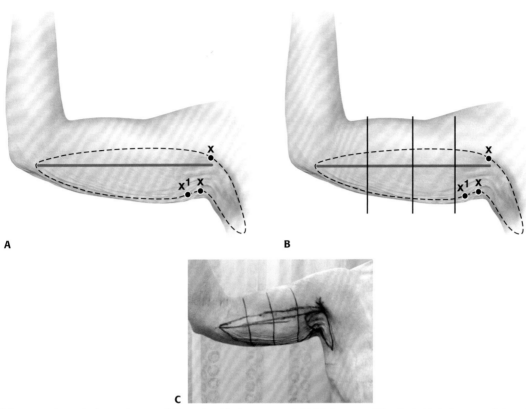

TECH FIG 1 • Markings for bicipital groove full scar brachioplasty. **A.** Mark bicipital groove (*blue line*). Mark the apex of the axilla (point x). Choose and mark point x′ to adequately distract the tissue upward and inward. Distract tissue downward to mark upper line. Using pinch technique, with x′ being pulled into x, to mark lower border. **B.** Place hash marks to line up the border. **C.** Preoperative markings.

- Using a heavy forceps, remark the x′ point. Make a vertical cut and inset to the high point in the axilla. Place 2 to 3 deep 0-Vicryl sutures from the axillary fascia to the deltopectoral fascia to avoid scar migration out of the axilla.[1]
- Resection must be performed in a segmental fashion to ensure closure. Starting at the most distal hash mark, use heavy forceps to mark the inferior excision point. Incise vertically, and staple the point. Continue this for all hash marks.
- Once appropriate tension has been set, mark the remainder of the inferior border and excise.

- Tailor tack the incision with staples. Do not leave the wound open for an extended period as swelling may occur, putting unnecessary tension on the closure or worse off, the inability to close.
- Lift arm up gently off the arm board to assess tension and appearance. Perform the procedure on the contralateral arm. When finished, compare both arms prior to closure for symmetry.
- If placing a drain, bring out from the lateral chest wall. In our practices, we have moved away from placing drains.
- Close the incision in layers.

PEARLS AND PITFALLS

Over-resection	▪ Always perform excision in a segmental fashion. Failure to do so may lead to an incision that cannot be closed.
Liposuction	▪ If performing liposuction in combination with a brachioplasty, be sure to do liposuction and the excision immediately afterward on one arm at a time (unless a two-team approach). Otherwise, swelling can lead to decreased ability to excise the desired tissue or can lead to failure to close the arm.
Scars	▪ Warn patients that the brachioplasty scars can heal red, raised, thickened, and/or cordlike. They can take up to 2 years to mature unlike other scars.
Staging	▪ For patients with significant residual adiposity, liposuction should be performed as a first stage to reduce the volume and then return for brachioplasty in at least 3 months. If the first stage is not performed, the patient will be left with a heavy arm. If all done in one stage, when the swelling subsides, the patient will likely have residual skin laxity.

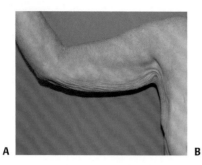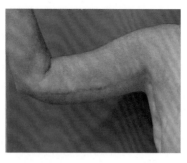

FIG 2 • A,B. Preoperative and postoperative view of male patient.

POSTOPERATIVE CARE

- Place the patient in an arm compression garment for 4 to 6 weeks.
- Keep arms elevated as much as possible.
- Do not exceed 90 degrees at the shoulder for 4 weeks.
- After 4 weeks, the patients can walk their fingers up the wall daily until full extension is reached.
- Begin massage therapy with the product of your liking and consider silicone gel or strips.

OUTCOMES

- Arm contour will immediately be improved (**FIGS 2** and **3**).
- Patient satisfaction with the shape of the arm is high; however, scars can take 1 to 2 years to mature and improve in color and texture.

COMPLICATIONS

- Seroma—fluid collection generally occurs near the elbow and may require serial aspirations in the office.
- Wound dehiscence—generally superficial in the axilla. Treat with dressing changes.
- Hematoma
- Infection
- Poor scarring—may require Kenalog injections.
- Over-resection can lead to failure to close the wound or total dehiscence postoperatively. Avoid by performing segmental excision at the time of procedure, and do not leave incision open for any meaningful period of time.
- Contracture across axilla—can cause pulling or banding in the axilla. May require a Z-plasty to recruit additional tissue to the area.
- Sensory loss
- Chronic swelling

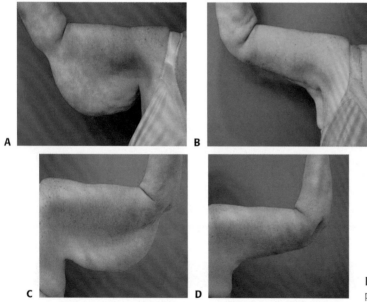

FIG 3 • A–D. Preoperative and postoperative view of female patient.

REFERENCES

1. Lockwood T. Brachioplasty with superficial fascial system suspension. *Plast Reconstr Surg.* 1995;96:912-920.
2. Downey S, Dross J. Lateral thoracic excisions in post massive weight loss patient. *Clin Plast Surg.* 2008;35:115-120.

Upper Thigh Lift

Michele A. Shermak

DEFINITION

- Upper thigh lift describes excision of lax and/or redundant thigh tissue to improve tautness, circumference, and/or shape of the thighs.
- This procedure is often included in approaching lower body lifting for individuals who have sustained massive weight loss.
- The procedure may be performed in combination with lifts of adjacent body regions such as the abdomen or back to globally improve the lower body region.

ANATOMY

- Anatomic details of the thigh are shown in **FIG 1**.
- The skin can demonstrate varying degrees of redundancy, vertical excess, laxity, and collagen strength. Thin skin may have greater recoil after surgery resulting in exacerbated loosening of the surgical result. Attention should be focused on the presence of varicose veins, and if there are many, referral to a vascular surgeon is prudent to minimize varicosities prior to embarking on thigh lift.
- Subcutaneous fat varies in thickness.
  - A thinner fat layer is more appropriate for thigh lift than a thick one, which would more optimally lead to a liposuction contouring procedure or recommendation for weight loss.
  - The fat between the anterior thigh and posterior thigh is different: anterior thigh fat is thinner and softer, whereas posterior fat tends to be thicker and fibrous.

- The final scar appearance may be impaired by the difference in fat characteristics in the medial anterior and posterior thigh with fullness and visibility, particularly if posterior fat is pulled anteriorly.
- Liposuction of the fat to be excised has been described to aid in better visualizing veins and lymphatics; however, liposuction may impair healing, and less is more may be the case here, with improved healing without liposuction performed in the area to be resected.
- Scarpa fascia is the pseudofascial plane in the subcutaneous fat that is located superior to the greater saphenous vein on the inner thigh. The depth of this fascial plane is short in the groin area where penetration can lead to potential injury of the saphenofemoral veins and femoral artery or nerve.
- Deep muscular fascia should be obscured by soft tissue with tissue undermining during thigh lift to help preserve the greater saphenous vein and lymphatics.
- Muscles in this should not be visualized as the muscular fascia is not penetrated; surgery only involves the skin and subcutaneous fat of the inner thigh.
- Patients seeking thigh lift may have superficial dilated varicose veins. The greater saphenous vein is important, because it is within the field of the vertical inner thigh lift and should not be traumatized, as injury may lead to distal extremity swelling. Perforators off the vein are ligated and cut. The saphenofemoral junction is close to the skin surface and may be seen and should be preserved.

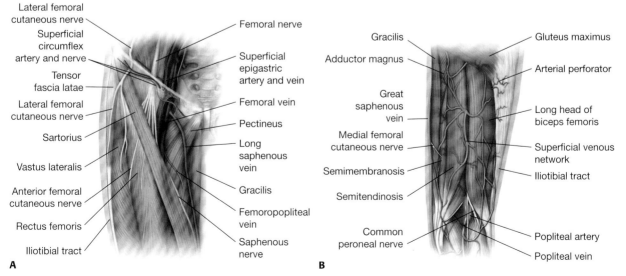

FIG 1 • **A,B.** Thigh anatomy is notable anteriorly for the saphenofemoral junction at the groin and the lymphatic collections at the groin and knee. External anatomy—skin quality, fat quantity, and superficial vein and varicosities—is variable in presentation.

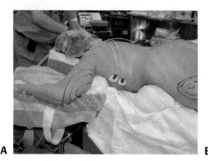
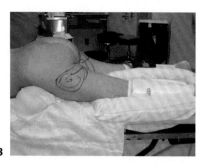

A **B**

FIG 2 • Prone positioning helps provide the best access to the posterior thigh, when performing APEX proximal thigh lift. Safety measures while the patient is in prone position include the following: **A.** Face in prone pillow with goggles protecting eyes from pressure and desiccation; arms are placed at 90 degrees, and gel bumps are placed under the chest and lumbar region. **B.** Bump under chest lumbar regions and forced warming blanket to avoid hypothermia.

- Dissected thigh tissue is always discarded, so arterial perforators are ligated and cauterized, and no major arteries are within the field of dissection. The femoral artery is close to the skin surface, and dissection should be carefully performed in the groin.
- Dissection deep to superficial fascia may result in injury to lymphatics, which travel close to the saphenous vein. Lymphoceles may develop postoperatively near the knee where lymphatics are dense.

PATHOGENESIS

- With skin laxity and/or weight loss of varying degrees, individuals can suffer from excess skin in the thigh.
  - This may be focally limited to the proximal aspect of the inner thigh with minimal skin change outside of this area, most often seen in younger massive weight loss patients.
  - On the other hand, others present with more diffuse, global changes in the inner thigh, with significant attenuation and redundancy of the skin, typically in the older, thinner patient who has experienced massive weight loss.
- A more extended approach to thigh lift in this patient population will reduce circumference and improve skin appearance all the way to the knee.

PATIENT HISTORY AND PHYSICAL FINDINGS

- Patient history should be probed for significant weight loss and, if present in the history, the mode and degree of weight loss, as well as nutritional challenges that may exist.
  - Weight should be stable at the time of surgery at least 3 months.
  - Medical conditions that may impact outcome of thigh lift surgery such as peripheral vascular disease, varicose veins, venous thromboembolism, diabetes, heart disease, sleep apnea, autoimmune and endocrinological disorders, and coagulation disorders and venous thromboembolic history should be queried.
  - Any history of surgery in the groin region must also be addressed, such as that performed for lymph node biopsy.
- Physical findings should note skin quality and degree of excess and redundancy and varicosities as well as adiposity.
  - Chronic calf swelling needs to be noted if present.
  - Adjacent body regions such as the mons pubis, abdomen, and back are examined to see if addressing these regions will improve overall lower body aesthetics.

SURGICAL MANAGEMENT
Preoperative Planning

- Preoperative planning with thigh lift includes addressing significant varicose veins ahead of surgery, as well as discussion of different thigh lift approaches with differing scar lengths.

- More focal proximal skin excess and good skin quality lend themselves well to proximal scar along groin crease, which is well hidden.
- More extended involvement to the knee with attenuated skin and cellulite may be better addressed with vertical incision along the length of the inner thigh.
- With existing calf swelling, the more limited proximal approach is preferable as the more extended thigh lift approach can exacerbate thigh swelling.
- Widened mons pubis may be treated at the time of thigh lift, with inclusion of lateral mons tissue within the zone of resection, paired with liposuction of the mons, as needed (see Chapter 19).

Positioning

- Positioning varies depending on the thigh lift approach.
- The proximal approach requires prone to supine positioning to treat posterior dog-ear and impact of result by extending excision into the infragluteal fold.
- Prone positioning precautions must be followed in the head and neck area and upper body, as well as the gluteal region and thighs.
  - Gel rolls are placed along the upper chest/axilla, and the neck is placed in a neutral position with head resting in prone pillow and eyes off-loaded.
  - Arms at elbow and axilla placed at no greater than 90 degrees with padding under arms and legs to protect pressure points (**FIG 2**).
- The more extended vertical inner thigh excision requires only supine positioning.
  - In the supine position, thigh lift is most easily performed with leg extension bars off the end of the operating room table to allow the surgeon to stand or sit between the legs, which are spread apart from each other.
- Positioning of the thighs in stirrups as seen in gynecological surgical procedures is not necessary and puts the patient at risk for venous thromboembolism (VTE) at the groin with flexion of the hip.

Approach

- Direct excision of the skin excess of the inner thigh is performed.
- Approach must be symmetrical and may include lateral mons pubis to reduce the pubis, which may be widened and full.
- Excision at the lower aspect of the pubis in the groin is most at risk for high tension, so a bottleneck in the excision is created at this point to avoid too much tension and predilection for wound healing problems or pull on the mons pubis or labia.
- Excisions marked should be equivalent bilaterally to aim for best, most symmetrical scar placement, and the ideal scar is hidden when the thighs come together.

■ Proximal "APEX" Thigh Lift

Posterior Portion

- The patient is marked while standing.
  - Posterior marking is made in the infragluteal fold, which the surgeon may have to choose with buttock deflation and multiple folds. This mark is connected to the anterior groin crease along the mons pubis (**TECH FIG 1A**).
  - A crescent is then marked more distally to define excision, aiming to avoid over-resection.
  - Skin is grasped and pulled tautly upward to determine skin excision.
  - The midline of the inner thigh should be marked vertically, and hatch marks may be marked posteriorly to guide closure.
- The patient is intubated on a stretcher and turned to the prone position with careful padding and protection of all potential pressure points.
- The patient is prepared with Betadine.
- If lower back lift is planned, that procedure should be performed first as the infragluteal fold marking may migrate superiorly and require revision.
- Incision is made in the gluteal fold, through the subcutaneous fat to deep fascia.
  - Vertical incision is made on the medial-most aspect of the thigh at the vertical marking.

- Dissection is then directed inferiorly toward the lower marked incision (**TECH FIG 1B**).
- Careful hemostasis is performed and the wound is irrigated.
- Local anesthetic is injected above and below the deep fascia; long-acting Marcaine is preferable.
- The amount of skin that may be safely excised is determined by pulling up on the skin flap and marking it, adjusting as needed from prior marking.
  - Local anesthetic, preferably long-acting Marcaine, is injected to the deep tissues in the wound.
- A braided no. 1 caliber suture is used to approximate the skin flap up to the ischial periosteum, which is encircled by the surgeon's fingers.
  - Proper placement in periosteum is ensured by pulling on the suture and seeing no movement in the buttock.
  - Lateral to the ischium, superficial fascia in the fat is approximated to the analogous gluteal fold fascia with 2-0 braided absorbable suture (**TECH FIG 1C**).
- The skin is closed with no. 3-0 monofilament absorbable suture to approximate deep dermis and running no. 4-0 monofilament absorbable suture as a running subcuticular suture.
- The skin is then better approximated with 4-0 nylon simple interrupted sutures (**TECH FIG 1D,E**).
- The wound is washed and dressed with cyanoacrylate glue.

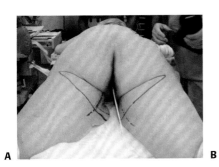
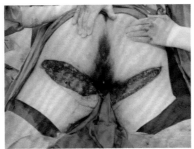
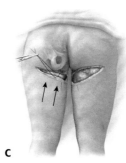

Sutures from thigh skin approximate to ischial periosteum reduce tension and create infragluteal crease

A **B** **C**

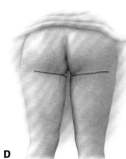

Posterior closure creates gluteal crease

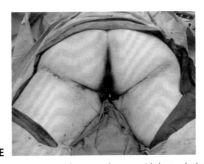

D **E**

TECH FIG 1 • A. Posterior marking is made in the infragluteal fold, which the surgeon may have to choose with buttock deflation and multiple folds. This mark is connected to the anterior groin crease along the mons pubis. A crescent is then marked to define the extent of excision. The midline of the inner thigh should be marked vertically, and hatch marks may be marked posteriorly to guide closure. **B.** Incision is made in the gluteal fold, through the subcutaneous fat to deep fascia. Vertical incision is made on the medial-most aspect of the thigh at the vertical marking. Dissection is then directed inferiorly toward the lower marked incision. **C.** Approximation of the posterior aspect of APEX thigh lift depends on deep suspension with multiple permanent sutures to ischial periosteum. **D,E.** Closure is completed superficially and defines the infragluteal crease.

Anterior Portion

- The patient is then turned supine, most safely performed by logrolling onto a stretcher with a roller on it and then pulling the patient back onto the OR bed (**TECH FIG 2A**).
  - Pillows are placed under the legs vertically to elevate the inner thigh up.
  - A small "bump" may be placed between the thighs.
  - The area is sterilized.
  - If abdominoplasty is planned, that is performed first.
- Incision in the inner thigh is continued along the groin crease, symmetric from the mons midline.
- The excision is begun from posterior to anterior in steps to assure there is no over-resection, with undermining of the marked skin quite superficially, by avoiding injury to veins and lymphatics in the groin area.

- The skin is sequentially cut, and the excision is tapered up to the lower abdomen to achieve lift of the upper anterior thigh.
  - Local anesthetic is injected to the wound and along the periosteum.
- The skin flap is approximated to pubic periosteum with no. 1 braided permanent sutures, again taking sufficient bite of periosteum to avoid labial pull and spread.
- More superior to the pelvis, approximation of superficial fascia along the upper groin and abdomen is performed with 2-0 braided absorbable suture, followed by 3-0 monofilament absorbable suture in deep dermis and running 4-0 monofilament absorbable subcuticular suture.
- The area is washed and dressed with cyanoacrylate glue (**TECH FIG 2B**).

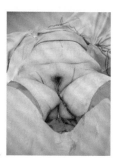 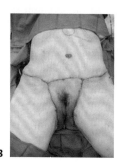

TECH FIG 2 • A. Remaining redundant inner thigh tissue is visible anteriorly in supine position. **B.** The excision proceeds from posterior to anterior with undermining of the thigh skin superficially. The skin flap is approximated to the pubic periosteum with multiple permanent sutures to avoid labial pull and spread.

▪ Extended Vertical Thigh Lift

- The patient is marked standing.
  - Skin is grasped and pulled taut toward midline of the thigh from the knee to the groin, and this area is marked as an ellipse that tapers distally to the knee and proximally along the lateral groin crease (**TECH FIG 3A,B**).
  - Cross-hatches are made to guide in closure.
- The patient is supine on the OR table, which is ideally fitted with padded leg extension boards, so the legs may be spread and allow a surgeon to stand or sit between them (**TECH FIG 3C**).

- Sterile Foley catheter is placed, and the patient is prepared with Betadine.
- Skin excision in stepwise fashion from distal to proximal using hatch marks as stop points.
  - The pinch test guides the extent of tissue removal (**TECH FIG 3D**).
  - Depth of excision should be just deep to superficial fascia to avoid injuring veins and lymphatics.
  - Perforating venous branches are ligated with clips. The skin is stapled with each stop point.

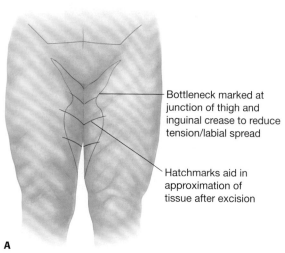

Bottleneck marked at junction of thigh and inguinal crease to reduce tension/labial spread

Hatchmarks aid in approximation of tissue after excision

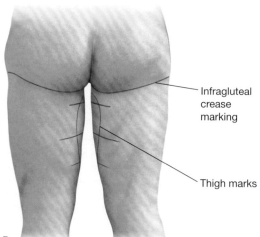

Infragluteal crease marking

Thigh marks

A   **B**

TECH FIG 3 • Extended vertical thigh lift. **A,B.** Skin markings.

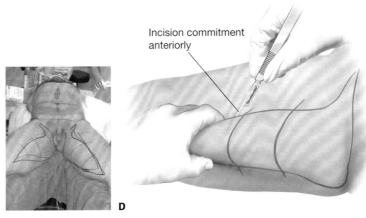

Incision commitment
anteriorly

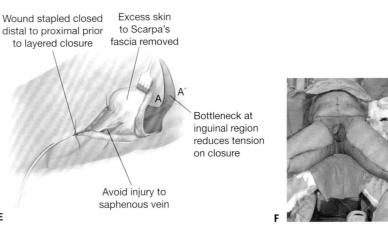

Wound stapled closed
distal to proximal prior
to layered closure

Excess skin
to Scarpa's
fascia removed

Bottleneck at
inguinal region
reduces tension
on closure

Avoid injury to
saphenous vein

TECH FIG 3 (Continued) • **C.** Patient positioning and markings. **D.** Tissue removal is guided by the pinch test. **E.** Skin excision proceeds in stepwise fashion from distal to proximal using hatch marks as stop points. Excess skin and Scarpa fascia are removed with progressive approximation from distal to proximal. Scarpa fascia is closed with 2-0 interrupted braided absorbable suture. The incision is closed over a drain. **F.** Closure in superficial fascia within the fat is performed with barbed continuous suture, and the skin is approximated in layers, dressed with cyanoacrylate glue.

- Once the pubic bone is reached, a bottleneck is made with smaller degree of skin excision to avoid tension.
  - Above this point, excision is very thin, skin only.
- A drain is passed from distal to proximal, exiting out the distal incision and fixed to the skin with 3-0 nylon suture (**TECH FIG 3E**).
  - The wound is approximated in the superficial fascial plane in fat with running barbed 0 PDO suture from midincision proximally and distally.

- The skin is closed with a 3-0 monofilament absorbable suture in deep dermis and running no. 4-0 monofilament absorbable subcuticular suture.
  - The area is washed and dressed with cyanoacrylate glue (**TECH FIG 3F**).
- The leg is wrapped from the toe to above knee with compression wrap to minimize swelling. The incision is protected by ABD pads.

PEARLS AND PITFALLS

Optimizing scar	■ The best scar results from reduction of tension on the wound, assured by limiting over-resection and by scar location and symmetry. Without gluteal augmentation, the gull wing scar leads the eye to a focused, well-contoured gluteal region. Maintaining adequate subcutaneous fat on the skin flap for autologous augmentation is critical to avoid wounds.
Optimizing wound healing	■ Avoid high tension closure and proactively address intraoperative issues such as hypothermia and anemia. Wounds are extremely common in the midportion of the incision at the lower sacrum and respond well to gentle cleansing and petrolatum application.
Avoiding lower extremity swelling	■ Avoid injury to the greater saphenous vein and lymphatic system by staying superficial to deep fascia while excising tissue. Swelling is particularly problematic with the extended vertical approach.
Avoid labial spread	■ Periosteal suspension with multiple braided permanent suture and avoidance of high tension closure are key to avoiding pull along the labia.
Improved efficiency of closure with barbed suture	■ Barbed suture works very well in the thigh because the tissues provide adequate coverage over the barbs. The quality and speed of closure are optimized by barbed suture.
Fluid collection management	■ Fluid collections near the knee are not uncommon with the extended vertical excision, as in the same region as the lymphatics in the leg. Most often, fluid collections are lymphoceles. They may be aspirated and compressed, and particularly, resistant ones can be opened and drained with a Penrose drain.

POSTOPERATIVE CARE

- Patients are followed on a weekly basis after surgery to assure optimal wound healing and drain care for the vertical approach.
  - Drains can be removed when drainage is 30 to 40 cc or less per day.
  - Compression of the leg from the toe to knee assists in preventing calf swelling.
  - If suspicious swelling develops, particularly unilaterally, ultrasound should be performed to rule out deep venous thrombosis.
- Strenuous activity may be resumed 4 to 6 weeks after surgery as long as healing is uncomplicated.
- Longer-term care is provided for scar management, including topical therapies to reduce scar visibility and massage to assist in dysesthesias and edema.

COMPLICATIONS

- Lymphedema: Best minimized by avoiding any interruption of lymphatics or veins. Compression from toe to knee and elevation may help. If swelling is asymmetrical, workup for venous thrombosis should be considered.
- Labial spread: With any procedure that creates some tension with tissue removal and lack of proper suspension of tissues around the mons. Multiple interrupted sutures suspending tissue to periosteum helps reduce risk.
- Wound healing problems are more of an issue with higher weight patients; undermining and adjunctive liposuction should be minimized. Permanent large caliber sutures around the groin may become infected with wound healing problems, necessitating removal of the exposed suture.

- Unsatisfactory scar: symmetrical treatment with sequential, stepwise tissue excision and avoidance of high tension closure assists in optimizing scar. Irregular contour of the inner thigh with vertical thigh lift is not uncommon as posterior thigh tissue is thicker than the anterior tissues, so it is important to not pull posterior tissue forward.
- Venous thromboembolism: It is necessary preoperatively to check on any history or elevated risk as per the modified Caprini scale. Patients must be encouraged to ambulate after surgery.
- Infection is not common, and risk can be reduced by optimizing surgical conditions like addressing efficiency with reduced operative time and hypothermia, as well as initial dose of antibiotics prior to making incision. Seromas can become sources of infection and should be treated.

SUGGESTED READINGS

Capella JF, Matarasso A. Management of the postbariatric medial thigh deformity. *Plast Reconstr Surg.* 2016;137(5):1434-1446.

Capella JF. The vertical medial thigh lift. *Clin Plast Surg.* 2014;41(4): 727-743.

Gusenoff JA, Coon D, Nayar H, et al. Medial thigh lift in the massive weight loss population: outcomes and complications. *Plast Reconstr Surg.* 2015;135(1):98-106.

Pannucci CJ, Barta RJ, Portschy PR, et al. Assessment of postoperative venous thromboembolism risk in plastic surgery patients using the 2005 and 2010 Caprini Risk score. *Plast Reconstr Surg.* 2012;130(2):343-353.

Richter DF, Stoff A. Circumferential body contouring: the lower body lift. *Clin Plast Surg.* 2014;41(4):775-788.

Shermak M, Shoo B, Deune EG. Prone positioning precautions in plastic surgery. *Plast Reconstr Surg.* 2006;117(5):1584-1588.

Shermak MA, Mallalieu J, Chang D. Does thigh plasty for upper thigh laxity after massive weight loss require a vertical incision? *Aesthet Surg J.* 2009;29(6):513-522.

Vertical Rectus Abdominis Myocutaneous Flap for Perineal Reconstruction

22
CHAPTER

Sahil K. Kapur and Charles E. Butler

DEFINITION

- The vertical rectus abdominis myocutaneous (VRAM) flap plays a beneficial role in improving postoperative outcomes for patients with defects created following abdominoperineal resection (APR) and pelvic exenteration (PE) surgery.
- Complications following APR and PE are related to large noncollapsible dead space, commonly irradiated dead space, with poor vascularity and bacterial contamination.[1]
- The flap provides healthy vascularized tissue to help obliterate the pelvic dead space—created after the resection. It serves as a barrier between the abdominal and pelvic cavity, as well as a source of skin and soft tissue for reconstructing and resurfacing the perineum.

ANATOMY

- The rectus abdominis muscle originates from the 6th, 7th, and 8th costal cartilages and inserts on the pubic bone. It measures approximately 6 cm in width at its origin and 3 cm in width at the insertion.
- It has a dual codominant blood supply (Type III Mathes/Nahai). Superiorly, it is supplied by the superior epigastric artery, a branch of the internal thoracic artery. Inferiorly, it is supplied by the deep inferior epigastric artery a branch of the external iliac artery.
- The deep inferior epigastric artery originates from the external iliac vessels at a point between the inguinal ligament to about 6 cm above it. The vessel enters the posterior rectus sheath at about the level of the ASIS and the arcuate line (4 to 6 cm above the pubic bone). This artery usually splits into a lateral and medial branch that supplies the lateral and medial row of myocutaneous perforators. Knowledge of perforator anatomy is important when attempting the fascial-sparing approach of VRAM harvest.
- The skin paddle for the VRAM flap is usually designed to include paraumbilical myocutaneous perforators. Extension of the skin paddle superiorly can be carried out without taking additional fascia (extended VRAM flap as described later). This is possible because the intercostal perforators supplying the extended portion have direct perforator-to-perforator connections with the epigastric perforators in the standard skin paddle.[2]

PATIENT HISTORY AND PHYSICAL FINDINGS

- Patients are assessed preoperatively to determine risk factors that would increase complication rates such as obesity, hernia, smoking, steroid treatment, and prior chemoradiation.
- A detailed surgical history is important to ensure that the patient has not had any prior surgeries that could have injured the deep inferior epigastric artery pedicle. Surgeries such as C-sections have a more medially placed scar and generally do not lead to pedicle injury. Prior abdominoplasty surgery is a relative contraindication to the use of a skin paddle because the perforators have been divided.
- Physical examination includes an examination of the abdomen and pelvic region for scars and assessment of hernias.

IMAGING

- Imaging involving CT or MRI is generally available because most patients have undergone an oncologic workup. CT images help determine the amount of diastasis, integrity and bulk of lateral abdominal musculature (in case a component separation is needed), and the presence of hernias.
- No special imaging to assess perforators is necessary for this reconstruction.

SURGICAL MANAGEMENT

Preoperative Planning

- Patients with pelvic or perineal defects benefit from pedicled VRAM flap reconstruction. The flap is based on the deep inferior epigastric artery. A skin paddle is used to provide skin resurfacing of the perineum. It can be de-epithelialized to provide bulk if necessary when the perineal skin is completely closed.

Positioning

- Patients are generally positioned in the lithotomy position by the resecting team. All areas of resection including the perineum and the abdomen beyond the level of the costal margin are prepped into the field.

Approach

- In general, two or more teams are involved. The reconstructive team will begin the operation if a fascial-sparing technique is to be used. The reconstructive team performs the laparotomy and spares the medial aspect of the anterior rectus sheath. Following the oncologic resection, the reconstructive team performs their portion of the procedure.
- The ostomy(s) are matured after the reconstruction is completed and the abdomen is closed.

■ Flap Harvest

- Make a midline skin incision, and dissect down to the linea alba (**TECH FIG 1A,B**).
- Once the rectus sheath is identified, begin dissecting laterally, superficial to the rectus sheath, to locate periumbilical and medial row perforators to the skin paddle.
- Incise the anterior rectus sheath 2 to 3 cm lateral to the midline but medial to the medial row perforators.
- Retract the rectus abdominis muscle laterally to expose the posterior rectus sheath.
- Incise the posterior rectus sheath 2 cm lateral to the midline to gain intraperitoneal access. Curve the incision back toward the linea alba at the arcuate line.
- Advance and suture the posterior rectus sheath to the anterior rectus sheath to protect the rectus abdominis muscle during the resection component of the procedure.
- Resume reconstruction once the resection has been completed. The ostomy is usually passed through the contralateral rectus abdominis muscle and matured by the primary team after the reconstruction and abdominal closure.
- Examine the perineal defect to estimate the bulk and nature of tissue needed. This information is used to decide if a skin paddle will be used or the perineal skin will be closed primarily over the flap.
- Design the skin paddle over the rectus abdominis muscle such that it will reach the defect once the muscle is transposed.

- Release the sutures that were previously placed between the anterior and posterior rectus sheath.
- Complete the soft tissue dissection to isolate the skin paddle.
- Dissect the flap from lateral to medial over the anterior rectus sheath to just lateral to the lateral row perforators.
- Incise the anterior sheath just lateral to the lateral row perforators.
- Dissect the lateral aspect of the anterior rectus sheath from the anterior surface of rectus abdominis muscle using a combination of finger dissection and electrocautery.
- Dissect carefully through areas of muscle inscriptions to prevent damage to the overlying rectus sheath or to the muscle itself.
- Dissect the rectus muscle off the posterior rectus sheath.
- Transect the rectus muscle cranial to the skin paddle and ensure the superior epigastric vascular pedicles are ligated.
- Rotate the flap medially and transpose it into the abdomen and pelvis.
- Ensure that the inferior epigastric artery and vein are dissected free from all soft tissue attachments to prevent compression and kinking of the pedicle.
- Leave the rectus muscle attached at its origin on the pelvis to prevent tension on the pedicle (**TECH FIG 1C**).
- The above described fascial-sparing approach is not advised when previous midline laparotomies, adjacent hernia sacs, and scarring prevent perforator identification.

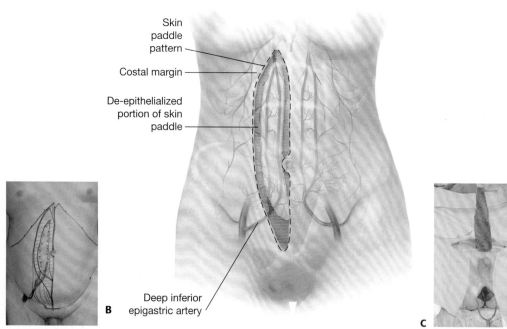

Skin paddle pattern

Costal margin

De-epithelialized portion of skin paddle

Deep inferior epigastric artery

TECH FIG 1 • Fascial-sparing approach to the harvest of a VRAM flap. **A.** The inner *solid lines* demonstrate the area of fascia harvested, *red dots* demonstrate the approximate location of perforators, and the area marked by *horizontal lines* demonstrates the area of fascial sparing. **B.** Important landmarks are indicated. **C.** VRAM flap after it has been elevated. The muscle is left connected to its origin at the pubis. (© Charles E. Butler, MD.)

Extended Skin Paddle Option

- In cases where additional bulk or length is needed, the skin paddle of the flap can be extended in the superolateral direction. Technique is described below:
  - Make a curvilinear incision starting from the superior-most aspect of the midline incision extending cephalad toward the inframamary fold and laterally toward the posterior axillary line. This line approximately parallels the general direction of the ribs. The inferior aspect of the extended skin paddle is based on the amount of laxity present to close the donor site (**TECH FIG 2**).
  - Do not incise any additional fascia with this superolateral extension. The extended portion of the flap is elevated in the subcutaneous plane.

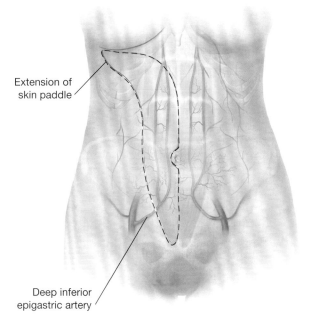

Extension of skin paddle

Deep inferior epigastric artery

TECH FIG 2 • Skin paddle design of the extended VRAM flap. (© Charles E. Butler, MD.)

Flap Inset

- After the flap has been elevated and transposed into the pelvis, place one or two 19-French round channel drains into the pelvic space.
- Inset the flap to maximize dead space fill and minimizes torque on the pedicle. If vaginal reconstruction is necessary then orient the flap with the skin paddle facing anteriorly. The skin paddle is oriented to face the anterior direction, the distalmost tip of the flap ends up posterior.
- De-epithelialize the skin paddle to the dimension necessary to reconstruct the skin defect. Use the rest of the epithelialized portion to close the perineal skin defect (**TECH FIG 3A,B**).
  - When the perineal skin is closed primarily without a skin paddle, the VRAM flap is completely de-epithelialized (**TECH FIG 3C–E**).
- Anchor the flap to remnant tissue in the pelvis using interrupted 2-0 resoluble sutures.
- Close the skin in a vest over pants fashion. Use 3-0 resorbable sutures for buried deep dermal sutures and 3-0 permanent monofilament sutures for the interrupted skin sutures.
- Two round channeled drains are used to drain the perineal space.

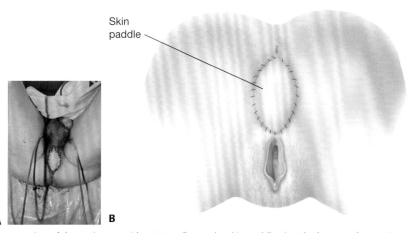

Skin paddle

A   **B**

TECH FIG 3 • **A,B.** Reconstruction of the perineum with a VRAM flap and a skin paddle. (© Charles E. Butler, MD.)

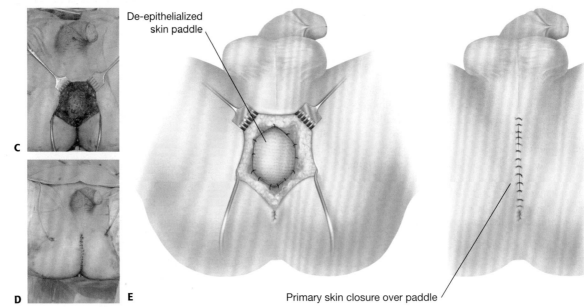

De-epithelialized skin paddle

Primary skin closure over paddle

TECH FIG 3 (Continued) • **C,D.** Reconstruction of perineum without a skin paddle. **E.** Flap in place with the skin paddle de-epithelialized. Primary closure of skin over the flap. (© Charles E. Butler, MD.)

■ Donor Site Closure

- If primary closure of the rectus sheath is not possible due to excessive tension, perform ipsilateral component separation by incising the external oblique aponeurosis and dissecting between the external and internal oblique muscles. If the fascial integrity is good, component separation will be enough (**TECH FIG 4**).
  - However, if the fascial integrity is poor or the fascial closure is tight then a mesh can be used to reinforce the closure.

- If primary closure is possible without excessive tension, suture rectus sheath using interrupted monofilament suture in figure-of-8 fashion. Include both the anterior and posterior sheath in the closure superior to the arcuate line.
- Place a round channel drain superficial to the rectus sheath to drain the subcutaneous space.
- Approximate the Scarpa fascia with interrupted 2-0 resorbable sutures.
- Approximate the skin with 3-0 resorbable sutures in a deep dermal fashion followed by a running subcuticular stitch with 4-0 resorbable sutures.

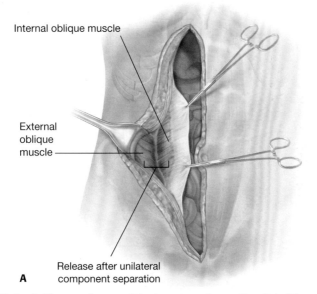

Internal oblique muscle

External oblique muscle

Release after unilateral component separation

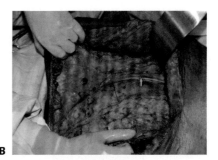

TECH FIG 4 • **A.** Diagram of open unilateral component separation. **B.** In this operative photograph, the *black line* demonstrates the extent of release. The *green arrow* indicates the fascial edge of the external oblique aponeurosis. (© Charles E. Butler, MD.)

PEARLS AND PITFALLS

Skin paddle design	■ Make sure the skin paddle is positioned appropriately such that it will include the periumbilical perforators and reach the distalmost aspect of the defect following muscle transposition. ■ If significant amount of bulk at the distal reach of the flap is required, then the extended skin paddle technique should be used as described in the techniques section.
Fascial-sparing technique	■ Fascial sparing is not advised when previous abdominal surgery, adjacent hernia sacs, and scarring prevent perforator identification.
Donor-site closure	■ Abdominal closure following VRAM harvest should be treated as a formal abdominal wall reconstruction. The scenario is more complex than encountered with a standard laparotomy. The central fascial defect on the side of the VRAM harvest, an ostomy on the contralateral side, and contamination from colon transection increase risk of wound complications and morbidity.

POSTOPERATIVE CARE

■ A foam thigh abduction pillow can be used to prevent adduction of the legs and compression of the skin paddle.

■ Patients are allowed to ambulate on the first postoperative day. No direct sitting is allowed for the first 3 weeks. Hospital stay ranges from 5 to 7 days.

OUTCOMES AND COMPLICATIONS

■ Perineal wound complication rate following APR ranges from 25% to 60%.[3]

■ Patients who undergo primary closure of APR defects have a much higher complication rate than those who undergo VRAM flap reconstruction (44% vs 16%).[4]

■ Time to perineal wound healing following wound complication is shorter for patients who undergo VRAM reconstruction compared to patients who undergo primary closure. (Average time: 65 vs 92 days).[4]

■ VRAM use is beneficial even if primary closure is possible in patients undergoing APR following chemoradiation. In these cases, patients who receive VRAM reconstruction have a significantly reduced rate of perineal abscess (9% vs 37%), wound dehiscence (9% vs 30%), and need for drainage procedures for fluid collections (3% vs 25%).[1]

■ Fascial-sparing techniques in VRAM harvest have reduced abdominal hernia rates from 11.5% to 1.5 %.[5]

■ Component separation technique for donor-site closure leads a threefold lower fascial dehiscence rate and a fourfold lower incisional hernia rate.[6]

■ The use of an underlay mesh in patients with poor fascial integrity has also reduced abdominal hernia rates (2.6% vs 5.5%).[5]

■ Reconstruction of perineal defects with the use of VRAM flaps has significant advantages over the use of thigh flaps in reducing complication rates (donor-site or recipient site cellulitis, pelvic abscess, and major wound dehiscence).[7]

REFERENCES

1. Butler CE, Gundeslioglu AO, Rodriguez-Bigas MA. Outcomes of immediate vertical rectus abdominis myocutaneous flap reconstruction for irradiated abdominoperineal resection defects. *J Am Coll Surg.* 2008;206(4):694-703.
2. Villa M, Saint-Cyr M, Wong C, Butler CE. Extended vertical rectus abdominis myocutaneous flap for pelvic reconstruction: three-dimensional and four-dimensional computed tomography angiographic perfusion study and clinical outcome analysis. *Plast Reconstr Surg.* 2011;127(1):200-209.
3. Butler CE, Rodriguez-Bigas MA. Pelvic reconstruction after abdominoperineal resection: is it worthwhile?. *Ann Surg Oncol.* 2005;12(2):91-94.
4. Chessin DB, Hartley J, Cohen AM, et al. Rectus flap reconstruction decreases perineal wound complications after pelvic chemoradiation and surgery: a cohort study. *Ann Surg Oncol.* 2005;12(2):104-110.
5. Campbell CA, Butler CE. Use of adjuvant techniques improves surgical outcomes of complex vertical rectus abdominis myocutaneous flap reconstructions of pelvic cancer defects. *Plast Reconstr Surg.* 2011;128(2):447-458.
6. Baumann DP, Butler CE. Component separation improves outcomes in VRAM flap donor sites with excessive fascial tension. *Plast Reconstr Surg.* 2010;126(5):1573-1580.
7. Nelson RA, Butler CE. Surgical outcomes of VRAM versus thigh flaps for immediate reconstruction of pelvic and perineal cancer resection defects. *Plast Reconstr Surg.* 2009;123(1):175-183.

23
CHAPTER

Gluteal Thigh Flap for Perineal Reconstruction

David Gerth and Christopher J. Salgado

DEFINITION

- Gluteal thigh flap is an axial fasciocutaneous flap based on the inferior gluteal artery.
- Usually raised as a pedicled flap, but free flap technique has been reported

ANATOMY (FIG 1)

- Blood supply: Descending branch of inferior gluteal artery[1]
  - Terminal branch of the internal iliac artery.
  - Course: exits the pelvis through the infrapiriform aperture
  - Supplies the lower aspect of the gluteus maximus muscle and overlying skin through musculocutaneous perforators[2]
    - These perforators combine with branches of the circumflex femoral arteries and obturator artery to create the cruciate anastomosis.
      - This anastomosis allows the posterior thigh to be adequately perfused even in the case of an absent inferior gluteal artery.
      - Recent study has shown that cutaneous branches supplying the distal gluteal and proximal posterior thigh can be more regularly identified.
      - 108 of 118 specimens had cutaneous branches derived from the descending branch of the inferior gluteal artery. Ten cases derived from medial or lateral circumflex femoral artery or from the profunda femoris.[3]
  - Pedicle is usually spared during radical pelvic ablations.
  - Pedicle is usually outside the area affected by pelvic radiation.[4]
- Venous drainage
  - Redundant
    - Deep system
      - Venae comitantes of inferior gluteal artery
      - Venae comitantes of deep femoral perforators
    - Superficial venous system
  - Due to substantial drainage, venous congestion rarely occurs.[5]
- Innervation: posterior femoral cutaneous nerves (S1-S3)
  - Many fascicles exit the sciatic foramen along with the inferior gluteal artery.
  - Fascicles converge to form a common trunk with the descending branch of the inferior gluteal artery.[4]

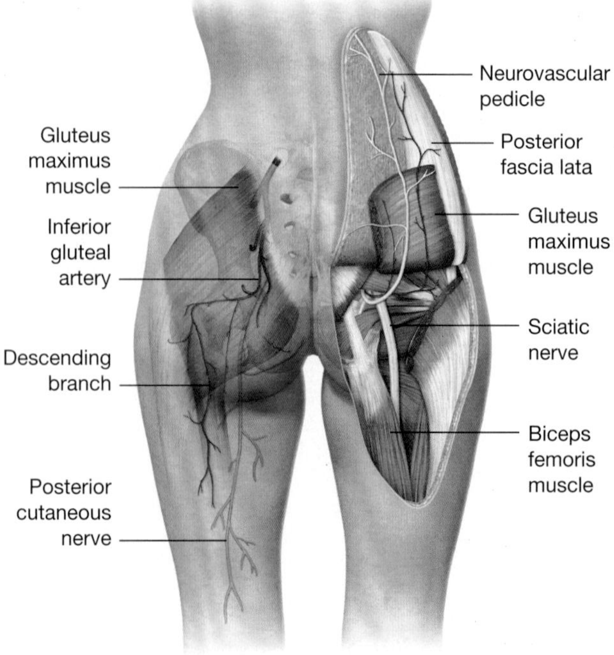

FIG 1 • Relevant surgical anatomy for the gluteal thigh flap. Note the relationship of the posterior femoral cutaneous nerve to the inferior gluteal artery. This classic relationship is not constant, however.

PATHOGENESIS

- Most common: Malignancy
- Infection
- Traumatic injury[6]

PATIENT HISTORY AND PHYSICAL FINDINGS

IMAGING

- No preoperative imaging is necessary.
- Viability of the flap can be assessed intraoperatively via quantitative fluoroangiography (**FIG 2**).

SURGICAL MANAGEMENT

- Goal of surgery
  - The process of perineal repair is especially difficult due to the necessity to preserve the anogenital triangle as well as to provide adequate skin coverage and tissue replacement.
  - Successful repair consists of appropriate reconstruction with vascularized tissue along with proper anogenital repair without leakage of feces or urine.
- Indications
  - Perineal or sacral wounds requiring resurfacing without the need of dead space closure

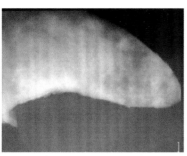

FIG 2 • Intraoperative quantitative fluoroangiography of harvested gluteal thigh flap. The patient is administered indocyanine green (ICG) intravenously, and then, after 3 minutes, the fluoroscope is placed over the flap. Within 120 seconds, adequate perfusion (if present) will register on the imaging. Certain systems may permit quantitation of perfusion relative to surrounding tissues.

- Preoperative planning
  - Before general anesthesia, the patient should be marked in an upright position.
  - The gluteal fold should be identified and marked.
  - The inferior gluteal artery can be located as it exits deep to the gluteus maximus with a mark halfway between the line from the ischial tuberosity to the greater trochanter of the femur. The course of the inferior gluteal artery can be verified with a Doppler probe.
- Positioning (**FIG 3**)

- The surgeon may position the patient in either prone or lithotomy position. The flap can be harvested in either position; positioning is dependent on location and size of the defect.
- Approach
  - The flap may be harvested as a pedicled rotation flap or as an island flap.
  - Flap size is directly contingent with thigh size and feasibility of donor-site closure.
  - The distal tip of the flap should not extend beyond the popliteal crease to minimize risk of scar deformity and scar contracture.

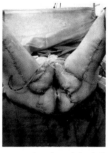

FIG 3 • Lithotomy positioning for gluteal thigh flap. Bilateral gluteal thigh flaps were harvested in this patient and inset for perineal reconstruction.

- Dissection begins at the distal aspect of the posterior thigh followed by subcutaneous tissue dissection with cauterization.
- The surgeon then dissects the flap distal to proximal. Limit is the inferior border of the gluteus maximus muscle. Proper proximal dissection with inclusion of the vascular pedicle is important for vitality. Care is taken to include the deep fascia within the contents of the flap.
- During flap elevation, the surgeon may place temporary sutures through the fascia and dermis to prevent shearing of the flap during mobilization. In the case of larger defects, bilateral flaps may be raised.[4]
- The posterior femoral cutaneous nerve is not a good reference for pedicle orientation due to its distal arborization.
- Division of the gluteus muscle inferior fibers allows for more proximal dissection of vessels and therefore a greater flap length, although this maneuver is rarely needed.
- Once fully mobilized, a deep subcutaneous tissue tunnel is created between the posterior thigh and the perineal defect. The flap is then passed through the tunnel.

- The surgeon will then mark and de-epithelialize the buried portion of the flap. Once completed, the flap is then inset into the defect.
- While avoiding the proximal vascular pedicle area, drains are placed in the pelvis and donor-site regions.
- Primary closure of the donor site can be performed or in other cases a skin graft may be necessary.[4]

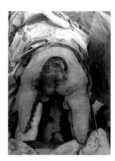

TECH FIG 1 • Elevation of bilateral gluteal thigh flaps. Patient placed in prone position.

TECHNIQUE (TECH FIG 1)

PEARLS AND PITFALLS

Technique	■ Avoid using the posterior femoral cutaneous nerve as a landmark for the vascular pedicle. ■ Divide distal fibers of the gluteus maximus to increase flap pedicle length and arc of rotation.
Postoperative care	■ Offload the perineum and the flap with no sitting for 2–3 weeks. ■ Use an air-fluidized mattress and frequent turns to decrease risk of pressure sores, especially in the case of a denervated femoral cutaneous nerve.

POSTOPERATIVE CARE

■ Due to the location of the flap and the location of the reconstruction as a whole, a 48-hour period of postoperative recovery is recommended before attempting any sort of strenuous leg movements such as walking.[4]

■ Patients should not sit at all for the first 2 to 3 postoperative weeks after which time they can gradually begin to sit again.[4]

■ A seating cushion with an open space in the middle may be used to offload the perineum while sitting.

■ Patients may experience pain up to several months after the surgery, which may impair their ability to sit.[7]

■ Routine drain care is followed, with care taken to observe output once the patient becomes mobile. The surgeon must be vigilant of any signs of infection, such as cloudy or foul-smelling drainage, increased erythema, or pain.

OUTCOMES

■ Walton et al. reported their case series of 46 patients, with 8 total complications.

■ There were two cases of flap failure:
  ▫ Thrombosed inferior gluteal artery
  ▫ Attempted free flap with subsequent venous thrombosis

■ Other case series have reported varying outcomes and complication rates, possibly due to small sample size:
  ▫ Achauer et al. reported two cases of delayed healing in seven flaps.[7]
  ▫ Friedman et al. reported their case series of 27 flaps.[4]
    • Only one failure was reported.
    • 10 of 19 patients experienced delayed wound healing.
  ▫ Saito et al. reported one case of total flap loss and two partial losses in their series of eight patients.[8]

COMPLICATIONS

■ Dysesthesia

▫ Dysesthesias may result from damage to the cutaneous nerve during surgery.[7] This loss of sensation combined with the limited mobility after surgery could lead to pressure sores. To decrease the chances of a pressure sore developing, some authors recommend placing patients on a pressure-reducing mattress.

■ Flap necrosis
  ▫ Though necrosis can result from either lack of blood flow or infection, it is relatively rare with this flap. Any fistulas that may develop need to be monitored and repaired.[8]
  ▫ When dealing with cancer patients who are undergoing radiation therapy, skin grafting may be necessary to promote wound healing.[4]

REFERENCES

1. Hurwitz DJ. Closure of a large defect of the pelvic cavity by an extended compound myocutaneous flap based on the inferior gluteal artery. *Br J Plast Surg*. 1980;33:256-261.
2. Hurwitz DJ, Swartz WM, Mathes SJ. The gluteal thigh flap: a reliable, sensate flap for the closure of buttock and perineal wounds. *Plast Reconstr Surg*. 1981;68:521-532.
3. Windhofer C, Brenner E, Moriggl B, Papp C. Relationship between the descending branch of the inferior gluteal artery and the posterior femoral cutaneous nerve applicable to flap surgery. *Surg Radiol Anat*. 2002;24:253-257, doi:10.1007/s00276-002-0064-z.
4. Friedman JD, Reece GR, Eldor L. The utility of the posterior thigh flap for complex pelvic and perineal reconstruction. *Plast Reconstr Surg*. 2010;126:146-155, doi:10.1097/PRS.0b013e3181da8769.
5. Scheufler O, et al. Anatomical basis and clinical application of the infragluteal perforator flap. *Plast Reconstr Surg*. 2006;118:1389-1400, doi:10.1097/01.prs.0000239533.39497.a9.
6. Mughal M, Baker RJ, Muneer A, Mosahebi A. Reconstruction of perineal defects. *Ann R Coll Surg Engl*. 2013;95:539-544.
7. Achauer BM, Turpin IM, Furnas DW. Gluteal thigh flap in reconstruction of complex pelvic wounds. *Arch Surg*. 1983;118:18-22.
8. Saito A. et al. Posterior thigh flap revisited: clinical use in oncology patients. *Surg Today*. 2014;44:1013-1017. doi:10.1007/s00595-013-0635-0.

Omental Flap for Pelvic Floor Reconstruction

Carrie K. Chu and Charles E. Butler

DEFINITION

- Pelvic floor defects may result from colorectal, urologic, and/or gynecologic extirpation (ie, abdominoperineal resection, pelvic exenteration) for oncologic, infectious, inflammatory, or traumatic indications.
- Goals of pelvic floor reconstruction include obliteration of dead space, prevention of pelvic and perineal hernia, avoidance of deep surgical site infection and pelvic sepsis, improved perineal wound healing, replacement of compromised perineal skin if necessary, and vaginal reconstruction when indicated.
- The omental flap can provide readily available vascularized tissue for achievement of many of these reconstructive goals with minimal donor-site morbidity and operative efficiency.[1–3]

ANATOMY

- The male pelvis is typically narrower throughout, from the pelvic brim through the outlet. The cavity is overall shaped like an inverted cone, in contrast to the wider female pelvis that more resembles a short, wide cylinder.

- The greater omentum, also called the gastrocolic omentum, is a curtain of adipose and lymphatic-rich tissue that extends from the greater curvature of the stomach and drapes over the large and small intestines while folding under itself toward the posterior abdominal wall. The posterior aspect of the reflection apposes the mesentery of the transverse colon (**FIG 1**).
- The vascular supply of the omentum derives from the right and left gastroepiploic arteries. The right gastroepiploic artery is a terminal branch of the gastroduodenal artery, which comes off of the common hepatic artery originating from the celiac axis. The left gastroepiploic artery is a branch of the splenic artery.
- Along the greater curvature of the stomach, gastric branches arise from both the right and left gastroepiploic arteries onto the anterior gastric wall, and the two vessels communicate in this manner. Multiple branches of these vessels supply the greater omentum (**FIG 2**).
- The flap may be based on either the right or left gastroepiploic artery. The pedicle should be selected based on the likelihood of maximal flap length to reach the pelvis following full mobilization. The right-sided vessel is often positioned more favorably for pelvic coverage.

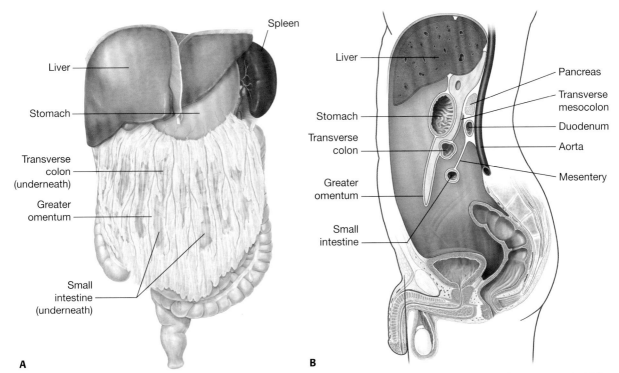

A

B

FIG 1 • **A,B.** The greater omentum extends from the greater curvature of the stomach and drapes over the large and small intestines while folding under itself toward the posterior abdominal wall. The posterior aspect of the reflection apposes the mesentery of the transverse colon.

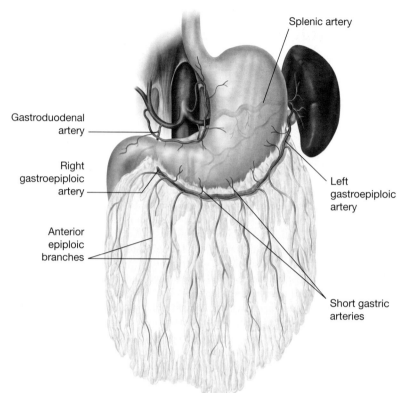

Splenic artery

Gastroduodenal artery

Right gastroepiploic artery

Anterior epiploic branches

Left gastroepiploic artery

Short gastric arteries

FIG 2 • The vascular anatomy and basis for the pedicled omental flap.

PATHOGENESIS

- Following removal of the rectum, the resultant void in the presacral space and pelvic outlet leaves noncollapsible dead space for fluid accumulation with infectious potential as well as a route for visceral herniation into the perineum. The volume of space is increased with additional resection of the bladder, prostate, uterus, and/or vagina.
- Secondary defects of the pelvic floor may occur from traumatic, obstetric, or iatrogenic etiologies.

PATIENT HISTORY AND PHYSICAL FINDINGS

- Special consideration should be given to the primary disease process and previous abdominal surgical surgery. Dense abdominal adhesions may render this flap unusable. Inflammatory processes or infectious complications may lead to distortion of the omental anatomy. Gynecologic oncologic surgeries often involve partial or total omentectomies. Prior procedures that may have compromised the source vessels of the right and left gastroepiploic vessels, including hepatectomy, pancreaticoduodenectomy, gastrectomy, and splenectomy, should all be noted.
- Physical examination should focus on body habitus, abdominal torso length, abdominal surgical scars, hernias, and evidence of intra-abdominal obesity.
- Pelvic radiotherapy may severely compromise the quality of the perineal skin.

IMAGING

- No routine imaging is necessary for preoperative planning for omental flap harvest. Computed tomography is of limited utility in assessing omental bulk, though well-timed contrast studies may facilitate visualization of branches of the celiac artery, superior mesenteric artery, and proximal gastroepiploic arteries. Magnetic resonance imaging may provide better depiction of omental volume.
- However, abdominal and pelvic cross-sectional imaging is often available as part of the primary disease workup. Review can yield useful information regarding dimensions of the pelvic inlet and outlet as well as the shape and depth of the presacrococcygeal space.

SURGICAL MANAGEMENT

- Omental flaps are most useful for filling of dead space in the pelvic cavity and separation of the intra-abdominal contents from the perineum. When perineal skin replacement is necessary due to disease involvement or radiation injury, omental flap alone will likely not suffice. Consideration should be given to use of a myocutaneous or fasciocutaneous flap instead of or in conjunction with the omental flap, depending on the size of the pelvic cavity.
- The omentum is also suitable for reconstruction of partial vaginectomy defects and can be used in conjunction with skin grafting for this purpose.[4]
- Pelvic floor reconstruction using pedicled omental flaps generally takes place at the time of the primary extirpative procedure. The usefulness of omental flap for secondary pelvic reconstruction in cases of delayed wound healing, pelvic abscess, or wound dehiscence can be limited.
- There is great individual variability in the bulk and dimensions of the greater omentum. Based on the characteristics of the omentum and the defect anatomy, each patient will require intraoperative evaluation and judgment regarding the appropriateness of this flap for pelvic reconstruction. The omentum may be used in combination with other myocutaneous flaps to accomplish the aforementioned goals.[5]

Preoperative Planning

- No routine preoperative imaging is indicated, but the aforementioned elements in the history and physical should be noted in preparation for surgery.
- Patients should be consented for thigh, gluteal, and abdominal wall donor-site alternatives, as the suitability of the flap is usually unable to be determined until the abdomen is opened.

Positioning

- There are no specific positioning requirements beyond the conventional lithotomy or, less frequently, supine positions used during primary resection, though consideration should

be given to prepping of alternative sites in case of inadequate omental mass or reach.

Approach

- A major advantage of this flap is its intra-abdominal location. Exposure beyond the extent performed by the primary surgeon is usually unnecessary. Superior extension of an infraumbilical laparotomy incision is sometimes required.
- In the setting of increasingly common laparoscopic or robotic procedures, the omentum can be similarly harvested using minimally invasive approaches with or without the assistance of a hand-assisted port for retraction.

■ Omental Flap Harvest With Right Gastroepiploic Pedicle

- Omental flaps for pelvic reconstruction are most commonly performed at the time of primary operation. Upon laparotomy, the integrity, mass, and length of the omentum are assessed for suitability for pelvic reconstruction.
- In reoperative cases, omental adhesions to the posterior abdominal wall and/or viscera may be released to preserve flap integrity.
- Following completion of the extirpative procedure, the size of the pelvic space, the dimensions of the pelvic outlet, and the extent of the perineal defect are examined. The ability of the omental flap to be mobilized into the pelvis is assessed.

Dissection

- Dissection of the omental flap begins with its mobilization off the transverse colon mesentery. The assistant gently lifts the transverse colon and retracts it inferiorly while the surgeon begins flap elevation with the cautery. Use of the surgeon's nondominant hand to lift the omentum away from the lesser sac with countertraction against the assistant motion will facilitate visualization of the appropriate plane (**TECH FIG 1**).
- The character of the globular omental fat differs in quality from the thick mesenteric fat, and care should be taken to maintain the avascular plane of separation to avoid injury to the mesentery. On the other hand, violation of the filmy attachments throughout the omentum, especially in thin patients, should be minimized as these can easily result in full-thickness defects through the omentum.
- The surgeon should be cognizant of the course of the middle colic artery, especially in reoperative abdomens, to avoid injury during flap elevation.
- The avascular plane between the omentum and the mesentery is easily taken down with cautery. However, any division of the omental tissue should be cautiously addressed and hemoclips or sutures used generously, as bleeding from the omentum can be insidious.
- As the dissection proceeds more posteriorly, the lesser sac posterior to the stomach is entered.

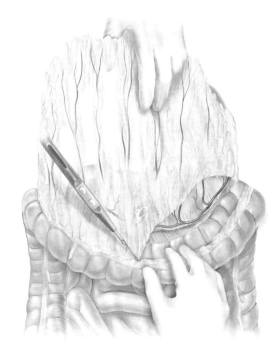

TECH FIG 1 • The omentum is dissected off the transverse colon mesentery through the avascular apposition plane, eventually entering the lesser sac.

- Once the omentum is elevated posteriorly, the mobilization is continued toward the left upper quadrant. Although it might be tempting to maximize the flap harvest in this region to increase flap length, extreme care should be taken to avoid injury to the short gastric vessels, the spleen, and the pancreatic tail. A conservative dissection leaving some omentum in the left upper quadrant is preferred to avoid injuring these vital structures.

Ligation and Division

- As the dissection approaches the proximal aspect of the greater curve, the left gastroepiploic artery will be encountered. Manual palpation can be used to confirm its position. The artery should be doubly ligated with hemoclips and/or ties prior to division (**TECH FIG 2A**).

TECHNIQUES

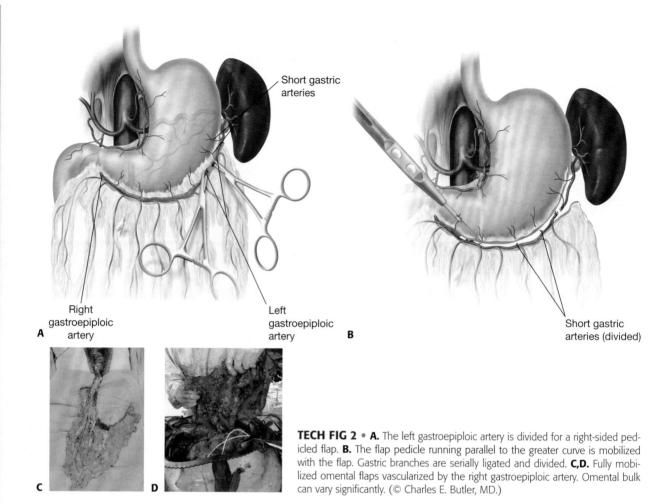

TECH FIG 2 • A. The left gastroepiploic artery is divided for a right-sided pedicled flap. **B.** The flap pedicle running parallel to the greater curve is mobilized with the flap. Gastric branches are serially ligated and divided. **C,D.** Fully mobilized omental flaps vascularized by the right gastroepiploic artery. Omental bulk can vary significantly. (© Charles E. Butler, MD.)

- The omentum is then sequentially separated from the greater curvature of the stomach. Serial gastric branches will require ligation and division.
- Bipolar energy-sealing system [Ligasure, Mansfield, MA] and ultrasonic coagulation (harmonic scalpel) are increasingly popular contact hemostatic tools used during this dissection. When larger vessels in excess of 3 mm are encountered, however, the conventional clamp-and-tie technique should be used as bleeding from one of these stumps can result in delayed catastrophic bleeding (**TECH FIG 2B**).
- When the thermal agents are used, meticulous care needs to be taken to avoid collateral injury to the adjacent gastric wall as well as the flap pedicle. The gastroepiploic arcade is located approximately one fingerbreath parallel to the greater curve and can be palpated for guidance.
- If concern arises regarding partial-thickness injury to the gastric serosa, oversewing can be performed due to the thickness of the gastric wall.
- Division is continued until the flap is of sufficient length to reach the pelvis without undue tension. For maximal safe length, the omentum can be safely mobilized just short of the pylorus, where the right gastroepiploic artery comes into direct contact with the stomach. The stomach is well vascularized via the remaining right and left gastric arteries from the lesser curve (**TECH FIG 2C,D**).

Flap Positioning

- A right-sided pedicled flap should generally be passed through the right paracolic gutter (**TECH FIG 3A**). If not already performed by the extirpative surgeon, to facilitate flap positioning, the ascending colon can be mobilized via release along the white line of Toldt.
- Alternatively, passage of the flap can be performed via the retrocolic plane through the transverse mesocolon to the right of the middle colic artery (**TECH FIG 3B**). The resultant mesocolonic defect should be repaired to prevent internal hernia.
- No suture fixation of the omentum is generally necessary in the pelvis. The flap should rest in the dependent position without excessive tension (**TECH FIG 3C**). Placement of the patient into the reverse Trendelenburg position may be useful for positioning.
- If question arises regarding viability of the distal aspect of the flap, options for flap assessment include handheld Doppler and fluorescein angiography.
- Should flap length be inadequate for reach into the pelvis without undue tension, the omentum may be transferred as a free flap using recipient vessels in the pelvis or lower abdomen.
- Additional perineal skin closure or flap reconstruction is performed as indicated.
- Laparotomy closure is performed as per routine.

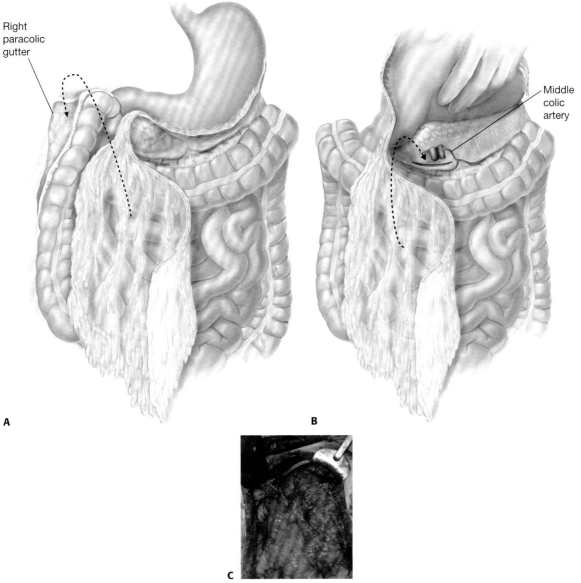

Right paracolic gutter

Middle colic artery

A

B

C

TECH FIG 3 • Inset of a right-sided pedicle flap. **A.** The omental flap may be passed through the paracolic gutter following mobilization of the white line of Toldt. **B.** Alternatively, the flap may also be passed via the retrocolic plane through the transverse or ileocolic mesocolon, across the sacrum, and into the pelvic defect. **C.** The pelvic defect is filled with the omental flap in position.

■ Omental Flap Harvest With Left Gastroepiploic Pedicle

- The flap is generally robust off either pedicle. Use of the left gastroepiploic artery can be required due to altered right upper quadrant anatomy or loss of the source vessels of the right gastroepiploic artery.
- Elevation of the omentum off the transverse colonic mesentery and into the lesser sac is performed in similar fashion as previously described.
- In the right upper quadrant, the flap is separated from the mesocolon of the hepatic flexure. As the gastroduodenal junction and the pylorus are encountered, the right gastroepiploic artery can be palpated. Secure ligation and division should be performed (**TECH FIG 4A**).

- Mobilization of the flap along the greater curvature can then proceed as described above toward the pedicle.
- The left gastroepiploic artery is the largest branch of the splenic artery. The gastric branches off of the left gastroepiploic should be taken down to no more than the middle third body of the stomach to avoid the splenic, short gastric, and pancreatic injuries as aforementioned.
- The mobilized flap can then be positioned along the left paracolic gutter into the pelvis or transmesocolonic as previously described. In the latter case, it can then be transposed to the left of the ligament of Treitz toward the pelvis (**TECH FIG 4B,C**).

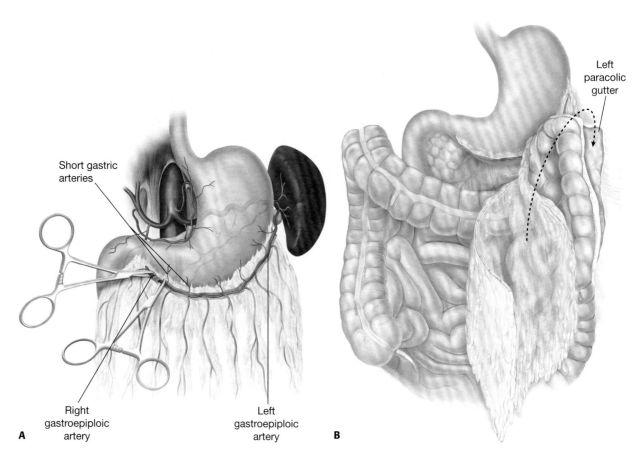

Short gastric
arteries

Right
gastroepiploic
artery

Left
gastroepiploic
artery

Left
paracolic
gutter

A

B

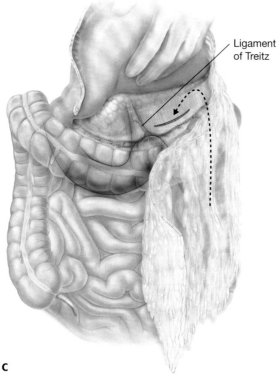

Ligament
of Treitz

C

TECH FIG 4 • A. For a left-sided pedicle, the right gastroepiploic artery is divided. **B.** Inset of a left-sided pedicle flap. For a left-sided pedicled flap, the flap can be transposed within the left paracolic gutter. The sigmoid colon and rectum have usually been mobilized. **C.** The flap may also be passed through the transverse colonic mesentery to the left of the middle colic artery and the ligament of Treitz.

■ Laparoscopic Harvest of Pedicled Omental Flap

- Laparoscopic or robotic-assisted pelvic surgery is increasingly common.
- The omentum can be harvested laparoscopically with one 10-mm periumbilical trocar and three additional 5-mm trocars in the lateral midabdomen to lower abdomen to allow for the concept of triangulation around the operative target with adequate retraction.[6] In some patients, placement of a hand port may facilitate retraction.
- The patient is placed into slight reverse Trendelenburg position. The abdomen is insufflated.
- While the assistant drives the camera with the nondominant hand and provides retraction of the transverse colon toward the patient's feet with a blunt grasper, the surgeon elevates the omentum toward the anterior abdominal wall. The hook cautery may be used to raise the flap off the transverse colon while the surgeons reposition graspers as needed to maintain adequate traction.
- Once the lesser sac is reached, the omentum is pulled down gently caudally, and a LigaSure or Harmonic device can be used to divide the omentum and to perform the release along the greater curve. Larger vessels are addressed with hemoclips, including the nonpedicle gastroepiploic vessel.
- During these steps, if a hand-assist port is in place in the lower abdominal midline, the surgeon's nondominant hand may be helpful for caudal retraction of the omentum with manual confirmation of the gastroepiploic arcade location.
- The flap can then be positioned in the pelvis as needed with the patient in reverse Trendelenburg position.

PEARLS AND PITFALLS

Preoperative considerations	■ Feasibility of the omental flap for pelvic floor reconstruction is typically assessed intraoperatively. The surgeon and patient should be prepared for alternative options from the abdominal wall, gluteal region, and thighs.
Flap elevation	■ Bleeding from the omentum can be difficult to control with conventional electrocautery and can be a source of postoperative hemorrhage. Threshold for secure hemoclip placement or surgical tying should be low.
	■ Correct use of thermal contact vascular sealing devices may be helpful in flap elevation.
	■ Awareness of the course of the middle colic artery is essential to avoid inadvertent injury.
	■ When the right gastroepiploic pedicle is used, mobilization of the omentum within the left upper quadrant should be cautiously and conservatively approached so as to avoid injury to the spleen and pancreatic tail.
Flap inset	■ If tension-free positioning within the pelvis cannot be achieved following full mobilization, an alternative flap must be considered. Partial flap necrosis due to excess tension can result in pelvic sepsis and perineal wound breakdown.

POSTOPERATIVE CARE

- Traditionally, the dogmatic practice of nasogastric decompression after omental flap mobilization is thought to decrease gastric distension and manage expected postoperative ileus. Prevention of gastric distention has also been theorized to reduce the risk of hemoclip dislodgement from the ligated stumps of the branches along the greater curve.
- However, enhanced recovery initiatives are now increasingly prevalent. Avoidance of empiric postoperative nasogastric tube use unless strictly indicated is in keeping with the early feeding regimens and prompt patient mobilization that facilitate quicker recovery without compromising patient outcomes.
- If patients become symptomatic with severe nausea, belching, emesis, and/or bloating, abdominal radiograph may be considered for gastric distension. Nasogastric tube insertion should then be performed as indicated.

OUTCOMES

- Comparison of complication rates in patients who were primarily closed following abdominoperineal resection or pelvic exenteration with those in patients who received omental flaps consistently demonstrates improved outcomes in the latter group. In a study of 29 patients with omental flaps either alone or in combination with another flap, and 41 without omental flaps, the incidence of major pelvic complications (abscess, dehiscence, hernia, bowel obstruction, fistula) was greater in the group that did not receive omental flap reconstruction (61% vs 21%, $P < .01$).[2,7]
- A systematic review of 14 studies (457 proctectomy patients with omental flap and 332 without) with median follow-up of 13.5 months demonstrated superior primary wound healing rate (66.8% vs 50.1%), shorter time to wound healing (24 vs 79 days), and lower wound infection rate (14.4% vs 18.5%) in patients who underwent omentoplasty.

COMPLICATIONS

- Bleeding
- Splenic injury
- Mesocolon injury, including disruption of the middle colic vessels
- Pedicle injury during mobilization along the greater curvature
- Gastric wall injury
- Partial flap loss
- Paralytic ileus
- Pancreatic injury
- Perineal delayed wound healing
- Perineal hernia
- Intestinal obstruction

REFERENCES

1. Hultman CS, Carlson GW, Losken A, et al. Utility of the omentum in the reconstruction of complex extra peritoneal wounds and defects. *Ann Surg.* 2002;235:782-795.
2. Hultman CS, Sherrill MA, Halvorson EG, et al. Utility of the omentum in pelvic floor reconstruction following resection of anorectal malignancy: patient selection, technical caveats, and clinical outcomes. *Ann Plast Surg.* 2010;64:559–562.
3. Momoh AO, Kamat AM, Butler CE. Reconstruction of the pelvic floor with human acellular dermal matrix and omental flap following anterior pelvic exenteration. *J Plast Reconstr Aesthet Surg.* 2010;63:2185-2187.
4. Kusiak JF, Rosenblum NG. Neovaginal reconstruction after exenteration using an omental flap and split-thickness skin graft. *Plast Reconstr Surg.* 1996;97:775-781.
5. Campbell CA, Butler CE. Use of adjuvant techniques improves surgical outcomes of complex vertical rectus abdominis myocutaneous flap reconstruction of pelvic cancer defects. *Plast Reconstr Surg.* 2011;128:447-458.
6. Kamei Y, Torii S, Hasegawa T, Nishizeki O. Endoscopic omental harvest. *Plast Reconstr Surg.* 1998;102:2450-2453.
7. Killeen S, Devaney A, Mannion M, et al. Omental pedicle flaps following proctectomy: a systematic review. *Colorectal Dis.* 2013;14:e634-e645.

Posterior Labial Artery Flap for Vulvar and Vaginal Reconstruction

CHAPTER 25

Chris A. Campbell

DEFINITION

- The posterior labial artery flap commonly known as the Singapore flap or pudendal thigh flap is a thin fasciocutaneous flap oriented along the groin crease within the perineum.[1]
- The flap's pedicle, the posterior labial artery, is a branch of the internal pudendal artery system.
- Unilateral or bilateral posterior labial artery flaps are commonly used for vulvar resurfacing and vaginal reconstruction.

ANATOMY

- The posterior labial artery flap is inferiorly based with its axis along the groin crease including the thin skin lateral to the labia majora medially and the medial thigh skin laterally.
- The flap's pedicle is the posterior labial artery, which courses above the deep perineal fascia, arising from the perineal artery as it pierces the Colles (superficial perineal) fascia. The perineal artery branches off of the internal pudendal artery that emerges from the pudendal canal located 1 cm medial and inferior to the ischial tuberosity.
- The flap's skin paddle can be up to 15 cm long by 6 cm wide in the adult with the base of the flap even with the posterior edge of the introitus.[2]
- The posterior labial branches of the pudendal nerve innervate the most posterior aspect of the skin paddle providing sensation to the reconstruction.

PATHOGENESIS

- Vulvar or vaginal defects resulting from resection of squamous cell carcinomas, extensive condyloma, lichen sclerosis, fistulas, necrotizing soft tissue infections, and other cutaneous conditions have been reconstructed with unilateral or bilateral posterior labial artery flaps.
- In the pediatric population, bilateral posterior labial artery flaps have been used for total vaginal reconstruction in cases of vaginal atresia.

PATIENT HISTORY AND PHYSICAL FINDINGS

- When approaching vulvar or vaginal reconstruction, evaluate the abdomen, thighs, and inguinal region to maintain rectus and thigh-based flap alternatives to the posterior labial artery flap, in the event significant tissue bulk is required.
- If the patient has had pelvic radiation to treat malignancy, the exam should focus on the quality of the groin and medial thigh skin to determine if it is within the radiated field. A severely radiated groin crease can increase the risk of partial flap loss and wound healing complications.

- Measure the surface area of vulvar skin or vaginal mucosa that requires resurfacing to ensure that this amount of groin crease skin is redundant to allow for closure of the donor site.

IMAGING

- Computed tomography of the pelvis will be part of the standard preoperative evaluation of patients requiring resection of vaginal abnormalities that will require subsequent reconstruction.
- The posterior labial artery flap lacks bulk and as such is used to resurface the posterior or circumferential vagina or vulvar skin.[3] Larger tumors that require pelvic exenteration will need alternative or additional flaps that provide soft tissue bulk in addition to skin resurfacing.

SURGICAL MANAGEMENT

- Unilateral or paired posterior labial artery flaps are used to reconstruct partial or circumferential vaginal defects, respectively, and to resurface vulvar defects with thin pliable skin.
- When total vaginal reconstruction is required, bilateral posterior labial artery flaps are sewn together and rotated into the pelvic defect producing a natural physiologic angle of inclination of the reconstructed vagina.[4]
- Key considerations for use of the posterior labial artery flap include the ability to cover the vaginal or vulvar defect surface area with adjacent available groin skin within the design of the Singapore flap and whether the skin paddles are within fields of significant pelvic radiation.

Preoperative Planning

- Pathology findings from prior biopsies and imaging studies should be reviewed to confirm the planned extirpation involving the vulva and/or vagina.
- All resections that include the vagina will be preceded by an examination under anesthesia to determine if there has been disease progression and to confirm the planned resection and reconstruction.
- A Foley catheter should be placed to protect urethral structures if total vaginectomy is required and to assist the patient with recovery.

Positioning

- The patient is placed in the lithotomy position on the operating table for both the extirpative portion of the operation and the vulvar and/or vaginal reconstruction with one or both posterior labial artery flaps (**FIG 1A**).

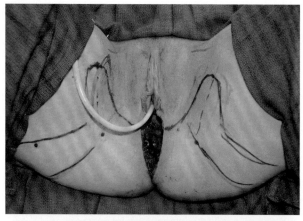

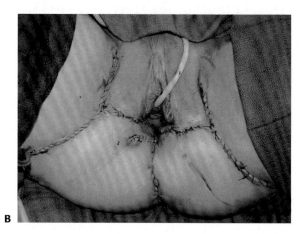

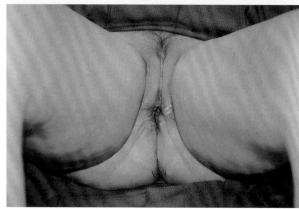

FIG 1 • Operative photos of bilateral posterior labial artery flaps for posterior vaginal reconstruction after rectal cancer resection. **A.** The patient is in lithotomy position with bilateral posterior labial artery flaps marked. Gluteal advancement flaps are also marked to obliterate the dead space from the abdominoperineal resection. **B.** Bilateral posterior labial artery flaps have been rotated into the pelvic defect to resurface the posterior and lateral surfaces of the vagina. **C.** Six months after surgery with donor-site incisions camouflaged within the groin creases and return of sexual function.

■ If other flap options are being considered for vulvar, vaginal, or perineal reconstruction, also prep the thighs down to the knees, lower buttocks, and lower abdomen to include abdominal, buttock, and thigh-based flap options.

Approach

■ For vulvar skin defects and vaginal defects where the wound interrupts the posterior introitus, the posterior labial artery flaps are rotated directly into the defect (**FIG 1B**).

■ For cases where the labial structures are not interrupted by the resection or in cases of vaginal atresia reconstruction, the posterior labial artery flaps are tunneled underneath posterolateral structures of the introitus as island flaps before inset.

T E C H N I Q U E S

■ Posterior Labial Artery Flap Design

■ The flap skin paddle is centered on the groin crease with the base of the flap being set at the most posterior point of the vaginal introitus.

■ Maximal flap length has been described as 15 cm in the adult female. A skin paddle that measures 6-cm wide can be closed primarily within the groin crease of the average adult.

■ Posterior Labial Artery Flap Elevation

■ Incise the skin of apex and medial and lateral edges of the planned skin paddle passing through subcutaneous fat and the deep perineal fascia and medial thigh fascia.

■ Elevate the flap from the anterior tip of the skin paddle and then proceed proximally in a subfascial plane to elevate the posterior labial artery with the flap. This dissection will continue until the posterior edge of the introitus is reached (**TECH FIG 1A**). The transverse fibers

of the superficial perineal musculature will provide resistance to further elevation of the deep fascia at this level.

■ For flaps elevated as an island flap intended to go underneath an intact edge of the introitus, additional dissection is performed posterior to the skin paddle. Dissect in the subcutaneous plane 4 cm beveling posteriorly to free the proximal edge of the skin paddle for medial tunneling into the defect (**TECH FIG 1B**). Do not violate the fascia on the posterior border of the skin paddle to avoid injury to the pedicle.

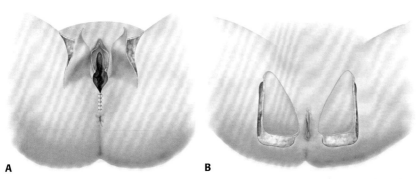

TECH FIG 1 • Bilateral posterior labial artery flap elevation. **A.** Skin paddles of posterior labial artery rotation flaps elevated in a subfascial plane from anterior to posterior stopping at the posterior edge of the introitus. **B.** For the design of bilateral posterior labial artery island flaps, a posterior incision is made through the skin with posteriorly beveled subcutaneous dissection for 4 cm. This additional posterior dissection allows the flap to be able to be tunneled under the intact posterolateral introitus to reach the pelvic defect.

■ Posterior Labial Artery Flap Rotation

- For defects that include a portion of the introitus, the posterior labial artery flaps are rotated directly into the defect (**TECH FIG 2A**). For vaginal reconstruction where the introital opening is intact, subcutaneous tunnels are created to pass the posterior labial artery flap as an island flap (**TECH FIG 2B**).

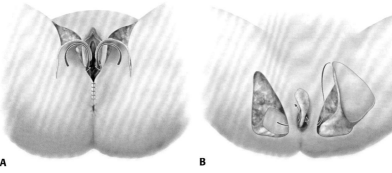

TECH FIG 2 • Bilateral posterior labial artery flap rotation: **A.** Bilateral posterior labial artery rotation flaps will be turned inward to reconstruct the vaginal defect. **B.** Bilateral posterior labial artery island flaps will be tunneled underneath intact skin flaps to reconstruct vaginal defects where the introitus is intact or in congenital cases such of vaginal atresia.

■ Posterior Labial Artery Flap Closure and Inset

- The medial edge of the skin paddles will be sewn to one another to create the posterior surface of the vaginal canal (**TECH FIG 3A**). For defects limited to posterior vaginal reconstruction, the lateral and distal edges of the combined skin paddle are sewn to the mucosal edges of the defect to complete the reconstruction.
- For total vaginal reconstruction, the lateral edges of the skin paddle are sewn to one another to create the anterior edge of the vaginal canal (**TECH FIG 3B**).
- Finally, the flap donor sites are closed in layers. The incision and resulting scar are camouflaged within the groin crease.

TECH FIG 3 • Bilateral posterior labial artery flap closure and inset. **A.** For total vaginal reconstruction, the medial edges of the skin paddles are sewn together to produce the posterior aspect of the vagina. **B.** The lateral edges of the skin paddles are sewn together to produce the anterior aspect of the vagina.

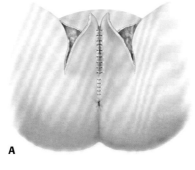
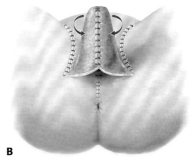

PEARLS AND PITFALLS

Preoperative evaluation	▪ It is critical to understand the extent of the planned resection to know if soft tissue bulk is required. Posterior labial artery flaps are thin pliable fasciocutaneous flaps. Therefore, another flap should be chosen for large volume defects.
Physical examination	▪ If the groin skin is firm and darkened from prior pelvic radiation, another flap should be chosen to avoid partial flap loss and wound dehiscence.
Technique—flap elevation	▪ The deep perineal fascia overlying the perineal musculature and the deep adductor fascia overlying the medial thigh should be elevated with the flap to avoid harm to the neurovascular pedicle.
Technique—bilateral flap rotation	▪ Subcutaneous dissection proximal to the skin paddle is required to allow for appropriate rotation of bilateral island flaps beneath the posterolateral introitus for total vaginal reconstruction. If not performed, the proximal portion of the skin paddles cannot be approximated without tension and will alter the incline of the resulting vaginal angle.
Postoperative care	▪ For patients requiring partial vaginal reconstruction in low estrogen states, consult with a gynecologic oncologist to determine if estrogen replacement or inserts may be required to prevent wound healing trouble due to vaginal mucosal atrophy.

POSTOPERATIVE CARE

▪ Maintain single shoulder's width leg positioning when lying or ambulating for the first 2 weeks after surgery.

▪ If the reconstruction only involves vaginal reconstruction, then brief episodes of sitting are permitted. A sidesaddle posture of favoring one buttock and then the other is encouraged. If there is also a perineal reconstruction with suture lines posterior to the introitus, then limiting head of bed to 45 degrees or less for 2 weeks without radiation and up to 4 weeks in the presence of preoperative radiation is required.

▪ The patient should wear dry gauze to the surgical site that is changed frequently to avoid skin maceration. The incision and resulting scar will be camouflaged within the groin crease (**FIG 1C**).

▪ Daily showering is recommended.

OUTCOMES

▪ Sexual adjustment after vaginal reconstruction is only successful in about half of women, with problems such as dryness, discomfort, or self-consciousness decreasing success.[5]

COMPLICATIONS

▪ Partial flap loss at the tip of the flap and wound dehiscence of the posterior vaginal closure and groin crease donor site are infrequent but do occur. Supportive dressing care is the mainstay of treatment.

▪ Premenopausal women following chemotherapy and postmenopausal patients with vaginal atrophy who require partial vaginal reconstruction may be more likely to exhibit remnant vaginal narrowing and skin flap dehiscence and may require estrogen replacement orally or in the form of vaginal inserts in the post-op period.

▪ Foreshortened reconstructed vaginas either due to cicatricial shortening or flap design may contribute to problems with sexual adjustment requiring vaginal dilatation.

REFERENCES

1. Wee JTK, Joseph VT. A new technique of vaginal reconstruction using neurovascular pudendal thigh flaps: a preliminary report. *Plast Reconstr Surg.* 1989;83:701-709.
2. Gleeson NC, Baile W, Roberts WS, et al. Pudendal thigh fasciocutaneous flaps for vaginal reconstruction in gynecologic oncology. *Gynecol Oncol.* 1994;54:269-274.
3. Cordeiro PG, Pusic AL, Disa JJ. A classification system and reconstructive algorithm for acquired vaginal defects. *Plast Reconstr Surg.* 2002;110(4):1058-1065
4. Woods JE, Alter G, Meland B, Podratz K. Experience with vaginal reconstruction utilizing the modified Singapore flap. *Plast Reconstr Surg.* 1992;90:270-274.
5. Mericli AF, Martin JP, Campbell CA. An algorithmic anatomical subunit approach to pelvic wound reconstruction. *Plast Reconstr Surg.* 2016;137(3):1004-1017.

Vertical Rectus Abdominis Flap for Perineal Reconstruction

Dhivya R. Srinivasa and Jeffrey H. Kozlow

DEFINITION

- Perineal reconstruction is often required after oncologic resections for anorectal, gynecologic, and/or genitourinary tumors. Other etiologies including inflammatory bowel disease (IBD), trauma, and necrotizing infections can also be treated in a similar fashion after control of the destructive process.
- The defect can be defined in two components: the internal pelvic outlet defect and the external skin/soft tissue defect.
- Because radiation therapy is an integral component of locoregional tumor management, the surgeon must consider the implications of radiation.
- Although multiple options are available to the reconstructive surgeon, a pedicled vertical rectus abdominis myocutaneous (VRAM) flap is one of the workhorse flaps for reconstruction of the perineum. The VRAM flap allows for harvest of varying combinations of the muscle, fascia, subcutaneous fat, and skin with tailoring of components to the acquired defect. The soft tissues of the VRAM are robust and reliable in anatomy, making this an attractive option for many reconstructive surgeons.

ANATOMY

- The surgeon must be well learned in pelvic and perineal anatomy including the following components:
  - Genitourinary: Bladder, seminal vesicles, and prostate
  - Gynecologic: Ovaries, uterus, cervix, and vagina
  - Colorectal: Rectum, levator muscles, and anus
- FIG 1 depicts a sagittal schematic of the male and female pelvis.
- In colorectal and perianal resections, the presence or absence of the levator musculature following extirpation can determine the need for pelvic outlet volume to fill the defect and close the pelvic floor. Removal of all the soft tissue in the pelvic outlet will result in a defect that will not collapse down due to the surrounding bony architecture, resulting in postresection "dead space."
- The abdomen is a readily available donor site for perineal reconstruction. It is remote from the zone of radiation, has a pedicle that originates close to the pelvis, and commonly has lax soft tissue.
- In most cases of perineal reconstruction, the donor site can be closed primarily. Component separation is a useful adjunct if needed to facilitate tension-free primary fascial closure.[1]
- The VRAM flap derives blood supply from the deep inferior epigastric artery (DIEA), a branch of the external iliac arterial system as depicted in FIG 2. Dissection of the flap pedicle

into the pelvis provides maximal arc of rotation. The DIEA and venae comitantes are predictably located on the underside of the rectus muscle, exiting into the pelvis along the lateral aspect of the muscle.

PATHOGENESIS

- Resection of anorectal and urogenital tumors is most often the impetus for perineal reconstruction. Although staging and management can be complex, a significant portion of these tumors undergo surgical therapy along with radiation for curative intent.
  - The use of neoadjuvant radiation portends approximately a 60% risk of complications including abscess, wound dehiscence, and enterocutaneous fistula. The introduction of vascularized, nonradiated tissue to the surgical site can significantly decrease the risk of major complications.[2]
  - Subsequent systematic reviews and meta-analyses have confirmed the benefits of local tissue transfer for perineal reconstruction.[3]
- In female patients, rectal tumors can also invade the posterior vagina requiring an even more complex reconstruction following extirpation. An example of this type of defect is pictured in FIG 3.
- Anal tumors are treated primarily with the Nigro protocol, of which radiation is a key component. However, salvage of recurrent disease requires abdominoperineal resection with a wide skin margin resulting in a more significant external defect. Primarily closing the perineal defect is often wrought with complications due to tension, pressure, and radiation injury. Thus, soft tissue reconstruction with regional flaps can improve wound healing and decrease complications.[4]
- Primary vulvar and vaginal tumors present similar challenges as do anorectal tumors but also require consideration of a functional reconstruction. Vulvar and vaginal tumors can be resected sans radiation, but locally advanced tumors, high-risk tumors, and positive margins can be treated with external beam radiation. Specifically for vulvovaginal reconstruction, restoration of appearance and function has quality of life benefits in addition to decreased wound healing complications.[5,6]
- IBD, namely Crohn disease, can present with fistulas and recurrent abscesses.
  - Recalcitrant disease that fails medical management is often treated surgically, and abdominoperineal resection is reserved for a severe disease affecting quality of life.

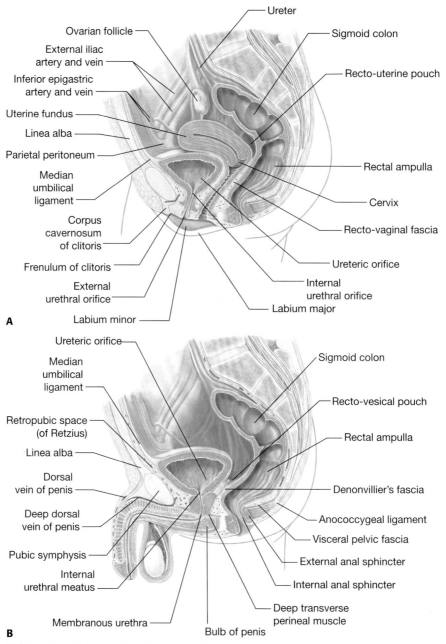

FIG 1 • **A.** Sagittal view of female anatomy. **B.** Sagittal view of male anatomy.

- Inherently, these patients are high risk for wound complications. Most have been on chronic immunosuppressive therapy with corticosteroids and other immune modulators. Further, the tissue has been inflamed for years, with notable friability.
- The introduction of healthy vascular tissue improves wound healing and decreased incidence of major complications.[7]
- Other etiologies for perineal defects include trauma and necrotizing infections, which require full debridement of nonviable tissue prior to reconstruction.

PATIENT HISTORY AND PHYSICAL FINDINGS

- Perineal reconstruction can be performed for a multitude of indications, and a thorough history should include pertinent information to each of these conditions.

- Prior to deciding on a reconstructive plan, the following information should be obtained.
  - Extent of planned defect focusing critically on:
    - Amount of external skin resection
    - Maintenance or resection of the levator complex
    - Vaginal involvement in anorectal tumors
    - Presence of fistulas, which may require extended resection margins
  - History of radiation or planned adjuvant radiation therapy
  - Past abdominal/pelvic surgery including approaches that may have sacrificed the DIEA such as a Maylard approach to gynecologic surgeries.
  - Patient goals: For resections involving the vagina, is restoration of sexual function possible and/or desired?

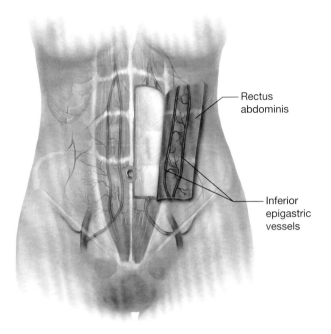

FIG 2 • Vascular anatomy of the deep inferior epigastric vessels.

■ Relevant surgical risk factors for delayed wound healing including:
  • Tobacco usage
  • Current or previous steroid use
  • Other immune modulator medications received or planned
■ Physical examination should include a thorough examination of the perineum and abdominal donor site.
  ■ Perineal examination should include evaluation of external structures, extent of radiation damage, and an understanding of the planned resection (including margins). Full examination of the genitalia and anus/rectum gives a better understanding of the planned resection, although ongoing radiation treatment may affect this estimate.
  ■ Donor-site examination should evaluate for previous surgical scars, tissue laxity, and skin quality of the anterior abdominal wall. The skin should be adequately lax for primary closure. A "pinch test" of the skin can offer a rough estimate of the maximum skin paddle width that will still be closed primarily. Previous or planned stomas should also be noted, along with the presence of any ventral hernias.

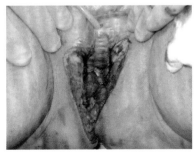

FIG 3 • Intraoperative defect involving the skin of the perineum, pelvic outlet soft tissue, and posterior wall of the vagina.

IMAGING

■ Preoperative imaging for cancer staging can offer details on degree of locoregional tumor involvement and necessary margins for resection. Imaging of the abdominal donor site is typically not necessary unless there is concern of DIEA patency.

SURGICAL MANAGEMENT

Preoperative Planning

■ Preoperative planning hinges on clear communication with the surgeon performing the resection. A discussion of planned margins, structures to be removed, the location of stoma(s), and adjuvant cancer therapies should be held prior to planning reconstruction.
■ Location of any previous and planned stomas can help guide which rectus is most amenable for flap harvest.
■ Discussion on port site locations for laparoscopic surgery is also important. Certain paramedian port sites may injure the DIEA vessel or rectus muscle.
■ Delayed reconstruction may be indicated if margins are likely to be positive.

Positioning

■ The patient will likely be positioned in lithotomy for the resection. The entire abdomen from below the nipples, including the perineum, and bilateral legs should be prepped to below the knee, exposing the medial and lateral thigh. The exposure should allow for alternative flap harvests as the ability to predict the defect is not always accurate preoperatively.
■ Appropriate padding of all pressure points is mandatory. Common peroneal and femoral nerve branches can develop neuropraxias with prolonged lithotomy positioning.
■ Bilateral lower extremity sequential compression devices (SCD) should be placed for deep venous thrombosis prophylaxis.
■ A safety belt should be used for all cases.
■ A warming blanket should be placed on the upper body to optimize normothermic core temperatures during the case.

Approach

■ Preoperative markings for a vertical rectus flap may not be necessary, but any midline or laparoscopic incisions should be discussed with the oncologic surgeon.
  ■ If a midline incision is used, it should be placed on the flap side of the umbilicus.
  ■ If laparoscopic incisions are used, discuss proximity of paramedian incision to the rectus and the deep inferior epigastric vessels. Move these incisions lateral to the rectus sheath if possible.
■ If a lower midline incision is used, the fascia (anterior sheath) is incised at the level of the medial row perforators cephalad to the existing incision to preserve as much fascia as possible.
■ The final skin paddle is often designed after the full nature of the defect is known. A pinch test can be used to confirm that the skin can be closed primarily, although typically 6 to 7 cm is the most needed and this can be harvested easily from most abdomens.

■ Incision

- The patient does not need specific markings preoperatively; however, incisions should be discussed with the oncologic surgeon.
- When a lower midline incision is used by the resecting surgeon, the cephalad extension of the incision through the fascia can be paramedian, at the level of the medial row perforators. This will allow adequate perfusion to the skin paddle but also preserve the fascia. This requires incision of the anterior sheath only as the muscle can be elevated off the posterior sheath.[8]
    - Design the skin paddle according to abdominal skin laxity and the size of the perineal defect (**TECH FIG 1**). This is typically designed such that the medial border of the flap is still in the midline.
    - An oblique skin paddle can be used, known as an oblique rectus abdominis myocutaneous flap, or ORAM, which is a semiarticulating skin and soft tissue paddle overlying the muscle. The incision then extends laterally below the costal margin. Here, the periumbilical perforators perfuse the oblique skin paddle and should be maintained as they pass through the rectus.

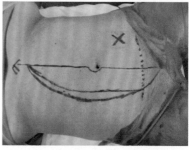

TECH FIG 1 • On-table markings for a VRAM flap. Note that the flap is situated on the contralateral side from the planned stoma. Further, the incision is on the flap side when curving around the umbilicus.

■ Elevation of Rectus and Skin Paddle

- Elevate the rectus from the posterior sheath. Keep in mind that the pedicle runs on the posterior surface of the muscle and should not be injured in this dissection. There will be lateral branches and the motor nerves that also must be divided.
- Transect the cephalad muscle and suture ligate the superior epigastric vessels.

- Once the entirety of the rectus and the overlying skin paddle is elevated, gently free the deep inferior epigastric pedicle as it exits the lateral border of the muscle. It will travel into the pelvis. Here, carefully ligate all small branches to avoid undue bleeding, which can be difficult to control in this region.
    - Incise the posterior rectus sheath for gentle curvature of the pedicle without undue kinking when the flap is passed into the perineal defect.

■ De-epithelization and Transposition of Skin Paddle

- In order to transpose the flap into the pelvis, the posterior sheath must be incised transverse inferiorly so that the pedicle is not kinked with transfer to the pelvis. This division of the posterior sheath is made well below the arcuate line, so there is little effect on closure strength.
    - **TECH FIG 1B** shows the elevated rectus with the skin paddle prior to inset (**TECH FIG 2**). The skin paddle can be de-epithelized inferiorly. For defect requiring both posterior vagina and perineum skin reconstruction, an hourglass skin paddle is designed by de-epithelization. This is best done prior to inset.
- The flap is then transposed into the pelvis with a gentle twist to allow the skin paddle to be used for external reconstruction.

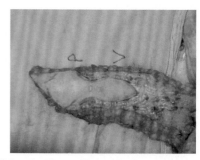

TECH FIG 2 • The skin paddle can be de-epithelialized in an hourglass pattern to allow for combined posterior vagina (*V*) and perineum skin reconstruction (*P*). The remainder of the de-epithelized flap provides bulk to fill the pelvic outlet.

Closure

- Abdominal donor-site closure requires approximation of the fascia and skin.
  - For fascial closure, primary tension-free approximation is best. If needed, an anterior component separation can be performed on the contralateral side with or without a mesh to decrease postoperative abdominal bulge or hernia.[9]
- The soft tissue should be closed in layers (Scarpa fascia, dermis, and skin).
- Inset of the flap should allow for tension-free closure as seen in **TECH FIG 1C** (**TECH FIG 3**).
  - The muscle should be used to fill the intra-abdominal pelvic defect.

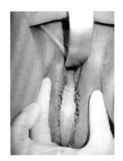

TECH FIG 3 • Inset of VRAM for perineal reconstruction. Part of the skin paddle was used to reconstruct the posterior wall of the vagina. The remainder of the skin paddle was used for the perineal incision.

PEARLS AND PITFALLS

Markings	■ Incisions should be discussed with the oncology surgeon. The incision should be placed on the side of the flap adjacent to the umbilicus
Spare fascia	■ The medial extent of the incision can be paramedian; to spare fascia, the anterior sheath can be incised at the level of the medial row perforators
Reduce hernia and abdominal bulge	■ Component separation can be used in patients where primary closure without tension is not possible ■ Fascia-sparing technique
Vaginal defects	■ The skin paddle can be tubed to reconstruct vaginal defects, whereas the muscle is used to fill in the intra-abdominal defect
Plan B	■ Alternative flaps should be available and prepped into the field. The thigh is a good alternative donor site (gracilis or ALT)
Tunnel for pedicled VRAM	■ Release the posterior sheath to allow passage of the flap without kinking

POSTOPERATIVE CARE

- Postoperative restrictions: For perineal reconstruction, it is important that the patient does not place direct pressure on the flap by sitting or lying directly supine. Orders should be written for turns every 2 hours, and the patient can lie on one side or the other, but not directly supine if this would put pressure on the flap. Foam wedges and bumps can be used to offload pressure as well.
- Care should also be taken to avoid hip abduction or complete hip flexion as this can put strain on or kink the pedicle.
- We allow patient ambulation on postoperative day 1 or 2 with the aid of physical therapy. However, sitting is not allowed for 3 weeks postoperatively and gradually advanced with proper cushioning.
- Drain management: Hematomas and seromas can place undue pressure on the flap and pedicle, therefore compromising flow. Pay careful attention to drain output, and any hematomas should be drained operatively.
- Flap monitoring: Nursing staff should monitor the flap overnight, with checks for capillary refill, color, and warmth every 2 to 4 hours. A Doppler stitch can be used if needed. Evidence of congestion or ischemia should be noted immediately. Sometimes, release of sutures can help if undue tension is the source of the problem. Concerns for

vascular compromise should prompt operative exploration to evaluate kinking or pressure on the pedicle.
- Review the pathology results to confirm margins are negative from the original resection for all oncologic procedures.

COMPLICATIONS

- Flap loss: Complete flap loss is due to compromise of the vascular pedicle. Ideally, this would be discovered soon postoperatively with subsequent operative salvage. However, in the case of irreversible flap loss, the tissue should be removed and other reconstructive options should be explored.
- Wounds: Delayed wound healing in the perineum is relatively common but can most often be managed nonoperatively. This would include debridement as needed, local wound care, and close monitoring.
- Infection: Most infections can be managed with antibiotics. Interventional drain placement is helpful for formed abscesses seen on imaging.
- Hematoma: Hematomas are possible at both the donor and recipient site. Drain output and physical examination are key. Hematomas should be drained surgically.
- Seroma: Late seromas can develop at the donor site. Most can be managed with drains.

REFERENCES

1. Espinosa-de-los-monteros A, Arista-de la torre L, Vergara-fernandez O, Salgado-nesme N. Contralateral component separation technique for abdominal wall closure in patients undergoing vertical rectus abdominis myocutaneous flap transposition for pelvic exenteration reconstruction. *Ann Plast Surg.* 2016;77(1):90-92.

2. Butler CE, Gündeslioglu AO, Rodriguez-bigas MA. Outcomes of immediate vertical rectus abdominis myocutaneous flap reconstruction for irradiated abdominoperineal resection defects. *J Am Coll Surg.* 2008;206(4):694-703.

3. Devulapalli C, Jia wei AT, Dibiagio JR, et al. Primary versus flap closure of perineal defects following oncologic resection: a systematic review and meta-analysis. *Plast Reconstr Surg.* 2016;137(5):1602-1613.

4. Sunesen KG, Buntzen S, Tei T, et al. Perineal healing and survival after anal cancer salvage surgery: 10-year experience with primary perineal reconstruction using the vertical rectus abdominis myocutaneous (VRAM) flap. *Ann Surg Oncol.* 2009;16(1):68-77.

5. Zhang W, Zeng A, Yang J, et al. Outcome of vulvar reconstruction by anterolateral thigh flap in patients with advanced and recurrent vulvar malignancy. *J Surg Oncol.* 2015;111(8):985-991.

6. Zeng A, Qiao Q, Zhao R, Song K, Long X. Anterolateral thigh flap-based reconstruction for oncologic vulvar defects. *Plast Reconstr Surg.* 2011;127(5):1939-1945.

7. Hurst RD, Gottlieb LJ, Crucitti P, et al. Primary closure of complicated perineal wounds with myocutaneous and fasciocutaneous flaps after proctectomy for Crohn's disease. *Surgery.* 2001;130(4):767-772.

8. Campbell CA, Butler CE. Use of adjuvant techniques improves surgical outcomes of complex vertical rectus abdominis myocutaneous flap reconstructions of pelvic cancer defects. *Plast Reconstr Surg.* 2011;128(2):447-458.

9. Baumann DP, Butler CE. Component separation improves outcomes in VRAM flap donor sites with excessive fascial tension. *Plast Reconstr Surg.* 2010;126(5):1573-1580.

Gracilis Flap for Perineal and Vaginal Reconstruction

Ajani G. Nugent, Yasmina Zoghbi, and Christopher J. Salgado

27
CHAPTER

DEFINITION

- Perineal defects reconstructed with gracilis flaps are applied after vulvovaginal resections or more extensive pelvic exenterations with considerable soft tissue loss, dead space, and distortion of the introitus.[1]
- Vaginal defects indicated for gracilis flap reconstruction are applied for partial or total circumferential full-thickness portions of the vaginal canal including mucosa and muscle layers.[1,2]
- The gracilis flap is a highly vascularized muscle or myocutaneous flap that provides regional tissue that has its own independent blood supply, fills in pelvic dead space, and separates abdominal contents from the perineal wound. The gracilis flap is often not in the potential radiation field.[1,3]

ANATOMY

- The gracilis muscle—one of the adductors of the leg—is found in the more superficial plane of the medial thigh muscles.
- Derived from the Latin word *gracile*, which means slender, the muscle is thin and straplike, measuring roughly 25 cm in length and tapering from superior to inferior from about 6 to 4 cm.[4]
- It takes origin from the ischiopubic ramus and inserts distally via the pes anserinus into the medial tibia inferior to the condyle. The muscle inserts posteromedially to the adductor longus and, along with its tendinous insertion, can be palpated with ease in thinner patients.
- The gracilis axis can be defined by drawing a line from the ischium to the medial condyle of the knee. Alternately, by palpating the adductor longus with the thigh abducted, the gracilis axis can be outlined 2 to 3 fingerbreadths posterior to the adductor longus.
- The gracilis flap is a type II muscle flap according to the classification of Mathes and Nahai. It has a dominant vascular pedicle from the medial femoral circumflex artery, a branch of the deep femoral system. Two secondary pedicles to the gracilis muscle can be found segmentally proximal and distal to the pedicle.[5]
- The neurovascular pedicle of the gracilis free flap is made up of a single arterial branch arising from the medial femoral circumflex artery, two vena comitantes, and the anterior branch of the obturator nerve.[6]
- On average, the vessel measures 1.6 mm in diameter and passes deep to the adductor longus and superficial to the adductor magnus to enter the proximal third of the gracilis.[5]
- The entry point of the vascular pedicle is typically found 8 to 10 cm inferior to the pubic tubercle.[6] The proximal attachment of the muscle is often not palpable, and the distal insertion is often used to aid in its identification.
- The anterior branch of the obturator nerve can measure up to 12 cm in length and is found approximately 6 cm from the pubic tubercle.[5]
- The muscle can be divided into two functioning units, owing to its motor nerve dividing into branches innervating the superior and inferior muscle separately.[7]
- Careful attention should be paid to the saphenous vein so that it is not injured during the dissection.

PATHOGENESIS

- Perineal defects
  - Perineal defects necessitating gracilis flap reconstruction are most often the result of extirpative oncologic surgeries but can be the result of infectious processes as well as trauma.[1]
  - Perineal malignancies most often occur in the colorectum or cervix and less commonly in the vagina, urinary tract, or anus.[1]
  - Total pelvic exenteration for recurrent or locally advanced carcinomas provides a potential oncologic cure that leaves a large pelvic defect.[8]
- Vaginal defects
  - Total circumferential acquired vaginal defects usually arise from perineal malignancies that require pelvic exenterations.[1]

NATURAL HISTORY

- Perineal defects
  - Management of perineal malignancies through resection or pelvic exenteration results in pelvic dead space.
  - Patients following pelvic exenteration often benefit from muscle or myocutaneous flap reconstruction to obliterate dead space and provide antibiotic delivery to these often large defects with high metabolic demands.[1]
  - With loss of perineal support, abdominal viscera may fall into the pelvic basin, leading to adhesions, obstructions, fistulas, or perineal hernias.[3] Gracilis flap reconstruction aids to decrease the risk of these sequelae.
  - Attempts of closing large perineal wounds, especially those previously irradiated, by primary or secondary intention, are at high risk of dehiscence and breakdown.
  - Perineal wounds that remain unhealed for over 6 months after surgery are predisposed to developing chronically draining perineal sinuses[3] and should be reconstructed with preferably locoregional flaps such as the gracilis flap, if available.

- Vaginal defects
  - Total vaginal resection without flap repair leads to prolonged healing, increased risk for complications, abnormal vaginal anatomy, and inadequate function.[9]

PATIENT HISTORY AND PHYSICAL FINDINGS

- Wound size
  - Evaluation of the defect size and shape is critical in determining if the wound should be managed through primary or secondary intention, debridement and packing, skin grafting, or flap utilization.[3]
- Radiation
  - Areas that have been previously radiated must be noted as they compromise the surgical site and occasionally may compromise the vascularity of potential flaps.
- Scars
  - Thorough preoperative examination includes evaluation for lower extremity scars, as prior surgery or trauma can influence flap selection.
- Femoral artery
  - With intentions of using the gracilis myocutaneous flap for perineal or vaginal repair, vascular status must be evaluated.
  - Physical exam should include palpation of the femoral, popliteal, posterior tibial, dorsalis pedis, and anterior tibial arteries.
  - Additional evaluations are capillary refill, skin color and turgor, and Doppler examination if pulses are not detected. Computed tomography angiography (CTA), magnetic resonance angiography, or even angiogram is necessary to ensure patency of arterial inflow. A venous phase with the CTA may be obtained to evaluate the venous outflow as well.
- Expectations
  - Typically, younger, sexually active women desire an anatomically similar, functioning reconstruction of the vagina to both be aesthetically pleasing and permit sexual activity after surgery.[1]
  - Conversely, much older patients who may be unlikely to resume intercourse after reconstruction may benefit from a more conservative approach with less risk of complications. Flap obliteration of the perineum without reconstruction of the vagina may yield a quicker and less complicated recovery for the patient.[1] Patients, however, often will request reconstruction of their vaginal canal.

IMAGING

- Imaging in the setting of perineal or vaginal reconstruction using the gracilis flap is generally not indicated in primary cases.
- Angiography, CTA, or MRA may be warranted in patients with a history of vascular disease, bypass graft involving the profunda femoris, multiple surgeries, or radiation.
- Postoperatively, a useful landmark to identify the gracilis flap on CT is the subcutaneous tunnel in the medial thigh that is used to transmit the flap.[10]
- If the muscular portion of the gracilis flap is denervated during harvest, it will show changes of atrophy, specifically smaller size and internal fat attenuation on CT.[10] Due to the increased fat content, this change will also be evident on MRI with increased signal on T1-weighed images.

- Changes associated with denervation will also be apparent on T2-weighted MRI due to increased cellular permeability leading to edema within the muscle. This should not be mistaken for inflammation or tumor infiltration within the flap, which would also increase the T2 signal intensity but would generally concurrently enlarge the flap.[10]

SURGICAL MANAGEMENT

Preoperative Planning

- As with any reconstructive procedure, a thorough understanding of pertinent local and regional anatomy is crucial, as well as remote anatomy in the event that free tissue options are to be considered.
- The anticipated reconstructive options are primarily guided by the nature of the defect. As such, detailed discussion with the resecting surgeon as it relates to margins and secondary deficits is crucial, in conjunction with review of preoperative imaging if available.
- After the anticipated defect is determined, preoperative optimization should be pursued. These measures include, but are not limited to, control of local infection if applicable with antibiotic therapy, nutritional optimization, and smoking cessation.

Positioning

- For vaginal/perineal reconstruction, the patient is usually in ideal positioning for gracilis harvest, which is usually lithotomy.
- It is important to note the rare, but reported, association of common peroneal nerve injury with prolonged immobilization in lithotomy. As such, appropriate padding of the fibular head should be carried out.
- Other positions ideal for gracilis harvest are supine, with thigh abduction (frog-leg); however, we have often found this position not useful for harvest.
- Rarely, for very posterior defects such as ischial pressure sores, the gracilis may be harvested from prone position.

Approach

- As mentioned above, gracilis harvest can be approached from both an anterior position (lithotomy or frog-leg) and less frequently posterior (prone) position (**FIG 1**).

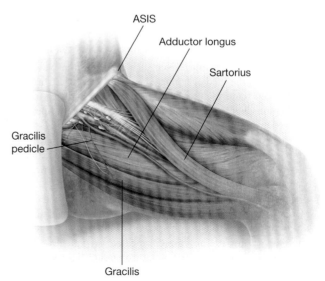

FIG 1 • Gracilis muscle anatomy.

■ Myocutaneous Gracilis Flap

- The skin paddle for the gracilis can be oriented either parallel or perpendicular (transverse) to the gracilis muscle, depending on the reconstructive needs of the flap. Both techniques rely on perforators coming from the proximal aspect of the muscle (**TECH FIG 1A**).
- Once the muscle is delineated, just medial to the palpable adductor longus muscle, an appropriately sized skin paddle is designed. Usually, a skin paddle width of 4 to 6 cm can be closed primarily without difficulty.
- Pencil Doppler is then used to identify the perforators, which will either be musculocutaneous (through the gracilis itself) or septocutaneous (in the septum between the gracilis and adductor longus muscle).
- An anterior incision is made through the skin, subcutaneous tissue, and into the fascia of the adductor longus muscle. Care is taken to bevel the cut away from the skin paddle and also to be cognizant of the saphenous vein.
- This fascia is then elevated from an anterior to posterior direction, until the intermuscular septum is encountered. Septocutaneous perforators will usually be identified here.
- Attention is then directed to making the posterior incision, once again incising down to the fascia, this time overlying the gracilis muscle. Once again, perforators are identified and preserved.
- The skin paddle is then elevated inclusive of fascia and the intermuscular septum.
- Once the skin paddle is dissected, attention is then directed to raising the remainder of the gracilis muscle.

- A continuation of the anterior skin paddle incision can be made, or a smaller distal incision can be made adjacent to the medial tibial condyle. This secondary incision is usually 3 to 4 cm in length.
- Dissection is carried out to the pes anserinus, at which point the tendons are identified.
- The gracilis can be differentiated from the sartorius muscle here using two techniques.
    - The gracilis is usually all tendinous at this point, whereas the sartorius will be more muscular.
    - If gracilis muscle fibers are present, they will usually be oriented in a longitudinal manner, whereas the sartorius muscle fibers will be oriented in an oblique manner.
- The gracilis tendon is then ligated once pulling on the muscle proximally will lead to tension of the muscle distally.
- A subcutaneous tunnel between the proximal incision and distal incision is created, and the muscle is passed from distal to proximal. This usually requires ligation of at least one minor pedicle coming from the superficial femoral artery. Attention is then directed proximally, where the adductor longus muscle can be retracted laterally and the vascular pedicle (medial femoral circumflex artery) is readily identified running superficially to the adductor magnus muscle.
- The pedicle is dissected from the surrounding fascial attachments as needed for tension-free inset. The flap is now ready to be inset proximally into the defect (**TECH FIG 1B**).
- If the creation of a vaginal canal is necessary, the skin paddle may be folded on itself as an "alpha-wrap" (**TECH FIG 1C**).

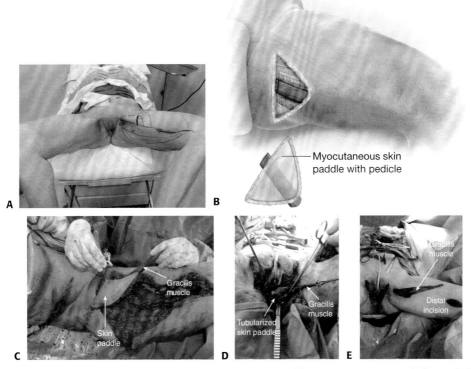

TECH FIG 1 • A. Surface markings of flap in frog-leg position. **B.** Transverse skin paddle. **C.** Myocutaneous gracilis flap ready for inset. **D.** Patient following Abbe-McIndoe procedure for vaginal reconstruction and left gracilis flap for anal sphincter and perineal restoration. **E.** Elevation of left gracilis muscle prior to alpha-wrap of incompetent anal sphincter for functional restoration and perineal reconstruction.

TECHNIQUES

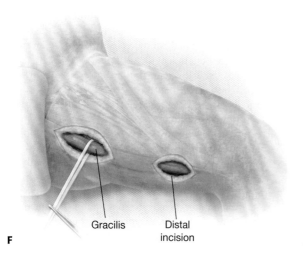

Gracilis   Distal
           incision

F

TECH FIG 1 (Continued) • **F.** Penrose drain around myofascial gracilis flap prior to distal disinsertion.

■ Myofascial Gracilis Flap

- The gracilis can be harvested as a myofascial flap only as well.
- In situations where epidermal lining is not needed, the pubic symphysis is palpated, and a corresponding line is drawn from there to the medial tibial condyle. This line usually corresponds to the adductor longus, which should be easily palpable as well. The gracilis muscle will be identified approximately 2 fingerbreadths posterior to this line.
- To prevent inadvertent trauma to the pedicle, an 8- to 10-cm demarcation from the pubic symphysis is made. This corresponds to the most proximal aspect of the harvest incision. Loupe magnification is advised to prevent injury to the pedicle. Identification of the pedicle to allow for maximum release of the muscle if needed.
- The incision is usually carried distally as needed for dissection of the proximal muscle. The incision is carried deep to subcutaneous tissue and fascia, once again, taking care to not violate the saphenous vein.
- The gracilis muscle will be seen as the most medial and thinnest muscle, just medial/posterior to the adductor longus (which will be bigger than the gracilis in this area).
- Dissection proceeds superficially and deep to the gracilis muscle, in a distal manner. As discussed above, a counterincision is then made distally by the medial condyle; dissection is continued accordingly.
- Drains are often placed in the donor thigh after harvest with passive drainage of the reconstructed site.

PEARLS AND PITFALLS

Hematoma	■ Meticulous hemostasis during flap elevation
Partial skin necrosis	■ Ensuring wide inclusion of the fascia and intermuscular septum
Flap loss	■ Meticulous dissection around the primary pedicle (medial femoral circumflex artery)
Postoperative foot drop	■ Proper padding of the lateral fibular head while in lithotomy position

POSTOPERATIVE CARE

- Reports in the literature on the length of follow-up vary, but there is some general agreement of a weekly follow-up for 1 month and twice monthly for the 2nd month until wounds are healed and then every 3 months afterward or as needed.[12] Median follow-up averages around 15 months.[13–15]
- Patients should be on bed rest for at least 48 hours. They may not sit up in bed; sitting up puts pressure on the perineal closure and flap, which can delay wound healing.
  - We have found air-fluidized beds to be beneficial to prevent pressure on the reconstruction and daily cleansing of the genital area to avoid bacterial overgrowth and infections.
  - After 48 hours, they may walk with the help of a physical therapist.
- Gram-positive and Gram-negative antimicrobial therapy is important as well as anaerobic coverage during the hospitalization.
- Dilation with soft vaginal conformers of the vaginal conduit is necessary to prevent stenosis. For total vaginal reconstruction, dilating the reconstructed canal 2 or 3 times daily with a dilator is sufficient.

- On the 2nd postoperative day, Burke et al. recommend starting a program of 3-times-daily perineal irrigation followed by 5 to 10 minutes of forced air-drying using a hair blower set at room temperature.
- The flap should be inspected daily to assess viability and primary healing. A complete examination of the flap, including speculum insertion and digital pelvic examination, should be performed about 1 week after surgery.
- Donor site drains can be removed in 5 days. Sutures should be left intact for about 7 days, and absorbable sutures, which we often use in the immediate genital area, may be left in place.
- Gradual resumption of physical and sexual activity is recommended as healing progresses[16] and is commonly at about 3 months after surgery.
- Hospital stay averages no more than 20 days.[16]

OUTCOMES

- Nelson and Butler prospectively analyzed 133 patients who underwent abdominoperineal resection or pelvic exenteration and immediate reconstruction with a pedicled VRAM (n = 114) or thigh flap (n = 19) between 1993 and 2007.[17]
- Thigh flaps were found to have significantly higher rates of major complications (42%), which included major wound dehiscence and pelvic abscess, than VRAM flaps (15%).[17]
- Thigh flap donor sites also had higher rates of infection than VRAM donor sites and required longer healing times than did VRAM donor sites. Furthermore, thigh flap recipient sites had higher rates of wound dehiscence, infection, and longer healing times than VRAM flap recipient sites.[17] The flap remains an excellent option, however, to avoid abdominal donor morbidity and in cases where the abdominal tissue is not usable.
- Casey et al. retrospectively reviewed 99 consecutive cases of vaginal reconstruction—this included 41 VRAM, 13 gracilis, and 45 modified Singapore flaps.
  - The overall complication rate was higher following the gracilis (61.5%) and Singapore flap (46.7%) than with the VRAM flap (31.7%).
  - The flap-specific complication rate was lowest in the VRAM group (22%) compared to the gracilis (53.8%) and Singapore flaps (37.8%).
  - It is important to note that 4 of the 13 gracilis flaps were used as salvage operations secondary to unsuccessful initial reconstruction, as opposed to none in the VRAM or Singapore flap groups.
  - There was no difference in length of stay between the three groups, and sexual function was adequate with all 3 types of reconstruction.[18]
- Vermaas et al. reported major and minor complication rates of 43% and 0%, respectively, in their study of reconstructions of 25 abdominoperineal resection and pelvic exenteration defects with pedicled gracilis myocutaneous flaps; however, they only included infection, abscess, hernia, and fistula in their analysis.[14]
- In a study on the use of bilateral gracilis myocutaneous flaps to repair total vaginal defects by Pusic and Mehrara, a 10% risk of pelvic abscess and a 10% to 20% incidence of skin loss were identified.[19]
- Wilson et al. conducted a review of the literature and found 87 gracilis flaps: 71 for persistent perineal sinus, 5 for fistulating

pelvic sepsis, and 4 for deep presacral sepsis. Of all flaps, 31 failed to heal within 12 months (success rate 64.4%).
  - The data suggest that around a quarter of flaps take longer than 3 months to heal.
  - The data did not show any pattern of failure with the pathology or type of flap used (muscle only or musculocutaneous).[20] This is a significant improvement to the era prior to flap reconstruction.

COMPLICATIONS

- Possible skin necrosis, which requires surgical debridement to achieve secondary healing, may be seen in the myocutaneous flap.[12,13]
  - There is a lower incidence of skin necrosis when the flap is smaller.[16]
  - The gracilis myofasciocutaneous advancement flap has great vascular supply to the cutaneous portion of the flap due to the inclusion of perforators from the gracilis muscle and the wide preservation of the fascia above the semitendinosus, semimembranosus, sartorius, and adductor muscles. Small septocutaneous perforators are kept intact, which allows a larger cutaneous territory to be harvested. This prevents the high partial flap necrosis.
- Partial or total flap loss
- Donor site complications include painful thigh wounds, sensory loss, abscess, and separation or infection (ie, local *Pseudomonas aeruginosa* infection).[14,16]
- Delayed ambulation due to medical complications related to respiratory distress and deep venous thrombosis[16]
- Seroma
- Perineal herniation[14]
- Perineal infection/abscess
- Perineal fistula
- Hematoma
- Wound dehiscence

ACKNOWLEDGMENTS

Natalie Joumblat
Denise Manfrini
Amir B. Behnam

REFERENCES

1. Salgado CJ, Chim H, Skowronski PP, et al. Reconstruction of acquired defects of the vagina and perineum. *Semin Plast Surg.* 2011;25(2):155-162.
2. Cordeiro PG, Pusic AL, Disa JJ. A classification system and reconstructive algorithm for acquired vaginal defects. *Plast Reconstr Surg.* 2002;110(4):1058-1065.
3. Woods JE, Beart RW Jr. Reconstruction of nonhealing perineal wounds with gracilis muscle flaps. *Ann Plast Surg.* 1983;11(6):513-516.
4. Azizzadeh B, Pettijohn KJ. The gracilis free flap. *Facial Plast Surg Clin North Am.* 2016;24(1):47-60.
5. Magden O, Tayfur V, Edizer M, Atabey A. Anatomy of gracilis muscle flap. *J Craniofac Surg.* 2010;21(6):1948-1950.
6. Papadopoulos O, Georgiou P, Christopoulos A, Sandris P. The gracilis flap revisited. *Eur J Plast Surg.* 2000;23(8):413-418.
7. Upadhyaya DN, Khanna V, Bhattacharya S, et al. The transversely split gracilis twin free flaps. *Indian J Plast Surg.* 2010;43(2):173-176.
8. Kaartinen IS, Vuento MH, Hyoty MK, et al. Reconstruction of the pelvic floor and the vagina after total pelvic exenteration using the transverse musculocutaneous gracilis flap. *J Plast Reconstr Aesthet Surg.* 2015;68(1):93-97.

9. McCraw JB, Massey FM, Shanklin KD, Horton CE. Vaginal reconstruction with gracilis myocutaneous flaps. *Plast Reconstr Surg.* 1976;58(2):176-183.

10. Sagebiel TL, Faria SC, Balachandran A, et al. Pelvic reconstruction with pedicled thigh flaps: indications, surgical techniques, and postoperative imaging. *AJR Am J Roentgenol.* 2014;202(3):593-601.

11. Kamath S, Venkatanarasimha N, Walsh MA, Hughes PM. MRI appearance of muscle denervation. *Skeletal Radiol.* 2008;37(5):397-404.

12. Vyas RM, Pomahac B. Use of a bilobed gracilis myocutaneous flap in perineal and genital reconstruction. *Ann Plast Surg.* 2010;65(2):225-227.

13. John HE, Jessop ZM, Di Candia M, et al. An algorithmic approach to perineal reconstruction after cancer resection—experience from two international centers. *Ann Plast Surg.* 2013;71(1):96-102.

14. Vermaas M, Ferenschild FT, Hofer SO, et al. Primary and secondary reconstruction after surgery of the irradiated pelvis using a gracilis muscle flap transposition. *Eur J Surg Oncol.* 2005;31(9):1000-1005.

15. Whetzel TP, Lechtman AN. The gracilis myofasciocutaneous flap: vascular anatomy and clinical application. *Plast Reconstr Surg.* 1997;99(6):1642-1652.

16. Burke TW, Morris M, Roh MS, et al. Perineal reconstruction using single gracilis myocutaneous flaps. *Gynecol Oncol.* 1995;57(2):221-225.

17. Nelson RA, Butler CE. Surgical outcomes of VRAM versus thigh flaps for immediate reconstruction of pelvic and perineal cancer resection defects. *Plast Reconstr Surg.* 2009;123(1):175-183.

18. Casey WJ III, Tran NV, Petty PM, et al. A comparison of 99 consecutive vaginal reconstructions: an outcome study. *Ann Plast Surg.* 2004;52(1):27-30.

19. Pusic AL, Mehrara BJ. Vaginal reconstruction: an algorithm approach to defect classification and flap reconstruction. *J Surg Oncol.* 2006;94(6):515-521.

20. Wilson TR, Welbourn H, Stanley P, Hartley JE. The success of rectus and gracilis muscle flaps in the treatment of chronic pelvic sepsis and persistent perineal sinus: a systematic review. *Colorectal Dis.* 2014;16(10):751-759.

Gender-Affirming Surgery

Katherine M. Gast and William M. Kuzon, Jr

DEFINITION

- Gender dysphoria is the incongruence between anatomic sex and gender identity. It is estimated to affect 1.4 million Americans, or about 0.3% of the population. Male-to-female transsexualism is 2 to 3 times more prevalent than female-to-male transsexualism.

ANATOMY

- Male
  - Penis—superficial to deep (**FIG 1**)
    - Skin
    - *Dartos* (superficial) fascia
    - *Buck* (deep) fascia
    - Neurovascular bundle: deep dorsal vein, dorsal artery, paired dorsal penile nerves
    - *Tunica albuginea* (surrounds each corpus individually)
    - Erectile tissue: paired corpora cavernosa, corpora spongiosum surrounds the urethra
  - Arterial supply
    - Internal pudendal artery branches into the perineal artery to the perineum and scrotum.
    - Common penile artery branches to the bulbourethral artery, dorsal artery, and deep cavernosal artery.
- Female (**FIG 2**)
  - Clitoris and clitoral hood
  - Labia minora and labia majora
  - Urethral meatus, just anterior to vestibule and introitus
  - Vagina

PATHOGENESIS

- Considerable evidence now supports a biological basis for determining one's gender identity.[1-4] Gender dysphoria remains a diagnosis in the DSM-5. It is noted that it is not a mental disorder requiring psychiatric treatment but an incongruence between the biologically determined gender identity and the patient's anatomic sex.
- There are two separate types of gender dysphoria.
  - Gender dysphoria of adolescence and adulthood (ICD10 302.85) often begins in early childhood and persists into adolescence and adulthood.
  - It is important to recognize that gender dysphoria of childhood (ICD10 302.6) is distinctly different. In the majority of these children, gender dysphoria is temporally limited and they will "desist" by adolescence.
    - Because these two scenarios appear to be distinct, considerable expertise is required to diagnose and treat gender-expansive children.

- When gender dysphoria of adolescence and adulthood is confirmed, puberty suppression is now the standard of care for young adolescents who exhibit significant distress with development of secondary sex characteristics. Puberty suppression is reversible and may or may not be followed by cross-hormone treatment.
- It is also important to note that gender dysphoria is distinct from disorders of sexual development (DSD), where there are congenital anomalies of the genitalia and/or are hormonally determined abnormalities of secondary sex development.
  - This has been a source of confusion in the past when DSD children were often assigned the gender most congruent with their anatomy or with the anatomy most easily reconstructed surgically.
  - This resulted in inappropriate assignment of gender with patients opting to surgically transition to their natal gender later in life. These patients were not gender dysphoric.
  - The management of patients with anomalous genitalia or hormonal development requires specialized, multidisciplinary expertise, and patients presenting with a self-reported diagnosis of DSD require appropriate evaluation and referral.

PATIENT HISTORY AND PHYSICAL FINDINGS

- Since plastic surgeons are not trained in the evaluation and management of gender dysphoria, internationally accepted standards of care (SOC) have been published by the World Professional Association for Transgender Health (WPATH). It is imperative that surgeons performing gender-affirming surgery are familiar with these guidelines and that they have in place mechanisms to assure that patients have met SOC before becoming surgical candidates.
  - Collaboration with local mental health providers who are familiar with this area is the most practical way of assuring the validity of the letters of readiness required by the SOC.
  - If that is not practical, then the surgeon must accept the responsibility of vetting the patient's preparation for surgery, including compliance with SOC.
- The WPATH SOC clinical guidelines address primary care, hormonal therapy, mental health services, and surgical treatment of transgender patients.
  - For chest surgery, patients must have one letter of readiness from a mental health professional, and 1 year of estrogen therapy is recommend for breast growth in male-to-female patients who desire breast augmentation.

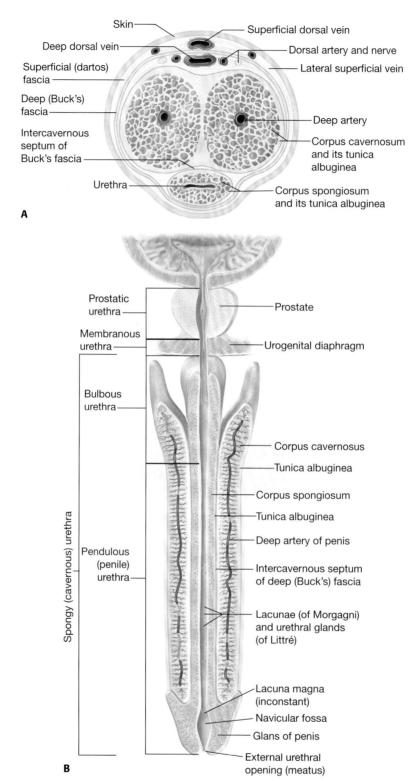

FIG 1 • A. Cross-sectional anatomy of the penis. Note the paired corpora cavernosum and the dorsal lying corpus spongiosum surrounding the urethra. The neurovascular bundle for the neoclitoris flap harvested from the glans is located on the ventral side of the penis and is deep to the Buck fascia. **B.** Longitudinal section of the male urethra.

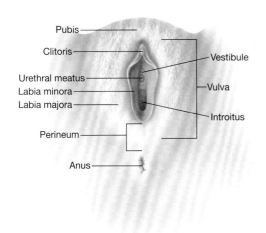

FIG 2 • External female genitalia.

- For genital surgery, or "bottom" surgery, patients must have two letters of readiness, have completed 1 year of hormonal therapy, and have completed 12 months of a "real-life experience" of living in congruent gender in all circumstances.
  - Ongoing, regular visits with a mental health professional are recommended. The WPATH SOC are meant to be flexible guidelines and may be modified for individual patients.
- Physical exam of male-to-female patients should document circumcision status, presence of any inguinal hernia, and examination of the testicles and spermatic cords. The central perineum must be examined for hair growth since this impacts surgical decision-making as described below.
- Physical exam of female-to-male patients should focus on the suitability of free flap donor sites suitable to provide tissue for phallic construction. The radial forearm flap is the most common donor site, so an Allen test of bilateral upper extremities is important. Since the flap must be double rolled into a phallus, the thickness of subcutaneous tissue of the radial forearm flap, the anterior lateral thigh flap, and the superficial circumflex iliac perforator flap should be documented.

IMAGING

- No diagnostic or radiologic studies are indicated.

SURGICAL MANAGEMENT

Penile Inversion Vaginoplasty

Preoperative Planning

- Hair removal: For male-to-female patients undergoing vaginoplasty, electrolysis or laser hair removal must be performed to remove hair of the perineum from anus to base of penis in midline of the scrotum. The reason for this is the perineal flap is used to widen the introitus and line the inferior posterior aspect of the neovagina.
  - The perineal flap can be defatted and follicles scraped from the dermis, but this compromises blood supply of the tissue.
  - In the event of a rectal injury, well-vascularized tissue over the direct repair is advantageous to prevent rectovaginal fistula.
- Hormone cessation: Estrogen therapy must be held 3 to 4 weeks prior to surgery. Estrogens are increase risk of perioperative thromboembolic disease. Hormones are resumed postoperatively when packing is removed and it can be determined that the patient will not require a repeat trip to the operating room. Spironolactone therapy may continue through the perioperative period.
- Bowel prep: A standard bowel prep to cleanse the colon and rectum of stool is performed the day prior to surgery. The patient is kept on a clear liquid diet 24 hours prior to surgery and then nothing by mouth for 6 hours prior to general anesthetic. In the event of a rectal injury, a repair is more durable if stool is not encountered immediately postoperatively.

Positioning

- Patient should be positioned in standard lithotomy position with sequential compression devices on bilateral lower extremities and pressure points appropriately padded. Arms can be tucked at patient's sides with padding at elbow and wrist.
- Patient should be prepped with Betadine including the lower abdomen, penis, scrotum, buttocks, and perineum.

Approach

- Penile inversion vaginoplasty with the penis skin tube lining the neovagina is the most commonly performed technique worldwide. The neovagina is often lengthened with full-thickness skin graft (FTSG) from the scrotum to a goal length of 14 to 16 cm in the operating room. The scrotal skin is fashioned into the labia majora. A portion of the dorsal glans penis is left on a dorsal neurovascular pedicle to create a sensate neoclitoris. Prepuce skin of the penis may be used to construct the labia minora in uncircumcised patients.
- Sigmoid colon vaginoplasty is a technique by which a segment of the colon is harvested by a general surgeon, secured to the sacrum to prevent prolapse, and then brought down into the pelvis and connected to the perineal reconstruction. Diversion colitis, excessive mucous discharge, and prolapse of the intestinal segment limit its widespread adoption as a primary method of vaginoplasty.

T
E
C
H
N
I
Q
U
E
S

■ Penile Inversion Vaginoplasty

Creation of the Perineal Flap

- The perineal flap is located anterior to the anus centered along the midline. The base of the flap is 3.5 cm wide and the flap is 10 cm in length. The flap is triangular shaped and is incised and raised ventral to dorsal with a 1-cm layer of subcutaneous fat, leaving it pedicled posteriorly adjacent to the anus (**TECH FIG 1A**). A vertical incision is then made through the scrotum up to the penile-scrotal junction. Dissection is carried down to the level of the bulbocavernosus muscle. The bulbocavernosus muscle is dissected free from overlying tissue along its length.
- A Foley catheter is placed.
- The origins of the bulbocavernosus muscles from the ischia are identified and dissected bilaterally circumferentially (**TECH FIG 1B**). The base of the bulbocavernosus muscles are clamped and divided on each side; 2-0 Vicryl suture ligatures are employed to control bleeding.
- The prerectal space is then dissected by dividing the plane between the bulbocavernosus and anal sphincter. Sharp dissection through the perineal body using cautery is used initially to the level of the urogenital diaphragm (**TECH FIG 1C**).
- Once the prerectal plane is entered, sharp and then blunt dissection is employed using digital dissection and a sponge stick following the Foley catheter.
- At the level of the prostate, the rectoprostatic fascia (Denonvilliers fascia) is detached from the tail of the prostate, and dissection proceeds anterior to Denonvilliers. This is done bluntly with the aid of a sponge stick, which is advanced slightly and then swept from anterior to posterior. Dissection is carried out to the level of the peritoneum, approximately 15 cm in depth.
- A moist sponge is placed in the neovaginal space. The rectum is filled with half-strength saline-Betadine solution. After 2 minutes, the laparotomy sponge is removed and inspected for Betadine. Bimanual examination with one finger in the rectum and one in the prerectal dissection and direct visualization of the anterior rectal wall is performed to ensure that no rectal injury occurred. The prostate is palpated and any abnormalities noted.
- The levator ani muscles are incised for about ½ cm on each side to widen the space for the neovagina.

Orchiectomy

- Bilateral orchiectomies are then performed in the usual fashion. The testicles are dissected free from the scrotal tissue in the plane just superficial to tunica vaginalis.
- The spermatic chords are dissected to the external inguinal ring.
- The vas deferens is separated from the remainder of the chord and ligated separately with 2-0 Vicryl ties, and the chord is suture ligated with 2-0 Vicryl at the level of the external ring. Careful attention must be paid to avoid retraction of bleeding vessels within the cord into the inguinal canal. The testicles are sent for pathologic examination.

Degloving of the penile shaft

- Two centimeters proximal to the corona, the skin is incised circumferentially and the shaft of the penis is degloved in a plane just superficial to the Buck fascia with Metzenbaum scissors. The prepuce or dorsal penile skin is left adjacent to the glans to serve as a clitoral hood and may be used to construct labia minora in patients who have not undergone circumcision. The penis is degloved to its base, and the penile shaft is pulled through the incision in the perineum used to raise the posterior flap.

Raising the Neurovascular, Neoclitoral Flap

- A "clitoral" flap is now raised from the dorsal area of the glans. A section of dorsal glans penis is marked out in an appropriate shape at the terminus of the dorsal neurovascular bundle. In addition, a portion of the distal dorsal and lateral penile skin is kept intact to serve as a clitoral hood. The 1-cm-wide portion of the glans will serve as the future neoclitoris. This may be shield shaped or M shaped and coned at inset.
- The neurovascular bundle consisting of the dorsal penile arteries, veins, and nerve is raised as a flap by dissecting them off the underlying corporal bodies. Dissection is begun at the midshaft of the penis, incising the Buck fascia along the midaxis of the penis on either side. Dissection is carried to the level of the tunica albuginea.
- The neurovascular bundle is now raised throughout its length from its base at the perineum to the glans portion, raising the Buck fascia and the neurovascular bundle off the underlying tunica using sharp, scissor dissection. The

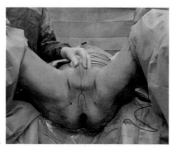
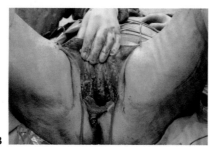
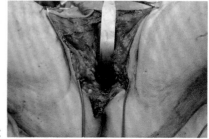

A   **B**   **C**

TECH FIG 1 • A. The perineal scrotal flap is marked with extension of the incision up the raphe of the scrotum. The perineal flap is used to widen the introitus to prevent a stricture. This area should be depilated prior to operation. **B.** The bulbocavernosus muscle is fully exposed and disinserted from the ischial tuberosities. **C.** The space for the neovagina is created anterior to the rectoprostatic fascia (Denonvilliers fascia). This is done sharply with cautery followed by blunt dissection with a sponge stick being careful to go slowly and gently, using a sweeping motion from anterior to posterior.

glans portion is then incised and raised with the neurovascular bundle, taking care to include some glans erectile tissue but to exclude the corpus cavernosum.

Resection of Corpus Cavernosa and Preparation of the Urethra

- Dissection of the corpus spongiosum away from the corpora cavernosa is performed in the midline cleft. The corpora cavernosa are then resected bilaterally. This is done to the level of the ischium on each side. Suture ligatures of 2-0 Vicryl are used to control the corporal vascular bundles.
- The corpus spongiosum is dissected up to the level of the urogenital diaphragm. The bulbocavernous muscle is split longitudinally and the muscle and the spongiosum are dissected off the urethra up to the level of the urogenital diaphragm (see **TECH FIG 1B**). The urethra is cut to leave about 10 cm in length distal to the urogenital diaphragm and the rest is discarded.

Creation of the Vulva and Inset of Neoclitoris

- The neoclitoris is formed by suturing the glans flap into a cone and by enveloping this with the dorsal penile skin as a clitoral hood (**TECH FIG 2A**). This is done with 3-0 Monocryl or chromic sutures. The neoclitoris is now inset. Prior to suturing the neoclitoris in place, the pedicle of the clitoral flap is looped anteriorly into the abdomen and stitched in place bilaterally using interrupted 2-0 Vicryl to prevent kinking, and the clitoris is anchored to deeper structures in the appropriate position using 3-0 Monocryl.

- Blake drains are now placed in the prerectal space dissection and in the lower abdomen and are brought out through separate stab incisions in the pubic hair.
- The penile pullback is now performed. The anchoring points are at the penile-scrotal junction on both sides of the former penile shaft. The degloved penis shaft is present between these two marks (**TECH FIG 2B**). These two points are then tacked posteriorly to the base of the perineal flap with deep dermal 2-0 Vicryl.
- Once the pullback has been done, an anterior Y-shaped incision is made in the skin anterior to the tube remaining from the degloving of the penis. The anterior portion of the Y is at the location of the neoclitoris, and the posterior portion is at the planned location of the urethral orifice.
- Tacking sutures are placed from the deep dermis of the penile pullback to the periosteum of the pelvis to anchor the central aspect of the new vulva down.
- The urethra is split along its ventral surface to about 2 cm distal to the urogenital diaphragm. Posterior stitches of 3-0 Vicryl in the neourethral orifice are placed between the posterior aspect of the Y-incision and the most anterior aspect of the ventral slit.
- The neoclitoris is inset into its new location using the Y-shaped incision to complete construction of the clitoral hood with the small central Y flap (**TECH FIG 2C**). This is inset using interrupted 3-0 chromic or Monocryl stitches.
- The urethral orifice is then inset using interrupted 3-0 Vicryl stitches from the posterior toward the anterior portion (**TECH FIG 2D**). The most anterior portion of the urethral mucosa abutted the neoclitoris. Careful attention must be made to bury any remnant erectile corpus spongiosa tissue; this will bleed postoperatively if exposed.

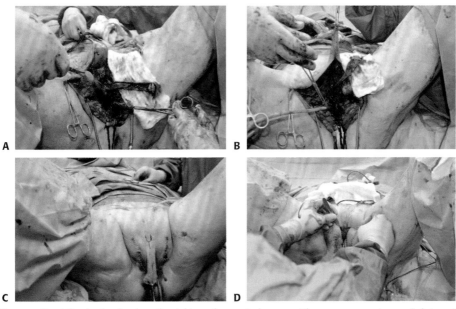

TECH FIG 2 • **A.** The neoclitoral flap is visualized on the right on the surgical sponge. The corpus spongiosum (inferior with Foley catheter in place) has been separated from the paired corpus cavernosa and remaining glans penis. The neoclitoral flap pedicle should be dissected to the pubic symphysis bone. **B.** The corpora cavernosa are amputated at the level of the perineum. Many surgeons prefer to leave a corporal stump and suture the two corpora together to provide a pedestal for the neoclitoris inset. Alternatively, one may choose to resect the corpora back to the ischium. **C.** A Y-shaped incision is made on the anterior most aspect of the penile skin tube for external inset of the neoclitoris and urethra. The penile skin tube is pulled back with anticipated inversion tension to estimate the location. **D.** Urethra inset. The corpus spongiosum is excised from the periphery of the urethra, and the mucosa is split longitudinally along the posterior surface. It is shaped into a diamond and inset as a fan to prevent a distal urethral stricture.

Creation of the Vaginal Vault

- A vaginal vault lining is constructed by insetting the posterior perineal flap into a longitudinal incision in the penile skin tube with running 3-0 chromic or Monocryl sutures (**TECH FIG 3A**). The labia majora are then constructed by pulling the deep scrotal contents posteriorly and anchoring them to the underlying tissue using interrupted 2-0 Vicryl stitches. The skin portion of the scrotum is then pulled posteriorly and laterally, and an ellipse is removed to create a labia shape. Do not over-resect the scrotal contents or skin.
- The vaginal vault is lengthened using FTSG from the resected scrotal skin (**TECH FIG 3B**). The preserved skin is defatted aggressively and sutured over a stent into a tube 10 cm in diameter and at least 5 cm in length. The size of the skin graft is 5 × 10 cm, and the tube of skin graft is now sutured to the end of the penile skin tube using 3-0 Monocryl sutures. The total vaginal length is now 14 to 16 cm.

- All remaining wounds are closed with interrupted and running 3-0 chromic or Monocryl stitches, leaving linear incisions on either side along the line of the labia majora.

Placement of Vaginal Pack

- The drains are connected to suction.
- A bacitracin ointment–impregnated vaginal packing is placed to maintain the new vaginal vault in position without undue pressure. The end of the vaginal pack is placed over the urethral and neoclitoral reconstruction in order to provide some dressing.
- The vaginal pack is held in place by through-and-through bolster stitches of 0 Prolene tied over silicone tubing lateral to the labia majora (**TECH FIG 4**).
- The wound is dressed with a perineal pad and mesh panties.
- The patient is taken out of lithotomy position.

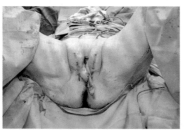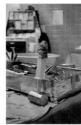

A   **B**

TECH FIG 3 • A. Skin graft sutured to penile skin, prior to inversion. The full-thickness skin graft tube is sutured to the penile skin tube and then inverted and placed into the prerectal space. **B.** Excess scrotal skin excised after constructing the labia majora is defatted on the back table and sutured over a 60-cc syringe to lengthen the neovagina. A skin graft is required in the majority of cases to provide lining for sufficient vaginal length.

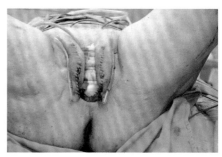

TECH FIG 4 • Final dressing. A large vaginal pack is placed in the neovaginal as a bolster for the full-thickness skin graft at the apex and allow adherence of the inverted skin tube. Spanning Prolene sutures with drain tubing prevents pressure on the labia majora skin.

■ Phalloplasty

Preoperative Planning

- There is no "standard" procedure for phalloplasty, and considerable variation in flap choice and in approach (one stage or two stage) is seen between and even within centers.
- Phalloplasty may be performed with radial forearm flap, SCIP flap, anterolateral thigh (ALT) flap, latissimus dorsi myocutaneous flap, or combination of the three to reconstruct an inner epithelialized urethra and outer roll of skin for the phallus.
- The phallus may be constructed from one flap in a "tube-in-a-tube" fashion (radial forearm flap most common), or the urethra and phallic skin may be reconstructed from two separate flaps (radial forearm flap or SCIP flap for the urethra with an ALT flap for the phallic skin most common).
- The choice of donor site is largely dependent on patient's body habitus and patient and surgeon preference.
- Permanent hair removal on the skin to be used for the neophallus and the neourethra should be completed to lower the risk of urethral strictures and fistulas.

- Allen test should be performed in bilateral upper extremities in preparation for radial forearm flap.

Positioning

- Patient should be positioned supine. If used, the upper extremity should be extended on hand table with sterile tourniquet.

Approach

- The tube within a tube may be accomplished by a double-roll technique of the radial forearm flap, but this is limited by subcutaneous fat thickness on the forearm (**FIG 3**). Alternatively, a thin radial forearm flap may be tubed and then surrounded by a pedicled ALT or SCIP flap in thin patients.
- In all techniques, vaginectomy is performed concomitantly by a gynecologist. It is also common to perform a hysterectomy and bilateral oophorectomy at the time of phalloplasty.

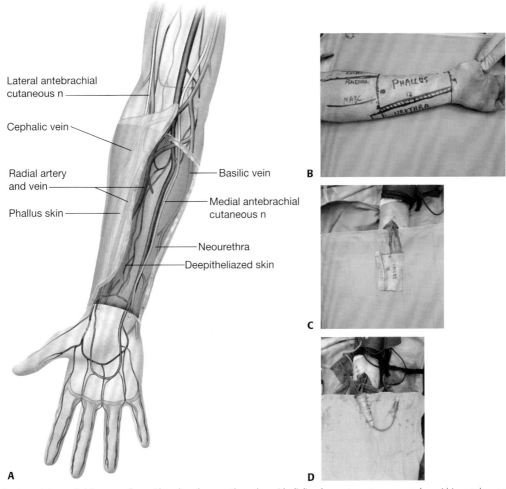

FIG 3 • A. Design of the radial forearm flap with volar ulnar urethra, de-epithelialized area to suture as a tube within a tube, and radial outer phallus. **B.** Markings for radial forearm flap phalloplasty. **C.** Radial forearm flap elevated. **D.** Radial forearm flap tubed on the forearm to create the urethra and phallus.

■ Radial Forearm Phalloplasty

- The patient is placed under general anesthesia in a supine position on the operating table. The perineum, both upper legs, and the left arm are prepped and draped in the usual sterile fashion.

Flap Dissection

- A preoperative Allen test confirmed that there is adequate ulnar artery flow to support the circulation of the hand without any need to reconstruct the radial artery. A radial forearm flap is then marked out over the axis of the radial artery. The flap is at least 20 cm wide and 15 cm long.
- A "tube-in-a-tube" method is used to construct the neophallus with a 3-cm-wide portion in the ulnar aspect (the most hairless part) of the flap serving as a neourethra and the external skin of the neophallus measuring 16 × 15 cm. The urethral skin strip is left approximately 2 cm longer than the remainder of the neophallus so the urethral coaptation will not lie directly subjacent to an external skin incision.

- The cephalic vein and the associated lateral antebrachial cutaneous nerve (LABC) are marked out, as is the location of the medial antebrachial cutaneous (MABC) nerve. It is sometimes possible to include the basilic vein with the flap for additional venous outflow.
- The arm is exsanguinated and a tourniquet is inflated for less than 120 minutes for this part of the dissection.
- Dissection is begun by incising the margin of the skin paddle of the radial forearm flap and dissecting distally to identify the radial artery and vena comitans. The radial artery and vena comitans are then divided distally at the volar wrist crease. Incisions along the radial and ulnar aspects of the flap are completed, and the flap is raised off the muscle fascia, which is left down.
- Dissection is continued until the brachioradialis on the radial aspect and flexor carpi radialis on the ulnar aspect of the flap are encountered. Proximally, the cephalic vein and its associated LABC are preserved. The MABC is identified and preserved.
- The interval between the brachioradialis and the flexor carpi radialis is opened proximally, and the radial artery

and its vena comitans are identified. The flap is now elevated from distal to proximal dissecting at the level of the deep fascia. This preserves the radial artery and its vena comitans is within the substance of the flap.

- The radial sensory nerve is dissected out of the substance of the flap on the radial distal aspect of the forearm and is preserved in total. Dissection is carried proximally until the flap is isolated on the two nerves, on two cutaneous veins, and on the radial artery and its vena comitans.
- A large communication between the cephalic vein and the vena comitans is almost always present in the proximal forearm. Preserving this communication allows a cephalic vein anastomosis to a recipient vein to drain both the deep and superficial venous systems within the flap. All of these structures are dissected proximally up to the antecubital fossa with side branches of all vessels being coagulated or clipped. The radial artery and its vena comitans are isolated right up to their takeoff at the bifurcation of the radial and ulnar vessels.
- The arm tourniquet is released and both the flap and the hand should have excellent perfusion as judged by capillary refill, color, and bleeding from cut edges. Hemostasis is obtained with bipolar electrocautery both the flap and the recipient bed.

Construction of Neourethra

- A neourethra is now constructed around no. 12 French Foley by tubing the ulnar portion of the radial forearm flap. A strip of skin between the urethra and phallus portion of the skin flap is de-epithelialized for suturing. The flap is tubed using interrupted and running 4-0 Monocryl.
- The reminder of the skin portion of the flap is now wrapped around the neourethra creating the external skin portion of the penis. This is sutured with 4-0 Monocryl deep dermal and subcuticular sutures, and the neourethra is sutured to the distal external phallus skin paddle using a running 4-0 Monocryl suture.
- A coronaplasty may be performed now or in a delayed fashion by making an incision 3 to 4 cm from the distal end of the phallus and advancing the distal edge, creating a roll. A narrow ring split-thickness skin graft (STSG) is placed behind the roll proximally, which can be harvested from the area of the flap that has been de-epithelialized.
- The flap is left perfused on the forearm at this time, covered with moist sponge, and attention is then turned to the perineum.
- Concurrently with the flap dissection, a gynecologist or urologist will perform the vaginectomy and preparation of the recipient urethra for anastomosis. A scrotoplasty using the labia majora can be done as well.

Preparation of the Recipient Site

- The recipient site is prepared, dissecting the perineal urethra. The clitoris is de-epithelialized and will be buried at the base of the neophallus. A short midline incision allows dissection of one of the dorsal clitoral nerves for later coaptation with the LABC; the other clitoral nerve is left intact. Because sensory reinnervation of the neophallic free flap is variable, this preserves a sensate, subcutaneous clitoris as an erogenous location.
- A curvilinear longitudinal incision 12 cm long is now made over the superficial femoral vessels in the left groin.

Dissection is carried down, and the superficial femoral vein, any venous side branches, and the saphenous vein are identified and prepared for microsurgery. The saphenous vein generally has a very large side branch just distal to its origin; this should be preserved.

- A subcutaneous tunnel is made between the perineal recipient site and the recipient vessels in the groin. The planned recipient artery is the superficial femoral via end-to-side anastomosis. If the radial artery will not reach, a vein graft can be employed, or better, an AV fistula can be created using the large, proximal branch of the saphenous vein anatomosed end to side to the femoral vein.
- The loop is then divided with the distal end of the loop serving as a vein graft for the arterial revascularization.

Flap Transfer, Vascular Anastomoses, and Nerve Coaptation

- Attention is turned back to the flap on the arm. The radial artery and its vena comitans are divided after ligaclipping the proximal vessels. The cephalic vein and LABC/MABC nerves are likewise divided.
- The neophallus is transferred to the perineum, and anchoring sutures are placed between the deep dermis portion of the flap and deep Scarpa layer of the suprapubic area. A coaptation of the neourethra in the flap to perineal urethra in the recipient site is performed with interrupted 4-0 Vicryl sutures. Anterior vaginal mucosal flaps, labia minora flaps, or even a gracilis muscle flap may be used to bolster the anastomosis.
- The no. 12 Foley catheter is in the neourethra and left in place for 2 weeks. A suprapubic catheter may or may not be used.
- An end-to-end neural coaptation is performed connecting the MABC to the ilioinguinal nerve and the LABC to one of the previously dissected dorsal clitoral nerves in an epineural fashion with 8-0 nylon sutures. This preservation of the innervated clitoris at the base of the phallus provides the potential for sensory and erogenous reinnervation of the neophallus while preserving a sensate clitoris.
- The recipient vessels are passed through into the right groin dissection through the tunnel made previously. The arterial anastomosis is done end to side to the femoral artery, possibly aided by vein grafts or an AV loop as described above. The cephalic vein is anastomosed end to end to a side branch of the femoral or saphenous vein.
- The clamps are released, and perfusion in the flap is evaluated by looking for good pulsation in the artery and good venous return. The flap should become pink and bleed from cut surfaces. The lie of the vessels is confirmed to be not kinked or redundant.
- The penile flap is now completely inset by tailoring the surrounding skin to inset the neophallus (**TECH FIG 5**). Inset of the flap is done using interrupted 3-0 Monocryl. The groin wound is now closed using interrupted 3-0 Vicryl stitches in the deep dermal layer and running sutures in the skin. At the end of the procedure, sterile dressings consisting of Xeroform fluff gauze and mesh pants are applied to the neophallus.

Closure of Donor Site and Dressings

- Attention is now turned to repairing the donor defect on the arm. Fascia was left down on the volar compartment with

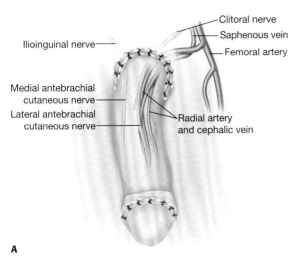

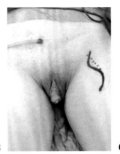

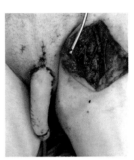

TECH FIG 5 • A. Schematic of plan for inset of the radial forearm phalloplasty with anastomosis to the saphenous vein and femoral artery. The lateral and medial antebrachial cutaneous nerves are coapted to the ilioinguinal nerve and one of the clitoral nerves. One clitoral nerve is left in situ to retain erogenous function of the clitoris, which is now buried beneath the neophallus. **B.** Recipient site planning. This patient has previously undergone metoidioplasty. **C.** Flap inset after urethral anastomosis and nerve coaptations and demonstrating vascular anastomoses.

the exception of between brachioradialis and flexor carpi radialis necessary to preserve the radial artery perforators.
- The proximal longitudinal exposure incision is closed with interrupted 3-0 Vicryl sutures in the deep dermal layer followed by 4-0 nylon for skin closure.
- A good quality, moderately thick (0.0012″–00.14″ thick) skin graft is harvested from the thigh and is meticulously sutured into the forearm donor site as a sheet graft. This is generally done with 4-0 chromic

sutures. Our preference is to place a dressing consisting of Xeroform, mineral oil–impregnated cotton batten, and a form-fitting, well-padded volar short-arm splint maintaining the hand and wrist in the intrinsic plus position, although a tie-over bolster may be used on the skin graft.
- After the dressings are placed on the arm and the Foley is connected to bag drainage, the patient is awakened and returned to the recovery area.

PEARLS AND PITFALLS

PENILE INVERSION VAGINOPLASTY

Rectal injury in vaginoplasty	■ The initial dissection through the perineal body, just posterior to the bulbocavernosus muscle, is sharp and performed with cautery. ■ Past the urogenital diaphragm, dissection should be performed bluntly with a sponge stick with gentle sweeping motion anterior to posterior. ■ Any injury to the rectum should be identified on exam and repaired in two layers.
Raising of neoclitoral flap in vaginoplasty	■ There is no defined plane between tunica albuginea and the dorsal penile bundle. ■ Dissection begins at the midaxis of the penis and using small Metzenbaum scissors carried dorsally in a lateral to medial on both sides. ■ You will notice a difference in fiber direction between bucks (longitudinal along the penis axis) and the more superficial investing fascia (diagonal and transverse). ■ This is tedious.
Placement of vaginal packing	■ Packing should extend into the apex of the neovagina. We use a vaginal pack coated in bacitracin ointment, but many surgeons use metronidazole gel. ■ An entire vaginal pack gauze should fit in the neovagina. ■ Sections of cut suction tubing are used as buttresses over the labia with 0-0 Prolene sutures to tamponade the packing in place.
Hemostasis in vaginoplasty	■ Estimated blood loss for this procedure averages 500 cc. ■ Patients should have two large-bore peripheral IVs and an active type and screen prior to surgical incision.

RADIAL FOREARM PHALLOPLASTY

Venous congestion	■ Positioning of the neophallus must keep distal aspect elevated. ■ AV fistula may be created in the distal phallus from end of radial artery and large vein.
Urethral fistula or stricture	■ A gracilis muscle flap may be used to bolster the urethral anastomosis at time of phalloplasty if there is significant concern for fistula. ■ Involvement of urologist is recommended for management of persistent fistula or strictures.

POSTOPERATIVE CARE

Penile Inversion Vaginoplasty

- The patient must remain on bed rest overnight until postoperative day 1.
- Examination on POD 1 should document swelling, labial incision integrity, labial skin viability, and neoclitoral viability. After this examination, patients are able to shuffle in their room and sit for limited periods in a well-padded chair, but activity is otherwise limited.
- Surgical drains and Foley catheter remain in place along with the vaginal packing until postoperative day 5 or 6.
- VTE prophylaxis is started 6 hours after surgery.
- Unless a rectal injury was noted and was repaired, patients are advanced to regular diet starting on postoperative day 1.
- Mesh underwear and Kerlix fluff are changed daily and as needed.
- On postoperative day 5 or 6, the vaginal packing is removed, and a speculum exam is performed to assess viability of the neovagina lining. The drains and Foley catheter are also removed at this time. Patients then begin vaginal rinses with 240 cc of normal saline using red Robinson catheter 3 times daily, are taught to perform twice-daily vaginal dilations with small-sized dilators, and are discharged from the hospital.
- Patients are examined again 10 to 14 days later to assess tissue viability and ensure they are managing dilation as instructed.
- Examination 4 to 6 weeks after the procedure should generally find nearly complete healing. At this point, the patient may progress to a larger vaginal dilator, begin relaxing activity restrictions, and return to work.
- Examination about 3 months postoperatively should document full healing before the patient is cleared for penetrative intercourse (**FIG 4**). Patients must understand the need to dilate daily indefinitely or to have penetrative intercourse to maintain vaginal depth.
- Patients must clearly understand that they still have a prostate gland and will still require surveillance for prostate disease as recommended by their PCP.

Phalloplasty

- Patient must remain on bed rest overnight until postoperative day 1.
- Surgical drains remain in for 5 to 7 days. Foley catheter remains in place for a minimum of 2 weeks.
- VTE prophylaxis is started 6 hours after surgery.
- Patients are advanced to regular diet starting on postoperative day 1.

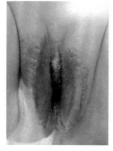

FIG 4 • Postoperative appearance at 3 months.

- Mesh underwear and Kerlix fluff are changed daily and as needed.
- Patients are allowed only very limited, in-room activity for 5 days. After this interval, they are mobilized over a 1- to 2-day period.
- A resting volar splint is kept in place for 5 to 7 days over the split-thickness skin graft on the radial forearm donor site. It is then removed and daily Xeroform dressing changes are performed. A removable splint is fashioned and worn for 3 weeks. After the graft has completely epithelialized, gentle active and passive range-of-motion exercises are initiated.
- Drains in the groin are removed 7 to 10 days postoperatively unless there is unusual high output, which may indicate a small lymph leak. They should then be left in place until output is less than 30 cc/d for 2 consecutive days.
- The Foley catheter remains in place for a minimum 2 weeks and a voiding trial is planned. If the patient is able to spontaneously void, then the suprapubic tube, if used, may be removed.
- The patient is seen 2 weeks postoperatively in clinic to assess surgical incisions, flap viability, and voiding function. They are then seen 3 months postoperatively at which time activity restrictions may be lifted and the patient may return to work.
- Delayed coronaplasty and glans tattooing may be performed after 3 months when all incisions are completely healed. Testicular implants may be placed at this time. Erectile prosthesis, either hydrolic or semirigid, may be placed after protective sensation is achieved in the neophallus, typically 1 year postoperatively.
- Erectile prosthesis may be placed after the neophallus regains protective sensation, at approximately 1 year. There is a high rate of erosion and ultimate explantation, approximately 50% within 5 years. Semirigid prostheses tend to be better tolerated than hydrolic devices. Necrosis of the phallus during placement of the erectile prosthesis has been described in the literature.

OUTCOMES

Penile Inversion Vaginoplasty

- Published case series have shown that transwomen who have undergone vaginoplasty are able to orgasm and have penetrative intercourse.
- A minority undergo revision labiaplasty to centralize the anterior commissure of the labia.
- With daily dilations, few transwomen need revisionary surgery to lengthen the vaginal vault postoperatively.
- Minor revisionary urethroplasties to address spraying or misdirection of the urinary stream are also moderately common.

Phalloplasty

- The goals of a phalloplasty are to urinate standing up and to provide a phallus for self-image (**FIG 5**).
- After development of protective sensation in 12 to 18 months, a semirigid erectile prosthesis may be implanted for sexual function. However, complications related to prostheses include necrosis of the phallus, infection, extrusion, and need for explantation. Newer prostheses, designed specifically for phalloplasty patients, may improve the complication rate.

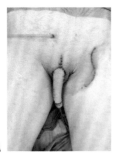 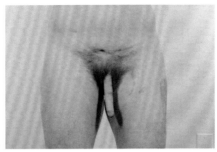 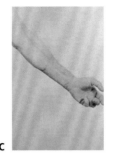

FIG 5 • **A.** Immediate postoperative result showing wound closure and suprapubic catheter. **B.** Appearance of the phallus at 3 months. **C.** Radial forearm flap donor site at 3 months.

COMPLICATIONS

Penile Inversion Vaginoplasty

- The most feared and serious complication is that of a rectovaginal fistula. We assess for undetected rectal injury using a Betadine enema in the operating room. If there is a tear in the rectum, it is repaired in two layers using 2-0 Vicryl. The patient is then left on a low-residue diet for several weeks.
  - If a rectovaginal fistula does develop, it is often managed with diverting ostomy, continued dilation of the neovagina, and watchful waiting. Assistance from a colorectal surgeon is necessary. A gracilis flap interposed between the rectum and neovagina may be necessary.
- Delayed bleeding from the corpus spongiosum deep to the urethral mucosa may be managed with sutures and/or direct pressure. At time of inset of urethra, attention must be paid to bury all erectile tissue under the mucosal closure.
- Delayed wound healing is relatively common, especially at the posterior aspect of the labia majora and inside the neovagina. Most will heal spontaneously without repeat intervention with meticulous hygiene and continued dilation.

Phalloplasty

- Venous congestion of the neophallus may be related to positioning the phallus in the dependent position. It should be elevated continuously for the first several postoperative days. If the phallus remains congested, venous outflow can be augmented with creation of an AV fistula at the distal end of the phallus between the ligated radial artery and vena comitans.
- Urethral fistulas and strictures are common (greater than 50% in many case series) and are difficult to manage. Involvement from a colleague from urology is necessary. Urinary diversion with Foley catheter or suprapubic catheter for an extended period may be necessary.
  - If a fistula remains after urinary diversion, superficial circumflex iliac perforator or pudendal perforator flap for coverage may be necessary. Cystoscopy may be required to assess and endoscopically treat urinary strictures.
  - Risks of urinary complications should be discussed with the patient preoperatively.

REFERENCES

1. Selvaggi G, Ceulemans P, De Cuypere G, et al. Gender identity disorder: general overview and surgical treatment for vaginoplasty in male-to-female transsexuals. *Plast Reconstr Surg.* 2005;116(6): 135e-145e.
2. Horbach SE, Bouman MB, Smit JM, et al. Outcome of vaginoplasty in male-to-female transgenders: a systematic review of surgical techniques. *J Sex Med.* 2015;12(6):1499-1512.
3. Monstrey S, Hoebeke P, Selvaggi G, et al. Penile reconstruction: is the radial forearm flap really the standard technique? *Plast Reconstr Surg.* 2009;124(2):510-518.
4. Monstrey SJ, Ceulemans P, Hoebeke P. Sex reassignment surgery in the female-to-male transsexual. *Semin Plast Surg.* 2011;25(3):229-244.

Section V: Reconstruction of Pressure Injuries
Gluteal Flaps for Sacral Pressure Injuries

Terri A. Zomerlei and Jeffrey E. Janis

DEFINITION

- Sacral pressure injuries are common in chronically supine patients.
- Patient populations most at risk include those in acute care settings, nursing home patients, and paraplegic populations.
- In addition to unrelieved pressure, the causes are multifactorial and may include incontinence/moisture, friction/shear force, and altered sensory perception.
- Characteristically, the appearance of the overlying skin represents only a small portion of the affected tissue ("the tip of the iceberg").

ANATOMY

- The sacrum is a large concave triangular bone at the base of the spine that is the fusion of sacral vertebrae S1-S5.
- A pressure injury develops as a result of unrelieved pressure between the sacral bone and the sitting or lying surface.
- The gluteus maximus muscle is a broad, thick, quadrangular muscle that forms the prominence of the buttocks.
  - The gluteus maximus originates along the posterior gluteal line of the ilium and the lateral aspect of the sacrum, coccyx, and sacral ligaments.
  - The superior portion of the muscle inserts along the iliotibial tract of the fascia lata, and the inferior portion of the muscle inserts into the greater trochanter of the femur.
  - It is a type III muscle with two dominant blood supplies, the superior and inferior gluteal arteries.
    - The vessels arise separately from the internal iliac artery.
    - The arteries exit the pelvis with their respective venae comitantes and the superior and inferior gluteal nerves.
- The anatomic landmarks for locating the neurovascular pedicles are the piriformis muscle, the posterior iliac spine, the greater trochanter, and the ischial tuberosity.
  - The superior gluteal artery exits above the piriformis one-third the distance from the posterior iliac spine along a tangent from the posterior iliac spine to the greater trochanter.
  - The inferior gluteal artery exits below the piriformis just lateral to a point half the distance between the posterior iliac spine and the ischial tuberosity (**FIG 1**).

PATHOGENESIS

- Primary mechanism of pressure injury is cellular ischemia.
  - Tissue pressure greater than the pressure of the microcirculation (32 mm Hg) causes ischemia.
  - If the ischemic period is long enough and repeated frequently, the eventual outcome is tissue necrosis.

- Pressure injuries (decubitus ulcers) almost invariably occur in the tissue over bony prominences in persons not able to change body position frequently.
- Pressure injuries overlying the sacrum are common in chronically supine patients.
- In acutely ill patients, third-space fluid may mechanically compromise the microvasculature.
- Etiologic considerations can be divided in extrinsic and intrinsic factors.
  - Extrinsic factors: Primarily mechanical forces on the soft tissues
    - Friction: Resistance that a surface encounters when moving over another; most often occurs with patient transfers
    - Moisture: Incontinence can lead to skin breakdown.
    - Pressure: Mechanical force that is applied perpendicular to a plane (ie, between a bony prominence and a chair or bed)
    - Shear: Mechanical stress parallel to the plane results in stretching and compression of the blood supply to the muscles and skin.
  - Intrinsic factors: Patient factors that affect the soft tissues
    - Altered level of consciousness: Results in lack of voluntary movements and protective reflexes that off-load pressure
    - Anemia: Can contribute to fatigue and weakness which can perpetuate immobility.
    - Autonomic control: Decreased levels result in spasms, perspiration with increased skin moisture, blood vessel

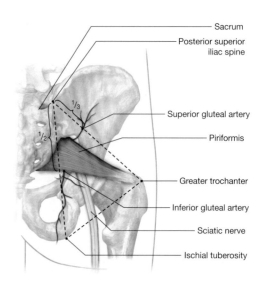

FIG 1 • Sacral anatomy.

engorgement with resulting tissue edema, and problems with bowel and bladder control.

- Age: Increasing age is associated with increased skin friability and decreased tensile strength.
- Diabetes: Poorly controlled blood glucose levels are associated with early recurrence of pressure injuries.
- Infection: Profoundly impairs wound healing abilities.
- Inflammation: Creates a hostile local milieu resulting in impaired healing, especially in the setting of chronic wounds.
- Malnutrition: Results in wasting and decreased muscle bulk and impairs wound healing abilities
- Sepsis: Can result in decreased tissue perfusion and ischemia
- Sensory loss: Patient is unable to experience the discomfort associated with prolonged pressure over prominences.

NATURAL HISTORY

- Pressure injuries are categorized according to the National Pressure Ulcer Advisory Panel Stages.
- Pressure injuries can progress through the following stages if extrinsic and intrinsic insults are not remedied (**FIG 2**).
  - Stage I: Intact skin with nonblanching erythema
  - Stage II: Partial thickness skin loss with exposed dermis
    - Presents as a blister, abrasion, or shallow open ulcer
  - Stage III: Full-thickness skin loss
    - Subcutaneous fat may be exposed.
    - Tunneling and undermining may be present.
  - Stage IV: Full-thickness skin and tissue loss
  - Unstageable: Full-thickness skin or soft tissue loss but depth is unknown usually due to the presence of an overlying eschar
  - Suspected deep tissue injury: Blood-filled blister or deep purple discoloration of intact skin may indicate deep tissue injury that needs to evolve prior to staging.

HISTORY AND PHYSICAL FINDINGS

- The preoperative evaluation of patients with any type of pressure injury includes a detailed assessment of the patient's medical history, social situation, and baseline health status and a comprehensive wound evaluation.[1]
- Patient history
  - How long has the pressure injury been present? Acute wounds may respond to conservative treatment, whereas chronic wounds tend to be more recalcitrant.

- What is the current wound care treatment? Changing local wound care regimens may help with improving the wound.
- What surgical options have been tried in the past? Obtain any and all operative reports as previous surgeries may limit surgical options.
- Is the patient ambulatory, or wheelchair or bed bound? Some flap procedures are not appropriate for ambulatory patients.
- What type of mattress and turning regimen is currently being used? Airflow mattresses offer the best protection, whereas normal mattresses offer little defense against pressure.
- Is fecal contamination a problem? A dressing or a temporary diverting ostomy may be prudent.
- Are there problems with urinary incontinence? A urinary diversion procedure (ie, suprapubic tube) or indwelling Foley catheter may be indicated.
- Does the patient have spasms? Optimize medications to control spasms.
- Does the patient have any fixed contractures?
- What is the baseline nutritional status of the patient?
- Social history is crucial to obtain in order to understand possible postoperative barriers to care and to thwart recurrence.
  - What is the social support/caregiver situation?
  - Do they have resources for obtaining durable medical equipment (low air loss bed, seat cushion if bed bound or wheelchair bound)?
  - Is there smoking or substance abuse history?
    - Active or prior nicotine use increases risk of poor wound healing.
    - A urine toxicology screen or urine cotinine test may be useful.
  - Is there a history of psychiatric illness?
  - Does the patient follow a specific diet (cardiac, diabetic)?
  - What is their daily protein intake?
  - What is the patient's compliance history?
- Laboratory studies
  - Complete blood count to assess for anemia or active infection
  - Albumin, prealbumin, and total protein to assess protein stores
  - Coagulation panel to assess for coagulopathies
  - Cultures that should be obtained with tissue or bone biopsies as wound swabs have little value due to chronic colonization. Cultures should be sent for quantitative analysis, and if the organism count is greater than 10^5, consideration should be given to systemic antibiotics and/or staged debridement and reconstruction.
  - Urinalysis

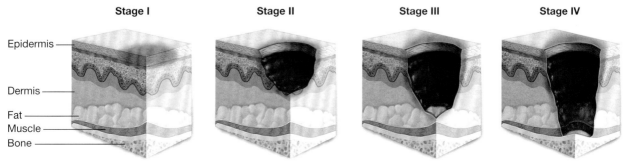

FIG 2 • Pressure injury staging.

Stage I   Stage II   Stage III   Stage IV

Epidermis

Dermis

Fat
Muscle
Bone

- Physical exam
  - *All wounds must be examined manually.*
  - Visual wound assessment alone is not sufficient to obtain necessary information about a wound.
  - Manually assess the size and depth of the wound, bony prominences, bursa, proximity to the rectum, and presence of tunneling (may need to use long cotton tip applicator to assess tunneling).
  - If an eschar is present, the wound cannot be accurately staged.
  - A limited bedside debridement may be useful, if the patient can tolerate this, so that the wound can be staged and to facilitate local wound care preoperatively.
  - From visual inspection, take note of any previous surgical scars as previous surgeries may preclude the use of a flap secondary to compromised vascular supply.
  - Muscle tone and bulk are assessed taking note of any spasticity or contraction of the extremities.
  - Assess the patient's sensation in the area of the wound.

IMAGING

- MRI is recommended for all stage IV pressure injuries to evaluate for osteomyelitis.
  - T2 hypersensitivity and low-intensity T1 is sensitive and specific for osteomyelitis (97% and 89%, respectively).
- If MRI is not available or the patient has conditions precluding its use, plain films and CT scan may be used. This imaging can be confirmatory for osteomyelitis but has low specificity.[2]

DIFFERENTIAL DIAGNOSIS

- Marjolin ulcer
- Burn
- Pilonidal disease
- Neoplasm with bony metastasis
- Soft tissue neoplasm with ulceration
- Chronic surgical wound
- Traumatic wound

NONOPERATIVE MANAGEMENT

- Relieve extrinsic pressure with frequent positional changes.
  - Turn every 2 hours when supine.
  - Lift for 10 seconds every 10 minutes when seated.
- Use proper mattress (low air loss) and cushion for seating and wheelchair (seat mapping).
- Minimize head of the bed elevation (less than 45 degrees).
- Optimize underlying medical status.
  - Address spasticity (baclofen, diazepam, dantrolene).
  - Optimize nutrition—protein intake of 1.5 to 3.0 g/kg/d.
- Local wound care in those who are poor surgical candidates or while optimizing a patient for surgery.
  - Dakin's ¼ strength for a limited time period (days up to 1 week) can be effective in decreasing wound colonization while preserving native tissues.[3]
  - Limited bedside debridement to remove any wet eschar to facilitate adequate packing and wound care may be warranted.
  - Enzymatic debridement is helpful when the wound has heavy slough.

SURGICAL MANAGEMENT

Preoperative Planning[4]

- The most crucial aspect of the surgical management of sacral pressure injuries is the preoperative and postoperative care.
- Do not operate on patients until their medical status is optimized and the underlying etiology determined.
- Obtain old operative reports to know what prior attempts at closure have been tried.
- Always consider future procedures in the operative planning so as to not "burn bridges."
- Review with the patient and all caregivers the postoperative expectations and restrictions to help ensure postoperative compliance.

Positioning

- To minimize repositioning, have anesthesia induced while the patient is supine on stretcher.
  - Ensure that anesthesia provider appropriately protects eyes, face, and endotracheal tube.
- Check OR table to ensure working properly (able to flex and extend at hips) prior to patient transfer.
- Position gel rolls for chest and hips onto OR table.
- Patient gown should be removed.
- With stretcher in locked position next to the OR table and with appropriate resources and careful choreography, roll patient to prone position.
- Pad all extremities with foam or gel pads; toes should be "floating" (consider a Wilson frame).
- Ensure that genitalia are free from compression.
- Arms should be on arm boards in "Superman" position.
- Check EKG pads, monitoring devices, grounding pads, and catheters to make sure they are not placing pressure on the skin and are outside of the operative field.
- Take care that any ostomies, if present, are free from compression.
- Ensure no traction on indwelling catheters.
- Secure patient to bed at both the trunk and lower legs.
- Apply warming blankets or forced air to the upper trunk.
- If the GI tract is still in continuity, an adhesive drape can be applied as a "mud flap" to exclude the rectum from the field.
- OR table can be flexed at the patient's hip level to improve exposure (**FIG 3**).

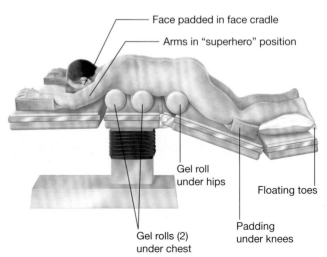

Face padded in face cradle
Arms in "superhero" position
Gel roll under hips
Floating toes
Gel rolls (2) under chest
Padding under knees

FIG 3 • Prone positioning.

Approach

- Gluteal rotation flap
  - Can be taken from either left or right gluteal area
  - Able to be readvanced as needed in the future
  - Available as a fasciocutaneous or musculocutaneous flap
    - Can be full or segmental (used in ambulators)
    - Musculocutaneous flaps have the advantage of additional bulk and robust blood supply
- V-Y advancement flap
  - Ipsilateral for small wounds
  - Bilateral for larger sacral wounds
- Sliding gluteal flap
  - A fasciocutaneous flap preferred for the ambulatory population
  - Can be unilateral or ipsilateral

■ Excisional Debridement

- Failure to adequately debride can lead to recurrent disease and poor wound healing.
- Probe wounds prior to debridement so all tunneling is addressed.
- Infiltration of the peribursal area with a wetting solution (1000 mL of normal saline plus 30 mL of 1% lidocaine, plus 1 ampule of epinephrine 1:1000) can assist with hydrodissection and decrease blood loss.[5]
- Coating the cavity with methylene blue applied with a cotton applicator can assist with bursa identification and verify the completeness of the debridement.

- Debridement removes necrotic tissue and biofilm and decreases bacterial count.
- Converts a chronic wound into an acute wound.
- Quantitative wound cultures should be obtained following debridement so that postoperative antibiotic coverage can be tailored appropriately.
- If the completeness of the debridement is ever in question, or the wound is severely contaminated, staged debridement and reconstruction can be performed, although outcomes may be similar to immediate reconstruction.[6]

■ Ostectomy

- Because most pressure injuries overlie bony prominences, and underlying osteomyelitis and unhealthy bone are likely, the bony prominence should be removed.

- The ostectomy should be performed only to lessen the prominence as radical removal may redistribute pressure points to adjacent tissue, result in excessive bleeding, and affect the origin and/or insertion of skeletal muscle.

■ Gluteal Rotation Flap

- Prep a wide field with Betadine and drape in the standard fashion (**TECH FIG 1A**).
- Mark key anatomic landmarks:
  - Posterior superior iliac spine
  - Greater trochanter
  - Ischial tuberosity
- Mark the locations of the vascular pedicles to the gluteus maximus.
  - Superior gluteal artery (SGA): Anticipated location is one-third the distance between the posterior superior iliac spine and the greater trochanter.
  - Inferior gluteal artery (IGA): Anticipated location is half the distance between the posterior superior iliac spine and the ischial tuberosity.
  - A handheld Doppler can be used to confirm location.
- Mark and elevate a larger flap than needed by 2 or 3 cm at least (**TECH FIG 1B**).
- The flap design can incorporate the SGA and its perforators and/or the IGA and perforators, depending on size needs (**TECH FIG 1C–E**).
- For a myocutaneous rotation flap, the incision is made with a scalpel and then deepened through the skin and subcutaneous tissues and muscle insertion with electrocautery.

- Take care to dissect straight down and not to undermine any of the subcutaneous tissue off of the muscle.
- Disinsert the gluteus at the lateral and inferior borders.
- Elevate the gluteus maximus in a superomedial direction in the areolar plane above the gluteus medius.
- Identify and protect the superior and/or inferior gluteal artery.
- Detach the gluteus maximus from its origin at the posterior superior iliac spine.
- Rotate the flap over the sacral defect (**TECH FIG 1F**).
  - A back-cut (Burow triangle) can be made at the inferolateral aspect to rotate tension-free (do not injure the IGA).
- Irrigate and obtain hemostasis.
- Suture the flap muscle to the contralateral gluteus maximus muscle without tension using monofilament long-acting absorbable suture.
- Insert drains into both donor and recipient site.
- Close the skin in layers with suture or suture plus staples.
- The flap can be rerotated at a later date should the need arise.
- A unilateral rotation flap can be used in conjunction with a contralateral V-Y advancement flap.

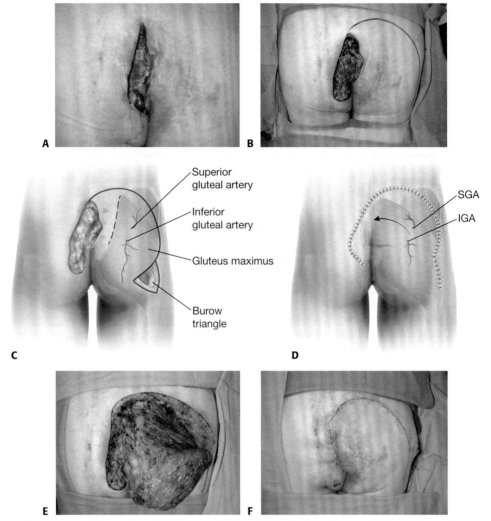

TECH FIG 1 • **A.** Sacral pressure injury prior to debridement. **B.** Wound following debridement. A right-sided gluteal rotation flap has been marked. **C,D.** Design of the gluteal rotation flap. **E.** A fasciocutaneous rotation flap based on the perforators of the inferior gluteal artery has been raised. **F.** The flap has been inset with absorbable suture. Note the back-cut or Burow triangle.

■ V-Y Advancement Flap

- Mark anatomic and vascular landmarks as described previously.
- Design and mark a skin paddle overlying the gluteus maximus (mark a flap larger than needed).
  - Flap is designed in a triangle shape and can be designed to incorporate the SGA, the IGA, or both (**TECH FIG 2A**).
- Incise the skin sharply, and use electrocautery to dissect down to the muscle beveling out to capture soft tissue.
- Do not undercut the skin paddle with dissection.
- Dissect from lateral to medial in the submuscular space after dividing the muscle laterally.

- Divide the muscle from the origin at the sacrum. Take care not to injure SGA or IGA.
- Once the muscle is fully divided around the skin paddle, the tissue should easily advance medially (**TECH FIG 2B**).
- Place drains into the donor and recipient sites.
- Suture the flap gluteus maximus to the contralateral muscle with absorbable sutures.
- Close the skin and subcutaneous tissues in layers with sutures or sutures and staples (**TECH FIG 2C**).
- The lateral donor site will close primarily (Y).
- This flap can be unilateral or bilateral and can be used in conjunction with a rotational flap.

TECHNIQUES

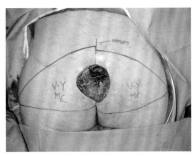 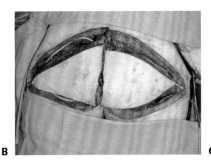 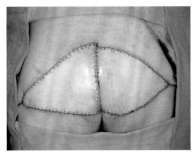

TECH FIG 2 • A. A sacral wound has been debrided, and bilateral myocutaneous V-Y flaps have been designed. **B.** The flaps easily advance to the midline, filling the defect. **C.** The flaps have been inset with suture.

■ Sliding Gluteal Flap (Fasciocutaneous)

- Mark anatomic and vascular landmarks as described previously (**TECH FIG 3A,B**).
- Design and mark a triangular skin paddle overlying the gluteus maximus (mark a flap larger than needed).
- Cutaneous skin island can reach up to T12 if needed.

- Incise the skin sharply and use electrocautery to dissect down to the muscle by beveling out to capture maximal soft tissue and preserve perforators.
- Do not undercut the skin paddle with dissection.
- Once skin paddle is "islandized," it should easily move medially.
- Insert drains into donor and recipient sites.
- Close donor and recipient sites with layered sutures or sutures and staples (**TECH FIG 3C**).

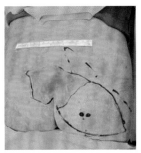 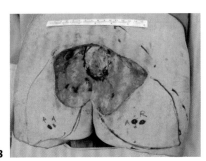 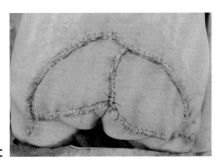

TECH FIG 3 • A. This ambulatory patient suffered a pressure injury during hospitalization for an acute injury. She developed a chronic wound and osteomyelitis. A fasciocutaneous flap based on the inferior gluteal artery perforators is planned. **B.** Following debridement, the wound is much larger than anticipated. Therefore, bilateral flaps were designed. The area of bone that will undergo ostectomy is outlined in methylene blue. Based on anatomic landmarks, "A" represents the "anticipated" location of the inferior gluteal artery. "R" represents the "real" location of the artery based on Doppler exam. **C.** The flaps are closed in a V-Y fashion. (Courtesy of R. Chandawarkar, MD.)

PEARLS AND PITFALLS

Preoperative planning	■ Evaluate extrinsic and intrinsic factors to determine wound etiology. ■ Ensure that the patient is medically optimized prior to their operation. ■ Engage social work to ensure that the patient has adequate social support and resources for the postoperative period. ■ Consult with appropriate consultants prior to reconstruction (colorectal for diverting ostomy, ID if osteomyelitis).
Positioning	■ Attention to choreography and team communication is crucial to position the patient safely in the prone position.
Operative strategy	■ Autonomic dysfunction in the patient can create difficulties for the anesthesia team, so communicate with your providers frequently. ■ Know the location of the blood supply to the flaps. Use a handheld Doppler if in doubt.
Postoperative care	■ Engage a multidisciplinary team including nursing, social work, and other consulting services as appropriate to ensure a safe discharge and to give the patient the "best chance" of preventing reoccurrence.[7]

POSTOPERATIVE CARE

- Patients are hospitalized for 1 to 2 weeks after surgery, and many patients will discharge to a rehabilitation hospital or an extended care facility for several weeks to receive a higher level of nursing care.
- A low air loss mattress should be ordered prior to the surgery and should be available to move the patient onto directly from the operating room table.
- The patient should limit the HOB to less than 10 degrees for 1 week.
- The patient should be repositioned every 2 hours, unless he or she is on an air-fluidized bed.
- The postoperative dressing should be left in place for 48 hours, after which time a light dressing can be applied to protect against shear and moisture or the wound can be left open to the air to allow for ease of wound monitoring.
- Bladder and bowel function should be controlled to prevent urinary or fecal contamination of the surgical site.
- Spasticity should be prevented with pharmacologic measures.
- Obtain a dietary consultation so that the patient can maintain a positive nitrogen balance.
- Meticulous drain care should be performed in the hospital and taught to all caregivers.
- Obtain an infectious disease consultation for any positive operative cultures to help guide antibiotic selection and duration of treatment.
- Evaluate need for long-term intravenous access for antibiotics.

OUTCOMES

- Recurrence rate is high.
- Local wound/incision problems are common and should be treated with local wound care.
- Anticipate further reconstruction options with every surgical intervention.

- Control for extrinsic and intrinsic factors that contributed to the initial pressure injury formation.

COMPLICATIONS

- Complications are not uncommon in those with significant preoperative comorbidities.
- Hematoma or seroma may occur.
  - If the patient is on anticoagulants, work closely with hematologist to determine when these can be safely held and resumed in the perioperative period.
  - One or more drains should be left under flaps for days to weeks to control for fluid accumulation.
- Small localized incisional breakdown should be treated with local wound care.
- Persistent infection can be minimized with thorough debridement and long-term antibiotics as deemed appropriate by infectious disease colleagues.
- Unless underlying medical problems and extrinsic factors are controlled, the recurrence rate is high.

REFERENCES

1. Marin J, Nixon J, Gorecki C. A systematic review of risk factors for the development of and recurrence of pressure ulcers in people with spinal cord injuries. *Spinal Cord.* 2013;51(7):522-527.
2. Huang AB, Schweitzer ME, Hume E, et al. Osteomyelitis of the hips/pelvis in paralyzed patients, accuracy and clinical utility of MRI. *J Comput Assist Tomogr.* 1998;22:437.
3. Heggers JP, Sazy JA, Stenberh BD, et al. Bactericidal and wound-healing properties of sodium hypochlorite solutions: The 1991 Lindberg Award. *J Burn Care Rehabil.* 1991;12:420.
4. Janis, JE, Kenkel, JM. Pressure Sores. *Selected Readings in Plast Surg.* 2003;9(39):1-42.
5. Han H, Fen J, Fine NA. Use of the tumescent technique in pressure ulcer closure. *Plast Reconstr Surg.* 2002;110:711.
6. Larson DL, Hudak KA, Waring WP, et al. Protocol management of late stage pressure ulcers: a 5-year retrospective study of 101 consecutive patients with 179 ulcers. *Plast Reconstr Surg.* 2012;129:897.
7. Bauer J, Phillips LG. Pressure sores. *Plast Reconstr Surg.* 2008;121:1-10.

Posterior Thigh and Hamstring Flaps for Ischial Ulcers

John Hulsen and Jeffrey E. Janis

DEFINITION

- A pressure injury is localized damage to the skin and soft tissue typically over a bony prominence.
- They occur as a result of prolonged pressure or pressure in combination with shear.
- National Pressure Ulcer Advisory Panel Stages[1] are shown in FIG 2 in Chapter 29.
- The ischial area is the most frequent site of development and recurrence of pressure ulcers.[2]
- Soft tissue overlying the bony prominence of the ischial tuberosity is particularly vulnerable to pressure injury especially in the wheelchair-bound/spinal cord injury patient.

ANATOMY

- The posterior thigh is a region bordered by the inferior gluteal fold superiorly, the iliotibial tract laterally, the thigh adductors medially, and the popliteal fossa inferiorly.
- The hamstring muscle group functions to flex, stabilize, and rotate the knee and are not expendable as a group in the ambulatory patient (**FIG 1**).[3]
  - Biceps femoris
  - Semimembranosus
  - Semitendinosus
- Blood supply of the posterior thigh skin:
  - The profunda femoris artery principally supplies the largest cutaneous area on the posterior thigh.[3]
  - It originates laterally from the femoral artery, gives off both medial and lateral circumflex femoral arteries, and then continues distally and traveling behind the adductor longus.
    - Medial branches enter into the adductor compartment.
    - Lateral branches (four profunda femoris artery perforating vessels) pierce the adductor magnus insertion and enter the posterior compartment of the thigh.
    - The fourth profunda femoris perforating artery is the termination of the profunda femoris artery.
    - Each profunda femoris perforating vessel perfuses musculocutaneous and/or septocutaneous perforators that contribute to the well-developed fascial plexus of the posterior thigh.
  - The inferior gluteal artery principally supplies the cutaneous vascular territory of the lower gluteal region.
    - It originates off the internal iliac artery and exits the pelvis to enter the gluteal region inferior to the piriformis with the sciatic and posterior cutaneous nerves. In 91% of patients, the inferior gluteal artery sends off a descending fasciocutaneous branch.[4]

- The descending branch of the inferior gluteal artery travels in a common sheath with the posterior cutaneous nerve in 72% of patients.
- Rather than singularly coursing down the thigh, the descending branch acts as a "relay artery," being reinforced along its length by myocutaneous and fasciocutaneous branches from the profunda femoris perforating vessels.[3]
- Anastomotic branches from the descending branch of the inferior gluteal artery join branches from the medial femoral circumflex artery, lateral femoral circumflex artery, and the first profunda perforating artery to form the cruciate anastomosis (**FIG 2**).[5]
- Each vessel that unites to form the cruciate anastomosis can provide collateral circulation to the longitudinally directed fascial plexus of the posterior thigh in the absence (or surgical ligation) of one of its constituents.[3,5]
- This accounts for the clinical reliability of the multitude of fasciocutaneous flap designs available from the posterior thigh.

PATHOGENESIS

- Pressure ulcers are the result of numerous factors, both extrinsic and intrinsic to the patient, that contribute to the development of a wound.
  - Pressure: Greatest areas found over bony prominences
    - Can produce tissue ischemia if applied in excess of 32 mm Hg (skin end capillary bed pressure)
    - The ischial tuberosities are particularly vulnerable to ulceration and recurrence as pressures over this region in the sitting position exceed 80 to 100 mm Hg.
    - Shearing: Sliding deformation of tissue caused by oppositely directed parallel forces
  - Friction: Contributes to abrasions and breakdown of the superficial skin barrier
  - Moisture: Contributes to maceration of the skin
  - Limited mobility: Inability to adequately off-load pressure points, potentially increasing friction and shearing forces
  - Altered sensation: Lack of protective sensory input
  - Spasticity: Interruption of supraspinal inhibitory pathways that may result in contractures that create new or altered pressure points
  - Altered level of consciousness: Unrecognized prolonged pressure with skin maceration/contamination from urine/fecal soilage

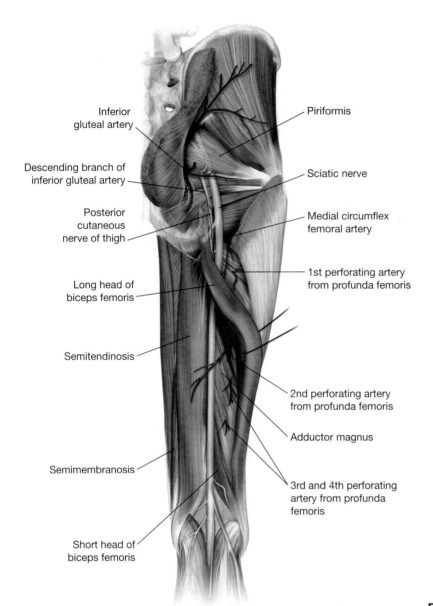

FIG 1 • Key posterior thigh anatomy.

Labels on figure:
- Inferior gluteal artery
- Descending branch of inferior gluteal artery
- Posterior cutaneous nerve of thigh
- Long head of biceps femoris
- Semitendinosis
- Semimembranosis
- Short head of biceps femoris
- Piriformis
- Sciatic nerve
- Medial circumflex femoral artery
- 1st perforating artery from profunda femoris
- 2nd perforating artery from profunda femoris
- Adductor magnus
- 3rd and 4th perforating artery from profunda femoris

- Tissue tolerance for pressure and shear forces is affected by microclimate, nutrition, perfusion, comorbidities, and condition of the soft tissue.[1]
- It is important to recognize, especially in the spinal cord injury patient, that all phases of wound healing are impaired in denervated tissue.

NATURAL HISTORY

- Skin hyperemia is seen within 30 minutes and is characterized by nonblanching erythema that resolves within 1 hour after pressure is alleviated.
- Tissue ischemia develops with sufficient continuous pressure for 2 to 6 hours, causing erythema that requires at least 36 hours to resolve after pressure cessation.
- Deep tissue injury/tissue necrosis can develop after 6 hours of unrelieved pressure and manifests as deep red, maroon, or purple skin discoloration with induration.
- Soft tissue ulceration over bony prominences occurs within 2 weeks after tissue necrosis occurs.

PATIENT HISTORY AND PHYSICAL FINDINGS

- Patient age, general health/functional status, medical comorbidities, nutritional intake, as well as the circumstances, etiology, chronology, and prior ulcer management should be documented.
  - Note any medications or therapy that impairs wound healing such as radiation and steroids.
  - Obtain reports from any previous surgical interventions that may influence ulcer reconstructive options.
  - Social history including tobacco use and a clear picture of the patient's support system should be obtained.
    - It is critical to identify the etiology that led to reconstructive failure when treating a recurrent ulcer.
    - Lack of compliance with postoperative care, lack of patient motivation, and inadequate resources for home care will doom even the best executed reconstruction and are critical to account for in determining whether a patient is a reconstructive candidate.

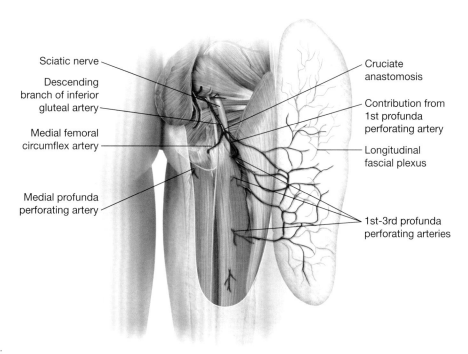

Sciatic nerve

Descending branch of inferior gluteal artery

Medial femoral circumflex artery

Medial profunda perforating artery

Cruciate anastomosis

Contribution from 1st profunda perforating artery

Longitudinal fascial plexus

1st-3rd profunda perforating arteries

FIG 2 • The cruciate anastomosis.

- Physical examination
  - General appearance, BMI, assessment of nutrition status: Does the patient appear well or fragile and emaciated?
  - Accurately assess location, dimensions (including tunneling), wound condition/odor, and stage/depth of ulcer.
  - Presence of diverting ostomy or suprapubic catheter
  - Presence of lower extremity fixed posturing or uncontrolled spasticity
  - Evaluate the posterior trunk and lower extremities for surgical scars from previous reconstructions while also assessing potential donor-site muscle bulk (diminished in spinal cord injury).

IMAGING AND OTHER DIAGNOSTIC STUDIES

- Preoperative laboratory studies
  - White blood cell count/differential and hemoglobin/hematocrit
  - Inflammatory markers: Erythrocyte sedimentation rate and C-reactive protein (especially if suspect osteomyelitis)
  - Glucose and HgbA1c: Ideally, good long-term glucose control in diabetics with a HgbA1c less than 6%[6]
- Nutrition studies
  - Accurate assessment of the nutritional status of the pressure ulcer patient is often compromised by proinflammatory factors that may preclude the use of typical serum protein values.
  - Ideal, and potentially unattainable, preoperative serum protein levels[7]:
    - Albumin: At least 3.5 g/dL with upward trend
    - Prealbumin: At least 20 g/dL with upward trend
- Unfortunately, there is little evidence that enteral or parenteral nutrition supplementation has any effect on healing existing pressure sores or the prevention of new ulcers.
- Data suggest that anemia, serum protein alterations, and markers of inflammation will actually normalize after surgical treatment of the ulcer.[8]

- These deficient values are viewed as the result of the ulcer rather than modifiable risk factors to optimize prior to surgery.
- Imaging studies
  - Used to assess for any undrained fluid collection and as noninvasive modality to detect osteomyelitis
  - MRI: 97% sensitive, 89% specific for diagnosis of osteomyelitis in the pelvis[9]
- Pathology/microbiology
  - Diagnostic standard for osteomyelitis is the pathology report of an aseptically obtained bone biopsy.

DIFFERENTIAL DIAGNOSIS

- Stage I to IV pressure ulcer, unstageable wound, or deep tissue injury
- Wound infection
- Acute or chronic osteomyelitis
- Malnutrition
- Muscle spasms
- Fecal and/or urinary incontinence
- Failed previous reconstruction

NONOPERATIVE MANAGEMENT

- Indications for nonoperative management include patients with stage I and II pressure ulcers as well as some patients with stage III and IV ulcers who are not candidates for reconstruction[7]:
  - Unmotivated patient
  - Inadequate home support or outpatient care
  - Comorbidities that place the patient at an unacceptable surgical or anesthesia risk
  - Unreconstructable defect
- In all pressure ulcer cases particular emphasis is placed on the prevention of wound complications and infections, halting ulcer progression, and reducing the risk of additional ulcers.

- If possible, the highest goal is a closed stable wound.
  - A closed wound is not an attainable goal for all patients.
  - The patient's social situation is just as important, if not more so, than any medical or surgical therapy.[7]
  - General treatment strategies for nonoperative management mirror those used in preoperative optimization of the pressure ulcer surgical candidate.
  - Offloading pressure points with specialty beds, seat mapping, and turning protocols every 2 hours.
  - Local skin and wound care to promote moist wound healing without maceration is essential.
    - Many passive and sophisticated active dressings are available; however, evidence is mixed regarding head-to-head superiority.
    - Fever/sepsis usually has a urinary or pulmonary source, not the open wound.
  - Negative-pressure wound therapy may be more comfortable to patients and effective in ulcers that fail to progress or as a bridge to surgery.
  - NPWT functions to increase wound perfusion and formation of granulation tissue while reducing bacterial load
  - A well-balanced diet is best to provide adequate nutrition for wound healing.
    - Supplements are beneficial only if there is a nutritional deficiency.[10]
    - Goal is 30 to 35 kcal/kg and 1.25 to 1.5 g protein/kg/d for adults with a pressure ulcer who are at risk for malnutrition.
    - Additional fluid should be provided to patients with heavily exudative wounds to prevent dehydration.
  - Management of muscular spasms helps to prevent new pressure points and reduces wound-shearing forces.

SURGICAL MANAGEMENT

- The presence of stage III and IV pressure ulcers alone is not an indication for surgical management.[7]
  - Optimization of medical comorbidities, modification of risk factors, assuring adequate home support, availability of medical equipment, access to outpatient care, assessment of patient compliance, and motivation to take an active role in self-care are essential for consideration of surgical candidacy.
  - The technical intraoperative aspects of pressure ulcer surgery are often the easiest facet of the patient's care.
- Goals of surgical management[7]:
  - Sharp debridement of all devitalized tissue (including complete excision of pseudobursa) to create a healthy bleeding wound bed
  - Ostectomy of devitalized bone to clinically hard bone with pinpoint bleeding and rasped smooth contour
  - Obtain soft tissue and bone biopsies following debridement under sterile conditions when indicated.
  - Provide tension-free soft tissue wound closure and obliterate dead space with judicious selection of large, well-vascularized flaps.
  - Avoid suture lines across pressure/seating surfaces.

- Selection of myocutaneous, fasciocutaneous, and perforator flap reconstruction is dependent on the location and dimensional characteristics of the ulcer, donor-site availability from prior surgery, ambulatory status of patient, and surgeon familiarity/preference.

Preoperative Planning

- Proactive coordination of multidisciplinary postoperative care and clear communication of expectations between the patient and team members prior to surgical intervention.
- Discuss temporary fecal diversion with the patient and general surgery (if incontinent or not compliant with a standard bowel regimen) if wound hygiene is a concern.
- Consider a urology consultation if there is concern for an occult urinary tract leak into the wound or uncontrolled urinary incontinence.
- Communicate in advance to the operating room staff the need for separate instruments for the contaminated debridement, sterile biopsy, and clean reconstructive portions of the case.

Positioning

- The patient is transferred to the operating room table in the prone position.
- Place the table in a moderate jack-knife position during flap inset to ensure adequate flap length while simulating tensile forces across the closure during the postoperative hip flexion protocol.
- Chest rolls are used to reduce breast and shoulder pressure.
- Assure adequate protective padding over the knees, legs, and feet.

Approach

- Ulcer excision is optimally approached after infiltration of epinephrine containing wetting solution around the pseudobursa/ulcer-healthy tissue interface and coating the cavity with dye.
  - This approach reduces blood loss and facilitates defining the ulcer for debridement.
- Despite attempts to standardize flap terminology, considerable variability exists in published literature and standard textbooks (with limited consensus even among practicing surgeons) regarding what is considered a "posterior thigh flap."
  - Numerous flaps (with common aliases), varying in type, anatomy, and clinical use are described in **Table 1**.
  - Regardless of nomenclature, it is vital to approach ulcer reconstruction with a sound understanding of the anatomical basis and constraints of each flap design.
    - Tailor flap choice to the patient's reconstructive needs, available donor sites, intact pedicles, and surgeon experience/preference.
    - Clear communication of your operative plan to the patient, surgical team, anesthesia staff, and rehabilitation team will allow for better coordination of OR resources and postoperative care

Table 1 Posterior Thigh Flaps

Flap Type	Names and Aliases	Muscles Sacrificed	Use in Ambulatory Patients?	Dominate Pedicle	Medial or Lateral Branch off Profunda Femoris Artery?
	Posterior thigh flap	None	Yes	Descending branch of inferior gluteal artery (if present) via cruciate anastamosis	None
	Posterior thigh fasciocutaneous flap	None	Yes	1st and 2nd profunda femoris perforator	Lateral
	Gluteal thigh flap Inferior gluteal thigh flap	None	Yes	1st and 2nd profunda femoris perforator + descending branch of inferior gluteal artery	Lateral
Fasciocutaneous	Posterior thigh flap Posterior thigh fasciocutaneous flap Posterior thigh rotation flap V-Y profunda femoris flap	None	Yes	1st and 2nd profunda femoris perforator +/− descending branch of inferior gluteal artery (if present and not previously divided)	Lateral
	Posterior thigh flap V-Y posterior thigh flap	None	Yes	Deeply based fasciocutaneous/septocutaneous perforators from posterior thigh compartment	Lateral
	Posterior thigh flap V-Y hamstring flap Biceps femoris flap Semicircular hamstring flap	Biceps femoris	Yes (potentially)[a]	1st perforating branch of profunda femoris artery	Lateral
Musculocutaneous	Posterior thigh flap V-Y hamstring flap Semicircular hamstring flap	Biceps femoris Semitendinosus Semimembranosus	No	1st perforating branch of profunda femoris artery	Lateral
	Posterior thigh flap Posterior thigh perforator flap	None	Yes	3rd perforating branch of profunda femoris artery	Lateral
Perforator	Posterior thigh flap Posterior thigh perforator flap Profunda artery perforator Flap PAP flap Adductor flap Adductor magnus perforator flap	None	Yes	1st medial branch of profunda femoris artery	Medial

[a]As an isolated muscle, it is expendable as a knee flexor except in certain athletic situations.

■ Ulcer and Pseudobursa Cavity Identification, Excision, and Bone

- The patient is prepped and draped with the ulcer cavity and flap donor sites exposed.
- Percutaneous access incisions are made within the rim of the planned ulcer excision as needed (**TECH FIG 1A,B**).
- Warmed wetting solution containing 30 mL of 1% plain lidocaine and 1 mL of 1:1000 epinephrine in 1000 mL of normal saline is injected circumferentially around the

entire cavity with a blunt-tipped infiltration cannula (**TECH FIG 1C**).

- Endpoints of wetting solution infiltration are increased skin turgor and adequate circumferential hydrodissection of the cavity from healthy tissue.
- Estimation of fluid volume used is 10 mL per 10 cm³ of pseudobursa cavity resection.[11]
- The epinephrine is allowed adequate time to achieve full hemostatic effect (no less than 7 minutes).

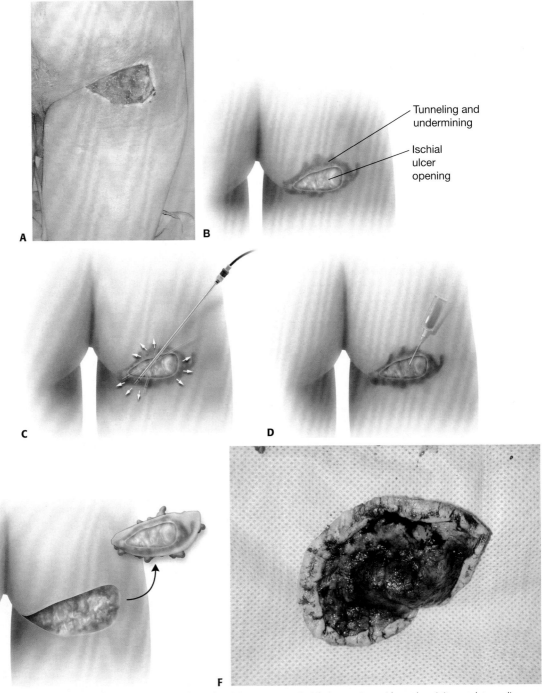

TECH FIG 1 • **A.** Stage III ischial pressure ulcer with undermining present. **B.** Ulcer opening with undermining and tunneling present. **C.** Infiltration of wetting solution containing epinephrine, "tumescent technique." **D.** Methylene blue is applied to the tunneling ulcer to identify all tissue to be excised. **E.** Clean, hemostatic wound, free from all ulcer/pseudobursa tissue. The true extent of the defect is now known. **F.** Pseudobursa and ulcer excised en bloc.

- The entire pseudobursa cavity is then coated with methylene blue dye (**TECH FIG 1D**).
  - Dye is loaded into a 10 mL syringe capped with a 14 g angiocath for clean application into tunneled areas.
- Borders of the ulcer, along a rim of any residual scar, are sharply incised.
- The rim of ulcer is grasped with an Allis or Kocher clamp for countertraction, and excision proceeds sharply through the hydrodissected planes with scissors and/or electrocautery. Endpoints are healthy, soft, bleeding tissue.
- The ulcer and pseudobursa cavity is excised en bloc, defining the new, larger defect (**TECH FIG 1E,F**).
- Ostectomy of exposed bony cortex proceeds, if indicated, using a sharp sterile osteotome.[12] Endpoints are hard, healthy, bleeding bone.
- A sterile rongeur is used to obtain a bone biopsy for culture.

Posterior Thigh Fasciocutaneous Rotation Flap With V-Y Closure

- Identify the midpoint between the ischial tuberosity and greater trochanter within the gluteal fold.
- A reference line is drawn from this point down the midaxis of the thigh to a distal point approximately 10 cm superior to the popliteal fossa.[5]
  - The most distal perforators are located approximately 10 cm proximal to the lateral femoral condyle.
- Outline the planned incisions for the V cutaneous island (**TECH FIG 2A**).
  - Medially, a curved line is drawn from the medial border of the ischial ulcer to the distal mark in the midaxis.
  - The lateral line curves cephalad from the distal mark toward the posterior border of the tensor fasciae latae terminating no higher than 10 cm inferior to the ischial tuberosity to preserve the first and second profunda perforators, which supply the flap with or without the descending branch of the inferior gluteal artery (if present) via the cruciate anastomosis.[5]
  - Primary closure of the donor site is possible with flap widths of 9 to 10 cm, otherwise plan for skin grafting.
- Carry incisions through marked outline into subcutaneous tissue and through the deep fascia of the posterior compartment just above the hamstring musculature.
- Begin elevation of the fasciocutaneous flap distally to protect the sciatic nerve, which, in this location, is deep to the biceps femoris.[5]
  - The posterior femoral cutaneous nerve arborizes distally and may not be a reliable reference for initial pedicle orientation.[13]
- The fasciocutaneous unit is easily and quickly raised off the posterior compartment muscles proximally with electrocautery.
  - The fascia is secured to the dermis of the skin paddle with suture to prevent shearing.[13]
- Identify and protect the sciatic nerve as it courses lateral and deep to the long head of the biceps femoris.[5]
  - The profunda femoris perforating vessels are encountered and usually preserved lateral to the sciatic nerve, approximately 10 cm inferior to the ischial tuberosity (**TECH FIG 2B**).
  - Perforators may be preserved or ligated and controlled with hemeclips/cautery if greater length is required and the inferior gluteal system/cruciate anastomosis is patent.
  - If the profunda perforating vessels are sacrificed, the dissection continues cephalad but does not extend superiorly beyond the level of the ischial tuberosity.
- The posterior thigh flap is then rotated into the ulcer/bursa defect.
- Redundant distal portion of the flap should be de-epithelialized and inset into the ulcer dead space and closed in a tension-free manner with long-acting absorbable monofilament suture over closed suction drains.
- The donor site is closed in a V-Y fashion over a drain (**TECH FIG 2C**).

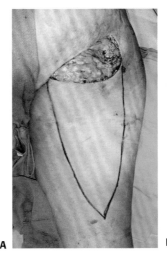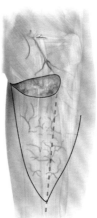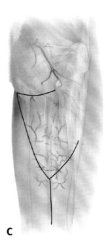

TECH FIG 2 • A. Clean ischial wound, all ulcer tissue excised. Posterior thigh/hamstring V-Y flap outlined. **B.** The profunda femoris perforating vessels are encountered lateral to the sciatic nerve, approximately 10 cm inferior to the ischial tuberosity. **C.** The flap is rotated into the defect, and the donor site is closed in a V-Y fashion.

A   B   C

- If primary closure is not possible, the donor site is closed with a meshed split-thickness skin graft over the intact hamstrings muscle wound bed.

Alternate Techniques

- Designing and raising the entire posterior thigh fasciocutaneous unit, with a distal V or U apex, to the base of the inferior border of the gluteus maximus has been shown to be reliable, as previously described (**TECH FIG 3**).[13]
- This technique relies on the presence of the descending branch of the inferior gluteal artery, and this system must be patent.[5]
- The descending branch of the inferior gluteal artery will supply the entire posterior thigh fascial plexus through the cruciate anastomosis.

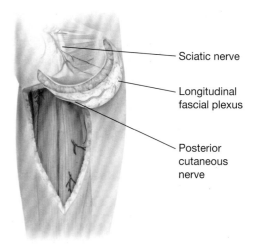

Sciatic nerve

Longitudinal fascial plexus

Posterior cutaneous nerve

TECH FIG 3 • The entire posterior thigh can be raised as a fasciocutaneous unit, the gluteal thigh flap.

■ Hamstring V-Y Flap[2]

- Identify the midpoint between the ischial tuberosity and greater trochanter within the gluteal fold.
- A reference line is drawn from this point down the midaxis of the thigh to a distal point approximately 10 cm superior to the popliteal fossa.[5]
  - The most distal perforators are located approximately 10 cm proximal to the lateral femoral condyle.
- Outline the planned incisions for the V cutaneous island.
  - Medially, a curved line is drawn from the medial border of the ischial ulcer to the distal mark in the midaxis.
  - The lateral line curves cephalad from the distal mark toward the lateral border of the pseudobursa/ulcer excision defect or the posterior border or the tensor fasciae latae.
  - A wide V design that encompasses the entire posterior thigh skin will reliably capture the underlying musculocutaneous and septocutaneous perforators without the concern of centering the skin paddle over the atrophied musculature.
    - Note: The posterior thigh muscles may be atrophied and difficult to identify, particularly in the spinal cord injury patient.
- Carry incisions through marked outline into subcutaneous tissue and through the deep fascia of the posterior compartment just above the hamstring musculature.
- Proximally, the hamstring muscle group has often been released from the ischial tuberosity during ulcer excision and limited ostectomy.
  - Separate any remaining attachments, in particular the deeper semimembranosus, with cautery.
- Laterally, identify the distal biceps femoris as it inserts onto the head of the fibula.
  - Divide the long head and deeper short head of the muscle at its musculotendinous junction just distal to the skin island with electrocautery.

- Medially, identify the distal semitendinosus and semimembranosus as they insert onto the medial condyle of the tibia.
  - The semitendinosus is the most posterior tendon of the pes anserinus, the conjoined tendon of the sartorius, gracilis, and semitendinosus.
  - Divide the remaining hamstring muscles at their musculotendinous junction, again just distal to the skin island, with electrocautery.
- Limited blunt undermining is performed laterally and medially to free the hamstrings from the posterior compartment; however, the profunda femoris perforator pedicles need not be skeletonized (**TECH FIG 4A,B**).
- The musculocutaneous unit is easily advanced 10 cm toward the defect.
- Meticulous hemostasis is achieved within the ulcer cavity and around the elevated flap with electrocautery.
- Hamstring muscle bulk and redundant distal fasciocutaneous flap is de-epithelialized and advanced into the ulcer dead space and inset over a drain in layers with long-lasting monofilament suture.
- The cutaneous donor site is closed in layers over a drain in a V-Y fashion (**TECH FIG 4C**).

Alternate Techniques

- Potential skin paddles include medial and laterally based semicircular rotation flaps with primary closure or split-thickness skin grafting of the donor site.
- A standard (deep-based) fasciocutaneous V-Y advancement flap may be used if limited advancement required.
  - Extend the lateral incision to the lateral base of the defect and dissecting down through the deep fascia.
  - Release in the subfascial plane around the cutaneous island borders for no more than 1 to 2 cm, leaving the hamstring musculature intact.
  - The fasciocutaneous unit is advanced into the defect and closed as above.

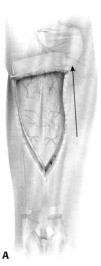 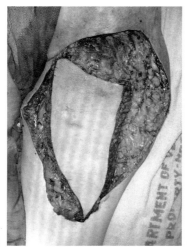 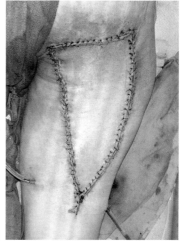

TECH FIG 4 • A. Hamstring complex is divided and the flap is freed to advance proximally. **B.** V-Y hamstring flap elevated laterally and medially following muscle division. **C.** The donor site is closed in a V-Y fashion, supporting the advanced skin island.

PEARLS AND PITFALLS

Patient selection and optimization	▪ Recognizing and addressing preoperative medical comorbidities as well as extrinsic and intrinsic etiologic factors in a compliant patient will improve chances of surgical success. ▪ In a young patient with recurrent ischial ulcers and multiple risk factors, chances of successful wound closure are essentially 0%.[6]
Technique	▪ Ulcer preparation with tumescent technique and methylene blue aids ulcer identification, dissection, excision, and hemostasis. ▪ Multiple flap options for reconstruction have been described; however, none have been shown to be superior. Plan your current flap design with future flaps in mind (including rerotation and/or readvancement).
Nutrition/glucose control	▪ Albumin less than 3.5 is a predictor of early ulcer recurrence; however, nutritional parameters may not improve until after ulcer reconstruction despite adequate intake. ▪ HgbA1c greater than 6 predictor of dehiscence and recurrence.
Postoperative care/ rehabilitation	▪ Monitor triggers for autonomic dysreflexia in spinal cord injuries at T6 or higher. ▪ Monitor sitting protocol closely for signs of undue pressure. Halt progression when indicated. ▪ Coach patient on proper pressure off-loading strategies on an up-to-date seat-mapped chair cushion.
Outcomes	▪ Despite medical and surgical advances, pressure ulcer recidivism remains very high. ▪ An engaged multidisciplinary team with a standard treatment protocol can improve outcomes and reduce costs. ▪ The social/psychological aspects of wound healing in the pressure ulcer population are likely more important than surgery.

POSTOPERATIVE CARE

▪ The patient is transferred to a pressure off-loading bed in the supine or prone position for a recovery period of flat bed rest.

   ▪ There is little consensus on the ideal duration (2–8 weeks) of flat immobilization or ideal setting of convalescence (inpatient hospitalization, acute care rehabilitation, home).

   ▪ Preoperative skin care, management of fecal/urinary incontinence, and regiments to control moisture, glucose level, and spasticity are continued throughout the postoperative course for the lifetime of the patient.

▪ Mobilization is initiated sequentially, with progression to each phase contingent upon tissue tolerance and uncomplicated wound healing.

   ▪ Immediate range of motion therapy for the unaffected limb

   ▪ Initiate range of motion therapy on the affected side at approximately week 5 (or nearing the initiation of planned sitting protocol)

   ▪ Sitting protocol, ideally in a seat-mapped cushion, is initiated at week 6.

      • Monitored sitting intervals beginning with 15-minute sessions 2 or 3 times a day on day 1.

- Evaluate the closure for any flap or incision line erythema concerning for undue pressure.
  - Absent incision/flap concerns, may continually progress intervals by 15 minutes each day (day 2, 30-minute intervals; day 2, 45-minute intervals; and so on) until able to tolerate 4 to 6 hours of sitting
- It is essential to coach the patient on adequate repositioning maneuvers when sitting to relieve pressure and maintain tissue perfusion.
  - Side-to-side shifting, lean forward, tilt backs
- Culture-directed antibiotic therapy should be initiated based on results of bone and deep tissue biopsies at the time of surgery.
- There should be clear coordination of outpatient care and social services as well as family member/caregiver education/instructions and follow-up prior to discharge.

OUTCOMES

- Wide variation exists in the reported outcomes for pressure ulcer reconstruction, which is likely attributable to the design of many studies in pressure ulcer literature, length of patient follow-up, and definitions of outcomes.
- Keys et al. assessed the predictors of pressure ulcer reconstructive failure in a retrospective review of 135 patients.[6]
  - 39% recurrence and 16% dehiscence rates were observed; 48% of recurrences occurred within the first year and 76% within the first 2 years.
  - Albumin less than 3.5, age less than 45, and previous same-site surgical failure predicted early recurrence within 2 years.
  - Ischial ulcer, age less than 45, and previous same-site surgical failure predicted late recurrence after 2 years.
  - Poor diabetes control (hemoglobin A1c greater than 6%) was a predictor of return to operating room for dehiscence as well as ulcer recurrence.
- Larson et al. described outcome of a single surgeon experience with a standard protocol of ulcer debridement with immediate reconstruction followed by inpatient hospital admission for 3 weeks in 101 patients.[12]
  - Ischial ulcers represented the most common ulcer at 49.7% of the series.
  - Recurrence rate of 16.8% and complication rate of 17.3% reported.
  - Primary closure was performed in 45.8% of ulcers, the remaining 54.2% underwent flap reconstruction. 17.8% had a V-Y biceps femoris flap and one patient had a hamstring myocutaneous flap.
  - Surgery was performed without preoperative consideration of nutritional status or osteomyelitis.
  - Outcomes for specific technique of reconstruction (primary closure vs flap reconstruction) or location of recurrence were not provided.
- Sameem et al. reviewed 55 articles in the pressure ulcer reconstruction literature covering each type of flap reconstruction and found no statistically significant difference in complication or recurrence rates between musculocutaneous, fasciocutaneous, and perforator-based flaps.[14]

- With no technique superior, consider the advantages and limitations of each approach rather than complication and recurrence rate.[14]

COMPLICATIONS

- Cellulitis
- Abscess
- Hematoma
- Seroma
- Urethral injury/leak
- Sciatic nerve injury
- Wound dehiscence
- Partial or total flap necrosis
- Ulcer recurrence

REFERENCES

1. National Pressure Ulcer Advisory Panel (NPUAP). Pressure Injury Stages. Available at: http://www.npuap.org/resources/educational-and-clinical-resources/npuap-pressure-injury-stages/Published 2016.
2. Hurteau JE, Bostwick J, Nahai F, et al. V-Y advancement of hamstring musculocuataneous flap for coverage of ischial pressure sores. *Plast Reconstr Surg.* 1981;68(4):539-542.
3. Cormack GC, Lamberty BG. The blood supply of thigh skin. Plast Reconstr Surg. 1985;75(3):342-354.
4. Windhofer C, Brenner E, Moriggl B, Papp C. Relationship between the descending branch of the inferior gluteal artery and the posterior femoral cutaneous nerve applicable to flap surgery. *Surg Radiol Anat.* 2002;24(5):253-257.
5. Rubin J, Whetzel T, Stevenson T. The posterior thigh fasciocutaneous flap: vascular anatomy and clinical application. *Plast Reconstr Surg.* 1995;95(7):1228-1239.
6. Keys KA, Daniali LN, Warner KJ, Mathes DW. Multivariate predictors of failure after flap coverage of pressure ulcers. *Plast Reconstr Surg.* 2010;125(6):1725-1734.
7. Larson JD, Altman AM, Bentz ML, Larson DL. Pressure ulcers and perineal reconstruction. *Plast Reconstr Surg.* 2014;133(1):39e-48e.
8. Scivoletto G, Fuoco U, Morganti B, et al. Pressure sores and blood and serum dysmetabolism in spinal cord injury patients. *Spinal Cord.* 2004;42(8):473-476.
9. Huang AB, Schweitzer ME, Hume E, Batte WG. Osteomyelitis of the pelvis/hips in paralyzed patients: accuracy and clinical utility of MRI. *J Comput Assist Tomogr.* 1998;22(3):437-443.
10. Harrison B, Khansa I, Janis JE. Evidence-based strategies to reduce postoperative complications in plastic surgery. *Plast Reconstr Surg.* 2016;137(1):351-360.
11. Han H, Few J, Fine NA. Use of the tumescent technique in pressure ulcer closure. *Plast Reconstr Surg.* 2002;110(2):711-712.
12. Larson DL, Hudak KA, Waring WP, et al. Protocol management of late-stage pressure ulcers: a 5-year retrospective study of 101 consecutive patients with 179 ulcers. *Plast Reconstr Surg.* 2012;129(4):897-904.
13. Friedman JD, Reece GR, Eldor L. The utility of the posterior thigh flap for complex pelvic and perineal reconstruction. *Plast Reconstr Surg.* 2010;126:146-155.
14. Sameem M, Au M, Wood T, et al. A systematic review of complication and recurrence rates of musculocutaneous, fasciocutaneous, and perforator-based flaps for treatment of pressure sores. *Plast Reconstr Surg.* 2012;130(1):67e-77e.

SUGGESTED READING

Posthauer ME, Banks M, Dorner B, Schols JM. The role of nutrition for pressure ulcer management: national pressure ulcer advisory panel, European pressure ulcer advisory panel, and pan pacific pressure injury alliance white paper. *Adv Skin Wound Care.* 2015;28(4):175-190.

Tensor Fascia Lata Flaps for Trochanteric Ulcers

Terri A. Zomerlei and Jeffrey E. Janis

DEFINITION

- Trochanteric ulcers are common in chronically bed-bound patients who lie in the lateral position.
- Patient populations most at risk include those in acute care settings, nursing home patients, paraplegic populations and those with hip flexion contractures.
- In addition to unrelieved pressure, other contributing factors include incontinence/moisture, friction/shear force, and altered sensory perception.
- Characteristically, the appearance of the overlying skin only represents a small portion of the affected tissue ("the tip of the iceberg").

ANATOMY

- The tensor fascia lata (TFL) is a thin, bandlike muscle located in the lateral thigh just distal to the greater trochanter. It functions as a lateral knee stabilizer (**FIG 1**).
  - Rectus femoris borders anteriorly
  - Biceps femoris borders posteriorly
  - Size: The muscle is 5 cm wide, 12 cm long, and 2 cm thick.
  - Origin: Anterior 5 cm of the lateral lip of the iliac crest and the lateral aspect of the anterosuperior iliac spine (ASIS). A small portion also originates from the greater trochanter.

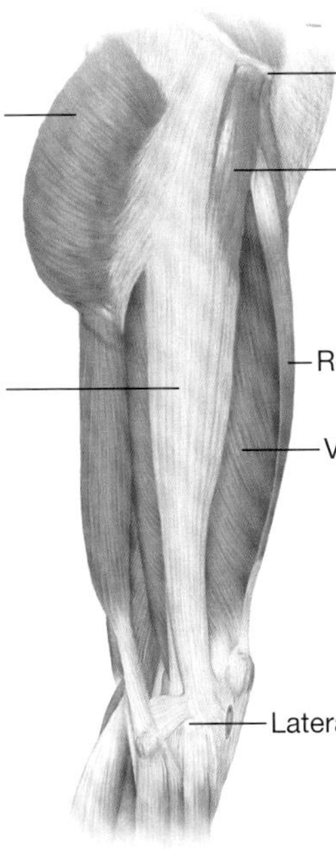

FIG 1 • Lateral leg anatomy.

- Insertion: The fascia lata is an extension of the TFL and inserts into the lateral condyle of the tibia.
- The aponeurosis of the superficial potion of the gluteus muscle, the aponeurosis of the TFL and the fascia lata are commonly referred to as the iliotibial tract.
  - When the iliotibial tract is taut, the knee is held in extension.
  - When tense, the iliotibial tract also stabilizes the hip and knee while standing.
  - Harvest of the TFL flap is associated with minimal functional morbidity.
- The TFL flap is a type I muscle with one dominant pedicle, the lateral circumflex femoral artery (LCFA).
  - The LCFA is a branch of the profunda femoris.
  - The LCFA passes deep to the sartorius and rectus femoris.
  - It gives rise to three branches: the ascending, the transverse, and the descending branches that supply the superior, mid, and inferior portions of the TFL respectively.
  - Two venae comitantes travel with the LCFA and join the femoral vein.
- The TFL receives its motor supply from the superior gluteal nerve, which has contributions from L4, L5 and S1. It enters the muscle in the middle third on the posterior aspect.
- The TFL sensory nerve supply is from the lateral cutaneous branch of T12, which provides sensory innervation to the most superior aspect of the muscle and its overlying skin.
- The lateral femoral cutaneous nerve with contributions from L2 and L3 innervates the remaining portion of the skin and muscle.

PATHOGENESIS

- Primary mechanism of pressure ulceration is cellular ischemia.
  - Tissue pressure higher than the pressure of the microcirculation (32 mm Hg) causes ischemia.
  - If the ischemic period is long enough and repeated frequently, the eventual outcome is tissue necrosis.
- Pressure sores (decubitus ulcers) almost invariably occur in the tissue over bony prominences in persons not able to change body position frequently.
- Pressure sores overlying the greater trochanter are common in those with hip flexion contractures who lie in the lateral position.
- In acutely ill patients, third-space fluid pressure may mechanically compromise the microvasculature.
- Etiologic considerations can be divided in extrinsic and intrinsic factors.
  - Extrinsic factors: Primarily mechanical forces of the soft tissues

- Friction: Resistance that a surface encounters when moving over another. Most often occurs with patient transfers
- Moisture: Incontinence can lead to skin breakdown.
- Pressure: Mechanical force that is applied perpendicular to a plane (ie, between a bony prominence and a chair or bed)
- Shear: Mechanical stress parallel to the plane results in stretching and compression of the blood supply to the muscles and skin.
  - Intrinsic factors: Patient factors that affect the soft tissues.
    - Altered level of consciousness: Results in lack of voluntary movements and protective reflexes that off-load pressure
    - Anemia: Can result in fatigue and weakness which can contribute to and perpetuate immobility. Also affects wound healing capabilities.
    - Autonomic control: Decreased levels result in spasms, perspiration with increased skin moisture, blood vessel engorgement and resulting tissue edema, and problems with bowel and bladder control.
    - Age: Increasing age is associated with increased skin friability and decreased tensile strength.
    - Infection: Profoundly impairs wound healing abilities
    - Inflammation: Creates a hostile local milieu resulting in impaired healing, especially in the setting of chronic wounds
    - Malnutrition: Results in wasting and decreased muscle bulk and impairs wound healing abilities
    - Sepsis: Can result in decreased tissue perfusion and ischemia
    - Sensory loss: Patient is unable to experience the discomfort associated with prolonged pressure over prominences

NATURAL HISTORY

- Pressure sores are categorized according to the National Pressure Ulcer Advisory Panel Stages (NPUAP 2016).
- Pressure sore can progress through the following stages if extrinsic and intrinsic insults are not remedied (see FIG 2 in Chapter 29).[1]
  - Stage I: Intact skin with nonblanching erythema
  - Stage II: Partial-thickness skin loss with exposed dermis
    - Presents as blister, abrasion, or shallow open ulcer
  - Stage III: Full-thickness skin loss
    - Subcutaneous fat may be exposed.
    - Tunneling and undermining may be present.
  - Stage IV: Full-thickness skin and tissue loss
  - Unstageable: Full-thickness skin or soft tissues loss but depth is unknown usually due to the presence of an overlying eschar
  - Suspected deep tissue injury: Persistent deep red, maroon, or purple discoloration of intact skin may indicate deep tissue injury that needs to evolve prior to staging.

PERTINENT HISTORY AND PHYSICAL FINDINGS

The preoperative evaluation of patients with pressure ulcers includes a detailed assessment of the patient's medical history, social situation, baseline health status, and a comprehensive wound evaluation.[2]

- Patient history
  - How long has the ulcer been present? Acute wounds may respond to conservative treatment while chronic wounds tend to be more recalcitrant.
  - What is the current wound care treatment? Changing local wound care regimens may help with improving the wound.
  - What surgical options have been tried in the past? Obtain any and all operative reports as previous surgeries may limit surgical options.
  - Is the patient ambulatory, wheelchair bound or bed bound?
  - What type of mattress and turning regimen is currently being used? Airflow mattresses offer the best protection while normal mattresses offer little defense against pressure.
  - Is fecal contamination a problem? A dressing or a temporary diverting ostomy may be prudent.
  - Are there problems with urinary incontinence? Does the patient require temporary or permanent urinary diversion?
  - Does the patient have spasms? Are their medications optimized to control spasms?
  - Does the patient have any fixed contractures?
  - What is the baseline nutritional status of the patient?
- Social history is crucial to obtain in order to understand possible postoperative barriers to care and to prevent recurrence.
  - Social support/caregiver situation
  - Resources for obtaining durable medical equipment (low air loss bed, seat cushion if bed bound or wheelchair bound)
  - Smoking or substance abuse history
    - Active or prior nicotine use increases risk of poor wound healing.
    - Consider urine cotinine testing.
  - Psychiatric illness
  - Diet, specifically amount of protein intake
  - Compliance history
- Laboratory studies
  - Complete blood count to assess for anemia or active infection
  - Albumin, prealbumin, and total protein to assess protein stores
  - Coagulation panel to assess for coagulopathies
  - Cultures that should be obtained with tissue or bone biopsies as wound swabs have little value due to chronic colonization. Cultures should be sent for quantitative analysis and if the organism count is greater than 105, consideration should be given to systemic antibiotics and/or staged debridement and reconstruction
  - Urinalysis
- Physical examination
  - All wounds must be examined manually.
  - Visual wound assessment alone is not sufficient to obtain necessary information about a wound.
  - Manually assess the size and depth of the wound, bony prominences, bursa, and presence of tunneling (may need to use long cotton tip applicator to assess tunneling).
    - If an eschar is present, the wound cannot be accurately staged.
    - A limited bedside debridement is useful to stage the wound and to facilitate local wound care preoperatively.

- From visual inspection, take note of any previous surgical scars because previous surgeries may preclude the use of a flap secondary to compromised vascular supply.
- Muscle tone and bulk are assessed, taking note of any spasticity or contraction of the extremities.
- Assess the patient's sensation in the area of the wound.

IMAGING

- MRI is recommended for all stage IV pressure ulcers to evaluate for osteomyelitis.
- T2 hypersensitivity and low-intensity T1 are sensitive and specific for osteomyelitis.
- CT scan or plain films have lower sensitivity but can be used if MRI not available or patient condition precludes its use.[3]

DIFFERENTIAL DIAGNOSIS

- Marjolin ulcer arising in a chronic wound
- Burn
- Soft tissue neoplasm with ulceration
- Chronic surgical wound
- Traumatic wound

NONOPERATIVE MANAGEMENT

- Relieve extrinsic pressure with frequent positional changes.
  - Turn every 2 hours when supine.
  - Lift for 10 seconds every 10 minutes when seated.
- Use proper mattress (low air loss) and cushion for seating and wheelchair (seat mapping).
- Minimize head of bed elevation (less than 45 degrees).
- Optimize underlying medical status.
  - Address spasticity (baclofen, diazepam, dantrolene).
  - Optimize nutrition.
- Local wound care in those who are poor surgical candidates or while optimizing patient for surgery
  - Dakin's one-fourth strength for a limited time period (up to 1 week) can be effective in decreasing wound colonization.[4]

SURGICAL MANAGEMENT

Preoperative Planning[5,6]

- The most crucial aspect of the surgical management of pressures ulcers is the preoperative and postoperative care.
- Do not operate on patients until their medical status is optimized and the underlying etiology determined.
- Obtain old operative reports to know what prior attempts at closure have been tried.
- Always consider future procedures in the operative planning so as to not "burn bridges."

Positioning

- The preferred patient position is the lateral decubitus position for ease of accessing the lateral thigh.
- Depending on patient body habitus, the TFL flap may be harvested with the patient in the supine position.
- Prior to patient transfer to the OR table, check OR table to ensure working properly.
- Place a "beanbag" body positioner on the OR table if available.

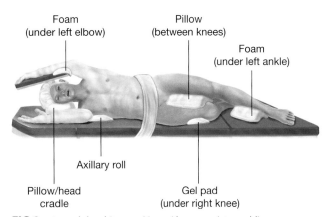

FIG 2 • Lateral decubitus position with appropriate padding.

- Patient is transferred to OR table, monitoring equipment is applied, and the patient is intubated. Ensure that tube is secure and eyes are protected.
- Patient gown should be removed.
- To place in the lateral position, with appropriate resources and careful choreography, the patient is shifted and rolled into the lateral decubitus position with the surgical site facing up (**FIG 2**).
- Make note of all pressure points and pad appropriately.
  - Head is placed in a doughnut or head cradle; ensure ear lobe and helix are not folded or compressed and eyes are protected.
  - The lower arm is placed on an arm board and pillows, or an additional arm board is placed for the upper arm.
  - The arms are secured with straps.
  - Pad the olecranon if needed.
  - A gel roll is placed as an axillary roll.
  - A gel pad is placed between the OR table and the "bottom leg" knee and ankle.
  - Foam or pillows are placed between the knees.
- Place foam or a pillow between the ankle malleoli.
- The beanbag positioner (if available) is "inflated" to help hold the patient in the lateral position.
- Ensure genitalia are free from compression.
- Check EKG pads, monitoring devices, grounding pads, and catheters to make sure they are not placing pressure on the skin and are outside of the operative field.
- Take care that any ostomies, if present, are free from compression.
- Ensure no traction on indwelling catheters.
- Secure patient to bed at both the trunk and lower legs.
- Apply warming blankets or forced air to upper trunk.

Approach

- To provide coverage for a greater trochanter pressure ulcer, the TFL flap is raised and advanced into position as a V-Y advancement flap.
- The flap is raised as a myocutaneous flap.
  - The V-Y advancement places the best perfused and bulkiest tissue into the defect.
  - In most cases, the donor site can be closed primarily.
  - If the flap is greater than 9 cm in width, the donor site may need to be skin grafted.

■ Excisional Debridement

- Failure to adequately debride can lead to recurrent disease and poor wound healing.
- Probe wound prior to debridement so all tunneling is addressed.
- Infiltration of the peribursal area with a wetting solution (1000 mL of normal saline plus 30 mL of 1% lidocaine, plus 1 ampule of epinephrine 1:1000) can assist with hydrodissection and decrease blood loss.[6]

- Coating the cavity with methylene blue applied with gauze or a cotton applicator can assist with bursa excision and verify the completeness of the debridement.
- Debridement removes necrotic tissue and biofilm and decreases bacterial count.
- Converts a chronic wound into an acute wound.
- Quantitative wound cultures should be obtained following debridement so that postoperative antibiotic coverage can be tailored appropriately.

■ Ostectomy

- Because most pressure sores are overlying bony prominences and underlying osteomyelitis and unhealthy bone is likely, the bony prominence should be eliminated (**TECH FIG 1**).

- The greater trochanter ostectomy should be performed conservatively to lessen the prominence because its radical removal may redistribute pressure points to adjacent tissue, result in excessive bleeding, and affect the origin and/or insertion of skeletal muscle.
- Send a portion of the ostectomy specimen as a bone biopsy to evaluate for osteomyelitis.

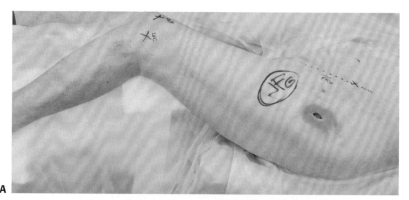

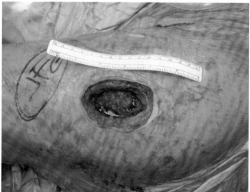

TECH FIG 1 • **A.** Left trochanteric ulcer prior to debridement. This ambulatory patient developed a pressure ulcer while recovering from a major surgery. **B.** Ulcer following debridement and ostectomy. (Courtesy of Noopur Gangophadyay, MD.)

■ Tensor Fascia Lata V-Y Advancement Flap

Markings and Flap Design

- Following debridement and limited ostectomy, begin with marking anatomical landmarks (**TECH FIG 2**).
  - ASIS.
  - Lateral femoral condyle.
  - Draw a line between these two landmarks—this line marks the anterior border of the muscle.

- The LCFA enters the TFL 7 to 12 cm distal to the ASIS.
  - Mark the position of the vascular pedicle.
  - This can be confirmed with handheld Doppler.
- Design the skin paddle so that is it centered over the TFL.
  - Mark a position on the iliac crest that is 3 cm posterior to the ASIS.
  - Draw a line from this point to the lateral condyle; this represents the midaxis of the TFL.
  - Measure a point on the midaxis that is 8 to 10 cm proximal to the lateral condyle—this marks the most distal extent that the flap can be designed.

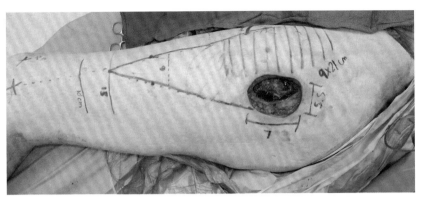

TECH FIG 2 • TFL anatomical markings and flap design. (Courtesy of Noopur Gangophadyay, MD.)

- The distal one-third of the skin territory is unreliable and the flap design should exclude this area if possible.
  - The flap width should be less than 9 cm if primary closure is desired.
  - The posterior marking of the flap incorporates the anterior portion of the debrided wound.

Flap Harvest and Inset

- The flap is harvested from distal to proximal.
- After the skin and fascia lata is incised inferiorly, it is helpful to suture these structures together temporarily to prevent shear.
- Dissection proceeds proximally in the subfascial plane (**TECH FIG 3A**).
- Anticipate the vascular pedicle starting 12 cm distal to the ASIS and proceed slowly when approaching this area.

- The lateral femoral cutaneous nerve is also located near the anterior aspect of the flap near the vascular pedicle; take care not to injure it.
- Near the point that the dissection approaches the pedicle, it is usually possible to advance the flap posteriorly into the defect.
- A back-cut may be necessary to improve the rotation and advancement into the defect.
- Drains are placed into the donor site and the recipient site.
- The flap is inset and the donor site closed with monofilament absorbable sutures and the skin is closed with sutures or staples (**TECH FIG 3B,C**).
- The advancement of the flap into the defect often produces a soft tissue "dog-ear" at the proximal part of the flap. This will flatten with time. Do not attempt to excise at this stage.

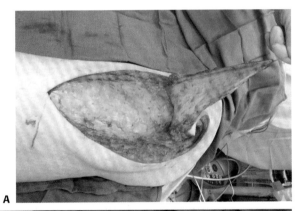

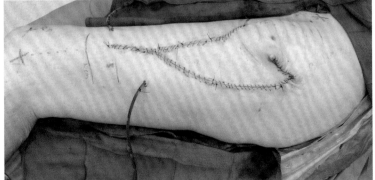

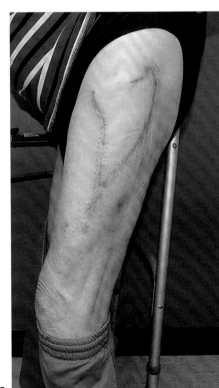

TECH FIG 3 • **A.** TFL flap dissection completed in the subfascial plane. **B.** Flap inset. Two drains were used. Donor site is closed primarily. **C.** TFL flap 3 months postoperatively. (Courtesy of Noopur Gangophadyay, MD.)

PEARLS AND PITFALLS

Preoperative Planning	▪ Correct any and all extrinsic and intrinsic factors that led to the pressure ulcer development. ▪ Sacrifice of the TFL could affect function in a patient who is an athlete.
Operative	▪ Avoid undue tension with flap inset; use a conservative back-cut if needed. ▪ The distal skin territory is unreliable; avoid excessive flap length. ▪ Primary donor-site closure is facilitated by undermining the fascia lata anteriorly and posteriorly.
Postoperative Care	▪ Engage a multidisciplinary team including nursing, social work, and other consulting services as appropriate to ensure a safe discharge and to the patient the "best chance" of preventing recurrence.

POSTOPERATIVE CARE

▪ Patients are hospitalized for 1 to 2 weeks following surgery, and many patients will discharge to a rehabilitation hospital or an extended care facility for several weeks to receive a higher level of nursing care.

▪ A low air loss mattress should be ordered prior to the surgery and should be available to move the patient onto the mattress directly from the operating room table.

▪ The patient should limit the HOB to less than 10 degrees for 1 week.

▪ The patient should be repositioned every 2 hours, and kept off the surgical site unless on an air fluidized bed.

▪ The postoperative dressing should be left in place for 48 hours; after that time, a light dressing can be applied to protect against shear and moisture or the wound can be left open to the air to allow for ease of wound monitoring.

▪ Bladder and bowel function should be controlled to prevent urinary or fecal contamination of the surgical site.

▪ Spasticity should be prevented with pharmacologic measures.

▪ Obtain a dietary consultation so that the patient can maintain a positive nitrogen balance.

▪ Meticulous drain care should be performed in the hospital and taught to all caregivers.

▪ Obtain an infectious disease consultation for any positive operative cultures to help guide antibiotic selection and duration of treatment.

▪ Evaluate need for long-term intravenous access for antibiotics.

OUTCOMES

▪ Recurrence rate is high, especially in those with hip flexion contractures.

▪ Local wound/incision problems are common and should be treated with local wound care.

▪ Anticipate further reconstruction options with every surgical intervention.

▪ Control for extrinsic and intrinsic factors that contributed to the initial pressure ulcer formation.

COMPLICATIONS

▪ Complications are not uncommon for those with significant preoperative comorbidities.

▪ Hematoma or seroma may occur.
  ▪ If patient is on anticoagulants, work closely with the hematologist to determine when these medications can be safely held and resumed in the perioperative period.
  ▪ One or more drains should be left under flaps for days to weeks to control for fluid accumulation.

▪ Small localized incisional breakdown should be treated with local wound care.

▪ Persistent infection can be minimized with thorough debridement and long-term antibiotics as deemed appropriate by infectious disease colleagues.

REFERENCES

1. National Pressure Ulcer Advisory Panel (NPUAP) Pressure Stages/Categories. 2016. Available at http://www.npuap.org/resources/educational-and-clinical-resources/npuap-pressure-injury-stages.
2. Marin J, Nixon J, Gorecki C. A systematic review of risk factors for the development of and recurrence of pressure ulcers in people with spinal cord injuries. *Spinal Cord.* 2013;51(7):522-527.
3. Huang AB, Schweitzer ME, Hume E, et al. Osteomyelitis of the hips/pelvis in paralyzed patients, accuracy and clinical utility of MRI. *J Comput Assist Tomogr.* 1998;22:437.
4. Heggers JP, Sazy JA, Stenberh BD, et al. Bacterialcidal and wound-healing properties of sodium hypochlorite solutions: The 1991 Lindberg Award. *J Burn Care Rehabil.* 1991;12:420.
5. Janis JE, Kenkel JM. Pressure Sores. *Sel Read Plast Surg.* 2003; 9(39):1-42.
6. Han H, Fen J, Fine NA. Use of the tumescent technique in pressure ulcer closure. *Plast Reconstr Surg.* 2002;110:711.
7. Bauer J, Phillips LG. MOC-PS(SM) CME Article: Pressure sores. *Plast Reconstr Surg.* 2008;121:1-10.

Repair of Flank and Lumbar Defects

CHAPTER 32

Sergey Y. Turin, Chad A. Purnell, and Gregory A. Dumanian

DEFINITION

- A defect in the flank/lumbar region of the abdominal wall can be a challenging problem as there is much discord in the literature regarding its etiology and management. Defined as an inability of the abdominal wall to properly contain the viscera and located lateral to the semilunar line, flank defects are encountered after surgeries requiring retroperitoneal access (transplant, vascular, urologic); these defects occurred fairly frequently, ranging from as low as 8% to 23% in the literature.[1-4] The etiology of these defects can be of two types—a hernia or a focal weakness of the abdominal wall, usually attributed to denervation injury. A true hernia implies violation of one or more of the layers of the abdominal wall musculature. In contrast, a bulge secondary to denervation injury leading to muscle attenuation and weakness implies continuity of all three layers of the abdominal wall. In our recent review of 31 patients, we found that 55% of patients had a disruption of the internal oblique and transversus abdominis muscles, whereas the external oblique muscle was intact—a type of "partial" hernia often confused with a denervation bulge. In 32%, all three abdominal wall layers were disrupted as true incisional hernias. In the remainder, the three layers of the abdominal

wall were intact but had a loss of tone due to denervation—true abdominal wall bulges.
- We present a reliable technique to repair the flank defects that is efficacious for true hernias and can be used for certain denervation injuries.

ANATOMY

- The lateral and lumbar abdominal wall is composed of three load-bearing muscular layers and their respective fascial envelopes—the external and internal oblique and the transversus abdominis. All three of these can be compromised by an incision for retroperitoneal access. Discontinuity of these layers would lead to a hernia defect. (See the chapter on "Synthetic and Biologic Mesh for Abdominal Wall Defects," **FIG 1**, for example.)
- The muscles of the abdominal wall are segmentally innervated by the 7th through 12th intercostal as well as the iliohypogastric and ilioinguinal nerves running between the transversus abdominis and the internal oblique muscles. In this plane, they are vulnerable to transection during a retroperitoneal approach for incisions that cross dermatomes. They are also susceptible to focal injuries from retractors, cautery, and abdominal wall full-thickness sutures (**FIG 1**).

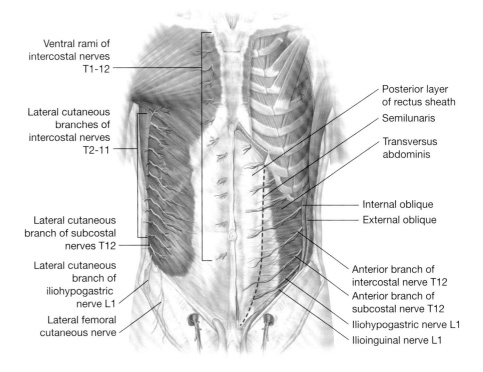

Ventral rami of intercostal nerves T1-12

Lateral cutaneous branches of intercostal nerves T2-11

Lateral cutaneous branch of subcostal nerves T12

Lateral cutaneous branch of iliohypogastric nerve L1

Lateral femoral cutaneous nerve

Posterior layer of rectus sheath

Semilunaris

Transversus abdominis

Internal oblique

External oblique

Anterior branch of intercostal nerve T12

Anterior branch of subcostal nerve T12

Iliohypogastric nerve L1

Ilioinguinal nerve L1

FIG 1 • Innervation of the abdominal wall.

PATHOGENESIS

- True hernias occur when the ultimate tensile strength of the repair is less than the forces applied. Acutely, the sutures can tear through the abdominal muscles during coughs and forceful movements and lead to a dehiscence or evisceration. Chronically, tissue located within the loop of suture becomes scar. When the strength of the scar, sutures, and foreign body reaction to those sutures is less than the forces applied, an incisional hernia develops. In comparison to incisional hernias, flank bulges are due to denervation of the abdominal wall. Narrow zones of denervation with loss of just one or two intercostal nerves during the original surgery do exist, often due to resection of spinal cord roots for exposure or tumors. Alternatively, there can be a large zone of denervation from a profound spinal injury. The larger the zone of injury, such as with a spinal cord injury, the less the techniques in this chapter apply.

- With maneuvers that are intended to stabilize the torso such as the Valsalva maneuver, the viscera instead distend the flank defect and cause a disagreeable and sometimes painful contour irregularity. Patients complain of discomfort due to an inability to raise their intra-abdominal pressure and altered torso mechanics—a loss of "core strength."

- See the chapter on "Abdominal Hernia Reconstruction" for a discussion of the biomechanics of the abdominal wall and the importance of evaluating abdominal wall compliance when dealing with these defects.

NATURAL HISTORY

- These defects can often be a cause of marked pain and lead to functional impairment with diminished quality of life.[5] The plastic surgeon will usually see the patient in a delayed setting, with the consultation being prompted by worsening symptoms.

PATIENT HISTORY AND PHYSICAL FINDINGS

- Patients are encouraged to obtain all the previous operative notes, and it is important to record if a rib was resected at the original procedure. Hernias present for many years are more difficult to close than a hernia less than 1 year from the index surgery. It is of great importance to discuss the medical history and comorbid conditions, such as COPD, diabetes, cardiac disease, and any rheumatoid conditions.

- Prior incisions are recorded, and an evaluation of skin quality and abdominal wall compliance is made. The patient is asked to stand as well as to lie in the lateral decubitus position to clarify the borders and size of the defect. Palpate the bulge with an eye toward feeling any muscle contraction or edge to the defect to gain an idea of whether the remaining muscle is innervated and continuous. Look for incisions of the midline back that denote spine pathology and possible denervation.

- A social history is important to appreciate the stresses on the torso required to return to work or important social activities.

IMAGING

- We routinely obtain a CT scan of the abdomen using oral and IV contrast to assess the layers of the abdominal wall, to measure the size of the defect, and to screen for any other intra-abdominal pathology (such as a recurrent cancer) as

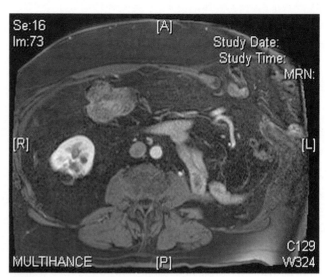

FIG 2 • CT Scan of a patient with a flank hernia.

dictated by the patient's history. Any midline hernias would be documented (though typically not addressed) at the time of the flank repair (**FIG 2**).

NONOPERATIVE MANAGEMENT

- If there is adequate soft tissue coverage over the viscera, we counsel the patient that closure of these large defects is indicated if they are symptomatic and the hernia affects their lifestyle and activities. Given the usually large size of these hernias, bowel incarceration is infrequent. Nonoperative management with binders or fajas is encouraged, but typically is only partially effective, and patients typically do not feel comfortable in these hot and heavy garments. Patients with significant medical problems and patients with large zones of denervation are often encouraged not to have repair in an effort to balance risks and benefits of the procedure.

SURGICAL MANAGEMENT

Preoperative Planning

- Patients are optimized for surgery with smoking cessation, weight loss, and improvement of exercise tolerance. A mechanical bowel prep with clear liquids, magnesium citrate, and bisacodyl tablets by mouth shrinks the bowel and improves the ability to perform the repair without changing the bowel flora.

- Use the Caprini risk-stratification model to assess the individual patient's risk for DVT/PE and assign chemoprophylaxis if appropriate.

- The lateral position required for repair of a flank hernia is not appropriate for other general surgery procedures with a single prepping and draping. Although midline hernias can be repaired simultaneously, we have tended to focus on one defect at a time.

Positioning

- The patient is positioned in a lateral decubitus position with the planned incision over the break in the operating table (**FIG 3**).

- Appropriate padding for the dependent extremities and an axillary support are placed.
- The operative field should extend from the level of the nipples to the level of the pubis and from the umbilicus anteriorly to the spinal column posteriorly (see **FIG 3**).

Approach

- We approach these repairs through the original incision and then trim back any excess soft tissue at the time of closing (**FIG 4**).

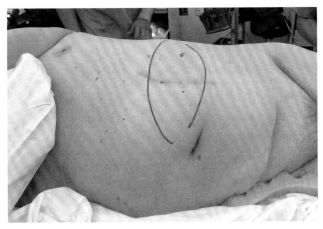

FIG 3 • Later decubitus positioning.

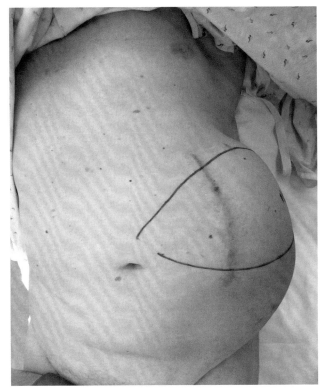

FIG 4 • Preoperative markings.

■ Approach and Development of Tissue Planes

- Make a generous incision through the original scar and extend it to facilitate later skin tailoring (**TECH FIG 1A,B**).
- Incise the abdominal wall and/or hernia sac through the prior scar to enter the abdomen and then clear the inner

aspect of the abdominal wall of omentum and bowel. At this point, raise skin flaps cranially and caudally to 4 cm past the level at which the abdominal musculature feels intact by a pinch test. The retracted internal oblique and transversus abdominis muscles can usually be palpated as a thickening of the abdominal wall layers.

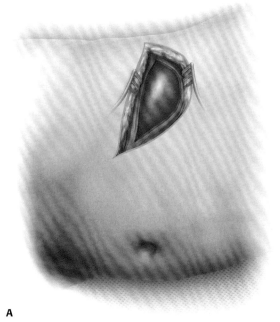

A

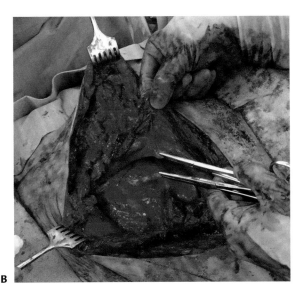

B

TECH FIG 1 • **A,B.** Incision and exposure of the hernia sac.

T E C H N I Q U E S

■ Determining Plane of Mesh Placement

- Grasping this thick aspect of the abdominal wall, assess how easily these two shelves of muscle tissue can be approximated once the operating table is placed in the reflex position. If they can be closed easily and the defect is relatively posterior, the two deep muscle layers are closed and mesh is placed deep to the external oblique as shown in **TECH FIG 2A**.

- If tissue quality is poor and the two deep muscle layers can only be closed with reflex positioning and tension, mesh is placed intraperitoneally as an underlay as shown in **TECH FIG 2B**.

- Mesh sutured repairs use strips of macroporous mesh as sutures to approximate layers of the abdominal wall work especially well in nonmidline defects and are especially helpful where the ribs or the iliac crest limit the ability to place even a narrow strip of mesh. The mesh sutures are introduced through the abdominal wall tissue with a sharp hemostat.

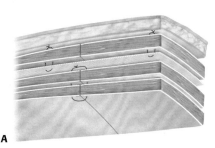
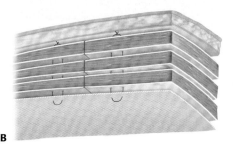

A   **B**

TECH FIG 2 • Mesh placement illustration. **A.** Mesh is placed deep to the external oblique if the deep muscle layers are brought together easily. **B.** Mesh is placed intraperitoneally if there is tension on the closure.

■ Mesh Placement and Muscle Approximation

- The more anterior the defect, the more likely intraperitoneal placement is required. The external oblique muscle and fascia thins at this anatomic area, and renders placement of mesh between the internal and external obliques quite problematic. Regardless of the plane, the technique of mesh placement is the same. We use a 7.5-cm-wide piece of soft midweight polypropylene mesh cut several centimeters longer than the defect with 4 cm bites on either side (**TECH FIG 3**).

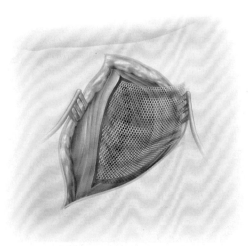

TECH FIG 3 • Mesh placement illustration—here, the internal oblique and the transversus abdominis are closed and the mesh is being placed deep to the external oblique.

- The mesh must be oriented so that tension across the mesh to close the defect will maintain the mesh pores open and macroporous. If the mesh has a smooth and rough side, place the smoother side facing the bowel if used intraperitoneally.

- When the mesh is placed deep to the external oblique, flex the table and close the internal oblique and transversus abdominis layers using a 2-0 polydioxanone suture.

- Place the mesh in the appropriate layer and then suture the mesh in place using interrupted 0 polypropylene sutures in a horizontal mattress fashion. Use transmuscular bites approximately 4 cm from the edges of the defect and 0.5 cm from the edge of the mesh. The sutures are spaced about 2 cm from each other (**TECH FIG 4**).

- The bites must be taken close to the edges of the mesh to minimize wrinkling of the mesh. We avoid bone anchors, transosseous suturing to the iliac crest, or sutures around ribs when possible. As the mesh is narrower (7.5 cm) than the distance between sutures on each side of the abdominal wall (4 cm × 2 = 8 cm), the lateral abdominal musculature falls together without tension along the axis of the mesh.

- Excise any redundant external oblique muscle, and close good quality muscle with figure-of-8 0 polypropylene sutures (**TECH FIG 5A,B**).

- This closure allows the mesh and abdominal wall suture lines to act as a load-sharing construct, distributing the forces of closure. This lowers the forces at each suture-tissue interface and minimizes suture pull-through, which is a primary cause of hernia recurrence.

TECHNIQUES

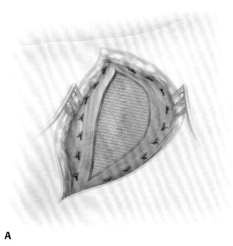
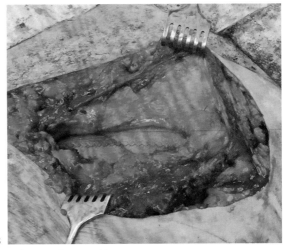

A   **B**

TECH FIG 4 • **A.** Diagram of mesh placement. **B.** Narrow mesh sutured into position.

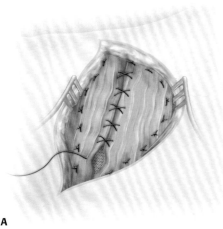
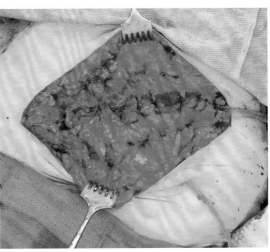

A   **B**

TECH FIG 5 • **A.** Diagram of closure of external oblique over mesh. Closure of muscular layer after mesh placement, creating three load-bearing suture lines. **B.** Patient with closed external oblique over mesh.

■ Closure

- Once the muscular layers of the abdominal wall are closed, redundant skin is excised to reduce dead space. Place one or two drains superficial to the external oblique (**TECH FIG 6**).

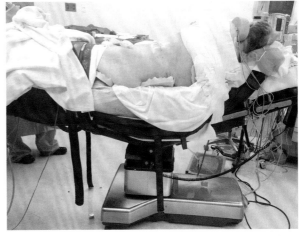

TECH FIG 6 • Final result using flexion of the table to facilitate closure.

PEARLS AND PITFALLS

Scar does not aid healing	■ Scar in the subcutaneous tissues, and even more so the scarred edges of the oblique muscles, may seem like strong tissue that can hold a stitch, but it is avascular and inelastic and has decreased potential to heal. With time, the suture will cheese wire through the noncompliant tissue leading to failure. We always excise all scar and make it a priority to close healthy tissue to healthy tissue.
Suture pull-through is the enemy	■ Not using enough suture fixation points to spread out the load of the closure along the suture lines will lead to disproportionately high force at the suture-tissue interface, leading to pull-through and surgical failure.
Mesh sutured repairs	■ These are efficacious and efficient means to close flank defects, though long-term follow-up does not yet exist for this novel closure method. The strips of mesh use the same concepts of force distribution and reduction of pull-through as tenants of successful abdominal wall surgery.

POSTOPERATIVE CARE

Diet management	We keep the patients NPO until return of bowel function. An aggressive antiemetic regimen is necessary to prevent emesis and the high abdominal wall stress associated with it.
Activity	Patients are instructed to ambulate on postoperative day #1. The same activity protocol exists as for midline hernias.
Pain management	We normally avoid the use of ketorolac given the fairly large dissection. Patients who we anticipate will have pain control difficulties undergo placement of an epidural catheter by the anesthesia pain team for the immediate postoperative period.
DVT Prophylaxis	DVT prophylaxis must be administered as dictated by patient risk stratification on the Caprini score.
Binders	Patients are placed into an abdominal binder to aid wound healing. They wear the binder for 1 month postoperatively to compress the soft tissues to help with healing.
Antibiotics	These are given preoperatively and for 24 hours after surgery.
Drains	Drains are removed when the patient has returned to normal activity and output is less than 30 mL/d.

OUTCOMES

■ In our recently published series of 31 patients[6] treated with the technique described above, 10 patients were found to have a hernia through all layers of the abdominal wall, 17 had a defect in the internal oblique and transversus abdominis with a continuous but bulging external abdominal oblique, and 4 had denervation injury with all the muscle layers in continuity. Mesh placement was intraperitoneal in 19 patients and extraperitoneal in 12 patients. There were no surgical sites infections, and with a mean follow-up time of 830 (± 1051) days, there were 3 recurrences—2 had small bulges, which were successfully repaired with an additional mesh layer between the internal and external oblique muscles, and one was a small asymptomatic hernia detected on a follow-up CT.

COMPLICATIONS

■ Abdominal compartment syndrome
■ Hematoma/Seroma
■ Infection
■ DVT/PE
■ Dehiscence

REFERENCES

1. Fahim DK, Kim SD, Cho D, et al. Avoiding abdominal flank bulge after anterolateral approaches to the thoracolumbar spine: cadaveric study and electrophysiological investigation. *J Neurosurg Spine.* 2011;15:532-540.
2. Ballard JL, Abou-Zamzam AM Jr, Teruya TH, et al. Retroperitoneal aortic aneurysm repair: long-term follow-up regarding wound complications and erectile dysfunction. *Ann Vasc Surg.* 2006;20:195-199.
3. Gardner GP, Josephs LG, Rosca M, et al. The retroperitoneal incision: an evaluation of postoperative flank 'bulge'. *Arch Surg.* 1994;129:753-756.
4. Honig MP, Mason RA, Giron F. Wound complications of the retroperitoneal approach to the aorta and iliac vessels. *J Vasc Surg.* 1992;15:28-33.
5. Chatterjee S, Nam R, Fleshner N, Klotz L. Permanent flank bulge is a consequence of flank incision for radical nephrectomy in one half of patients. *Urol Oncol.* 2004;22:36-39.
6. Purnell CA, Park E, Turin SY, Dumanian GA. Postoperative flank defects, hernias, and bulges: a reliable method for repair. *Plast Reconstr Surg.* 2016;137(3):994-1001.

Section VI: Posterior Trunk Reconstruction
Erector Spinae (Paraspinous) Muscle Flap

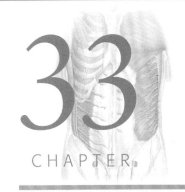

Lauren M. Mioton and Gregory A. Dumanian

DEFINITION

- The erector spinae muscle flap is used for coverage of spinal wounds.

ANATOMY

- The erector spinae, also known as the paraspinous muscles, are paired structures comprised of the iliocostalis (most medial), longissimus, and spinalis muscles (most lateral).
- The iliocostalis muscle originates from the sacrum, erector spinae aponeurosis, and iliac crest, with insertions onto the ribs and transverse processes of C6-C4. It contributes to extension and lateral flexion of the vertebral column.
- The longissimus muscle is the largest of the erector spinae with varying portions originating from the sacrum and transverse processes of the lumbar and thoracic vertebra. It inserts into the transverse processes of lumbar, thoracic, and cervical vertebrae. It contributes to extension and lateral flexion of the vertebral column.
- The spinalis muscle originates from and inserts into the spinous process of lumbar and thoracic vertebrae. It aids with extension of the vertebral column.
- The erector spinae muscles are round and large along the inferior aspect of the lumbar region but become thinner more superiorly along the underside of the trapezius.
  - They have a convex shape with segmental blood vessels originating from the thoracic and abdominal aorta, entering on the lateral and deep aspects of the longissimus and iliocostalis muscles. There are typically both lateral and medial vessels entering the erector spinae, and all of the muscle will stay viable just on its lateral blood flow. In the thorax, these vessels travel through the lateral border of the erector spinae to be the minor pedicle of the latissimus muscle.

PATIENT HISTORY AND PHYSICAL FINDINGS

- Past medical and surgical history with attention to the back is necessary. Prior spine incisions, their location, a history of radiation, and a history of prior infections should be sought. A focused physical examination documenting prior incisions and the suppleness of the posterior soft tissues should be performed. A history of spina bifida, a cord lipoma, or lack of fusion of the posterior spinal tube implies a lack of development and/or small size of the erector spinae inferiorly.
- A prior, or planned, lateral approach to the spine may lead to transection of the erector spinae muscles and eliminate it as a flap option.

IMAGING

- No preoperative imaging is warranted in preparation for this flap.

SURGICAL MANAGEMENT

- The erector spinae muscles are no longer functional for spine extension and flexion and seen as expendable following spine fusion.
- It is an appropriate flap for wounds ranging from the high cervical to low lumbar region.
  - It may not provide coverage of high occipital or the sacral recess (between the sacrum and lumbar spine).

Preoperative Planning

- The patient's medical history should be reviewed as prior to any planned surgery.

Positioning

- The patient is placed in the prone position for the erector spinae flap procedure. Arms may be tucked at the patient's side or abducted with elbows at 90 degrees.

Approach

- The spinal wound, especially if chronic in nature, should be appropriately excised and debrided prior to reconstruction.
- Patients who have undergone prior spine surgery may have notable scar tissue in the wound bed. Clearing the surgical bed of this fibrous tissue will reduce the likelihood of postoperative wound complications as well as allow the surgeon to properly identify the erector spinae muscles and dissection planes.
- Spinal closures are performed prophylactically after spine instrumentation to help achieve a durable closure (especially after multiple prior surgeries) and also for treatment of acute postoperative spinal hardware infections. In the latter, the hardware should be assessed for stability and maintained if it feels stable. Switching out of components of the hardware and rendering it less prominent is at the discretion of the spine team. Loose nonincorporated bone graft should be removed, but it is not necessary to remove every piece of bone graft.

■ Erector Spinae Muscle Flap

- Skin flaps are elevated on either side of the wound either deep or superficial to the thoracolumbar fascia, allowing the latissimus and trapezius muscles to stay attached to the skin.
  - Retractors can be placed on the soft tissues, and cautery can be used to enter the granulation tissue prior to bluntly dissecting in the appropriate plane.
  - The cutaneous perforators and dorsal sensory nerves can often be identified and preserved during elevation of the skin flaps.
  - Over undermining should be avoided to decrease the change of marginal skin vascularity and to limit dead space.
- When the dissection plane is initially superficial to the thoracolumbar fascia, palpation of the lateral border of the erector spinae should reveal its lateral border clearly. The lateral blood supply enters the muscle along this lateral line, and perforators extending to the latissimus and skin are often identified. Near this lateral border, the thoracolumbar fascia is incised along its length to allow it to mobilize medially (**TECH FIG 1A,B**).
- With the skin still retracted, dissection proceeds along the medial and deep aspects of the erector spinae muscles (**TECH FIG 1C,D**).
  - Division of the medial row of blood vessels entering the erector spinae muscles is necessary for full mobilization of the erector spinae muscles. One places dissecting fingers on the lateral border of the muscle, and one should limit the deep dissection so that the muscle maintains its lateral attachments and lateral segmental blood supply.
  - Following this dissection on both its deep and superficial surfaces allows the erector spinae muscles unfold, changing shape from a rounded muscle mass to a more elliptical form (**TECH FIG 1E**).
- With the tissues fully mobilized, stiff and inflamed tissue along the medial aspect of the skin, subcutaneous tissue, and paraspinous muscles should be sharply debrided.

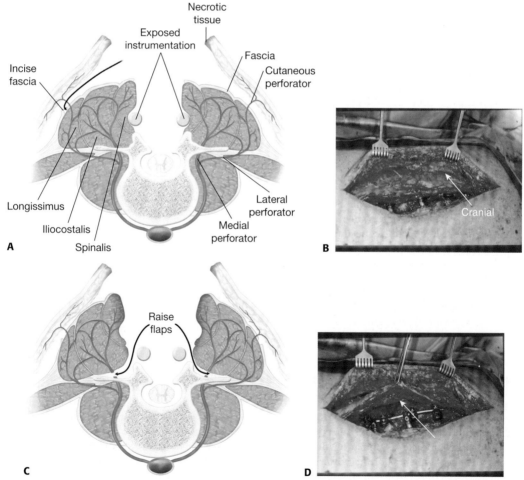

TECH FIG 1 • **A.** Cross-sectional anatomy of superficial aspect of dissection for creation of erector spinae muscle flaps. **B.** Superficial dissection performed in a patient with a postoperative spinal fusion procedure infection. *Arrow* shows incised thoracolumbar fascia. A nerve can be seen passing through the muscle to reach the overlying skin, and it can be preserved. **C.** Cross-sectional anatomy of deep aspect of dissection for creation of erector spinae muscle flaps. **D.** Deep dissection performed in a patient with a postoperative spinal fusion procedure infection. *Arrow* shows lateral-most dissection along deep surface of the erector spinae muscle.

- The erector spinae muscles should be reapproximated in the midline with two or more drains placed both deep and superficial to muscles (**TECH FIG 1F**).
- Drains should be placed both deep to the muscle closure and between the muscle closure and the undermined

skin. The exit sites for the drains should not be on bony prominences of the back. Quilting sutures help to avoid troublesome seromas.

- The overlying skin is then closed with interrupted monofilament sutures.

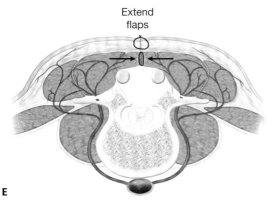
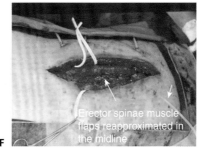

TECH FIG 1 (Continued) • **E.** Cross-sectional anatomy of erector spinae flaps mobilized and approximated in the midline. Note the shape change that occurs in the muscles. **F.** Erector spinae muscle flaps used to close a postoperative spinal fusion procedure infection. Multiple drains placed above and below the muscle closure.

PEARLS AND PITFALLS

Technique	■ Lateral release of the erector spinae muscle alone allows the muscle to move only an estimated 30% of its full potential.
	■ When proceeding with the medial dissection of the erector spinae muscles, place your nondominant hand on the lateral aspect of the muscle along the lateral row of vessels to ensure they are protected.
Outcomes	■ When the erector spinae muscle closure is of good quality, there should be no need for a second overlying muscle flap.

POSTOPERATIVE CARE

- The patient is placed under physical activity restrictions based on the location of spinal fusion. These are often coordinated between plastic surgery and spine surgery services.
  - Patients with high-level fusions often have upper arm restrictions, including limitations in shoulder abduction and forward flexion, that are kept in place for 6 weeks.
- The surgical dressing is kept in place for 72 hours following surgery. Once removed, the incision can be left open to the air.
- When appropriate, patients should be walking and working with physical therapy on postoperative day 1, pending approval by the spine surgery team.
- The largest and lowest closures require the patients to be on a pressure-relief bed to allow the skin and muscle flaps to be directly lied on and compressed.
- Drains are left in place until drainage reaches less than 30 cc a day for 2 days in row.

OUTCOMES[1-3]

- A systematic review of the evidence regarding prophylactic and therapeutic use of flaps for coverage of complex spinal defects revealed that the erector spinae muscle flap was

the most commonly used flap for reconstruction of spinal wounds (56% of cases).
  - Use of such flaps in a prophylactic setting in patients undergoing spinal instrumentation with spinal neoplasms led to a markedly decreased postoperative complication rate when compared to those who did not receive prophylactic flap coverage (20% vs 45%).

COMPLICATIONS

- Skin flap or muscle flap dehiscence
- Seroma
- Hematoma
- Abscess
- Hardware extrusion
- Osteomyelitis

REFERENCES

1. Chieng LO, Hubbard Z, Salgado CJ, et al. Reconstruction of open wounds as a complication of spinal surgery with flaps: a systematic review. *Neurosurg Focus.* 2015;39(4):e17.
2. Dumanian GA, Ondra SL, Liu J, et al. Muscle flap salvage of spine wounds with soft tissue defects or infection. *Spine.* 2003;28:1203-1211.
3. Wilhelmi BJ, Snyder N, Colquhoun T, et al. Bipedicle paraspinous muscle flaps for spinal wound closure: an anatomic and clinical study. *Plast Reconstr Surg.* 2000;106:1305-1311.

34

CHAPTER

Trapezius Muscle Flap

Lauren M. Mioton and Gregory A. Dumanian

DEFINITION

- The trapezius muscle flap is a reliable option for coverage of the posterior trunk and for defects of the head and neck.

ANATOMY

- The trapezius muscle, which has a unique triangular shape, is the most superficial muscle on the posterior neck and thorax (**FIG 1**).
- It is composed of three parts: descending, transverse, and ascending portions.
  - The descending or superior part originates from the occiput and inserts into the lateral third of the clavicle. It acts to elevate the scapula.
  - The transverse or middle part originates from the spinous processes of the 1st to 5th thoracic vertebra and inserts into the acromion. It acts to retract the scapula.
  - The ascending or inferior part originates from the spinous processes of the 6th to 12th thoracic vertebra and inserts into the spine of the scapula. It acts to depress the scapula.
- There are three arterial supplies to the trapezius muscle. The relative importance and the origin of these vessels are quite variable.
  - The upper one-third of the muscle receives its blood predominantly from the transverse cervical artery, which itself is a branch of the thyrocervical trunk or the suprascapular artery almost 80% of the time. It passes through the posterior triangle of the neck to the anterior border of the levator scapulae muscle before dividing into two main branches.
- The branch entering the upper trapezius is termed the superficial cervical artery, or the superficial branch of the transverse cervical.
- The dorsal scapular artery (DSA) supplies the middle one-third of the trapezius.
- In 75% of cases, the DSA originates off the subclavian artery and passes between the upper and middle (or middle and lower) trunks of the brachial plexus before coursing through the rhomboids.
- A branch emerging from between the rhomboid muscles serves as the perforator to the inferior trapezius. It also supplies the skin paddle above and lateral to the overlying latissimus.
- The third source of blood to the inferior-most trapezius is from segmental, posterior intercostal arteries 3 to 6. Due to these numerous small perforators and a dominant larger perforator, most classify this muscle as Mathes and Nahai type V.
- Dominance of one source vessel tends to cause a lack of development of the adjacent vascular territory.
- The entry point of the transverse cervical is cephalad and medial in location to the entry point of the DSA.
  - The trapezius muscle is innervated by the spinal accessory nerve (CN XI).
  - It accompanies the superficial branch of the transverse cervical artery in the superior portion of the muscle and the dorsal scapular artery in the inferior portion. It crosses superficial to the superficial cervical artery in a majority of cases.
- The levator scapulae, rhomboid minor, rhomboid major, and latissimus dorsi muscles all lie deep to the trapezius.
  - The levator scapulae extend from the 1st to the 4th cervical vertebrae and insert on the superior angle of the scapula.
  - The rhomboid minor originates from the spinous process of the 6th and 7th cervical vertebrae and inserts into the medial aspect of the scapula.
  - The rhomboid major begins off the spinous processes of the 1st to 4th thoracic vertebrae and inserts into the medial border of the scapula, below the spine of the scapula.

PATIENT HISTORY AND PHYSICAL FINDINGS

- The medical evaluation of patients is based on their preexisting medical conditions. No special considerations are needed for this procedure. Importance of shoulder abduction for work may lead to the choice of an alternate reconstruction.

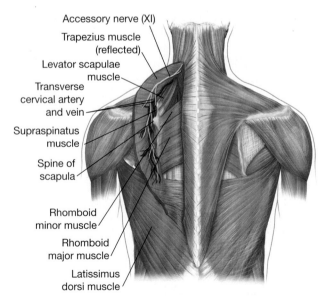

Accessory nerve (XI)
Trapezius muscle (reflected)
Levator scapulae muscle
Transverse cervical artery and vein
Supraspinatus muscle
Spine of scapula
Rhomboid minor muscle
Rhomboid major muscle
Latissimus dorsi muscle

FIG 1 • Regional anatomy of the back.

- Physical examination
  - The skin is examined for scars or previous incision sites. If a previous radical neck dissection or instrumentation of the subclavian artery has been performed, a preoperative evaluation of the transverse cervical artery and the dorsal scapular artery with duplex ultrasound or even arteriogram may be necessary to determine vascular patency.
  - A functional assessment of the shoulder and arm mobility should be performed with baseline function documented.

IMAGING

- Imaging, such as CT or MR angiography, is often not performed in the preoperative evaluation for a trapezius muscle flap.

SURGICAL MANAGEMENT

- The trapezius muscle flap can be used for coverage of the posterior back or for soft tissue defects of the head and neck.
- The decision to use such a flap should be based on the location of the defect and tissue required.
- Smaller defects of the posterior trunk that only require the muscle supplied by the dorsal scapular artery (descending branch) can be performed without significant arm dysfunction, as the upper and middle aspects of the muscle remain present to help with shoulder stability. However, mobilization of the entire muscle to reach the neck, face, and anterior trunk is associated with a sizeable donor site morbidity including limited arm elevation and pain. It should only be considered when other flap options have been eliminated, microsurgery is not an option, or the accessory nerve has already been divided during tumor resection.

Preoperative Planning

- Oncologic history, including radiation, should be well documented.
- One should be aware of the location and type of hardware involved.
- Any pulmonary conditions or other baseline medical comorbidities that would prohibit lateral decubitus or prone positioning should be noted.

Positioning

- Patient positioning will depend on the recipient site.
  - Trapezius muscle flap coverage of occipital, posterior neck or spinal wounds can be done in the prone position. The ipsilateral arm should be prepped into the field, and the arms should remain abducted (at 90 degrees) with the shoulder dropped to move the scapula laterally.
  - The patient may be placed in the lateral decubitus position for cases requiring coverage of the anterior head, neck, or axilla. The ipsilateral arm should be prepped in so that it remains flexible and allows the surgeon to manipulate the scapula.

Approach

- The upper trapezius muscle flap is based on the transverse cervical artery and the lower on the dorsal scapular artery. The latter is the more common. The upper (descending) portion of the trapezius based on the occipital artery and the lower-most trapezius based on segmental intercostal perforators are rarely utilized on their own.
- The entire trapezius muscle flap can be based on the transverse cervical artery, though the most distal aspects of the flap may not remain viable.
  - A trapezius flap based on the branches of the transverse cervical can support the transversely oriented fibers of the muscle and can be harvested as a myocutaneous or osteocutaneous flap if need be.
  - This flap can be utilized for soft tissue defects of the anterior neck and lower face, back, axilla, posterior neck, and occipital regions.
- Trapezius muscle flap based on the DSA
  - The inferior segment of the trapezius can be elevated leaving the rest of the muscle alone based on the dorsal scapular artery with limited morbidity. It is ideal for coverage of hardware in the upper thoracic and lower cervical spine area. This flap is ideal for soft tissue defects of the midface and orbital region as well as defects of the anterior neck, lower face, back, axilla, posterior neck, and occipital region.
- Preoperative markings are best done with the patient sitting or standing with the arms adducted, with a clear mark placed over the tip of the scapula and the scapular spine.

■ Trapezius Flap Based on the DSA

- The inferior portion of the trapezius can be isolated and harvested alone based on the dorsal scapular artery (**TECH FIG 1**).
- The lower part of the trapezius muscle and scapula should be marked.
- The medial border of the scapula and the rhomboid muscles are outlined to identify the perforating point of the pedicle artery. A handheld ultrasound Doppler can be used to mark the putative entry point of the DSA into the trapezius. The main pedicle of the inferior trapezius from the DSA enters the muscle 7 to 8 cm on its deep aspect lateral to the midline at the level of the C7 spinous process.

- A skin island, if planned, should be designed so that at least one-third of its diameter overlies the distal border of the muscle. It must not lie more than 10 cm distal to the inferior angle of the scapula. Extensions of skin distal to the muscle are notoriously unreliably, and alternatives to this flap design including skin grafts placed on the muscle flap should be considered.
- Identify the distal and inferior triangular portion of the trapezius as it overlies the latissimus dorsi muscle. The crossing muscle fiber directions of these two muscles allow for easier distinction.
- Identification of a blood vessel on the lateral border of the inferior trapezius, termed the superficial dorsal scapular artery, can make more reliable carrying of a skin paddle.

- The skin lying lateral and cephalad to the skin paddle can be elevated off of the trapezius.
- An inferior-to-superior muscle elevation is performed until one reaches this perforator entering the deep substance of the muscle.
- Dissection around the medial attachments may be most unclear given the thickness of the attachments, whereas the lateral border of the muscle is clearly distinct from the deeper back muscles. Therefore, the medial attachments are divided only after the muscle has been elevated off of the back. As one nears the scapular spine, the lateral border also becomes indistinct. It is acceptable to divide the tendinous lateral border of the trapezius rather than continuing to follow it further laterally toward the posterior axially line.
- With the main perforator identified and under direct view, the muscle flap can be turned into an island for greater arc of rotation. The DSA pedicle itself can be mobilized to facilitate movement.
- For extreme cephalad mobilization, the DSA can be temporarily clamped with a vascular bulldog, and flow from the transverse cervical system can be assessed. A viable muscle flap with the DSA clamped can allow for further muscle mobilization up to the transverse cervical vessel to harvest an extremely large flap. Caveats to creation of a flap based on the entire trapezius include the following:
  - The higher the dissection proceeds, the greater the postoperative morbidity due to shoulder drop.

The morbidity is attributed to both pain and dysfunction.

- The donor site should be closed directly, if possible, over a normal suction drain in two layers. Quilting sutures may help to limit troublesome seromas that often accompany muscle elevation.

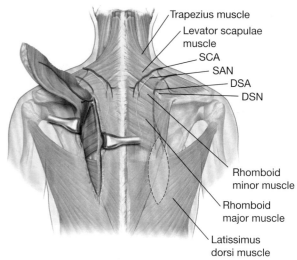

TECH FIG 1 • Trapezius myocutaneous flap based on the dorsal scapular artery. SCA, superficial cervical artery; SAN, spinal accessory artery; DSN, dorsal scapular nerve.

■ Trapezius Flap Based on the Transverse Cervical (Superficial Cervical Artery)

- A smaller portion of the trapezius muscle, the transverse portion in particular, can be harvested on the superficial cervical artery (**TECH FIG 2**).
- The anterior border of the trapezius muscle; the scapula, including the spine of the scapula; and the acromion are marked. A handheld ultrasound Doppler can be used to mark the position and course of the course of the arteries.
- The acromion should be left intact. If a cutaneous component is planned, the skin island should be marked transversely with the distal aspect overlying the scapular spine. It should not extend over the middle of the scapula to ensure inclusion of the vascular pedicle.
- To allow for direct closure of the donor site, skin islands should not extend beyond 8 cm vertically and 6 cm transversely.

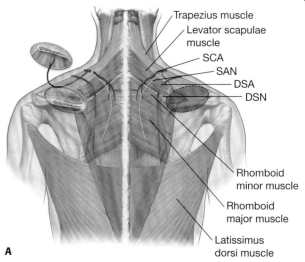

A

TECH FIG 2 • **A.** Elevated trapezius myocutaneous flap based on the superficial cervical artery. SCA, superficial cervical artery; SAN, spinal accessory artery; DSN, dorsal scapular nerve.

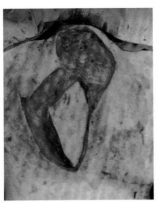 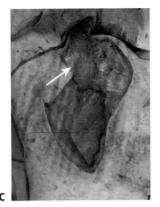

TECH FIG 2 (Continued) • **B.** Incised myocutaneous trapezius flap based on the SCA. The skin paddle was oriented at the inferior aspect of the muscle. The patient had a cervical wound following excision of a metastatic neuroendocrine tumor. **C.** The trapezius flap inset with a 180-degree twist (*arrow*). The superficial dorsal scapular artery was not included with this flap, resulting in mild hypoperfusion of the skin paddle.

PEARLS AND PITFALLS

Technique	■ The higher the dissection proceeds along the lateral muscle dissection, the greater the arc of rotation but the greater the postoperative morbidity due to shoulder drop.
Therapy	■ Physiotherapy is needed to strengthen shoulder muscle agonists.

POSTOPERATIVE CARE

- The ipsilateral shoulder should be immobilized in an adducted position for 1 to 2 weeks if the donor site incision is more cephalad in location. Lower incisions, such as those seen with trapezius flaps based off the DSA, do not require immobilization for healing.
- The flap (either muscle or skin island) should be monitored for the first 5 days.
- No particular anticoagulation regimen is warranted.
- It is important to avoid pressure on the pedicle vessels.
- Beds with air cushions may offload pressure on posterior recipient sites, including occipital, posterior neck, and cervical and thoracic spine regions.
- Physiotherapy is recommended to strengthen the muscle agonists.

OUTCOMES

- Donor site function is acceptable when the accessory nerve is preserved and muscle function—the upper and middle parts of the muscle in particular—is maintained.

- Aesthetically, a trapezius myocutaneous flap has an appropriate skin match for posterior recipient sites but may prove lighter than surrounding skin in anterior head and neck sites. The long scars over the back are often visible and cosmetically unappealing.

COMPLICATIONS

- Loss of scapula stabilization (winged scapula) weakens shoulder and arm elevation.
- Skin necrosis (in cases of skin paddles placed very distally)
- Donor site seroma

SUGGESTED READINGS

Haas F, Weiglein A, Schwarzl F, Scharnagl E. The lower trapezius musculocutaneous flap from pedicled to free flap: anatomical basis and clinical applications based on the dorsal scapular artery. *Plast Reconstr Surg.* 2004;113:1580-1590.

Huelke DF. A study of the transverse cervical and dorsal scapular arteries. *Anat Rec.* 1958;132:233-245.

Yang D, Morris SF. Trapezius muscle: anatomic basis for flap design. *Ann Plast Surg.* 1998;41:52-57.

35
CHAPTER

Superior Gluteal Artery Perforator Flap

Lauren M. Mioton and Gregory A. Dumanian

DEFINITION

- The superior gluteal artery flap is relevant to the treatment of pressure ulcers, coverage of the lower lumbar spine, and breast reconstruction.

ANATOMY

- The superior gluteal artery is a continuation of the posterior division of the internal iliac artery (**FIG 1**).
  - It runs between the lumbosacral trunk and the first sacral nerve.
  - It exits the pelvis above the piriformis and immediately divides into superficial and deep branches.
    - The deep branch passes between the gluteus medius and the iliac bone.
    - The superficial branch continues on to supply the upper portion of the gluteus muscle and overlying fat and skin.
- The superior gluteal nerve supplies this flap.
  - It arises from the dorsal divisions of the 4th and 5th lumbar and 1st sacral nerves.
  - It exits the pelvis through the greater sciatic foramen with the superior gluteal vessels.

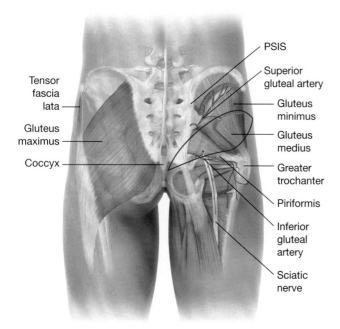

FIG 1 • Anatomic landmarks of piriformis, superior gluteal artery, and superior cluneal nerve.

PATIENT HISTORY AND PHYSICAL FINDINGS

- A thorough history and physical examination should be performed on the patient in the preoperative setting.
  - Prior lower surgery in the gluteal region should be noted as it may preclude the use of the SGAP flap. A history of spina bifida could be associated with lack of formation, small size, or aberrant location of the superior gluteal artery.

IMAGING

- Specific preoperative imaging is not standard workup for SGAP flaps, though it could be performed with a computed tomography angiography.

SURGICAL MANAGEMENT

- The SGAP flap can be used for pressure ulcer reconstruction. Additionally, it is a dependable option for autologous breast reconstruction when abdominal tissue is not available.
- When designing the SGAP flap, the incisions can be in an oblique or more horizontal orientation. A horizontal scar is often deemed more cosmetically acceptable.
- Beveling on dissection creates more dead space and can therefore lead to greater seroma development. Positioning the SGAP more superiorly on the buttock allows for beveling more superiorly and is often associated with decreased revision rates and contour deformities.
- Perforators designed more laterally will lead to longer pedicles.
- The average height and length of the SGAP flap are 10 and 24 cm.

Preoperative Planning

- Patients should undergo additional medical clearance pending their comorbidities.
- The SGAP flap should be avoided in severely obese patients.

Positioning

- Positioning for an SGAP flap depends on the area to be reconstructed.
  - For pressure sore reconstruction or bilateral breast reconstruction, the patient should be placed in the prone position with the arms tucked.
  - In the cases that an SGAP flap is being used for unilateral breast reconstruction, the patient may be in the lateral decubitus position.
    - In both bilateral and unilateral breast reconstruction cases, the patient is subsequently rolled supine for final flap inset. They should be re-prepped and draped during the position change.

Approach

- Markings are placed on the patients in the position that they will be in the OR.
- A line is drawn from the posterosuperior iliac spine (PSIS) to the superior portion of the greater trochanter of the femur. The superior gluteal artery exits the greater sciatic foramen and enters the buttock at the junction of the proximal and middle thirds of this line. The location is confirmed with a handheld Doppler probe.

- Another line is drawn from the PSIS to the coccyx. The intersection of this line with the superior edge of the greater trochanter helps identify the position of the piriformis.
- Perforators located just superior to the piriformis should be considered for flap harvesting.
- The skin paddle is marked to include these perforators.

■ Superior Gluteal Artery Flap

- With the patient properly marked, prepped, and positioned, the previously drawn marks are incised (**TECH FIG 1A,B**).
- Electrocautery is then used to divide the fat to the level of the gluteal fascia.
  - The fat can be beveled superiorly and inferiorly to include as much fat as necessary for the reconstruction.
  - Avoid harvesting of soft tissue over the ischium to avoid painful sitting.
- The cluneal nerves are encountered after dissection through the superficial fascia at the cranial aspect of the flap.
- The gluteal fascia is then incised laterally, and dissection proceeds in a subfascial manner lateral to medial (**TECH FIG 1C,D**). The patient should be paralyzed to reduce the likelihood of movement and possible damage to the pedicle during dissection.
- Perforators with an artery of 1 mm or more in diameter are traced through the muscle. The muscle is split longitudinally to reveal the proximal aspect of the perforator.
- The perforator is freed through both blunt and sharp dissection, and the deep aspect of the gluteus maximus and its associated anterior fascia are reached (**TECH FIG 1E,F**).

- The dissection can terminate at this level for pedicled SGAP flaps with appropriate pedicle length.
- If a longer pedicle is desired for either a pedicled or free flap, the fascia is incised to expose the subgluteal fat pad. The pedicle is traced as medially as required into the pelvis.
  - There is a delicate vascular network in this region that requires broad exposure and careful dissection. The fascia is strong, rendering blunt dissection quite difficult.
  - The flap is detached from the gluteus muscle in the suprafascial plane, and the pedicle is sectioned off.
- Once the pedicled flap or free flap is placed into the recipient site, the donor site may be closed in multiple layers over a drain (**TECH FIG 1G,H**).
  - The skin is undermined and the hip can be extended to reduce tension on the closure.
  - The dermal edges of the donor site are often reapproximated with interrupted mattress or simple sutures in patients requiring a SGAP flap for sacral wound coverage.
  - When the SGAP is utilized as a free flap for breast reconstruction, the donor site epidermis may be closed with a running subcuticular suture.

T E C H N I Q U E S

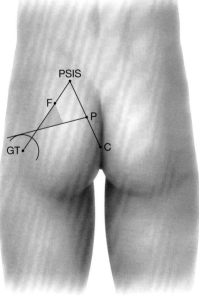

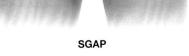

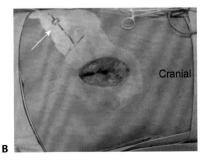

TECH FIG 1 • **A.** Surface landmarks for identification of superior gluteal artery entrance into the upper buttock soft tissues. **B.** Lumbosacral wound 3 weeks after placement of spinal instrumentation and with postoperative infection. A superior gluteal artery perforator turnover flap is to be used to fill the defect. *Arrow* points to Doppler signal present on left buttock from the superior gluteal artery system.

TECHNIQUES

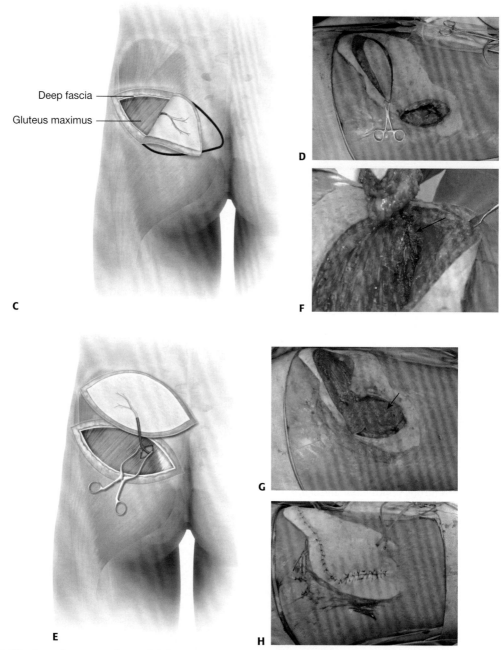

TECH FIG 1 (Continued) • **C.** Lateral to medial dissection of the flap, bringing the deep fascia of the gluteus muscle with the elevated soft tissues. **D.** Superior gluteal artery perforator flap incised to include pedicle, with distal tip of flap pointed toward the greater trochanter. **E.** Dissection of the pedicle through the gluteus maximus muscle. **F.** Superior gluteal artery pedicle (*arrow*) dissected free from gluteus muscle. **G.** Turnover flap easily reaches and fills the lumbosacral defect. The skin paddle is deepithelialized and inset into the spinal defect (*arrow*). **H.** Skin closed over the flap in the midline and primary closure of donor site.

PEARLS AND PITFALLS

Incision placement	■ More horizontal incisions leave fewer contour deformities and are more cosmetically acceptable.
Technique	■ Beveling superiorly, inferiorly, and laterally can allow you to obtain more fat and soft tissue. Avoid beveling medially over the ischium. ■ More lateral perforators lead to a longer pedicle.

POSTOPERATIVE CARE

- Free flaps
    - The patient will be monitored in the intensive care unit for at least 24 hours with flap arterial and venous Doppler checks every hour.
    - Once discharged to a floor bed, the flap will be checked every 4 hours.
    - If the patient is ambulatory at baseline, patient is out of bed and ambulatory on the first postoperative day.
    - Patients often return to work or normal activity 4 weeks following surgery.
- Pedicled flaps for pressure sore reconstruction
    - The patient should remain inpatient, and pressure should be offloaded from the SGAP flap for 2 weeks. This can be facilitated by the use of a special air mattress or by having the patient in the prone position.

OUTCOMES

- A small retrospective review comparing SGAP free flaps to DIEP flaps for breast reconstruction reviewed equivalent flap and donor-site complication rates.[1,2]
- Another study comparing functional outcomes after SGAP-based breast to DIEP-based breast reconstruction showed no significant lower extremity functional scores.[3]

COMPLICATIONS

- Donor Site Complications
    - Seroma
    - Hematoma
    - Contour deformities
    - Donor site pain
- Flap complications
    - Artery or venous occlusion
    - Venous congestion
    - Hematoma
    - Seroma
    - Partial necrosis
    - Infection

REFERENCES

1. Gagnon AR, Blondeel PN. Superior gluteal artery perforator flap. *Semin Plast Surg.* 2006;20:79-88.
2. Hur K, Ohkuma R, Bellamy JL, et al. Patient-reported assessment of functional gait outcomes following superior gluteal artery perforator reconstruction. *Plast Reconstr Surg Glob Open.* 2013;10:e31.
3. Hunter C, Moody L, Luan A, et al. Superior gluteal artery perforator flap: the beauty of the buttock. *Ann Plast Surg.* 2016;76:S191-S195.

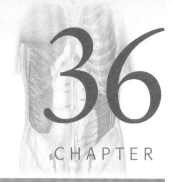

36 CHAPTER

Tissue Expansion for Trunk Defects

Ibrahim Khansa and Jeffrey E. Janis

DEFINITION

- Tissue expansion is the mechanical increase of the surface area of tissue. It relies on two phenomena:
  - Creep: deformation of the tissue in response to stress
  - Stress relaxation: gradual decrease in the amount of force required to stretch the tissue over time

ANATOMY

- In the trunk, the tissues most commonly expanded for wound coverage are the skin and subcutaneous tissue.

PATHOGENESIS

- As the skin and subcutaneous tissue are expanded, all layers get thinner, except for the epidermis, which undergoes cellular hyperplasia via mitosis.[1]
- After removal of the tissue expander, all layers return to normal thickness, except the adipose layer, which permanently thins.
- Expanded skin has improved vascularity compared to nonexpanded skin.
- Around the tissue expander, a capsule forms, consisting of collagen and fibroblasts. The zone between the native tissue and the capsule is highly vascular.

PATIENT HISTORY AND PHYSICAL FINDINGS

- Tissue expansion is indicated when there is a local deficiency of soft tissue coverage over a wound, with healthy tissue in the surrounding zone that is able to be expanded.
- Ask about history of radiation, because this makes radiated tissues much more stiff and difficult to expand and increases the risk of tissue expander exposure, infection, and/or loss.
- On physical examination, look for infection/contamination, as this increases risk of complications with tissue expansion.
- In the lower abdominal wall, regional transfer of tissues from the anterolateral thigh may be a better option for soft tissue coverage than tissue expansion. However, in the epigastric region, those flaps may not have sufficient reach. In addition, the epigastric region often has a scarcity of soft tissue, which increases the usefulness of tissue expansion in this area.

IMAGING

- No imaging is required specifically for tissue expansion.

SURGICAL MANAGEMENT

Preoperative Planning

- Control contamination
  - Mupirocin nasal ointment and chlorhexidine baths for 5 days preoperatively in patients at risk for methicillin-resistant *Staphylococcus aureus* (MRSA) or who are known MRSA carriers.
    - This protocol has been shown to reduce surgical site infections in total joint arthroplasties.[2]
- Optimize the patient to lower complication rates:
  - Glucose control: Hemoglobin A1c should be ≤7.4%.[3]
  - Nutrition: Albumin should be 3.25 g/dL or higher, and prealbumin should be 15 mg/dL or higher.[3,4]
  - Obesity: BMI should be 42 or lower and preferably below 40.[3]
  - Tobacco usage: Patients should quit all tobacco products for 4 weeks preoperatively and 4 weeks postoperatively.[3]
- Tissue expander selection
  - Choose largest tissue expander that can be placed in the pocket.
  - Length of the expander should be at least as long as the defect.
  - Crescentic and rectangular tissue expanders tend to be best suited for abdominal wall defects. Rectangular expanders tend to have the highest yield.[5]
  - Remote port tissue expanders are preferred.

Positioning

- Supine with arms abducted 90 degrees, with all pressure points padded

Approach

- The planned flap movement should be designed before tissue expansion is begun. The incision to insert a tissue expander is usually made very close to the border of the soft tissue defect. This helps minimize the amount of tissue between the leading border of the flap and the wound, which will be discarded, and provide for expansion of uninjured/unscarred tissue to transpose later directly to the defect.

Subcutaneous Tissue Expander Insertion Into the Abdomen

- Prep the skin with alcohol-containing prep (chlorhexidine and alcohol or iodine and alcohol).[3,6] If a wound is present, use iodine alone.
- Design an advancement or rotation flap, which, when expanded, will cover the defect. The leading edge of the flap should be along one of the edges of the defect (**TECH FIG 1A**).
- Make an incision within 3 to 5 mm of the edge of the defect. This will serve as the insertion access for the tissue expander and the leading edge of the flap. The incision should not be made immediately at the edge of the wound, as this incision will need to be closed and requires healthy tissue to obtain a closure robust enough to protect the tissue expander (see **TECH FIG 1A,D**). However, minimize the amount of tissue between the edge of the wound and the incision, as this tissue will be discarded.
- Dissect down to the anterior rectus sheath, and elevate the skin and subcutaneous tissue off the rectus sheath from medial to lateral. The length and width of the undermining should correspond precisely to the dimensions of the tissue expander (**TECH FIG 1B**).
- Once the precise pocket is dissected, create an additional small pocket for the remote port. Through the dissected expander pocket, choose a location for the remote port adjacent to the expander. The location should be chosen so that the remote port is distant enough from the expander to avoid expander puncture during fills, where the subcutaneous tissue is thinnest in order to facilitate palpation of the port during fills, and preferably over a bony area to provide support during needle access/insertion during fills. Dissect a small pocket that will precisely fit the remote port. Do not overdissect, as this could result in port migration or rotation.
- Obtain hemostasis and irrigate with warm normal saline and triple antibiotic solution.
- A closed-suction drain is inserted into the pocket through a separate stab incision laterally.
- Use no-touch technique to insert the tissue expander:[7]
  - Re-prep the skin with Betadine and allow to try.
  - Use triple antibiotic irrigation (1 g cefazolin, 80 mg gentamicin, 50,000 units bacitracin in 500 cc of normal saline to irrigate the pocket and immerse the tissue expander).[8]
  - Only one person touches the tissue expander. That person puts on new talc-free gloves.
  - New retractors are used. They should be immersed in triple antibiotic solution before use.
  - The skin is retracted using the new retractors, and the tissue expander is inserted into the pocket without touching the skin (**TECH FIG 1C**).
- The remote port can be sutured to the fascia if there is concern that it will rotate or migrate.
- The incision is closed in three layers using absorbable sutures (Scarpa fascia, deep dermis, subcuticular), and dressings are applied (cyanoacrylate or Xeroform) (**TECH FIG 1D**).

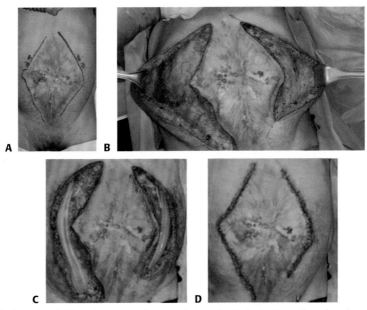

TECH FIG 1 • Tissue expander insertion. **A.** The advancement flaps are designed, with the incisions along the edges of the defect. **B.** Subcutaneous pockets are dissected to precisely fit the tissue expanders. **C.** The tissue expanders are inserted into the subcutaneous pockets. **D.** Meticulous layered closure is performed.

T E C H N I Q U E S

■ Tissue Expander Fill

- Filling the tissue expander is begun 2 to 3 weeks after insertion (assuming no wound healing problems). Fills are performed weekly.
- The fill is performed after prepping the skin with chlorhexidine-alcohol. The end points of filling are (a) patient pain and (b) skin blanching.

- Filling is continued until the length of the flap overlying the tissue expander is at least equal to the wound diameter plus the base width of the expander. Judicious overfilling is preferable.

■ Tissue Expander Removal and Flap Advancement

- The advancement or rotation flap is designed (**TECH FIG 2A**).
- Before excising the wound or the skin graft on bowel, the previous incision (for tissue expander insertion) is recreated along its full length, along with any additional back cuts necessary to advance or rotate the flap.
- The tissue expander and fill port are removed, and the pocket is irrigated with warm normal saline.
- The flap is advanced, transposed, or rotated as designed, and its ability to close the defect is assessed.
- If the flap cannot reach the distal end of the defect, several options are available.
  - In a rotation flap, perform a back-cut, or Burow triangle, in order to increase the rotation of the flap. The triangle should be designed to avoid incising into the base of the flap, which may compromise vascularity.
    - Another maneuver is to incise the fascia underneath the intact skin at the point of maximal tension, which will allow for further excursion.

- In an advancement flap, undermine farther laterally to increase advancement. This should be performed carefully as it will decrease the vascularity of the flap. Back-cuts can also be performed unilaterally or bilaterally.[9]
- Perform capsulotomies in the tissue expander capsule. These should be performed perpendicular to the desired direction of advancement (**TECH FIG 2B**). They should be performed carefully, incising through capsule only and avoiding injuring the flap itself. Multiple capsulotomies can be performed, spaced approximately 1 cm from each other. Extrapolating from galeal scoring in scalp reconstruction, the tension should be checked after each capsulotomy, and additional capsulotomies performed if more advancement is needed.[10] Capsulectomies are not recommended, as they can decrease flap vascularity.
- Only excise part of the wound, and leave the remainder for a later serial excision or second round of expansion.
- After the reach of the flap is verified, the wound is excised (partially or fully, depending on flap reach), and the flap is advanced/rotated and inset. A closed-suction drain should be placed under the flap (the capsule will tend to form a seroma unless the pocket is drained).

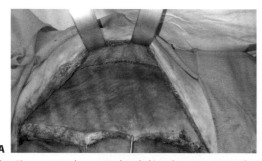 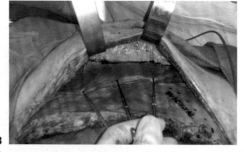

TECH FIG 2 • Tissue expander removal and skin advancement. **A.** The advancement flap is re-elevated, and the tissue expander is removed. **B.** Capsulotomies perpendicular to the advancement vector can be performed to increase flap excursion.

■ Other Techniques

- Some authors have described expansion of the external oblique,[11] of the internal oblique-external oblique complex,[12,13] or of the entire abdominal wall musculofascia using intraperitoneal tissue expanders.[14] However, these techniques lead to thinning and attenuation of the musculofascial layer and have not gained widespread use.

PEARLS AND PITFALLS

Planning	■ The planned flap movement should be designed before the incision for the insertion of the tissue expander is made.
	■ Most patients require multiple tissue expanders to be placed. In most cases, one tissue expander can be placed on either side of the wound, and filling of both expanders can be performed concurrently.
Surgical technique	■ The capsule is highly vascular. Performing a capsulectomy at the time of tissue expander removal and flap advancement risks skin flap compromise and hematoma formation. Capsulotomies can be performed perpendicular to the desired advancement vector to increase flap excursion.
	■ Infection and extrusion are major complications that can result in sabotage of the expander-based reconstruction due to need for tissue expander removal. Therefore, meticulous attention to patient selection, sterile technique (both in the OR and during postoperative expansion), and adherence to end points of tissue expansion are paramount.

POSTOPERATIVE CARE

■ After tissue expander insertion
  ▪ The drain should be kept in until its output is less than 20 cc/day for 2 consecutive days with the patient ambulatory. This end point may not be reached until tissue expander fills are begun, as the tissue expander starts to fill the dead space.
  ▪ Many surgeons keep patients on antibiotics to cover skin flora while the drain is still present and in contact with the tissue expander. There is no evidence to support or contradict this practice, and the published evidence is inconclusive.[15,16]
■ After tissue expander removal and flap advancement
  ▪ The drain should be kept in until its output is less than 20 cc/day for 2 consecutive days with the patient ambulatory.

OUTCOMES

■ Outcomes are generally good, even in the presence of ostomies or enterocutaneous fistulas. These can increase the rate of infection and add morbidity and reoperations. Despite that most patients can usually complete the expansion process successfully.[17–20]

COMPLICATIONS

■ Tissue expander infection
  ▪ If mild cellulitis with no systemic symptoms, attempt treatment with oral or intravenous antibiotics.
  ▪ If severe or with systemic symptoms, requires surgical washout and tissue expander removal.
■ Tissue expander exposure
  ▪ Usually requires washout and tissue expander removal. If infection is present, no new expander should be inserted. If no infection is present, a new tissue expander can potentially be inserted after washout.
■ Seroma
  ▪ If threatening skin flap viability, aspirate or perform interventional radiology drain insertion
  ▪ If not causing a problem and not infected, can potentially observe and wait for resolution
■ Hematoma
  ▪ Requires washout as hematomas that are not evacuated will lead to capsular scarring, which would make flap movement very difficult

■ Skin flap necrosis
  ▪ If causing tissue expander exposure, requires washout and debridement and expander removal
  ▪ If occurs after tissue expander removal and flap advancement/rotation, can usually treat with local wound care until demarcated and then may require debridement

REFERENCES

1. Johnson PE, Kernahan DA, Bauer BS. Dermal and epidermal response to soft-tissue expansion in the pig. *Plast Reconstr Surg.* 1988;81:390-397.
2. Sporer SM, Rogers T, Abella L. Methicillin-resistant and methicillin-sensitive *Staphylococcus aureus* screening and decolonization to reduce surgical site infection in elective total joint arthroplasty. *J Arthroplasty.* 2016;31:144-147.
3. Harrison B, Khansa I, Janis JE. Evidence-based strategies to reduce postoperative complications in plastic surgery. *Plast Reconstr Surg.* 2016;137:351-360.
4. Kudsk KA, Tolley EA, DeWitt RC, et al. Preoperative albumin and surgical site identify surgical risk for major postoperative complications. *J Parenter Enteral Nutr.* 2003;27:1-9.
5. van Rappard JHA, Molenaar J, van Doorn K, et al. Surface-area increase in tissue expansion. *Plast Reconstr Surg.* 1988;82:833-837.
6. Darouiche RO, Wall MJ, Itani KM, et al. Chlorhexidine-alcohol versus povidone-iodine for surgical-site antisepsis. *N Engl J Med.* 2010;362:18-26.
7. Mladick RA. "No-touch" submuscular saline breast augmentation technique. *Aesthetic Plast Surg.* 1993;17:183-192.
8. Khansa I, Hendrick RG, Boehmler JH, et al. Breast reconstruction with tissue expanders: implementation of a standardized best-practices protocol to reduce infection rates. *Plast Reconstr Surg.* 2014;134:11-18.
9. Zide BM, Karp NS. Maximizing gain from rectangular tissue expanders. *Plast Reconstr Surg.* 1992;90:500-504.
10. Leedy JE, Janis JE, Rohrich RJ. Reconstruction of acquired scalp defects: an algorithmic approach. *Plast Reconstr Surg.* 2005;116:54e-72e.
11. Jacobsen MW, Petty PM, Bite U, Johnson CH. Massive abdominal-wall hernia reconstruction with expanded external/internal oblique and transversalis musculofascia. *Plast Reconstr Surg.* 1997;100:326-335.
12. Byrd HS, Hobar PC. Abdominal wall expansion in congenital defects. *Plast Reconstr Surg.* 1989;84:347-352.
13. Hobar PC, Rohrich RJ, Byrd HS. Abdominal-wall reconstruction with expanded musculofascial tissue in a posttraumatic defect. *Plast Reconstr Surg.* 1994;94:379-383.
14. Marin-Gutzke M, Mirelis E, Sanchez-Olaso A, et al. Restoring the abdominal cavity space by intraabdominal and extraabdominal tissue expansion. *Plast Reconstr Surg.* 2008;121:359-360.
15. Phillips BT, Fourman MS, Bui DT, et al. Are prophylactic postoperative antibiotics necessary for immediate breast reconstruction? Results of a prospective randomized clinical trial. *J Am Coll Surg.* 2016;222:1116-1124.

16. Wong A, Lee S, Sbitany H, et al. Postoperative prophylactic antibiotic use following ventral hernia repair with placement of surgical drains reduces the postoperative surgical-site infection rate. *Plast Reconstr Surg*. 2016;137:285-294.

17. Paletta CT, Huang DB, Dehghan K, Kelly C. The use of tissue expanders in staged abdominal wall reconstruction. *Ann Plast Surg*. 1999;42:259-265.

18. Carr JA. Tissue expander-assisted ventral hernia repair for the skin-grafted damage control abdomen. *World J Surg*. 2014;38:782-787.

19. Kuokkanen H. Tissue expander-assisted ventral hernia repair for the skin-grafted damage control abdomen. *World J Surg*. 2014;38:788-789.

20. Watson MJ, Kundu N, Coppa C, et al. Role of tissue expanders in patients with loss of abdominal domain awaiting intestinal transplantation. *Transpl Int*. 2013;26:1184-1190.

Keystone Flaps

Theodore A. Kung and Peter Neligan

DEFINITION

- The keystone flap is a versatile fasciocutaneous flap that transfers available soft tissue to an adjacent defect and can be designed anywhere on the body where perforators are present. It serves as a reliable alternative to more complex forms of reconstruction, such as free tissue transfer, and can be used for large as well as small defects.
- Advantages of keystone flaps include simple and rapid dissection that results in relatively shorter operative times compared to alternative reconstructive options, techniques that are easily reproducible and teachable, and reconstruction with local tissue of similar quality. In addition, although keystone flaps are based on perforating vessels, there is no need to perform a meticulous perforator dissection.
- Appropriate use of a keystone flap over other choices of reconstruction (eg, muscle flap with skin graft, myocutaneous flap, free flap) can minimize donor-site morbidity and facilitate a more expeditious postsurgical recovery.

ANATOMY

- The keystone flap is a fasciocutaneous advancement flap. The donor-site secondary defect is addressed by performing two V-Y closures.
- Knowledge of the location of musculocutaneous and septocutaneous perforators can facilitate design of well-vascularized keystone flaps (**FIG 1**).
- Anteriorly, perforators from the internal mammary, intercostal, and epigastric systems can supply keystone flaps for chest and abdominal reconstruction.
- Posteriorly, midline closures may take advantage of paravertebral intercostal perforators. Multiple perforators arising from the subscapular system may be used to design keystone flaps for the mid and upper back. Lower back and buttock keystone flaps can include perforators from the posterior intercostal, lumbar, and gluteal systems.
- In upper and lower extremities, numerous perforators from the major longitudinal vessels can supply keystone flaps of various sizes. For larger defects, named perforators can be used to ensure adequate vascularity to the flap (eg, perforators from the descending branch of the lateral circumflex femoral artery), whereas smaller defects may depend on randomly distributed perforating vessels emanating from the underlying fascia and muscle.
- One notable location where keystone flaps may fail is the scalp due to its axial blood supply and relatively unyielding quality.
- In principle, to close a defect with a keystone flap, the volume of the keystone flap needs to be redistributed in order to fill nearly all of the primary and the secondary defect (the total defect size, primary plus secondary, is modestly reduced during closure due to advancement of the wound margins). Thus, the keystone flap is not an ideal choice to fill large concave defects. In those instances, one should consider reconstructive options that provide additional tissue volume.

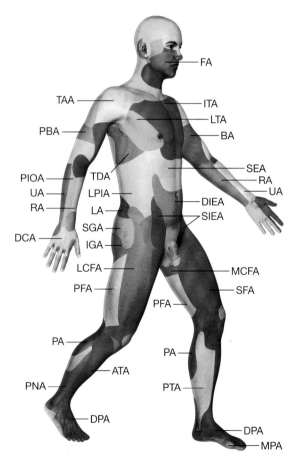

FIG 1 • Keystone flaps may be designed based on knowledge of the location of major perforators and their vascular territories. ATA, anterior tibial artery; BA, brachial artery; DCA, dorsal carpal arch; DIEA, deep inferior epigastric artery; DPA, dorsalis pedis artery; FA, facial artery; IGA, inferior gluteal artery; ITA, internal thoracic (mammary) artery; LA, lumbar arteries; LPIA, lateral branches of posterior intercostal arteries; LTA, lateral thoracic artery; MCFA, medial circumflex femoral artery; MPA, medial plantar artery; PA, popliteal artery; PBA, profunda brachial artery; PFA, profunda femoris artery; PIOA, posterior interosseous artery; PNA, peroneal artery; PTA, posterior tibial artery; RA, radial artery; SEA, superior epigastric artery; SFA, superficial femoral artery; SGA, superior gluteal artery; SIEA, superficial inferior epigastric artery; TAA, thoracoacromial artery; TDA, thoracodorsal artery; UA, ulnar artery.

- More than one keystone flap can be designed around a defect in order to distribute the tension burden of secondary defect closure.

HISTORY

- As described by Behan in 2003, the keystone flap is a trapezoidal perforator advancement flap. The name is derived from the flap's resemblance to the shape of an architectural keystone within an ancient Roman arch.[1]
- The keystone flap has been successfully applied to a vast array of clinical scenarios, including reconstruction of the trunk, head and neck, extremities, and perineum.[2-7]
- Multiple variations of the keystone flap have been described. These include the use of more than one keystone flap, a rotational keystone flap, and an omega-variant technique.[1,8]

PATIENT HISTORY AND PHYSICAL FINDINGS

- The potential use of a keystone flap can be noted preoperatively during physical examination. Patients should be counseled that flap selection is ultimately based upon the dimensions of the defect as well as the laxity of the surrounding tissues. Therefore, other possible reconstructive options should also be reviewed with the patient before surgery.
- For reconstruction after tumor extirpation, knowledge of the necessary surgical margins is helpful to predict if adequate local tissue will be available for design of a keystone flap. Extensive surgical margins commonly result in a wide concave defect that demands a significant amount of volume replacement. On these occasions, the keystone flap may not provide sufficient volume for coverage.
- The need for preoperative or postoperative radiation therapy should be noted. A keystone flap using soft tissues that have been previously radiated can demonstrate significantly decreased laxity and may not adequately advance into the defect. When postoperative radiotherapy is planned, the well-vascularized keystone flap can be expected to sustain radiation without major complications.

IMAGING

- Imaging studies are not required for successful design of a keystone flap, but oftentimes, preoperative CT scans obtained for surgical planning are helpful to identify perforators.
- Use of a handheld pencil Doppler probe can assist in identifying perforators to help design the keystone flap. Smaller keystone flaps supplied by random perforating vessels may not demonstrate Doppler signals but can still be used successfully.
- Although the viability of the keystone flap can be readily determined by clinical examination alone, if there is any question about the vascularity of the flap after harvest, intraoperative fluorescent angiography can be used to confirm both arterial inflow and venous outflow. A fluorescent dye such as indocyanine green is injected intravenously, and arterial inflow is confirmed within 30 seconds as the dye flows into the keystone flap. After about 20 minutes, venous outflow can also be confirmed by observing the absence of dye within the flap.

SURGICAL MANAGEMENT

- Keystone flaps are commonly utilized in the reconstruction of tumor extirpation defects. These flaps provide durable soft tissue coverage and well-vascularized tissue capable of sustaining adjuvant radiation therapy.
- Some resection defects are quite large and involve full-thickness removal of skin, fat, muscle, and bone (eg, sarcoma excision) (**FIG 2**). Many of these defects would otherwise require the use of a pedicled muscle-based reconstruction method or a free flap. Alternatively, resection defects can be small but located on difficult locations, such as the hand or foot and ankle, where reliable soft tissue coverage is needed to protect underlying tendon and bone (**FIG 3**).
- In the trunk and proximal extremities, where multiple robust perforators are known to exist, the keystone flap should always be a reconstructive option, especially when there is substantial soft tissue laxity adjacent to the defect.

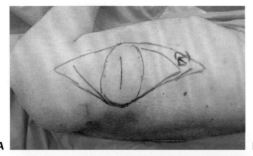

A

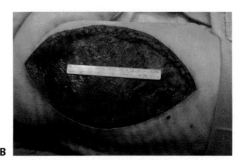

B

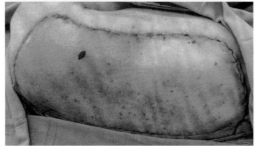

C

FIG 2 • A–C. Wide excision of a sarcoma of the lateral back. A large keystone flap was used to advance skin and soft tissue from a posterior to lateral direction. Adequate exposure is critical to designing a keystone flap of sufficient size to fill such a large defect.

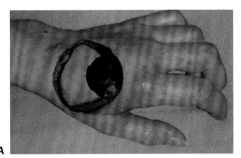 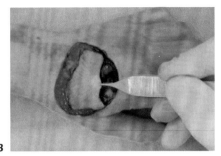

A   **B**

FIG 3 • A,B. Smaller defects can also be closed using keystone flaps. A dorsal hand wound resulting from excision of a melanoma is closed with a keystone flap based on underlying perforators of the dorsal metacarpal arteries. Importantly, no undermining should be attempted to preserve vascularity for smaller keystone flaps.

- For more distal defects, such as those on the hand or foot, a keystone flap may still be used; however, one must be particularly careful not to undermine the flap in an effort to preserve vascularity.
- A keystone flap can be used in conjunction with another local flap to close especially large defects.
- Secondary defects resulting from harvest of another flap can be closed with a keystone flap. For example, when a wide flap containing skin (eg, radial forearm, parascapular, anterolateral thigh, etc.) is needed for reconstruction and the donor site cannot be approximately primarily, a keystone flap can be designed to permit closure of the secondary defect.

Preoperative Planning

- In the vast majority of cases, a keystone flap can be designed based upon knowing the location of key perforators near the site of the defect. Thus, there is rarely a need for dedicated preoperative imaging for the sake of the keystone flap.

- A handheld pencil Doppler probe can be used to confirm the presence of major perforators.
- Alternatively, intraoperative fluorescent angiography can be performed to identify the location of perforators.

Positioning

- When a keystone flap is to be performed after tumor extirpation, coordination with the oncologic surgeon is critical to determine the optimal positioning for reconstruction.
- Adequate exposure of the surrounding tissues is critical to properly design a keystone flap.

Approach

- Design of a keystone flap is individualized to each patient and requires consideration of the shape and size of the defect, the surrounding soft tissue quality and laxity, and the most favorable placement of scars.

■ Technique for Keystone Flap Design

- The skin and soft tissue around the defect are palpated to determine the areas of maximum laxity.
- Classically, for an elliptical defect, each limb of the keystone flap is drawn at a 90-degree angle to each end of the defect (**TECH FIG 1A**). For a circular defect, these limbs must be designed such that the inner corners of the keystone flap are not excessively narrow in order to optimize vascularity and advancement (**TECH FIG 1B**). Alternatively, a circular defect can be first converted into an elliptical defect, or, the keystone flap may be modified to obviate the need for excision of normal tissue (**TECH FIG 1C**).
- The width of the keystone flap should be equal to or slightly greater than the width of the defect.
- All edges of the keystone flap are incised, and dissection is carried down through the underlying deep fascia. The deep fascia must be completely incised to maximize flap mobility.
- Normally, the perforators that feed the keystone flap are not visualized.
- If adequate mobility permits, the inner corners of the keystone flap may be trimmed away in a rounded fashion.

- Closure begins by placing a stitch at the point of maximum tension. Next, the outer corners of the keystone flap are closed in a V-Y fashion. Finally, the halving principle is used for the remainder of the closure to distribute the tension.
- If there is excessive tightness during closure, several strategies can be considered:
  - Check that the deep fascia at the margins of the keystone flap has been adequately incised.
  - Perform limited undermining of the keystone flap while preserving any visualized perforators.
  - Superficially incise the underlying muscle at the edges of the keystone flap to gain additional mobility.
  - Undermine the soft tissues surrounding the defect to recruit more laxity at the point of maximum tension.
  - Turn the inner corners of the keystone flap toward the defect so that the tips of these corners become the leading edge of the keystone flap. This technique is possible only if the inner corners are sufficiently vascularized (ie, if the tips are not excessively narrow).
  - Consider performing a second keystone flap on the other side of the defect.

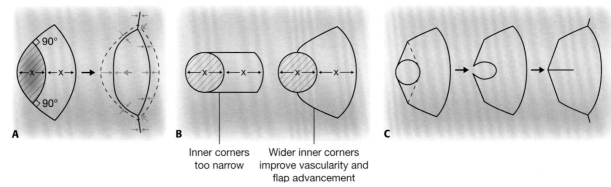

TECH FIG 1 • A. Keystone flap closure of an elliptical defect. The donor site is closed in a V-Y fashion, and this aids in flap advancement. **B.** With a circular defect, the inner corners of the defect must not be excessively narrow. Wider inner corners will result in improved vascularity and a larger keystone flap, which facilitates flap advancement. If adequate mobility permits, the inner corners may be trimmed away in a rounded fashion. **C.** As an alternative to converting a circular defect into an elliptical defect, the keystone flap may be modified to avoid excising normal tissue.

Keystone Flap for Back Reconstruction

- Midline back defects are especially amenable to bilateral keystone flap closure (**TECH FIG 2**).

- Each flap is supplied by robust perforators, and the advancement requirement for tension-free closure is shared by the two flaps.

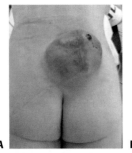 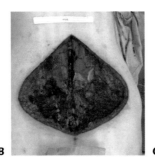 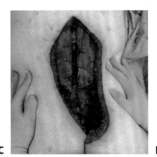 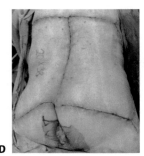

TECH FIG 2 • A–D. Excision of a large sarcoma from the midline lower back resulting in a large defect that cannot be reapproximated. Tension-free closure was achieved by performing bilateral keystone flaps.

Keystone Flap for Foot Reconstruction

- A keystone flap can be used on glabrous skin of the hand or foot (**TECH FIG 3**).
- In these locations, the skin is firmly adherent to the underlying fascia. Complete release of the fascia is mandatory to maximize flap advancement.

- If necessary, tissue scissors can be used to spread in a vertical fashion perpendicular to the plane of the skin. This technique releases the multiple subcutaneous septa and results in greater flap mobility.

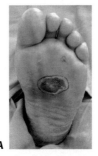 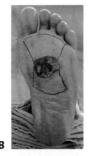 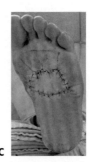

TECH FIG 3 • A–C. An ulcerating plantar foot lesion is excised, resulting in exposure of the plantar fascia. Due to the adherent nature of plantar skin, two opposing keystone flaps were planned. However, after complete release of the plantar fascia and vertical spreading along the margins of the flap, the defect was successfully closed with only one keystone flap.

Keystone Flap to Close a Donor-site Defect

- When reconstruction calls for a large fasciocutaneous or musculocutaneous flap involving a wide skin paddle, the secondary defect may not close primarily.

- As an alternative to skin grafting, which results in poor appearance and may lead to contour deformity, a keystone flap can be designed to fill the donor-site defect (**TECH FIG 4**).

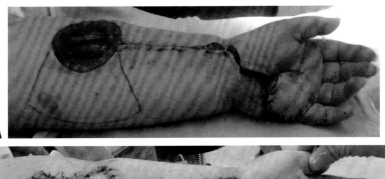

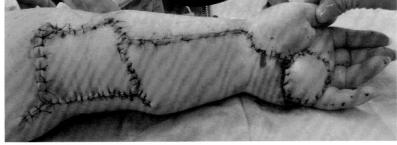

TECH FIG 4 • A,B. A keystone flap can be used to close a secondary defect after harvest of a fasciocutaneous or musculocutaneous flap. A radial forearm flap was harvested for coverage of a palmar hand defect following resection of a sarcoma. The resultant donor-site defect could not be closed primarily. Therefore, a keystone flap was designed to transfer mobile volar forearm skin and soft tissue to achieve closure of the secondary defect.

PEARLS AND PITFALLS

Design	■ The dimensions of the keystone flap must be of sufficient size to close the intended defect.
	■ The width of the keystone flap must approximate the width of the defect, or else closure may be excessively tight or even impossible.
	■ A large keystone flap will ensure inclusion of more perforators.
	■ The V-Y closures of the keystone flap should be designed to maximize advancement of the flap into the primary defect.
Technique	■ A handheld pencil Doppler probe may be used to help identify perforators.
	■ In rare instances, the keystone flap requires cautious undermining. If so, every effort should be taken to preserve perforators.
	■ Underlying muscle may be superficially incised along the borders of the keystone flap to permit additional advancement, if necessary.
	■ The first closure stitch should serve to close the primary defect. Subsequently, the secondary defect is closed using the halving principle in order to even distribute tension.
Postoperative	■ Patients should be placed on appropriate activity restrictions specific to the anatomic region where a keystone flap was performed. This will minimize the rate of dehiscence.
	■ Superficial wounds can be treated conservatively with dressing changes. These minor wounds should not delay any planned postoperative adjuvant radiation.

POSTOPERATIVE CARE

- The patient is restricted from any movements that increase tension on the keystone flap, especially along the short axis of the flap. A postoperative splint may be beneficial for a short period of time when the reconstruction is on an extremity.
- Physical therapy consultation is helpful for some patients after reconstruction of large lower extremity defects.
- Non–weight bearing for about 2 weeks after foot and ankle keystones
- The patient is seen within 1 week after discharge and then for suture removal at the 2-week postoperative visit.

OUTCOMES

- Keystone flaps have been utilized to close a wide variety of defects and boasts a success rate of 97% to 100%.[2,6]
- Major complications requiring a secondary operation are rare; minor complications commonly involve superficial wound dehiscence that can be treated conservatively.
- Compared to other coverage options, such as muscle-based flaps or free flaps, appropriate selection of a keystone flap for reconstruction can result in shorter operative time, shorter inpatient stay, and shorter time to patient mobilization.

COMPLICATIONS

- Delayed wound healing can occur at points of relative tension along the keystone flap incisions. In the vast majority of cases, these wounds are superficial and can be treated with dressing changes.
- Frequently, planned postoperative adjuvant radiation therapy is not initiated until the reconstruction has sufficiently healed. Superficial wounds should not delay initiation of radiation therapy. For larger wounds, secondary

interventions such as split-thickness skin grafting may be considered to hasten wound closure in anticipation of radiation therapy.
- Rarely, keystone flaps may demonstrate venous congestion in the immediate postoperative period. Consider releasing some sutures to relieve tension, application of nitropaste, or the use of leeches. Also, evaluate if patient position and mobility is contributing to the problem.
- Seromas are a rare occurrence after keystone flaps because undermining of the surrounding tissues is generally not necessary.

REFERENCES

1. Behan FC. The keystone design perforator island flap in reconstructive surgery. *ANZ J Surg.* 2003;73:112-120.
2. Khouri JS, Egeland BM, Daily SD, et al. The keystone island flap: use in large defects of the trunk and extremities in soft tissue reconstruction. *Plast Reconstr Surg.* 2011;127:1212-1221.
3. Behan FC, Rozen WM, Azer S, Grant P. 'Perineal keystone design perforator island flap' for perineal and vulval reconstruction. *ANZ J Surg.* 2012;82:381-382.
4. Moncrieff MD, Bowen F, Thompson JF, et al. Keystone flap reconstruction of primary melanoma excision defects of the leg: the end of the skin graft?. *Ann Surg Oncol.* 2008;15:2867-2873.
5. Behan F, Sizeland A, Gilmour F, et al. Use of the keystone island flap for advanced head and neck cancer in the elderly: a principle of amelioration. *J Plast Reconstr Aesthet Surg.* 2010;63:739-745.
6. Mohan AT, Rammos CK, Akhavan AA, et al. Evolving concepts of keystone perforator island flaps (KPIF): principles of perforator anatomy, design modifications, and extended clinical applications. *Plast Reconstr Surg.* 2016;137:1909-1920.
7. Pelissier P, Gardet H, Pinsolle V, et al. The keystone design perforator island flap. Part II: clinical applications. *J Plast Reconstr Aesthet Surg.* 2007;60:888-891.
8. Behan FC, Rozen WM, Lo CH, Findlay M. The omega - Ω - variant designs (types A and B) of the keystone perforator island flap. *ANZ J Surg.* 2011;81:650-652.

Treatment of Axillary Hyperhidrosis

David L. Larson

DEFINITION

- Hyperhidrosis is excessive sweating beyond the normal physiologic response to heat or emotional stimuli.
- Any such sweating is excessive when it so negatively affects the daily life of individuals that their normal interactions with the world around them are compromised.

ANATOMY

- The greatest concentration of eccrine (sweat-producing) glands is in the palms, axilla, and soles of the feet, where only about 5% of the glands are normally active at any one time.[1]
- These glands are located in the subcutaneous tissue of the axilla and *not* in the dermis (**FIG 1**)—a fact that is of particular significance when considering the rationale for and effectiveness of axillary shaving in the treatment of hyperhidrosis.

PATHOGENESIS

- Primary hyperhidrosis is not psychological in nature, is not self-limiting, and can significantly impact quality of life (QOL), as validated by QOL scales, showing it to be comparable to end-stage renal disease, rheumatoid arthritis, multiple sclerosis, and severe psoriasis.[2,3]

- Secondary hyperhidrosis is associated with many *common diseases* (eg, Parkinson's, hyperthyroidism, gout), *conditions* (eg, pregnancy, obesity, menopause), and *drugs* (eg, neuropsychiatric, antimicrobials, urologic) that can cause diaphoresis. Once these etiologies have been ruled out by history and/or pattern of sweating, a diagnosis of primary or idiopathic hyperhidrosis should be entertained.

NATURAL HISTORY

- Though previously viewed as a benign condition, it is now recognized as a potentially extremely debilitating disease, impairing the social interactions and occupational activities of those affected.
- Affecting 1.4% of the US population, axillary hyperhidrosis generally appears spontaneously in puberty or early adulthood (less than 30 years old). About one-third of these patients will be so negatively affected by the embarrassment, need of frequent change of clothes, and/or malodor that it may eliminate careers such as education, sales, and marketing.

PATIENT HISTORY AND PHYSICAL FINDINGS

- Many patients (over 40%) will not seek medical aid because of embarrassment, the thought that nothing can be done, or misdirection by caregivers (eg, "learn to live with it").

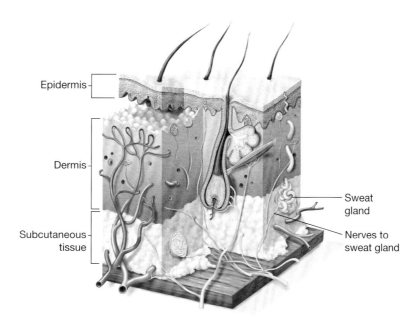

Epidermis

Dermis

Subcutaneous tissue

Sweat gland

Nerves to sweat gland

FIG 1 • Anatomy of the skin and its adnexa.

- Diagnosis is made primarily by history, which includes focal, visible, excessive sweating of at least 6 months duration without apparent cause. In addition, there must be at least two of the following characteristics: bilateral and symmetric, impairment of daily activities, at least one episode weekly, onset in youth (eg, 13 to 25 years old), positive family history (usually positive in 25% of patients), and cessation of sweating during sleep. Many times, all of these findings are noted.
- The only physical finding is excessive moisture in the affected area.

IMAGING/DIAGNOSIS

- Diagnosis can be confirmed by measuring the transepidermal water loss (g/m²/h) using a VapoMeter (Delfin Technologies, Stamford, Connecticut) (**FIG 2**).[4]
- Alternatively, the Minor test (starch-iodine test) can be used for confirmation:
  - Clean and thoroughly dry the axilla.
  - Paint the entire underarm with iodine solution or povidone-iodine.
  - Use a makeup brush, sifter, or gauze pad to evenly dust the site with fine starch powder.
  - After 10 to 15 minutes, areas of sweat will turn the mixture dark purple-blue, which should be documented with a photo.

DIFFERENTIAL DIAGNOSIS

- N/A

NONOPERATIVE MANAGEMENT[5]

- Topical antiperspirants: "clinical-grade" topical deodorants have usually been initiated by the patient. Locally applied powder can also be used, but Drysol (prescription item) only lasts 3 to 4 days, is messy, is difficult to apply, and causes local skin irritation.
- Oral anticholinergics: Robinul (1 mg bid and increase 1 mg q 2 weeks until effective) or oxybutynin (2.5 mg daily ×

7 days, then 2.5 mg bid × 5 weeks) is sometimes effective. Generally, side effects (eg, blurred vision, dry mouth, constipation, etc.) limit the effectiveness, but these should still be the initial treatment.
- Botox injection (50 units per axilla) is very effective but expensive and lasts only 4 to 6 months.
- When conservative management has been used for 2 to 3 months and found wanting, surgical management is justified to both the patient and the insurer.

SURGICAL MANAGEMENT[6–9]

Preoperative Planning

- As the offending sweat glands are only associated with the hair-bearing area of the axilla, this area is outlined in the holding area of the ambulatory.
- Although it might seem reasonable to consider use of a local anesthesia with sedation, this is not advised. The potential movement of the patient while using a powered, rotating instrument blindly in the axilla is very real. A short, general anesthetic will also expedite the efficiency and ensure the safety of this 60-minute procedure.
- This is, at the very least, a two-person operation. Though the surgeon and a scrub nurse will suffice, an additional assistant will significantly aid in providing the essential maximum lateral tension on the surgical field.
- Following induction, the hair-bearing area is outlined and shaved. Taking care to mark a 1-cm access incision within the axillary fold prior, superficially inject (producing a wheal) about 20 to 30 mL of 0.5 % Xylocaine with 1/200 000 epinephrine within the outlined area (**FIG 3**).

Positioning

- In the supine position, the patient's arms are abducted at about a 100-degree angle and secured.
- The surgeon then preps for surgery concurrent with the patient's prep, hereby adding to the hemostatic effect of the local anesthetic.

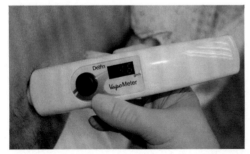

FIG 2 • VapoMeter provides practical, reproducible, and rapid measurement of sweating in g/m²/h (Delfin Technologies, Stamford, Connecticut).

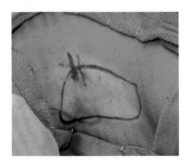

FIG 3 • The hair-bearing area is shaved and injected for local hemostasis, and the 1-cm access incision in the anterior axillary line is marked.

- After draping the axilla, the surgeon takes a place at the head of the table above the arm board and the abducted arm.
- The assistants provide maximal lateral tension to the surgical field to facilitate elevation of the axillary tissue safely and efficiently (**TECH FIG 1A**).
- The previously placed anterior axillary fold mark is incised. Using curved Metzenbaum dissecting scissors, the previously outlined hair-bearing area is elevated in the most superficial subcutaneous plane possible by leaving fatty tissue on the elevated flap. This dissection is typically rapid and bloodless.
- The suction-assisted cartilage shaver, a Stryker CORE Powered Instrument Driver, is brought on to the surgical field (**TECH FIG 1B**). This shaver, commonly used in endoscopic orthopedic cartilage shaving of joints, consists of two concentric metal cannulas, one smaller than the other. At its tip, the outer larger cannula has a half-opened portion that protects the sharp, inner, oscillating cannula, thus allowing continuous curettage and suction drainage (**TECH FIG 1C**).

- With the handpiece setting placed at its lowest setting (900 rpm or less), the shaving tip is inserted into the previously created subcutaneous tunnel, taking care to ALWAYS hold the open cannula toward the undersurface of the elevated flap and keeping the shaver moving.
- With the flap under maximal tension by the assistants, the shaver is slowly passed in a systematic, gridlike fashion over the undersurface of the flap, thereby aspirating the subcutaneous fat and permanently damaging/aspirating the offending sweat glands (**TECH FIG 1D**). Care must be taken to keep the shaver moving to prevent perforation of the flap by the shaver. The hair follicles are always preserved, as is innervation of the surgical area.
- At completion of the shaving, the skin is everted to verify total removal of the subcutaneous tissue and preservation of the axillary skin (**TECH FIG 1E**).
- Wound suction and external pressure is obtained with placement of a small-caliber drain through the incision and an externally applied surgical sponge (**TECH FIG 1F**). The skin is closed with simple nylon sutures.

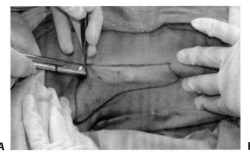
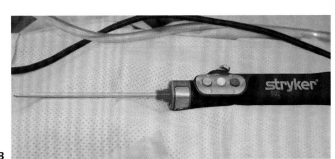

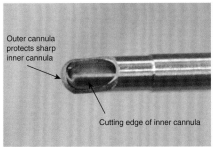

Outer cannula protects sharp inner cannula

Cutting edge of inner cannula

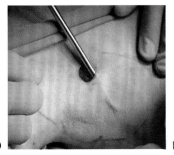
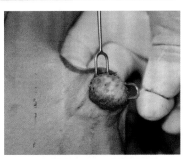

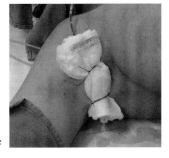

TECH FIG 1 • **A.** Maximal lateral tension by assistants greatly facilitates subcutaneous dissection. **B.** The Stryker suction-assisted cartilage shaver. **C.** The double-lumen cannula that provides continuous curettage and simultaneous suction. **D.** Aspiration of the subcutaneous fat. **E.** Eversion of the now shaved axillary tissue reveals the hair follicles devoid of fat tissue, which is synonymous with ablation of the sweat glands. **F.** Secure compression on the flap plus a small drain helps prevent seroma formation.

TECHNIQUES

PEARLS AND PITFALLS

Diagnosis	■ Most patients present with the same, classic history, and signs and symptoms.
	■ Any positive starch test or VapoMeter reading greater than 100 mL/m²/h is diagnostic of hyperhidrosis.
	■ Initially, use nonoperative, conservative approach (anticholinergic).
	■ Provide insurer with thorough description of symptoms, failure to respond to conservative therapy, and a photo of positive axillary starch test or VapoMeter data.
	■ This operation is equally effective when the primary complaint is offending malodor +/– sweating.
Technique	■ If possible, use two assistants (four hands) to provide lateral traction on the axilla while elevating and shaving the flap.
	■ Keep moving the shaver while exerting gentle upward pressure on the flap while assistants provide tension.
	■ If a perforation of the axillary skin occurs, close it with a fast-absorbing suture; it heals quite kindly.
	■ Using retraction and overhead light, transilluminate the flap to verify a "clean" shaving that preserves only the bulb of the axillary hair follicles.

POSTOPERATIVE CARE

- The external dressing and drain are removed the next day; the permanent sutures are left in place 5 to 7 days, as dehiscence occurs if removed earlier.
- There is very little pain associated with the operation.
- When the dressing is removed, the patient almost always notes total cessation of sweating, which is permanent in greater than 95% of patients.
- Patients should limit arm abduction for one week postoperatively and are typically absent from out-of-home employment about 4 days.

OUTCOMES

- Over 95% of patients have no recurrence of sweating and are quite pleased.
- If sweating does recur, it is usually nominal and managed with conservative methods.
- There is no compensatory sweating (new appearance of hyperhidrosis in another area).

COMPLICATIONS

- There has been one hematoma and one infection in my series. Both responded to conservative measures.

- In the very uncommon occurrence of a recurrence of significant symptoms, the procedure has been repeated without consequence and with a successful outcome (2×/8 years).

REFERENCES

1. Sato K, Kang WH, Saga KT. Biology of sweat glands and their disorders: I. Normal sweat gland function. *J Am Acad Dermatol.* 1989;20(4):537-563.
2. Amir M, Arish A, Weinstein Y, et al. Impairment in quality of life among patients seeking surgery for hyperhidrosis: preliminary results. *Isr J Psychiatry Relat Sci.* 2000;37(1):25-31.
3. Cina CS, Clase CM. The illness intrusiveness rating scale: a measure of severity in individuals with hyperhidrosis. *Qual Life Res.* 1999;8(8):693-698.
4. DePaepe K, Houben E, Adam R, et al. Validation of the VapoMeter, a closed unventilated chamber system to assess transepidermal water loss vs. the open chamber Tewameter. *Skin Res Technol.* 2005;11:61-19.
5. Walling HW, Swick BL. Treatment options for hyperhidrosis. *J Am Acad Dermatol.* 2011;12(5):285-295.
6. Larson D. Definitive diagnosis and management of axillary hyperhidrosis: the VapoMeter and suction-assisted arthroscopic shaving. *Aesthet Surg J.* 2011;31(5):552-559.
7. Bechara FG, Altmeyer P, Sand M, Hoffmann K. Surgical treatment of hyperhidrosis. *Br J Dermatol.* 2007;156:398-399.
8. Tung T. Endoscopic shaver with liposuction for treatment of axillary bromhidrosis. *Ann Plast Surg.* 2001;46:400-408.
9. Arneja JS, Hayakawa TEJ, Singh GB, et al. Axillary hyperhidrosis: a 5 year review of treatment efficacy and recurrence rates using a new arthroscopic shaver technique. *Plast Reconstr Surg.* 2007;119:562-567.

Index